Young Adult Mental Health

Editorial Advisory Board

Naomi A. Fineberg, M.A., M.B.B.S., M.R.C.Psych.
Consultant Psychiatrist and Visiting Professor
University of Hertfordshire Postgraduate Medical School
National OCD Specialist Service
Hertfordshire Partnership NHS Foundation Trust
Queen Elizabeth II Hospital
Welwyn Garden City
United Kingdom

Linda C. Mayes, M.D.
Arnold Gesell Professor
Child Psychiatry, Pediatrics, and Psychology
Yale Child Study Center
New Haven, CT

Peter E. Nathan, Ph.D.
Professor of Community and Behavioral Health
University of Iowa Foundation Distinguished Professor Emeritus of Psychology
    and Public Health
Iowa City, IA

Dan J. Stein, M.D., Ph.D.
Professor and Chair
Department of Psychiatry and Mental Health
University of Cape Town
Cape Town, South Africa

Hermano Tavares, M.D., Ph.D.
Faculty of Medicine
University of Sao Paulo
Sao Paulo, Brazil

Young Adult Mental Health

Edited by
Jon E. Grant
and
Marc N. Potenza

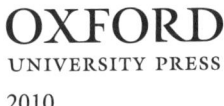
2010

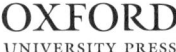

Oxford University Press, Inc., publishes works that further
Oxford University's objective of excellence
in research, scholarship, and education.

Oxford   New York
Auckland   Cape Town   Dar es Salaam   Hong Kong   Karachi
Kuala Lumpur   Madrid   Melbourne   Mexico City   Nairobi
New Delhi   Shanghai   Taipei   Toronto

With offices in
Argentina   Austria   Brazil   Chile   Czech Republic   France   Greece
Guatemala   Hungary   Italy   Japan   Poland   Portugal   Singapore
South Korea   Switzerland   Thailand   Turkey   Ukraine   Vietnam

Copyright © 2010 by Oxford University Press, Inc.

Published by Oxford University Press, Inc.
198 Madison Avenue, New York, New York 10016

www.oup.com

Oxford is a registered trademark of Oxford University Press

All rights reserved. No part of this publication may be reproduced,
stored in a retrieval system, or transmitted, in any form or by any means,
electronic, mechanical, photocopying, recording, or otherwise,
without the prior permission of Oxford University Press.

Library of Congress Cataloging-in-Publication Data
Young adult mental health / edited by Jon E. Grant & Marc N. Potenza.
    p.   ;   cm.
Includes bibliographical references and index.
ISBN 978-0-19-533271-1
1. Young adults—Mental health.   2. Adolescent psychiatry.   I. Grant, Jon E.
II. Potenza, Marc N., 1965–
[DNLM: 1. Mental Disorders.   2. Mental Health.   3. Young Adult.
WM 140 Y68 2010]
RJ503.Y675 2010
616.8900835—dc22
                                                2009001729

9 8 7 6 5 4 3 2 1

Printed in the United States of America
on acid-free paper

Contents

Contributors   vii

    Introduction   3
    Jon E. Grant & Marc N. Potenza

1. Development in the Transition to Adulthood: Vulnerabilities and Opportunities   5
   Keith B. Burt & Ann S. Masten

2. Adolescence: On the Neural Path to Adulthood   19
   Monique Ernst & Julie L. Fudge

3. Risk-Taking Behaviors across the Transition from Adolescence to Young Adulthood   40
   Elizabeth K. Reynolds, Jessica F. Magidson, Linda C. Mayes & Carl W. Lejuez

4. Impact of Childhood Mental Health Problems   64
   Leslie A. Hulvershorn, Craig A. Erickson & R. Andrew Chambers

5. College and Career   80
   Jessica M. Cronce & William R. Corbin

6. Gender Issues: Modern Models of Young Male Resilient Mental Health   96
   William S. Pollack

7. Cultural and Ethnic Considerations in Young Adult Mental Health   110
   Declan T. Barry & Mark Beitel

8. Body Image   126
   Jennifer L. Greenberg, Sherrie S. Delinsky, Hannah E. Reese, Ulrike Buhlmann & Sabine Wilhelm

9. Coping with Stress and Trauma in Young Adulthood   143
   Scott M. Hyman, Steven N. Gold & Rajita Sinha

10. Intimate Romantic Relationships in Young Adulthood: A Biodevelopmental Perspective   158
    Beth A. Auslander & Susan L. Rosenthal

11. Marriage in Young Adulthood   169
    Hui Liu, Sinikka Elliott & Debra J. Umberson

12. Developmental Pathways to Parenting *Thomas J. McMahon*	181
13. Barriers to Mental Health Service Use in Young Adulthood *Deborah A. Perlick, Yariv Hofstein & Lesley A. Michael*	195
14. Psychiatric Disorders in Young Adults: Depression Assessment and Treatment *Carlos A. Zarate, Jr.*	206
15. Anxiety Disorders *Brian L. Odlaug, Waqar Mahmud, Andrew Goddard & Jon E. Grant*	231
16. Obsessive-Compulsive Disorder in Young Adults *Maria C. Mancebo, Jane Eisen & Steven A. Rasmussen*	255
17. Tobacco Use and Nicotine Dependence *Anne E. Smith & Suchitra Krishnan-Sarin*	272
18. Alcohol Use Disorders in Young Adulthood *Andrew K. Littlefield & Kenneth J. Sher*	292
19. Drug Use Disorders among Young Adults: Evaluation and Treatment *Edward V. Nunes*	311
20. Impulse Control Disorders *Jon E. Grant & Marc N. Potenza*	335
21. Attention-Deficit/Hyperactivity Disorder in Young Adults *Joel V. Oberstar & George M. Realmuto*	352
22. Schizophrenia in Adolescents and Young Adults *Afshan Anjum, Priyanka Gait, Kathryn R. Cullen & Tonya White*	362
23. Bipolar Disorder in Early Adulthood: Clinical Challenges and Emerging Evidence *Alan C. Swann*	379
24. Eating Disorders in Young Adults *Scott J. Crow*	397
25. Pervasive Developmental Disorders *Noha F. Minshawi, Naomi B. Swiezy, Stacie L. Pozdol, Melissa Stuart & Christopher J. McDougle*	406
26. Personality Disorders *Donald W. Black & Nancee Blum*	424
Index	441

Contributors

Afshan Anjum, M.D.
University of Minnesota Medical School
Department of Psychiatry
Division of Child and Adolescent Psychiatry
Minneapolis, MN

Beth A. Auslander, Ph.D.
Division of Adolescent and Behavioral Health
Department of Pediatrics
University of Texas Medical Branch
   at Galveston
Galveston, TX

Declan T. Barry, Ph.D.
Associate Research Scientist
Department of Psychiatry
Yale University School of Medicine
New Haven, CT

Mark Beitel, Ph.D.
Assistant Clinical Professor
Department of Psychiatry
Yale University School of Medicine
New Haven, CT

Donald W. Black, M.D.
Professor of Psychiatry
University of Iowa
Roy J. and Lucille A. Carver College
   of Medicine
Iowa City, IA

Nancee Blum, M.S.W.
Clinical Instructor of Psychiatry
University of Iowa
Roy J. and Lucille A. Carver College
   of Medicine
Iowa City, IA

Ulrike Buhlmann, Ph.D.
Postdoctoral Research Fellow
Humboldt University Berlin
Berlin, Germany

Keith B. Burt, Ph.D.
Assistant Professor
Department of Psychology
University of Vermont
Burlington, VT

R. Andrew Chambers, M.D.
Lab for Translational Neuroscience of Dual
   Diagnosis & Development
Department of Psychiatry
Indiana University School of Medicine
Indianapolis, IN

William R. Corbin, Ph.D.
Department of Psychology
Yale University
New Haven, CT

Jessica M. Cronce, M.S., M.Phil.
Department of Psychology
Yale University
New Haven, CT

Scott J. Crow, M.D.
Professor of Psychiatry
University of Minnesota
Minneapolis, MN

Kathryn R. Cullen, M.D.
University of Minnesota Medical School
Department of Psychiatry
Division of Child and Adolescent Psychiatry
Minneapolis, MN

Sherrie S. Delinsky, Ph.D.
McLean Hospital
Belmont, MA

Jane Eisen, M.D.
Associate Professor
Department of Psychiatry and Human Behavior
Warren Alpert Medical School
Brown University
Providence, RI

Sinikka Elliott, Ph.D.
Assistant Professor
Department of Sociology and Anthropology
North Carolina State University
Raleigh, NC

Craig A. Erickson, M.D.
Riley Hospital Child & Adolescent
  Psychiatry Clinic
Department of Psychiatry
Indiana University School of Medicine
Indianapolis, IN

Monique Ernst, M.D., Ph.D.
Head of Neurodevelopment of
  Reward Systems
Emotional Development and Affective
  Neuroscience Branch (EDAN)
Mood and Anxiety Disorders Program
National Institute of Mental Health
Bethesda, MD

Julie L. Fudge, M.D.
Associate Professor of Psychiatry and Neurobiology
  and Anatomy
University of Rochester Medical Center
Rochester, NY

Priyanka Gait, M.D.
Resident
Department of Psychiatry
University of Minnesota
Minneapolis, MN

Andrew Goddard, M.D.
Professor of Psychiatry & Radiology
Indiana University School of Medicine
Director, Adult Psychiatry Clinic &
  Study Center
Director, Adult Anxiety Program
University Hospital
Indianapolis, IN

Steven N. Gold, Ph.D.
Professor, Center for Psychological Studies
Director, Trauma Resolution & Integration Program
Nova Southeastern University
Fort Lauderdale-Davie, FL

Jon E. Grant, M.D., J.D., M.P.H.
Associate Professor of Psychiatry
University of Minnesota
Minneapolis, MN

Jennifer L. Greenberg, Psy.D.
Clinical & Research Fellow in Psychology
  (Psychiatry)
Massachusetts General Hospital and Harvard
  Medical School
Boston, MA

Yariv Hofstein, M.S.
University of Massachusetts
Amherst, MA

Leslie A. Hulvershorn, M.D., M.Sc.
New York University Child Study Center
New York University School of Medicine
New York, NY

Scott M. Hyman, Ph.D.
Associate Research Scientist
Yale Stress Center
Yale University School of Medicine
New Haven, CT

Suchitra Krishnan-Sarin, Ph.D.
Associate Professor of Psychiatry
Yale University School of Medicine
New Haven, CT

Carl W. Lejuez, Ph.D.
Associate Professor
Center for Addictions, Personality, and Emotion
  Research
University of Maryland
College Park, MD
Adjunct Professor
Yale Child Study Center
New Haven, CT

Andrew K. Littlefield, M.A.
University of Missouri-Columbia
Columbia, MO

Contributors

Hui Liu, Ph.D.
Assistant Professor
Sociology Department
Michigan State University
East Lansing, MI

Jessica F. Magidson, B.A.
Center for Addictions, Personality, and Emotion Research
University of Maryland
College Park, MD

Waqar Mahmud, M.D.
Department of Psychiatry.
Indiana University School of Medicine,
Indianapolis, IN

Maria C. Mancebo, Ph.D.
Assistant Professor (Research)
Warren Alpert Medical School of Brown University
Providence, RI

Ann S. Masten, Ph.D.
Distinguished McKnight University Professor
Institute of Child Development
University of Minnesota
Minneapolis, MN

Linda C. Mayes, M.D.
Arnold Gesell Professor
Child Psychiatry, Pediatrics, and Psychology
Yale Child Study Center
New Haven, CT

Christopher J. McDougle, M.D.
Albert E. Sterne Professor and Chairman
Department of Psychiatry
Indiana University School of Medicine
Indianapolis, IN

Thomas J. McMahon, Ph.D.
Yale University School of Medicine
Departments of Psychiatry and Child Study
New Haven, CT

Lesley A. Michael, B.A.
Mount Sinai School of Medicine
New York, NY

Noha F. Minshawi, Ph.D.
Assistant Professor of Clinical Psychology in Clinical Psychiatry
Indiana University School of Medicine
Department of Psychiatry and Christian Sarkine Autism Treatment Center
James Whitcomb Riley Hospital for Children
Indianapolis, IN

Edward V. Nunes, M.D.
Professor of Clinical Psychiatry
Columbia University College of Physicians and Surgeons
New York, NY

Joel V. Oberstar, M.D.
Assistant Professor of Psychiatry
Associate Director, Child & Adolescent Psychiatry Fellowship
University of Minnesota Medical School
Minneapolis, MN

Brian L. Odlaug, B.A.
University of Minnesota
Ambulatory Research Center
Department of Psychiatry
Minneapolis, MN

Deborah A. Perlick, Ph.D.
Associate Professor of Psychiatry
Mount Sinai School of Medicine
New York, NY

William S. Pollack, Ph.D.
Director, Centers for Men & Young Men
McLean Hospital
Assistant Clinical Professor of Psychology
Department of Psychiatry
Harvard Medical School
Founder/Director, Real Boys® Educational Programs
Boston, MA

Marc N. Potenza, M.D., Ph.D.
Associate Professor of Psychiatry and Child Study
Yale University School of Medicine
New Haven, CT

Stacie L. Pozdol, M.S., L.M.H.C.
Lead Behavioral Specialist
Christian Sarkine Autism Treatment Center
Riley Hospital for Children and IU School of Medicine
Indianapolis, IN

Steven A. Rasmussen, M.D.
Associate Professor of Psychiatry
Warren Alpert School of Medicine at Brown University
Medical Director, Butler Hospital
Providence RI

George M. Realmuto, M.D.
Professor of Psychiatry
University of Minnesota
Medical Director of State Operated Services for Child and Adolescent Behavioral Health Services of the State of Minnesota
Minneapolis, MN

Hannah E. Reese, M.A.
Harvard University
Cambridge, MA

Elizabeth K. Reynolds, M.S.
Center for Addictions, Personality, and Emotion Research
University of Maryland
College Park, MD

Susan L. Rosenthal, Ph.D.
Division of Adolescent and Behavioral Health
Department of Pediatrics
University of Texas Medical Branch at Galveston
Galveston, TX

Kenneth J. Sher, Ph.D.
Curators' Professor of Psychological Sciences
University of Missouri
Columbia, MO

Rajita Sinha, Ph.D.
Professor of Psychiatry
Director, Yale Stress Center
Yale University School of Medicine
New Haven, CT

Anne E. Smith, Ph.D.
Yale University School of Medicine
New Haven, CT

Melissa Stuart, M.S.
Behavioral Research Specialist
Department of Psychiatry
Indiana University School of Medicine
Indianapolis, IN

Alan C. Swann, M.D.
Professor and Vice Chair for Research
Department of Psychiatry and Behavioral Sciences
The University of Texas Health Science Center at Houston
Houston, TX

Naomi B. Swiezy, Ph.D., H.S.P.P.
Alan H. Cohen Family Scholar of Psychiatry
Associate Professor of Clinical Psychology in Clinical Psychiatry
Clinical Director, Christian Sarkine Autism Treatment Center
Program Director, HANDS in Autism
Riley Hospital for Children and IU School of Medicine
Indianapolis, IN

Debra J. Umberson, Ph.D.
Professor
Sociology Department and Population Research Center
The University of Texas at Austin
Austin, TX

Tonya White, M.D.
University of Minnesota Medical School
Department of Psychiatry
Division of Child and Adolescent Psychiatry
Minneapolis, MN

Sabine Wilhelm, Ph.D.
Associate Professor, Harvard Medical School
Director, OCD and Related Disorders Program
Massachusetts General Hospital
Boston, MA

Carlos A. Zarate, Jr., M.D.
Chief Experimental Therapeutics
Mood and Anxiety Disorders Program
National Institute of Mental Health
Bethesda, MD

Young Adult Mental Health

Introduction

Jon E. Grant and Marc N. Potenza

Young adults, typically defined as individuals aged 18 to 29 years, constitute a unique population with regard to mental health issues and care. Evidence suggests that not only do many mental health problems in adolescence persist into young adulthood, but also a wide range of mental health concerns begin in young adulthood. The severity of emotional problems for young adults is evidenced by the findings that one out of four young adults will experience a depressive episode by age 24 (American Psychiatric Association, 2009), and when left untreated, mortality from suicide is almost three times greater among young adults than among adolescents (National Center for Injury Prevention and Control, 2008).

Young adults with mental health problems encounter multiple barriers to accessing appropriate medical care. One such barrier is gaps in insurance coverage, given that children once covered by public health insurance or private family plans become ineligible as they enter young adulthood (Yu, Adams, Burns, Brindis, & Irwin, 2008), and almost half of employed young adults work in jobs that provide no insurance (Callahan & Cooper, 2004). Young adulthood is a transitional epoch, and the transitional nature of this developmental period makes it difficult to establish appropriate support systems that would ensure consistent mental health care. For mental health needs, there is often little support provided to ensure that young adults will continue to receive health services or seek care from an adult provider (Davis & Sondheimer, 2005).

Compared to prior decades, the time from 18 to 29 years of age has become an extended period of personal exploration bridging the period of adolescence to the acquisition of more stably defined routines of middle adulthood. Young adulthood is a time of decisions regarding one's identity—"Who am I? What do I want out of work, school, and intimate relations?" With these questions come a range of personal, social, and cultural pressures. Risk-taking behaviors, including substance use, typically peak during this time period in part due to neurobiological development, identity exploration, and social interactions. Young adult women and men face unique challenges that the psychiatric field has largely ignored. Most major psychiatric disorders develop during young adulthood and may present differently in young adults. As such, specific prevention and treatment strategies are important for this age group.

Over the last 5 years, the volume of research on young adult mental health has grown significantly. Although the great body of research in mental health has historically been based on adults or children and adolescents, until recently the research had largely failed to address the important transitional period between adolescence and established adulthood and how that transition integrally influences the clinical presentation and treatment of various disorders. Clinicians in the United States and elsewhere in the world encounter young adults with various psychiatric problems but often have no clear understanding of the issues faced by this age cohort, how psychiatric disorders present differently in this age group, or how the available treatment options differ. This book will provide the latest knowledge about young adult mental health issues, review the strength of the evidence, and provide treatment options for readers in an easily accessible format. For mental health researchers, knowledge about how disorders present differently in young adults may provide insight into possible psychological and neurobiological processes during development.

The 26 chapters of this book are grouped into three sections focusing on developmental issues unique to the transition from adolescence to young adulthood, mental health issues of young adulthood, and the assessment and treatment of psychiatric disorders in this age group.

The first section of this text highlights the important aspects of transition from adolescence to young adulthood. The first three chapters (Chapter 1: Individuation and Psychological Aspects of Becoming and Adult Childhood; Chapter 2: Brain Development and Neuropsychological Development; and Chapter 3: Risk-Taking Behaviors) provide comprehensive examinations of the psychological and neurobiological development of this age group. Chapter 4 (Impact of Childhood Mental Health Problems) describes the influence of childhood mental health problems on this transitional period into adulthood.

A primary aim of this book is also to present mental health as well as mental illness concerns of young adults. As such, the second section of this text addresses areas of healthy psychological development unique to this age group. This section includes developmental topics often paramount during this time period (Chapter 5: College and Career; Chapter 10: Sexuality, Intimacy and Relationships; Chapter 11: Marriage; Chapter 12: Parenting), as well as sociocultural issues of particular salience to young adulthood (Chapter 6: Gender Differences; Chapter 7: Cultural and Ethnics Consideration; Chapter 8: Body Image; Chapter 9: Coping with Stress and Trauma).

When young adults present with psychiatric disorders, clinicians often assume that the presentation and treatment will be similar to what is seen either with adolescents or older adults. Certain psychiatric disorders, however, may not begin until young adulthood, may present differently for this age cohort, and may necessitate different treatment approaches. Because young adults with psychiatric disorders often go untreated, the third section of this text begins with the problems of access to care (Chapter 13: Access to Mental Health Care). The remainder of this section addresses the major mental health issues facing young adults as they consider seeking help for their mental health problems and what clinicians may do to address these concerns.

In summary, young adult mental health represents an important and yet largely neglected area of clinical care. As the chapters of this volume eloquently attest, extraordinary progress has been made regarding how young adults with various psychiatric disorders present differently and how treatment interventions may need to be modified based on the unique developmental features of this age group. This volume presents a multidisciplinary perspective on young adult mental health by addressing developmental considerations, exploring psychosocial topics salient to young adults, and presenting treatment options for a wide array of psychiatric disorders occurring during young adulthood. We hope that clinicians who wish to better understand how they can make informed decisions regarding the mental health and well-being of young adults will find this text valuable.

References

American Psychiatric Association. (2009). *College mental health statistics.* Retrieved February 16, 2009, from http://www.healthyminds.org/collegestats.cfm

Callahan, S. T., & Cooper, W. O. (2004). Gender and uninsurance among young adults in the United States. *Pediatrics, 113,* 291–297.

Davis, M., & Sondheimer, D. L. (2005). State child mental health efforts to support youth in transition to adulthood. *Journal of Behavioral Health Services Research, 32,* 27–42.

National Center for Injury Prevention and Control. (2008). *Mortality reports database,* US Department of Health and Human Services, Centers for Disease Control and Prevention. Retrieved February 16, 2009, from http://www.cdc.gov/ncipc/wisqars

Yu, J. W., Adams, S., Burns, J., Brindis, C., & Irwin, C. E., Jr. (2008). Use of mental health counseling as adolescents become young adults. *Journal of Adolescent Health, 43,* 268–276.

Chapter 1

Development in the Transition to Adulthood: Vulnerabilities and Opportunities

Keith B. Burt and Ann S. Masten

There are many accounts of young people from risky backgrounds whose lives go astray in adolescence, but some of these adolescents manage to turn their lives around during the transition to adulthood. The life of Michael Maddaus provides a dramatic example of this "late bloomer" pattern of resilience (Masten, Obradović, & Burt, 2006). Maddaus experienced a chaotic early caregiving environment that included a mother with chronic alcohol problems and a physically abusive stepfather. By early adolescence, Maddaus was chronically truant from school and hanging around with delinquent peers. He reports that he was arrested two dozen times as a juvenile. Yet, as he approached the age of majority and evaluated his prospects, Maddaus decided to join the Navy. This was the first step on a road that would eventually lead him to medical school. But the road was not entirely straight and smooth. Serving in the military during the Vietnam War, Maddaus continued to struggle with substance abuse. Nonetheless, he managed to complete his service with an honorary discharge. He pursued a high school equivalency degree after his return home and the G.I. Bill made it possible for him to attend community college. Still, it was a drunk-driving accident in his early twenties that motivated Maddaus to take charge of his life and plan for a better future. Soon mentors, including a physician, took an interest in this bright young man with the troubled background. Maddaus was encouraged to pursue his interests in medicine and eventually attended medical school at the University of Minnesota, where he became a highly successful surgeon who now trains surgery residents. Although his path was unique, the life story of Maddaus exemplifies many of the risks and protective factors that have been the focus of resilience research. Clearly, his own talents, thinking, motivation, planning, and actions were pivotal, and it is likely that brain maturation played a role in the improvements in his decision making about his life. But opportunities also mattered, such as the chance to join the military, return to school, get funding for community college, and enter medical school, all despite his juvenile delinquency. Moreover, mentors outside Maddaus's family played a key role in opening doors, encouraging him, and providing support for positive change. The Maddaus story illustrates how the transition to adulthood is a time of opportunity and change.

The young adult years offer a unique window into issues of development and mental health that have profound implications for theory, intervention, and policy. Until recently, however, research informed by a developmental psychopathology orientation, in which normal and abnormal functioning are seen as mutually informative, has centered largely on infancy, childhood, and adolescence. This relative neglect of the early adult years occurred even though a developmental psychopathology perspective has clear implications and applications across the full life span (Cicchetti, 2006; Rutter & Sroufe, 2000). The goal of this chapter is to review the status of research on young adult development from a developmental psychopathology perspective, particularly with respect to psychosocial competence and problems in adaptive function. We begin by discussing developmental task theory in the young adult years, noting the importance of integrating behavioral and biological research with the study of developmental context. Following a general review of research on competence and resilience in this developmental period, we discuss Arnett's (2000) concept of emerging adulthood as a distinct developmental period and its implications for young adult mental health. Finally, we review recent empirical work on competence and resilience through the transition to adulthood, drawing on findings from the Project Competence studies of adaptation in a normative community cohort as well as related research from high-risk samples. Our goal is to highlight issues and findings that inform emerging science and practice related to successful and unsuccessful adaptation through the transition to adulthood and key categories of psychological disorder.

Developmental Tasks and the Transition to Adulthood

Developmental task theory has deep historical roots in psychoanalytic stage theories as well as Erikson's theory of psychosocial development (Masten, Burt, & Coatsworth, 2006). However, contemporary perspectives on developmental tasks are most closely aligned with the concepts delineated by Havighurst (1972). Working from an applied educational perspective, Havighurst observed that societies create a series of graded expectations that vary by age and are used to judge whether a given individual is considered to be successful. Subsequent theorists have noted that mastery of age-salient developmental tasks can itself be taken as evidence of self-organizing systems in human development (Sroufe, 1979; Waters & Sroufe, 1983). In essence, individuals gain particular skills at different ages and these interacting skills are then are put to the test in subsequent developmental challenges.

Lists of salient developmental tasks have been proposed by a variety of scholars for different age periods (Masten & Coatsworth, 1998).

Developmental tasks wax and wane in significance across time as individual development, contexts, and expectations change. In most societies, during the years when children and youth are expected to acquire the education needed for adult life, young people are expected to go to school and meet societal expectations for academic skills, while at the same time they are expected to behave appropriately and get along with peers and teachers. As youth mature, new tasks emerge, often in the form of expectations for forming romantic relationships, establishing families, and work, either at home or in gainful employment. Adults are also expected to contribute to the common good of the community through civic engagement (Obradović & Masten, 2007). The salience of the work, romantic, and civic engagement domains in the transition to adulthood is demonstrated in part by their expected, and confirmed, associations with trajectories of well-being (Schulenberg, Bryant, & O'Malley, 2004). Eventually, the salience of academic achievement as a developmental task fades, as the tasks of work, romantic relationships, parenting, and/or community contributions become more prominent.

Developmental task criteria for successful adaptation also may include psychological achievements. During adolescence and early adulthood, the most common psychological tasks pertain to the concepts of *identity* and *autonomy*. In Erikson's theory of the life cycle, for example, achieving a coherent identity was the central issue of adolescence (Erikson, 1968). Identity as a developmental task may not be as salient in cultures or subcultural ethnic or community groups that emphasize belonging and collectivism over autonomy and individualism (Masten & Coatsworth, 1998).

Examples of common developmental tasks of emerging or early adulthood are presented in Table 1.1. There are salient tasks originating in younger years that remain important for many young adults. Academic attainment remains salient for many young adults in modern societies, and it also remains important to have friends. In both cases, the expectations for the quality or level of achievement would be higher than expected for a much younger person, such as a young adolescent. Similarly, behaving according to the rules and laws of the

Table 1-1. Developmental Task Examples from Adolescence to Adulthood

Age Period	Task
Adolescence	Successful transition to secondary schooling
	Academic achievement
	Forming close friendships
	Forming a cohesive sense of self / identity
	Rule-abiding conduct
Emerging adulthood through young adulthood	(Maintaining competence in adolescent tasks)
	Forming close romantic relationships
	Work competence (in jobs or in the home)
	Effective parenting (if a parent)
	Emerging task example: Civic engagement

community or context continue to play an important role in evaluations of competence or success in this period. Domains rising in salience in comparison to young adolescents are the tasks of establishing positive intimate relationships and achieving successful employment and engagement in work. Although these domains center on an individual's engagement with the outside world, they have close connections to traditional ideas of developing autonomy, intimacy, and psychological individuation as key tasks of young adulthood. Family formation and effective parenting are also frequently expected tasks of the early adult years, though in many societies this domain is more varied in expectations and options. Having children may not be necessarily "expected." Nonetheless, once an adult has a child, typically there are expectations for responsible parenting. In a sense, then, parenting is a conditional developmental task, triggered by the birth of a child.

Developmental tasks reflect both universal features of human development as well as unique perspectives grounded in particular cultures, communities, or historical contexts. Learning to talk is an enduring developmental task of early childhood, reflecting the typical development of the human species, while learning to hunt bison is an example of a task more unique to a geographical, cultural, and historical context. Thus, cohort changes and the larger structure of society would be expected to have effects on which domains are emphasized as key developmental tasks. As discussed below in the section on emerging adulthood, broad demographic changes in postindustrial societies have changed the makeup of what constitutes a typical young adult developmental pathway in the twenty-first century.

Developmental task expectations likely reflect accumulated observations and knowledge about human development and pathways to adult success across generations. At the same time, these expectations will shape individual development in a given culture and context. Stakeholders in human development notice and respond to success in these tasks, including parents, prospective employers, neighbors, and the person himself or herself. Communities also structure opportunities and contexts to promote achievement in these tasks. The contexts of development change quite dramatically during the transition to adulthood. For example, while the majority of American children and adolescents both live with their family of origin and participate in formal schooling full time, during the transition to adulthood many American youth have opportunities to pursue different lifestyles as well as greater geographic and economic mobility.

Developmental tasks would be expected to track not only the course of typical individual development but also the gradual changes in societies and the nature of human development across generations. For example, the changes of body, behavior, and context associated with adolescence clearly play a role in our expectations for adolescents. Adolescents undergo many dramatic changes at the levels of biology and brain development, from hormonal activation and pubertal changes to continuing development of executive functioning structures (Masten, 2007a, 2007b; Steinberg et al., 2006; see also Ernst, Chapter 2, this volume). These changes are extremely complex, interactive, multilevel, and also vary by individual and context, making summary statements extremely difficult. However, researchers in the developmental psychopathology of adolescence have highlighted the rise of emotion regulation structures throughout this period, with the corollary that adolescents are also quite vulnerable to disorders of mood, appetite, and behavior regulation (Steinberg et al., 2006).

Even more important, the crucial changes in biology and brain functioning themselves interact with the unique contexts of adolescent development, and these contexts are themselves moving targets. Over the past century or so, there appear to be important changes in the timing and course of adolescent development, along with dramatic changes in the contexts and opportunities of adolescent life, such as media and schooling. Physical changes of puberty are observed at younger ages, particularly among girls, while education and training opportunities have extended into the twenties and opened for increasing numbers of girls and minority youth. Such cohort trends in development across generations would be expected to influence developmental task expectations in communities or societies where they occur.

Defining and Assessing Competence and Resilience

The history of research on competence and resilience crosses diverse disciplines and theoretical orientations, informing basic and applied research on childhood and adult development. Here we briefly review some key points from this literature; for a more in-depth treatment of these issues the reader is referred to Luthar (2006), Masten, Burt, and Coatsworth (2006), and Masten (2007b). Although different researchers and theorists have proposed varying definitions, we have defined competence as the manifested capacity for effective adaptation in one's environment, often inferred from a track record in age-salient developmental tasks, and always embedded in developmental, cultural, and historical context (Masten et al., 2006). Key debates on defining and assessing competence have focused on issues such as the following: who makes the judgments and how (e.g., who decides the criteria, which informants, what measures) or when (e.g., timing or duration concerns); the scope of function to include (e.g., broad or narrow domains of life); and the nature of evidence (e.g., how capacity versus actual performance is weighed). Strict consensus on these questions is not necessarily desirable, although many researchers are in agreement that accurate judgments of competence require information from more than one informant about functioning in more than one domain of adaptation over some period of time, rather than the immediate present or a single instance.

Resilience in human development refers to positive adaptation or development in the context of significant threats to the life or function of the person. Definitions of resilience also vary across disciplines and investigators, although a consensus is emerging in support of a broad definition that could serve to integrate research across levels of analysis (from cells to global climate) and also unify work in the behavioral sciences with ecology and other fields. From a general systems theory perspective, resilience refers to "the capacity of dynamic systems to withstand or recover from significance disturbances" (Masten, 2007b, p. 923). Definitions of resilience, both conceptual and operational, always require two elements: the criteria for identifying positive adaptation and the criteria for assessing threat or adversity, the indicators of risks or challenges to positive adaptation (Luthar, 2006; Masten & Coatsworth, 1998).

Resilience research encompasses a wide variety of phenomena, studied in many different ways. These include research on recovery from maltreatment, trauma, war and disasters, good functioning in disadvantaged families or neighborhoods, and adaptation following common negative life experiences such as divorce or death of a parent. Diverse research topics with great relevance to young adult mental health include studies of desistance following delinquency, mental illness, or substance abuse; successful aging out of foster care or other kinds of institutions; successful parenting by adults mistreated as children; positive adaptation of refugee youth; rehabilitation of child soldiers; and recovery from assault in young adults. This body of work encompasses many kinds of risk or adversity, and just as research on competence has engendered debates over definitions, measurement, and analytic techniques, the assessment and judgment of risk and adversity is an area of research of its own (Obradović, Shaffer, & Masten, in press).

Emerging Adulthood: Theory and Empirical Support

In an influential article published in 2000, Arnett proposed that changes in modern postindustrial societies and individuals growing up in these societies have resulted in a new era of development spanning adolescence and adulthood, which he named *emerging adulthood*. He argued that cohort trends observed in multiple societies, including extended timeframes for education and exploratory work or travel, delays in the timing of traditional adult roles such as marriage and parenthood, as well as other social forces have created a distinct and lengthy period of transition to adulthood, from around 18 to around 25 years of age. Arnett distinguished this period both from adolescence and adulthood in terms of youth self-perceptions as well as the role of youth in families and communities. Proponents of emerging adulthood were quick to note that it is in many ways a culturally bound phenomenon, and there is small a growing research base on aspects of emerging adulthood in cultural minority groups (e.g., Cheah & Nelson, 2004), ethnic identity in emerging adulthood (Phinney, 2006), and emerging adulthood outside of North America (e.g., Buhl & Lanz, 2007; see also Arnett & Eisenberg, 2007).

Arnett presented data suggesting that many youth in this age range tend to self-identify as neither fully adult nor fully adolescent. Behaviorally, there is a high degree of variability in how emerging adults live their lives and spend their time, with many youth exploring different work contexts and romantic relationship patterns for shorter periods of time, moving in and out of their home of origin, and receiving varying degrees of continued financial support from parents (Arnett, 2000). In fact, longitudinal growth-curve analyses of "transition level" (quantified independence ratings) in the domains of romance, work, finances, and parenting have shown dramatic within-person variability over time through the emerging adulthood years (Cohen, Kasen, Chen, Hartmark, & Gordon, 2003).

A recent edited volume (Arnett & Tanner, 2006), which summarized existing research on emerging adulthood, focused on changes in individual behavior during this developmental period (e.g., symptoms, skills, social competence), as well as changes in contexts and relationships of individuals with others in these contexts (e.g., changes in family, friendships and romantic relationships, education, work, and the media). The majority of researchers working in emerging adulthood have been experts on individual development in adolescence who are following youth forward through the transition to adulthood; increasingly, however, scientists specializing in marriage and family theory and research have been focusing research attention on the antecedents of healthy adult functioning, with growing contributions to the emerging adulthood knowledge base. For example, one recent investigation from a family research perspective highlights the importance of the "marital horizon"—broadly referring to whether emerging adults consider marriage to be a near-term versus long-term prospect—for predicting substance use and sexual behavior (Carroll, Willoughby, Badger, Barry, & Madsen, 2007).

Recent research on brain development and cognition, meanwhile, is documenting notable gains in executive function, planning, and decision making that coincide with the functionality and connectivity of neural systems and the rather late myelination of neurons in parts of the brain, including the prefrontal cortex, which extend well into the twenties (Dahl & Spear, 2004; Giedd et al., 1999; Spear, 2007; Steinberg et al., 2006). This raises interesting questions of how changes in structural brain development interact with the recent contextual changes encapsulated by the theory of emerging adulthood. Although research on competence and resilience in this age period rarely includes direct assessment of brain functioning through neuroimaging and related techniques, such methods are entirely consistent with a developmental psychopathology framework. There are growing calls for integration of biologic and neuroscience perspectives and methods with behavioral studies and strategies, both broadly in developmental psychopathology (Cicchetti & Curtis, 2006), and also more specifically in research on competence and resilience (Cicchetti & Curtis, 2007; Lester, Masten, & McEwan, 2006). At the same time, existing research on neurobiological changes during adolescence suggests that changes in brain structure and function result in changing sensitivity of adolescents to variation in their larger context, with problematic consequences for some adolescents in the areas of emotional and behavioral regulation (Dahl & Spear, 2004; Steinberg et al., 2006).

Competence and Resilience Research in the Transition to Adulthood

Evidence on what influences the development of competence and resilience throughout the transition to adulthood has taken different forms. These include broad longitudinal investigations as well as more focused studies on particular risk populations.

Broad Longitudinal Investigations

Several unique datasets, spanning varied cohorts and contexts, have followed at-risk or normative groups from childhood or adolescence into young adulthood. In general, research on this transition has highlighted "turning point" opportunities, such as potential changes in romantic or other close relationships, career openings, and religious or spiritual conversion, as well as interpersonal and cognitive qualities that aid in one's taking advantage of such contextual opportunities. For example, work on age trends in crime and delinquency has consistently noted the effects of stable work and positive romantic relationships on predicting a turn away from antisocial behavior during the transition to adulthood (e.g., Moffitt, Caspi, Harrington, & Milne, 2002; Sampson & Laub, 1993), including youth at high risk for persistent offending due to an early history of behavior problems (Roisman, Aguilar, & Egeland, 2004). In addition to work engagement, staying in school has also been associated with desistance in serious delinquent offending in the Pittsburgh Youth Study through the emerging adulthood years (Stouthamer-Loeber, Wei, Loeber, & Masten, 2004).

In a similar vein, studies focused specifically on resilience following adverse experiences have noted the possibility of turning points and windows of recovery through the emerging adulthood years. Results from the well-known Kauai longitudinal study suggested that "second-chance opportunities," including positive marriages as well as work and school opportunities, predicted a positive transition to adulthood (Werner & Smith, 1992, 2001). In addition, participants in the Kauai study from a multiple-risk background who were doing well by age 18 tended to continue experiencing successful outcomes into young adulthood and beyond. Thus, their data also showed evidence for continuity of resilient adaptation over time.

Other longitudinal studies, informed by sociological as well as psychological perspectives, have focused on the timing of entry into various adult roles and responsibilities relative to one's cohort, with results that also emphasize the importance of salient developmental task domains. In this vein, Wickrama, Conger, Wallace, and Elder (2003) tested mediational models predicting young adult physical health from childhood disadvantage and adversity through adolescent and emerging adult transitions. Although their model highlights multiple complex pathways to young adult health, their results suggest that early entry into family responsibilities and shortened educational attainment (relative to peers) were mediators of associations between past family stress and childhood problem behavior, on the one hand, and compromised adult physical health on the other.

Our own work and that of our colleagues in the Project Competence studies of risk and resilience indicate similar patterns of continuity and change. The Project Competence longitudinal study, initiated by Norman Garmezy and Auke Tellegen in the late 1970s, followed a normative cohort of children across adolescence and the transition to adulthood (Masten et al., 1995, 1999, 2004). This body of research is consistent with much of the work noted above in drawing attention to the personal, family, and community contexts that foster and maintain resilience throughout this period. In particular, this study brought early and enduring attention to the central importance of assessing multiple dimensions of competence in age-appropriate ways over the course of development. In a series of articles on assessment of and continuity and change in competence, various investigators in the Project Competence study have developed reliable measures for multiple informants of competence across multiple domains of age-salient developmental tasks, eventually testing the concurrent and predictive validity of competence constructs, along with stability and change (e.g., Burt, Obradović, Long, & Masten, 2008; Gest, Sesma, Masten, & Tellegen, 2006; Masten, Morison, & Pellegrini, 1985; Masten et al., 1995, 1999, 2005; Obradović & Masten, 2007; Roisman, Masten, Coatsworth, & Tellegen, 2004).

This body of work has also served to test hypotheses generated by developmental task theory. For example, focusing on links within and between broad competence domains over time, Roisman et al. (2004) tested the basic premise that success in salient tasks in one period of development serve to set the stage favorably for success in future salient tasks, including newly emerging tasks in different but related domains of functioning. They confirmed the expectation that manifested competence in core developmental tasks of adolescence, particularly in relation to quality of friendships, rule-abiding conduct, and academic achievement, would predict not only functioning in the corresponding domains 10 years later but also the newly salient domains of romantic relationships and work. In contrast, early success during adolescence in the adult tasks of achieving and maintaining high-quality romantic relationships and work success (at a time when these tasks are in emergent form) did not show comparable predictive validity. These findings of heterotypic rather than homotypic continuity in competence domains are consistent both with the emphasis of waxing and waning salience for various developmental tasks over time and with the emerging adulthood emphasis on the changing nature of romantic relationships and work during the transition-to-adulthood years.

In addition to work focused on continuity in competence over time, investigators from Project Competence have examined resilience in the transition to adulthood (see Masten et al., 2004). Following other studies using this dataset, this work has made use of both variable- and person-centered analytic approaches to answer questions about predicting positive and negative turnarounds through this crucial developmental period. Variable-focused analyses, for example, have examined how attributes of an individual or family and various indices of negative life experiences are related to manifested competence over time. Both main effects (of attribute and adversity index) and interactions (testing for moderating effects of adversity by attribute) have been tested, in an effort to discover what helps individuals overcome adversity to succeed in life. The person-focused approach typically involves identification of groups of people of interest according to diagnostic criteria who are then compared. For example, participants in the Project Competence longitudinal study were classified after the 10-year follow-up assessments (when the cohort were ages 17 to 23) into nine mutually exclusive groups according to their life history of adversity (low, medium/mixed, or high) and their recent track record of success in age-salient developmental tasks (poor, mixed, or good). People were classified as "OK" in competence if their scores on all three core developmental task composites (social competence, conduct, academic attainment) fell in the average range or better of the normative sample, whereas they were classified as not doing well if they fell below this range on at least two of the three domains. Similarly, comprehensive life adversity scores were created using ratings of detailed life history charts created from longitudinal assessments (see Gest, Reed, & Masten, 1999), classifying people into three groups of low, mixed/medium, or high lifetime adversity.

The cross-classification of competence and adversity yielded nine possible categories, with a focus on the "corner" groups, labeled as *resilient* (high adversity and OK on competence), *competent/unchallenged* (low adversity and OK competence), *vulnerable/unchallenged* (low adversity and poor competence), and *maladaptive* (high adversity and poor competence). Then specific groups could be compared on a set of key "adaptive resources" measured in childhood (10 years earlier), adolescence (3 years earlier), concurrently (emerging adulthood), or even subsequently (10 years later, when the 20-year follow-up was completed). It was interesting to find that one category, low adversity with poor competence, was nearly empty of people (only 3 people from a cohort of 205), suggesting that this pattern is unusual in a cohort recruited from a normative school population. This pattern could reflect a nonnormal organism or a false-negative adversity score. Nonetheless, it is noteworthy that adaptation in developmental tasks tends to be good when risk or adversity exposure is low.

In the Project Competence analyses focused on the role of resources in the person or their social resources for competence and resilience over the transition to adulthood, we examined patterns with both variable- and person-centered approaches (Masten et al., 2004). Based on the literature on predictors of change, we tested whether measures of planfulness/future motivation, behavioral and emotional autonomy, adult support, and coping skills would predict adult competence 10 years later, taking current competence, adversity, and other differences into account. We also examined whether the small group of individuals who moved from the maladaptive to the resilient category during this 10-year period differed from peers who remained maladaptive on these attributes. Results of the two strategies were congruent in suggesting that while competence and resilience tended to endure the transition to adulthood (as expected), favorable movement toward adult competence was forecasted by indications of planfulness, autonomy, and motivation to change, along with support from adults beyond one's parents. The small group of individuals who would dramatically turn their lives around during emerging adulthood already differed in revealing ways from young people who would continue along a maladaptive path of life.

Looking at results for particular domains of competence, results suggested that different adaptive resources made predictive contributions to different domains in a theoretically meaningful manner. Variable-centered analyses highlight such differences. In hierarchical multiple regression analyses, a variable indexing planfulness and motivation for future success was a significant predictor of academic competence controlling for prior academic success, IQ, gender, age, and SES (Masten et al., 2004). In contrast, behavioral and emotional autonomy predicted romantic relationship competence over and above the same control variables. As noted above, romantic competence itself in emerging adulthood was not a good predictor of the same construct 10 years later (Roisman et al., 2004). A somewhat more complex relationship was observed for competence in the work domain, in which it was the common variance shared among emerging adulthood adaptive resources that was the best independent predictor, possibly reflecting the complex nature of the combined skills required for success in the work domain.

Additional research from the Project Competence longitudinal data has examined the interaction of risk and competence over time through semiparametric mixture modeling, a methodology that essentially seeks to represent subgroups of a sample who may display particular patterns of variation over time (Nagin & Tremblay, 1999). Using global ratings of adaptation as the outcome variable, this work also emphasizes that the emerging adulthood years can be a period of potential change both for better and for worse (Obradović, Burt, & Masten, 2006). In this analysis, a subgroup of participants who were classified on an improving adaptation trajectory scored higher on emerging adulthood ratings of reality of goals and commitment and persistence toward meeting those goals than a subgroup who were similarly rated in adolescence but who showed a declining trajectory through the transition to adulthood. In addition, male participants appeared to be at greater overall risk of membership in a declining adaptation trajectory over the transition-to-adulthood years.

Studies of Specific Risk Populations

Although resilience investigations have classified people according to their cumulative risk on multiple factors (e.g., the Kauai study by Werner & Smith), other research has focused on populations at specific risk for a particular negative outcome. In these studies, investigators examine youth who manage well in the transition to adulthood despite their risk for a specific kind of problem. As an example, Hussong and

Chassin (2004) examined differences in coping strategies among youth at risk of substance abuse problems, the adolescent children of alcoholics, compared to low-risk peers, using latent trajectory modeling. Although their findings were complex, results echo some of the Project Competence findings described above. Hussong and Chassin (2004) noted that individuals who demonstrated planful coping engaged in less heavy drinking and drug use in young adulthood. Other work focusing on youth with a history of substance abuse has shown that the interaction of higher levels of social and academic competence predicted less marijuana use in the emerging adulthood years (Clingempeel, Henggeler, Pickrel, Brondino, & Randall, 2005).

Research following more seriously disturbed youth into adulthood has documented both continuity and change over time in individuals who were on both adaptive and maladaptive paths through the transition years. Gralinski-Bakker, Hauser, Stott, Billings, and Allen (2004; see also Hauser, Allen, & Golden, 2006) report a follow-up into the thirties of a cohort of youth who were hospitalized for nonpsychotic mental illness in adolescence. Using a fairly stringent definition of resilience that incorporated indices of both external and internal adaptation, the authors report a small percentage of their high-risk sample (~13%) categorized as competent in developmental task domains, free of psychiatric diagnosis, and having a sense of internal well-being. However, substantially larger percentages of the sample met each of these criteria considered separately, with roughly 60% of the sample not meeting criteria for psychiatric diagnosis in adulthood. Their results provide evidence of diversity in developmental pathways over the transition to adulthood and the potential for resilience even among extremely vulnerable youth in adolescence. At the same time, their results provide evidence of continuity in adaptation through the young adult years and the rarity of simultaneously maintaining both external and internal well-being when faced with dramatic developmental risk.

A large body of specific-risk literature has arisen in the area of juvenile delinquency and general externalizing problems, with substantial focus on the emerging adult years due to the well-documented "age–crime curve" showing aggregate population increases in antisocial behaviors through the adolescent years with a peak and subsequent decline of overall offending through emerging and young adulthood (e.g., Laub & Sampson, 2001). As with any developmental phenomenon, this age-related decline or desistance itself is not explanatory but rather invites explanation. Although a full discussion of the delinquency literature is beyond the scope of this chapter, from a resilience standpoint it is noteworthy that recent investigations have attempted to identify predictors of desistance from delinquent offending. Despite great difficulty in operationalizing and measuring desistance, some consistent findings have emerged. In particular, there is evidence that positive engagement in salient developmental tasks, especially work and romantic relationships, is related to desistance from juvenile delinquency (e.g., Farrington, 1995; Moffitt et al., 2002). In analyzing a wide variety of risk, protective, and promotive factors using data from the oldest cohort of the Pittsburgh Youth Study (PYS), a longitudinal study of serious delinquency in three cohorts of males, Stouthamer-Loeber et al. (2004) found that being employed or in school during emerging adulthood was a significant predictor of desistance. Similarly, other life-course data on juvenile offenders (e.g., Laub, Nagin, & Sampson, 1998) suggests that prosocial, cohesive marriages exert gradual but cumulative effects over time toward desistance from crime. Given effects of assortative mating, it is important to distinguish the character and quality of romantic relationships in such studies, because only positive or prosocial relationships would be expected to encourage desistance (see Rhule-Louie & McMahon, 2007, for related discussion). Desistance in the transition to adulthood is also predictable from variables assessed earlier in childhood and adolescence, with deviant peer association and interpersonal callousness related to less likelihood of desistance in the youngest cohort of the PYS (Loeber, Pardini, Stouthamer-Loeber, & Raine, 2007).

Finally, the emerging adulthood years can be seen as a particularly vulnerable window for the development of binge drinking behavior and alcohol use disorders (Masten, Faden, Zucker, & Spear, 2008; Zucker, 2006). This is concerning because even moderate trajectories of binge drinking are associated with increased risk for alcohol use disorders (e.g., Chassin, Pitts, & Prost, 2002), prevalences of which show clear age-related increases and decreases through the emerging adult and young adult years (Brown et al., 2008; Masten et al., 2008). Problematic alcohol use in the transition to adulthood is related to a variety of other potential problems in living and in relationships (Sher & Gotham, 1999). Moreover, evidence is growing that brain development and function during adolescence and emerging adulthood may be differentially sensitive to alcohol effects and consequences, interacting in complex ways with the particular contexts of emerging adulthood drinking (Brown et al., 2008).

In findings reminiscent of research on delinquency, some binge drinking research has shown that the factors related to initiation of binge drinking differ from those related to its maintenance or desistance. For example, Schulenberg, Wadsworth, O'Malley, Bachman, and Johnston (1996) used national panel survey data to follow high school students into the transitional years, finding that male gender, low social conservatism, and drinking to get drunk were robust risk factors for onset and continuance of binge drinking over time. However, when comparing subgroups of youth who persisted versus desisted in their binge drinking by age 24, they also found that work role readiness and self-efficacy (their variable being related to planfulness) differentiated the two groups (Schulenberg et al., 1996). Of note, delinquent behavior and problematic alcohol use have themselves been linked empirically and in theories focused on generalized undercontrol and poor connection to social institutions (Jessor, Donovan, & Costa, 1991).

Summary and Conclusion

Research from a variety of populations and focused on a variety of risks and outcomes converges on the transition to adulthood as a window of both vulnerability and opportunity. As the perspective of emerging adulthood has emphasized, the transition to adulthood in twenty-first century America and similar cultures is dramatically different than even 30 years previously, with a widening of the intermediary period between economic and residential dependence on one's family of origin and various markers of independent adult functioning. In part because of these secular societal trends, youth in some countries are faced with a dizzying array of choices and pathways in the domains of academics, work, romantic relationships, friendships, and living arrangements. Many young people appear to use the emerging adult years as a time to explore such opportunities and continue the processes of individuation and autonomy that began in adolescence. Investigations of competence in various developmental tasks show strong continuity in adaptation over time despite often dramatic within-person variability in a given setting or context. The salient tasks of adolescence, including performing well in school, getting along well with others, and maintaining rule-abiding conduct, are powerful predictors of the new work and romantic relationship contexts of young adulthood.

For youth at risk for psychopathology, research on adversity and resilience suggests that while there is broad continuity in adaptation over the emerging adulthood years, this period can be a window of opportunity for improvement. Internal (e.g., planfulness, emotional autonomy) and external (e.g., support from a trusted adult) factors appear to play a powerful potential role for a small but compelling group of youth who dramatically turn things around from a pathway of poor adaptation and psychopathology to competent adult functioning, as evidenced by the life history of Dr. Michael Maddaus described in the opening case vignette of this chapter. Resilience research suggests that recovery and positive change evident during the transition to adulthood may reflect changes in fundamental but powerful adaptive systems in the person and their interactions with the environment that generate a new capacity for change (Masten, 2001; Masten et al., 2006). However, these processes may take time to manifest and are themselves vulnerable to disruption.

At the same time, the transition to adulthood is also a period of heightened vulnerability for many different aspects of psychopathology, especially disorders of impulse control and emotion regulation. Even for adolescents and young adults who are free from diagnosed mental disorder, research on the deleterious consequences of binge drinking and on the "snares" (e.g., incarceration, drug use initiation, motor vehicle accidents) present for some individuals in even mild antisocial behavior suggests that the transition years are fraught with potential difficulty.

The nature of the transition from adolescence to adulthood itself is developing and transforming in many societies. The nature of challenges and opportunities and the timing and duration of time allotted for this transition appear to have shifted, and the concomitant changes in brain development and their role in the transitional processes are still being charted by neuroscientists. Nonetheless, it is clear that insights from basic research on competence and resilience will be informative for prevention and intervention efforts targeted toward youth who are at risk for, or who are already manifesting problems in, young adulthood.

KEY POINTS

- In many contemporary societies, the transition years spanning adolescence to adulthood have increased in duration and complexity, yielding an important window of opportunity and challenge.
- There is continuity in the overall adaptation of individuals across the transition to adulthood, yet there is great variability during this developmental period, both individual differences among people the same age and changes over time within a specific person.
- Many behavioral and mental health problems surge, peak, or decline in prevalence during the transition years from adolescence into adulthood.
- Success in developmental tasks of adolescence set the stage for successful transitions to adulthood, although some young people with a history of adversity and problems turn their lives around in this period of development, manifesting resilience.

PRACTICE GUIDELINES

- For adolescents, early entry into the adult roles of work and romantic relationships does not predict competence in those domains in adulthood. Accomplishments in age-appropriate developmental tasks such as academics and peer activities are the strongest markers of later success in adulthood. Thus, it is important to assess competence in developmental tasks as well as symptoms of problems.
- It is important to consider changes in the contexts of a young person's life in addition to individual-targeted interventions because enduring change is more likely when interventions are coordinated across levels of a person's life, including family or peer relationships, the contexts of work or community, and the level of the individual person.
- Intervening to promote competence in important domains of function and attachments to prosocial people and institutions can help reduce problem behavior in addition to promoting positive development.

References

Arnett, J. J. (2000). Emerging adulthood: A theory of development from the late teens through the twenties. *American Psychologist, 55*, 469–480.

Arnett, J. J., & Eisenberg, N. (2007). Introduction to the special section: Emerging adulthood around the world. *Child Development Perspectives, 1*(2), 66–67.

Arnett, J. J., & Tanner, J. L. (Eds.). (2006). *Emerging adults in America: Coming of age in the 21st century*. Washington, DC: American Psychological Association.

Brown, S., McGue, M., Maggs, J., Schulenberg, J., Hingson, R., Swartzwelder, S., Martin, C., Chung, T., Tapert, S. F., Sher, K., Winters, K. C., Lowman, C., & Murphy, S.. (2008). A developmental perspective on alcohol and youth: Ages 16-20. *Pediatrics, 121*(Suppl. 4), S290–S310.

Buhl, H. M., & Lanz, M. (2007). Emerging adulthood in Europe: Common traits and variability across five European countries. *Journal of Adolescent Research, 22*, 439–443.

Burt, K. B., Obradović, J., Long, J. D., & Masten, A. S. (2008). The interplay of social competence and psychopathology over 20 years: Testing transactional and cascade models. *Child Development, 79*(2), 359–374.

Carroll, J. S., Willoughby, B., Badger, S., Barry, C. M., & Madsen, S. D. (2007). So close, yet so far away: The impact of varying marital horizons on emerging adulthood. *Journal of Adolescent Research, 22*, 219–247.

Chassin, L., Pitts, S. C., & Prost, J. (2002). Binge drinking trajectories from adolescence to emerging adulthood in a high-risk sample: Predictors and substance abuse outcomes. *Journal of Consulting and Clinical Psychology, 70*, 67–78.

Cheah, C. S. L., & Nelson, L. J. (2004). The role of acculturation in the emerging adulthood of aboriginal college students. *International Journal of Behavioral Development, 28*, 495–507.

Cicchetti, D. (2006). Development and psychopathology. In D. Cicchetti & D. J. Cohen (Eds.), *Developmental psychopathology* (2nd ed., Vol. 1, pp. 1–23). New York: Wiley.

Cicchetti, D., & Curtis, W. J. (2006). The developing brain and neural plasticity: Implications for normality, psychopathology, and resilience. In D. Cicchetti & D. J. Cohen (Eds.), *Developmental psychopathology* (2nd ed., Vol. 2, pp. 1–64). New York: Wiley.

Cicchetti, D., & Curtis, W. J. (2007). Multilevel perspectives on pathways to resilient functioning [Special issue]. *Development and Psychopathology, 19*(3), 627–629.

Clingempeel, W. G., Henggeler, S. W., Pickrel, S. G., Brondino, M. J., & Randall, J. (2005). Beyond treatment effects: Predicting emerging adult alcohol and marijuana use among substance-abusing delinquents. *American Journal of Orthopsychiatry, 75*, 540–552.

Cohen, P., Kasen, S., Chen, H., Hartmark, C., & Gordon, K. (2003). Variations in patterns of developmental transitions in the emerging adulthood period. *Developmental Psychology, 39*, 657–669.

Dahl, R. E., & Spear, L. (2004). Adolescent brain development: Vulnerabilities and opportunities. *Annals of the New York Academy of Sciences, 1021*, 1–22.

Erikson, E. H. (1968). *Identity, youth and crisis*. New York: Norton.

Farrington, D. P. (1995). The development of offending and antisocial behaviour from childhood: Key findings from the Cambridge Study in Delinquent Development. *Journal of Child Psychology and Psychiatry, 36*, 929–964.

Gest, S. D., Reed, M.-G. J., & Masten, A. S. (1999). Measuring developmental changes in exposure to adversity: A life chart and rating scale approach. *Development and Psychopathology, 11*, 171–192.

Gest, S. D., Sesma, A., Masten, A. S., & Tellegen, A. (2006). Childhood peer reputation as a predictor of competence and symptoms 10 years later. *Journal of Abnormal Child Psychology, 34*, 509–526.

Giedd, J. N., Blumenthal, J., Jeffries, N. O., Castellanos, F. X., Liu, H., Zijdenbos, A., Paus, T., Evans, A. C., & Rapoport, J. L.. (1999). Brain development during childhood and adolescence: A longitudinal MRI study. *Nature Neuroscience, 2*, 861–863.

Gralinski-Bakker, J. H., Hauser, S. T., Stott, C., Billings, R. L., & Allen, J. P. (2004). Markers of resilience and risk: Adult lives in a vulnerable population. *Research in Human Development, 1*(4), 291–326.

Hauser, S. T., Allen, J. P., & Golden, E. (2006). *Out of the woods: Tales of resilient teens*. Cambridge, MA: Harvard University Press.

Havighurst, R. J. (1972). *Developmental tasks and education* (3rd ed.). New York: David McKay.

Hussong, A. M., & Chassin, L. (2004). Stress and coping among children of alcoholic parents through the young adult transition. *Development and Psychopathology, 16*, 985–1006.

Jessor, R., Donovan, J. E., & Costa, F. M. (1991). *Beyond adolescence: Problem behavior and young adult development*. Cambridge, England: Cambridge University Press.

Laub, J. H., Nagin, D. S., & Sampson, R. J. (1998). Trajectories of change in criminal offending: Good marriages and the desistance process. *American Sociological Review, 63*, 225–238.

Laub, J. H., & Sampson, R. J. (2001). Understanding desistance from crime. *Crime and Justice: A Review of Research, 28*, 1–69.

Lester, B. M., Masten, A. S., & McEwan, B. S. (Eds.). (2006). *Resilience in children* (Annals of the New York Academy of Sciences series). Malden, MA: Blackwell.

Loeber, R., Pardini, D., Stouthamer-Loeber, M., & Raine, A. (2007). Do cognitive, physiological, and psychosocial risk and promotive factors predict desistance from delinquency in males? *Development and Psychopathology, 19*, 867–887.

Luthar, S. S. (2006). Resilience in development: A synthesis of research across five decades. In D. Cicchetti & D. J. Cohen (Eds.), *Developmental psychopathology* (2nd ed., Vol. 3, pp. 739–795). New York: Wiley.

Masten, A. S. (2001). Ordinary magic: Resilience processes in development. *American Psychologist, 56*, 227–238.

Masten, A. S. (2007a). Competence, resilience, and development in adolescence: Clues for prevention science. In D. Romer & E. F. Walker (Eds.), *Adolescent psychopathology and the developing brain* (pp. 31–52): Oxford University Press.

Masten, A. S. (2007b). Resilience in developing systems: Progress and promise as the fourth wave rises. *Development and Psychopathology, 19*, 921–930.

Masten, A. S., Burt, K. B., & Coatsworth, J. D. (2006). Competence and psychopathology in development. In D. Cicchetti & D. J. Cohen (Eds.), *Developmental psychopathology* (2nd ed., Vol. 3, pp. 696–738). New York: Wiley.

Masten, A. S., Burt, K. B., Roisman, G. I., Obradovic, J., Long, J. D., & Tellegen, A. (2004). Resources and resilience in the transition to adulthood: Continuity and change. *Development and Psychopathology, 16*, 1071–1094.

Masten, A. S., & Coatsworth, J. D. (1998). The development of competence in favorable and unfavorable environments: Lessons from research on successful children. *American Psychologist, 53*(2), 205–220.

Masten, A. S., Coatsworth, J. D., Neeman, J., Gest, S. D., Tellegen, A., & Garmezy, N. (1995). The structure and coherence of competence from childhood through adolescence. *Child Development, 66*, 1635–1659.

Masten, A. S., Faden, V. B., Zucker, R. A., & Spear, L. P. (2008). Underage drinking: A developmental framework. *Pediatrics, 121* (Suppl. 4), 235–251.

Masten, A. S., Hubbard, J. J., Gest, S. D., Tellegen, A., Garmezy, N., & Ramirez, M. (1999). Competence in the context of adversity: Pathways to resilience and maladaptation from childhood to late adolescence. *Development & Psychopathology, 11*(1), 143–169.

Masten, A. S., Morison, P., & Pellegrini, D. S. (1985). A revised class play method of peer assessment. *Developmental Psychology, 21*, 523–533.

Masten, A. S., Obradović, J., & Burt, K. B. (2006). Resilience in emerging adulthood: Developmental perspectives on continuity and transformation. In J. J. Arnett & J. L. Tanner (Eds.), *Emerging adults in America: Coming of age in the 21st century* (pp. 173–192). Washington, DC: American Psychological Association.

Masten, A. S., Roisman, G. I., Long, J. D., Burt, K. B., Obradović, J., Riley, J. R., Boelcke-Stennes, K., & Tellegen, A. (2005). Developmental cascades: Linking academic achievement, externalizing and internalizing symptoms over 20 years. *Developmental Psychology, 41*, 733–746.

Moffitt, T. E., Caspi, A., Harrington, H., & Milne, B. J. (2002). Males on the life-course-persistent and adolescence-limited antisocial pathways: Follow-up at age 26 years. *Development and Psychopathology, 14*, 179–207.

Nagin, D. S., & Tremblay, R. E. (1999). Trajectories of boys' physical aggression, opposition, and hyperactivity on the path to physically violent and nonviolent juvenile delinquency. *Child Development, 70*(5), 1181–1196.

Obradović, J., Burt, K. B., & Masten, A. S. (2006). Pathways of adaptation from adolescence to young adulthood: Antecedents and correlates. *Annals of the New York Academy of Sciences, 1094*, 340–344.

Obradović, J., & Masten, A. S. (2007). Developmental antecedents of young adult civic engagement. *Applied Developmental Science, 11*, 2–19.

Obradović, J., Shaffer, A., & Masten, A. S. (in press). Risk in developmental psychopathology: Progress and future directions. In L. C. Mayes & M. Lewis (Eds.), *A developmental environment measures handbook*. Cambridge, England: Cambridge University Press.

Phinney, J. S. (2006). Ethnic identity exploration in emerging adulthood. In J. J. Arnett & J. L. Tanner (Eds.), *Emerging adults in America: Coming of age in the 21st century* (pp. 117–134). Washington, DC: American Psychological Association.

Rhule-Louie, D. M., & McMahon, R. J. (2007). Problem behavior and romantic relationships: Assortative mating, behavior contagion, and desistance. *Clinical Child and Family Psychology Review, 10*, 53–100.

Roisman, G. I., Aguilar, B., & Egeland, B. (2004). Antisocial behavior in the transition to adulthood: The independent and interactive roles of developmental history and emerging developmental tasks. *Development and Psychopathology, 16*, 857–871.

Roisman, G. I., Masten, A. S., Coatsworth, J. D., & Tellegen, A. (2004). Salient and emerging developmental tasks in the transition to adulthood. *Child Development, 75,* 123–133.

Rutter, M., & Sroufe, L. A. (2000). Developmental psychopathology: Concepts and challenges. *Developmental Psychopathology, 12,* 265–296.

Sampson, R. J., & Laub, J. H. (1993). *Crime in the making: Pathways and turning points through life.* Cambridge, MA: Harvard University Press.

Schulenberg, J. E., Bryant, A. L., & O'Malley, P. M. (2004). Taking hold of some kind of life: How developmental tasks relate to trajectories of well-being during the transition to adulthood. *Development and Psychopathology, 16,* 1119–1140.

Schulenberg, J. E., Wadsworth, K. N., O'Malley, P. M., Bachman, J. G., & Johnston, L. D. (1996). Adolescent risk factors for binge drinking during the transition to adulthood: Variable- and pattern-centered approaches to change. *Developmental Psychology, 32,* 659–674.

Sher, K. J., & Gotham, H. J. (1999). Pathological alcohol involvement: A developmental disorder of young adulthood. *Development and Psychopathology, 11,* 933–956.

Spear, L. P. (2007). The developing brain and adolescent-typical behavior patterns: An evolutionary approach. In D. Romer & E. F. Walker (Eds.), *Adolescent psychopathology and the developing brain: Integrating brain and prevention science* (pp. 9–30). New York: Oxford University Press.

Sroufe, L. A. (1979). The coherence of individual development: Early care, attachment, and subsequent developmental issues. *American Psychologist, 34,* 834–841.

Steinberg, L., Dahl, R. E., Keating, D., Kupfer, D. J., Masten, A. S., & Pine, D. (2006). The study of developmental psychopathology in adolescence: Integrating affective neuroscience with the study of context. In D. Cicchetti & D. J. Cohen (Eds.), *Developmental psychopathology* (2nd ed., Vol. 2, pp. 710–741). New York: Wiley.

Stouthamer-Loeber, M., Wei, E., Loeber, R., & Masten, A. S. (2004). Desistance from persistent serious delinquency in the transition to adulthood. *Development and Psychopathology, 16,* 897–918.

Waters, E., & Sroufe, L. A. (1983). Social competence as a developmental construct. *Developmental Review, 3,* 79–97.

Werner, E. E., & Smith, R. S. (1992). *Overcoming the odds: High risk children from birth to adulthood.* Ithaca, NY: Cornell University Press.

Werner, E. E., & Smith, R. S. (2001). *Journeys from childhood to midlife: Risk, resilience, and recovery.* Ithaca, NY: Cornell University Press.

Wickrama, K. A. S., Conger, R. D., Wallace, L. E., & Elder, G. H. (2003). Linking early social risks to impaired physical health during the transition to adulthood. *Journal of Health and Social Behavior, 44,* 61–74.

Zucker, R. A. (2006). Alcohol use and the alcohol use disorders: A developmental biopsychosocial systems formulation covering the life course. In D. Cicchetti & D. J. Cohen (Eds.), *Developmental Psychopathology* (2nd ed., Vol. 3, pp. 620–656). New York: Wiley.

Chapter 2

Adolescence: On the Neural Path to Adulthood

Anatomy, connectivity, and ontogeny of the nodes of the triadic model

Monique Ernst and Julie L. Fudge

As soon as his eyes fall on Maria, Tony experiences the most intense yearning to approach her. The surrounding world vanishes, except for Maria. They meet, they talk. Maria enters the spell. Braving familial and societal interdicts, Maria and Tony decide that they can change the world and be together. First and last love. Their desire leads to their destruction.

This vignette is a prototype of classical love stories told for centuries and across cultures. *Romeo and Juliet*, *West Side Story*, and *Werther*, among many extraordinary pieces of art, all draw the extremes of emotional intensity that move adolescents. They also portray the almost delusional aspect of these emotional states, which are characterized by a sense of invulnerability, disregard for danger, separation from a safe environment (i.e., family), and the most powerful drive to approach the object of desire. At the same time, the cognitive capacity for planning and navigating through complex situations is intact, if not exceptional. The ability to appreciate delayed rewards or anticipate loss may be deficient.

This vignette serves to introduce the unique conundrum of adolescence: peak of cognitive skills and remarkably poor decision making, which is held responsible for the unusual high rate of morbidity and mortality during this period. This chapter is dedicated to what is known at present of the neural underpinnings of adolescent motivated behavior, a mixture of greatness and awfulness.

Introduction to Adolescence

Young adulthood embodies the realization of the vulnerabilities and opportunities that characterize adolescence. What are the predictors of a successful transition from adolescence to adulthood? What can prevent the development, maintenance, or worsening of behavioral difficulties in the young adult? What can foster the fulfillment of the promises carried through adolescence? How can adolescent history inform treatment interventions for young adults? For example, problems with substance use that are preceded by depression in adolescence may benefit from a different approach than when preceded with attention-deficit/hyperactivity disorder. These questions beg an understanding of the factors that move adolescence into adulthood. These factors are multiple and encompass genetic, biological, and environmental determinants that act both separately and interactively. This chapter is focused on the contribution of brain ontogeny. More specifically, it is concerned with a dynamic neurobiological model of adolescence and presents a description of what is known of the anatomical and connectivity development of the three key cerebral structures of this model, that is, amygdala, striatum, and prefrontal cortex. These three neural nodes are proposed to interact in the processing of incoming information about stimuli that should be either approached, avoided, or just ignored. As discussed in length below, the amygdala, striatum, and prefrontal cortex each contribute to the final behavioral output, with the amygdala circuits playing a privileged, but not selective, role in avoidance, striatum circuits in approach, and prefrontal cortex in regulating approach versus avoidance.

Adolescence is the transition period during which individuals acquire and refine cognitive, emotional, and social skills in preparation for moving into responsible, independent, and sexually mature adults. Typical physical and behavioral changes take place during this period. These changes result from the interplay of biological and environmental factors, which map onto the classical nature–nurture scheme. The biological factors arise from genetic, hormonal, and neural domains. These factors promote changes that occur along a set timeline governed by a "developmental clock." A number of processes contribute interactively to this developmental clock, including the role of clock genes and the cumulative effects of hormonal and neural maturational changes that result in sharp irreversible new states.

Puberty is one of these new states. Some confusion between the boundaries of adolescence and puberty often occurs, because puberty is the most conspicuous event of this period. Here, we define puberty from an endocrine perspective as the activation of the hypothalamic-pituitary-gonadal axis and its consequences on physical growth and sexual maturation (Dorn, Dahl, Woodward, & Biro, 2006; Sisk & Foster, 2004).

Sexual maturation is accompanied by behavioral and social changes, which permit the adolescent to transit into his/her new role as an independent, reproductively mature, and socially competent adult. Together, these changes conform to the evolutionary fitness scheme (Steinberg & Belsky, 1996), which serves the ultimate goal of optimal species reproduction. Adolescents need to move away from the familial net and explore new territories to ultimately conserve genetic diversity and avoid genetic inbreeding. Behaviors that facilitate emigration include novelty seeking, risk taking, and a social shift from family to peer primacy.

The evolutionary-driven selection of these behaviors, which serve the ultimate goal of species conservation, comes at a high cost.

Adolescents, despite being at their lifetime peak of health, experience a considerable increase in rates of morbidity and mortality, which is attributed to emotional and behavioral perturbations. Particularly, a number of psychiatric disorders, such as substance use disorders, anxiety, and depression, exhibit their peak onset during adolescence (Arnett, 1992; Costello et al., 2002; Dahl, 2004; Ernst & Spear, 2008; Ernst, Pine, & Hardin, 2006; Masten, 2004; Pine, Cohen, Gurley, Brook, & Ma, 1998). Adolescence is thus recognized as a unique period of vulnerability for psychopathology and of opportunity for new life experiences and learning. Understanding the mechanisms underlying these critical behavioral and emotional changes may provide approaches for interventions that could reduce cost without altering benefit.

We will focus this review on the anatomy and neurodevelopmental changes of three major structures that form a triadic system and are associated with the regulation of goal-directed behavior (Fig. 2-1) (Ernst et al., 2005). Based on this system, we describe a heuristic model that can help formulate specific mechanistic hypotheses regarding the neural basis of typical developmental changes in goal-directed behavior, particularly relevant to adolescent risk-taking proclivity. By design, this model is simple and at present does not include factors such as hormones, genes, or environment. These excluded factors will need to be considered in future, more comprehensive renditions of the model. In addition, despite the well-recognized neurogenic role of neurotransmitter systems during development, particularly dopamine and serotonin, and their critical role in modulating the function of the triadic nodes, this review will not cover neurotransmitter systems, mainly due to space constraints. Readers are referred to discussion in the following references (Carlezon, Mague, & Andersen, 2003; Chambers, Taylor, & Potenza, 2003; Gaspar, Cases, & Maroteaux, 2003; Laviola, Adriani, Terranova, & Gerra, 1999; Ohtani, Goto, Waeber, & Bhide, 2003).

First, we will describe the triadic model. Second, we will review the anatomical and functional organization of the components of this model. A brief description of what is known of their ontogenic changes will also be provided.

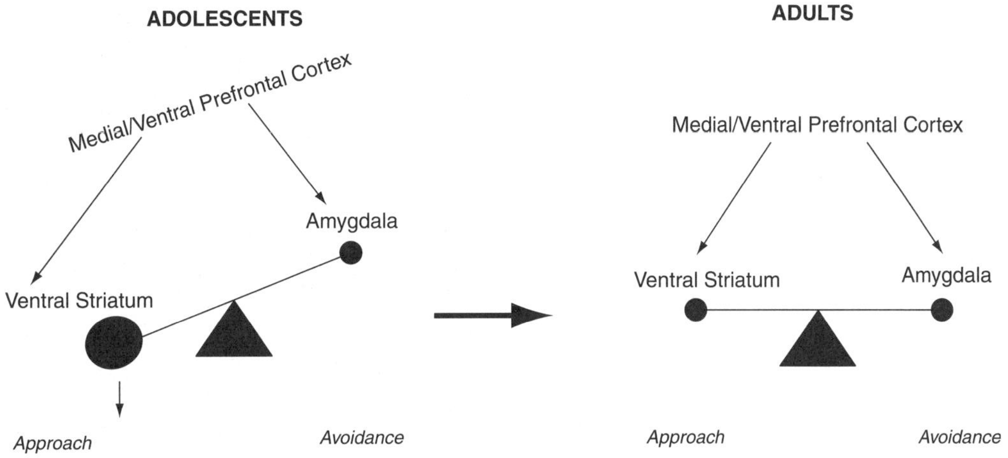

Figure 2-1. *Triadic model.* The balance between approach and avoidance systems is tilted toward approach behavior in adolescents relative to adults. The prefrontal cortex is not yet modulating this balance in a mature pattern. (This figure is also used in Ernst M, & Spear L. Development of reward systems in adolescence. In Michelle de Haan & Megan R. Gunnar (Eds.), *Handbook of Developmental Social Neuroscience*, Guilford Press, in press.)

The most striking feature of the latter is the dearth of data pertaining to the adolescent period. This section is designed not only to inform the theoretical foundation of the model but also to aid in the interpretation of the rapidly growing body of functional neuroimaging work dedicated to normal brain development. Third, we will integrate knowledge about these structures with the triadic model and identify questions and lines of research in most need of research for providing clinical applications.

The Triadic Neural Developmental Model

The triadic model provides a simple dynamic scheme of brain function that underlies goal-directed behavior (Fig. 2-1). This scheme was developed to understand how different patterns of regional brain maturation can explain different patterns of goal-directed behaviors.

Two lines of advances in cognitive and developmental neuroscience have inspired this model. First, goal-directed behaviors can be decomposed into component processes (e.g., approach, avoidance) that map onto distinct functional neural circuits (e.g., ventral striatum, amygdala). Reward-related processes are associated with approach responses, and aversive-related processes with withdrawal responses. Any goal-directed action emerges from the resolution of an impetus to move toward, to move away, or not to move. This resolution can be achieved through the integration of activity in the neural systems underlying approach and avoidance, and the supervision of this integration by a higher order system. Second, recent work shows that different brain regions undergo maturational changes along unique temporal trajectories, although most of these findings are reported for cortical regions (Casey, Jones, & Hare, 2008; Galvan et al., 2006; Giedd et al., 1999; Gogtay et al., 2004; Sowell, Trauner, Gamst, & Jernigan, 2002). Consequently, for similar input information, different end-point behaviors may arise at different points in time during development as a function of the functional balance among systems controlling behavioral responses. Particularly, in adolescence, this balance would favor approach behavior.

The three neural systems that constitute the triadic model underlie approach/reward behavior, avoidance/withdrawal behavior, and the regulation and fine-tuning of the balance between these two behavioral systems. These functional systems map onto discreet neural networks, which show some overlap with one another. At this early stage of the model, only three key structures, representative of each system, are considered: *amygdala* as the representative of the network supporting avoidance/withdrawal behavior, *nucleus accumbens* as the representative of the network supporting approach behavior, and *prefrontal cortex* as the representative of regulatory control. Of note, the role attributed to these structures is not absolute. This qualifier is important because it will need to be considered in future iterations of the model.

Indeed, the amygdala and nucleus accumbens both contribute to the processing of positively valenced (e.g., reward) and negatively valenced (e.g., punishment, threat) stimuli. However, a distinct functional dominance, which is best demonstrated with lesion studies, characterizes these structures: lesions of the amygdala typically are associated with reduced avoidance behaviors in the nonhuman primate, such as the reduced avoidance of snake (Aggleton, 2000; Bauman, Lavenex, Mason, Capitanio, & Amaral, 2004; Emery et al., 2001; Izquierdo, Suda, & Murray, 2005; Kalin, Shelton, Davidson, & Kelley, 2001; Kluver & Bucy, 1997; Machado & Bachevalier, 2006; Meunier, Bachevalier, Murray, Malkova, & Mishkin, 1999; Prather et al., 2001; Stefanacci, Clark, & Zola, 2003; Zola-Morgan, Squire, Alvarez-Royo, & Clower, 1991). Similar reduced fear response is reported in neurological patients with amygdala lesions (Adolphs, 2002; Bechara et al., 1995; LaBar, LeDoux, Spencer, & Phelps, 1995), and unique amygdalar sensitivity to threat stimuli has been documented in functional neuroimaging studies (for review, see Whalen, 1998).

In contrast, excitotoxic lesions of the nucleus accumbens "core" induces risk-averse choice in rats (Cardinal & Howes, 2005) and lesions of the nucleus accumbens "shell" region result in hypoactivity and attenuated response to the normally activating effects of amphetamine (Parkinson, Olmstead, Burns, Robbins, & Everitt, 1999). However, lesions of the nucleus core have also shown enhanced behavioral responses to amphetamine, reflecting functional heterogeneity of this structure (Parkinson et al., 1999). Chemical dopamine lesions of the nucleus accumbens in adult rodents result in difficulties switching fluidly from one behavior to another (Koob, Riley, Smith, & Robbins, 1978). By analogy, Parkinson disease is also associated with deficits in reward responses, particularly in "changing sets" to achieve a goal (Lewis, Dove, Robbins, Barker, & Owen, 2003; Taylor & Saint-Cyr, 1990).

Finally, the prefrontal cortex is a large functionally heterogeneous region, which comprises several areas involved in cognitive control (Miller, 2000). Medial prefrontal structures, including anterior cingulate cortex and medial prefrontal pole (Ridderinkhof, Ullsperger, Crone, & Nieuwenhuis, 2004) are probably the regions most closely associated with maintaining an adaptive balance between approach and avoidance behavioral responses. The triadic model is based on a unique functional balance among these three systems as a function of brain maturation.

The functional dominance of one system over the other could originate from *(1)* either a developmentally appropriate set-point, that determines the threshold for approach versus withdrawal behavior and is maintained by the regulatory control system, *(2)* a delayed maturation of one system relative to the other, *(3)* a delayed maturation of functional connectivity among these systems, *(4)* or any combination of the above. Much work needs to be done to clarify these possible underlying mechanisms.

The next section, by describing the anatomy and connectivity of the triadic nodes (amygdala, nucleus accumbens, and prefrontal cortex), may begin to provide some clues for the direction that research should take to examine these questions. A last caveat is about functional specificity. This chapter focuses on the neural mechanisms that underlie typical adolescent behavior, mainly novelty seeking and risk taking. The structures reviewed below contribute to a number of functions, not all directly at the service of goal-directed behavior. For example, processes such as emotional memory or conditioning depend heavily on the integrity of amygdalar and striatal structures. Conceivably, developmental changes may affect differently the various functions carried by a given network system, for example, mature conditioning versus immature approach behavior. This specificity needs to be kept in mind in the following discussion.

Anatomy, Connectivity, and Ontogeny of the Triadic Nodes

As far as we know, reviews of neurobiological models of behavior have not focused on detailed anatomy and connectivity of attendant neural structures, mainly because the current tools to investigate these structures in humans do not possess sufficient spatial resolution to provide such information (i.e., functional neuroimaging techniques). Here, we detail the anatomy and connectivity of each structure involved in the triadic model in the hope of strengthening the foundation of the model and to permit a more differentiated account of its mode of action.

Amygdala

Anatomy and Connectivity. The amygdala is a heterogeneous structure composed of highly interconnected nuclei (Price & Russchen, 1987) (Fig. 2-2). These nuclei can be functionally distinguished based on gene expression patterns, which correlate with unique embryologic origins for specific subdivisions (Zirlinger, Kreiman, & Anderson, 2001).

The cortical-like, or deep, nuclei of the amygdala form the greater part of this structure. These large nuclei resemble the cortex, without the apparent layering: they contain glutamatergic projection neurons in the form of pyramidal cells, are interconnected with the cortex, and project to the same striatal sectors as their reciprocal cortical targets (Van Hoesen, Yeterian, & Lavizzo-Mourey, 1981). The cortical-like nuclei are the main receiving nuclei, onto which converge inputs from sensory association cortex and hippocampus (Carmichael & Price, 1996; Ghashghaei & Barbas, 2002; Rosene & Van

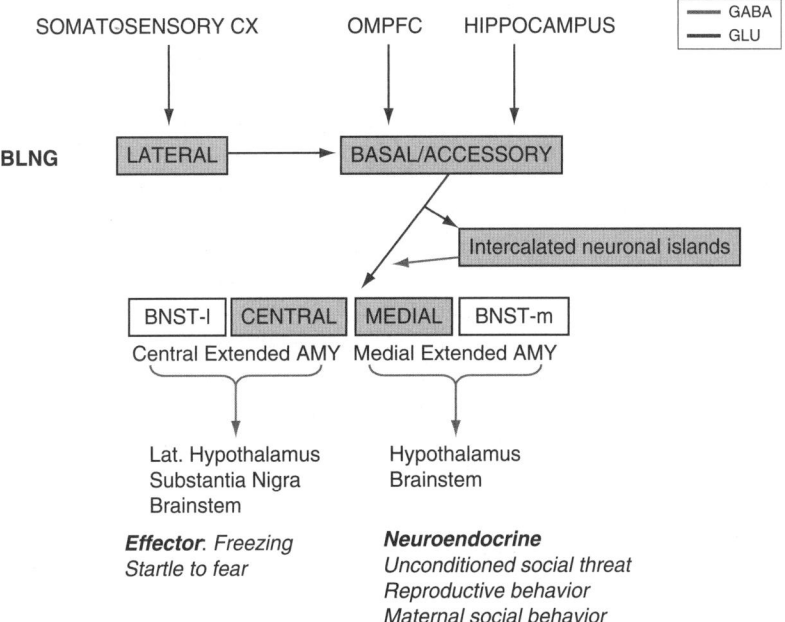

Figure 2-2. *Anatomy and connectivity of the amygdala.* Filled areas are nuclei of the amygdala. The medial extended amygdala is composed of the medial nucleus, the medial subdivision of the bed nucleus of the stria terminalis (BNST-m), and the near-continuous islands of cells that link them in the basal forebrain. The central extended amygdala includes the central nucleus, lateral BNST (BNST-I), and the chain of cell clusters intersperse between them in the basal forebrain. AMY, amygdala; BLNG, basolateral nuclear group; OMPFC, orbital and medial prefrontal cortex; BNST-m, medial subdivision of the bed nucleus of the stria terminalis; BNST-I, lateral subdivision of the bed nucleus of the stria terminalis. Arrows are glutamatergic projections, and GABAergic projections.

Hoesen, 1977; Saunders, Rosene, & Van Hoesen, 1988; Stefanacci & Amaral, 2000; Turner, Mishkin, & Knapp, 1980). They include the lateral, basal, and accessory basal nuclei, and they are often collectively referred to as the *basolateral nuclear group (BLNG)*.

Within the BLNG, information flows via distinct paths. Sensory association cortices project to the lateral nucleus following a general topography determined by sensory modality (Pitkanen & Amaral, 1998; Stefanacci & Amaral, 2000; Turner et al., 1980) The lateral nucleus, in turn, projects to the basal and accessory basal nuclei. In primates, the basal and accessory basal nuclei receive the majority of inputs from the hippocampus and orbital and medial prefrontal cortex (OMPFC) (Carmichael & Price, 1995; Saunders et al., 1988; Stefanacci & Amaral, 2000), areas that mediate information about the emotional context (via hippocampus) and incentive value (via OMPFC) of a stimulus.

Embedded in fibers surrounding the glutamatergic BLNG are islands of small GABAergic cells, known as the intercalated islands. These neuron clusters play an important role in setting the inhibitory tone of amygdala pathways (Pare, Royer, Smith, & Lang, 2003). The intercalated islands modulate the passage of information from the BLNG to the central nucleus in a feed-forward inhibitory mechanism by which excitatory fibers stimulating the central nucleus send collaterals to the intercalated islands. This has the effect of driving inhibitory output of the intercalated islands, which in turn modulate the central nucleus (Fig. 2-2). Anatomical studies in nonhuman primates indicate that these internal modulators of amygdala output themselves are strongly influenced by the caudal orbitofrontal cortex (Ghashghaei & Barbas, 2002) and the serotonin system (Bauman & Amaral, 2005; O'Rourke & Fudge, 2006). In rats, anterior cingulate may also play a role, since its stimulation dampens amygdala output and results in increased expression of neural activation markers (e.g., detected by c-fos expression) in the intercalated islands (Berretta, Pantazopoulos, Caldera, Pantazopoulos, & Pare, 2005; Quirk, Likhtik, Pelletier, & Pare, 2003). These studies suggest that cortical inhibition of amygdala outputs via the central nucleus is at least partly mediated through projections to the intercalated islands.

In contrast to the BLNG, the medial and central nucleus are relatively smaller nuclei that belong to a larger macrostructure known as the *extended amygdala* (Alheid & Heimer, 1988). The extended amygdala receives massive BLNG output, channeling this information to the hypothalamus and brain stem, modulating autonomic, visceral, and reflexive responses to rapidly changing environmental stimuli. Animal studies show that the extended amygdala is involved in responses to both positive and negative environmental cues.

The extended amygdala is further divided into a medial and a lateral component (Fig. 2-2). In rodent studies, the medial extended amygdala is involved in unconditioned responses to social threat (Blanchard, Canteras, Markham, Pentkowski, & Blanchard, 2005; Kollack-Walker, Watson, & Akil, 1997) along with reproductive and maternal social behaviors (Numan, Numan, Marzella, & Palumbo, 1998; Parfitt & Newman, 1998). The *central extended amygdala* is considered an effector of motor and autonomic responses such as freezing and startle to fear stimuli (Hitchcock & Davis, 1991; Parfitt & Newman, 1998; Wilensky, Schafe, Kristensen, & LeDoux, 2006;), but it is also involved in balancing approach and avoidance of stimuli during changes in the predictive value of environmental cues (Holland & Gallagher, 2006; Killcross, Robbins, & Everitt, 1997; Petrovich et al., 2006). These latter effects may be partly mediated through inputs to the dopamine neurons of the substantia nigra, which modulate striatal and cortical function (Fudge & Haber, 2000; Lee et al., 2005; Lee et al., 2006). As can be seen, the developmental stage and emotional processing capacity of the amygdala will have important downstream effects on neuroendocrine and social defensive behaviors (medial extended amygdala) mediated through the hypothalamus, and fear/approach behaviors (central extended amygdala) mediated through the dopamine system in the developing animal or human.

Ontogeny. The amygdala is the earliest formed structure of the telencephalon, and its nuclear subdivisions can be appreciated by 8–9 weeks gestational age in the human (Macchi, 1951; Muller & O'Rahilly, 1990). Development continues over the ensuing gestation, with differential developmental trajectories for specific nuclei (Kordower, Piecinski, & Rakic, 1992; Kornack & Rakic, 1998).

Whether and how the primate amygdala matures over human postnatal life is not well studied. MRI studies in children show that the amygdala enlarges in a linear fashion relative to temporal lobe volume more in boys than girls (Giedd et al., 1996). However, there is large variability in individual growth, suggesting the need for very large sample sizes to draw conclusions. Microscopic studies indicate that immature neurons persist throughout postnatal life and beyond in both humans and monkeys (Bernier, Bedard, Vinet, Levesque, & Parent, 2002; Crosby & Humphrey, 1941; Fudge, 2004; Fudge & Haber, 2002; Millhouse, 1986). These immature cells are specifically distributed in the paralaminar nucleus (located in the remnant of the germinal zone) and in fiber bundles of the stria terminalis that pass through this region. Their presence suggests that the postnatal primate amygdala has the capacity for neuroplastic changes well into adulthood. What is not understood is whether these cells integrate into existing amygdala circuits and, if so, when this occurs.

Since the time of Kluver-Bucy, newer lesioning techniques have helped define the role of the amygdala and its function over development. These studies support the idea that the amygdala matures postnatally, since ibotenic acid lesions placed in infancy result in different behavioral profiles in adulthood (Bauman et al., 2004; Prather et al., 2001). Both adult and infants with amygdala lesions have blunted fear responses to non-social cues, such as snakes (Izquierdo et al., 2005; Kalin et al., 2001; Meunier et al., 1999; Prather et al., 2001; Stefanacci et al., 2003). This suggests a role in signaling nonsocial, perhaps hard-wired, fear responses in both adulthood and infancy. Unchanging fear responses to cues that are always dangerous would clearly be an adaptive function. At the same time, new studies show that responses to *social* cues (the presence of other animals) is altered depending on the age of the animal at the time of lesioning and testing.

For example, amygdala-lesioned adult monkeys show increased excitability and exploratory behaviors with other animals, suggesting a loss of learned fear associations (Emery et al., 2001; Machado & Bachevalier, 2006). However, lesioned infant monkeys show more fear behaviors and lower aggression to novel animals, and normal proximity responses to familiar caregivers present since birth (Bauman & Amaral, 2005; Goursaud & Bachevalier, 2007; Prather et al. 2001; Thompson & Towfighi, 1976). These data suggest that the infant amygdala mediates social emotional learning, laying down engrams of what is familiar and safe, what is familiar and dangerous, and what is unknown and therefore potentially dangerous in the social environment. Human studies of children with Williams syndrome, a genetic neurodevelopmental disorder that results in increased amygdala volume and hypersociability, indicate that these children have abnormally low amygdala responses to social threat compared to normal children (Meyer-Lindenberg et al., 2005; Reiss et al., 2004).

Virtually no animal studies have examined the developmental trajectories, encompassing the adolescent period, of the structures and connections of the amygdala. However, there is clear evidence that dynamic changes in connectivity occur between infancy and adulthood (Webster, Ungerleider, & Bachevalier, 1991). Functionally, neuroimaging work in humans is beginning to identify differences in amygdala responses to affective stimuli in adolescents compared to adults. Overall, the amygdala seems to be more responsive in adolescents than in adults during identification of negatively valenced social face stimuli (Guyer et al., 2008; Killgore & Yurgelun-Todd, 2004; Monk et al., 2003) but less influenced by processes involved in negative monetary outcomes (Ernst et al., 2005). This functional pattern suggests either lower modulation of this structure by regulatory systems mainly originating from prefrontal regions (immaturity of top-down modulatory systems) or intrinsic cellular/molecular/neurochemical immaturity within the structure. Although highly speculative, it is conceivable that the medial extended amygdala, which is associated more specifically with social threat, matures differently across adolescence than the central extended amygdala, which mediates freezing response to threat. This functional dichotomy would explain the differences in adolescent-adult contrasts of amygdala responses to social threat versus nonsocial aversive stimuli.

Striatum

Anatomy and Connectivity. The striatum (caudate and putamen) is largely composed of medium-spiny neurons (Graveland & DiFiglia, 1985), which send information through basal ganglia circuits. The striatum and the globus pallidus are referred to as the basal ganglia. Information flows from the cortex, to the striatum, where it is channeled to the globus pallidus, then the thalamus and finally back to the cortex (Fig. 2-3). In fact, the corticostriatal projection is one of the major projections from the prefrontal cortex in primates (Goldman & Nauta, 1977; Kemp & Powell, 1970). The highly specialized medium-spiny neurons are recipients of a large number of excitatory afferent fibers from the prefrontal cortex and amygdala, which terminate mainly on the many spine heads covering each dendrite (Lapper, Smith, Sadikot, Parent, & Bolam, 1992). This anatomic arrangement allows for multiple cortical inputs to modulate individual striatal cells and, in turn, determine basal ganglia output. The midbrain dopamine neurons also send afferents throughout the striatum and regulate which cortical inputs ultimately result in striatal cell firing (Grace, Floresco, Goto, & Lodge, 2007) (see below).

The topography of striatal inputs from the limbic, association, and motor-related regions of the prefrontal cortex has led to the idea that the striatum can be divided into discrete functional domains. Yet significant debate exists as to whether cortical inputs to the striatum are organized in a strictly topographic manner (Alexander & Crutcher, 1990) or whether there are opportunities for convergence of information from different functional regions of cortex (Haber, Kim, Mailly, & Calzavara, 2006).

In general, the amygdala and those cortical regions most directly influenced by the amygdala ("limbic-related") project to the ventral striatum. This region includes the "shell" and "core" of the nucleus accumbens, and the ventromedial caudate and putamen. Cortical regions involved in sensorimotor processes project to the dorsolateral striatum. Associative, or "cognitive-related," regions such as the dorsolateral prefrontal cortex (Brodmann areas 46, 9) project to central regions of the striatum that lie interposed between the ventral striatum and dorsolateral striatum.

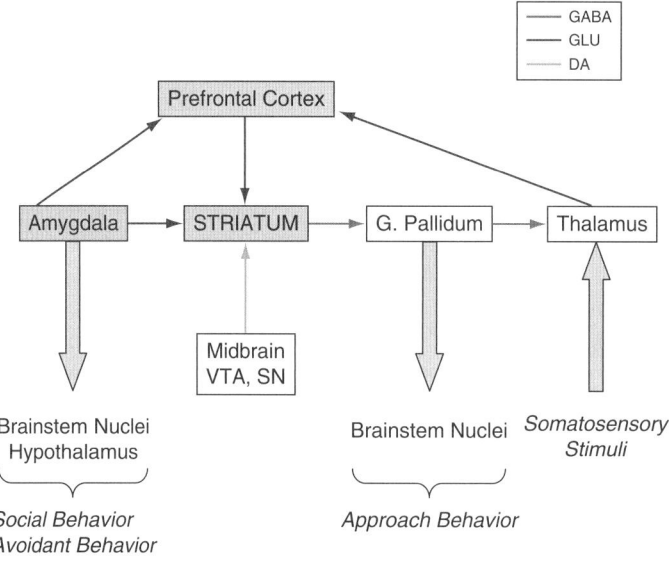

Figure 2-3. *Anatomy and connectivity of the striatum.* VTA, ventral tegmental area; SN, substantia nigra; G. Pallidum, globus pallidum; DA, dopamine; GLU, glutamate.

However, recent evidence shows that inputs from diverse functional domains of the cortex converge in patches in the striatum, creating hot spots where information can be integrated (Haber et al., 2006). Thus, for example, afferent fibers from limbic-related and associative areas converge in patches within the central striatum (Haber et al., 2006). It is not yet known whether such foci of cortical afferent convergence correlate with cellular islands that arise during development (see below), or how and when such convergence occurs. In summary, while the concept of a "functional topography" of the striatum based on segregated cortical inputs has heuristic value, new data indicate that this scheme may be overly simplistic.

The overall functional topography of the striatum exists along the entire rostrocaudal extent of the striatum, a fact which has been under-appreciated. Thus, the functional gradient traditionally attached to the rostral striatum (anterior to the decussation of the commissure) extends caudally. In a series of elegant experiments, Selemon demonstrated that cortical projections terminate along the ventromedial (limbic) to dorsolateral (sensorimotor) gradient following the entire rostrocaudal extent of the striatum (Selemon & Goldman-Rakic, 1985). In addition, anterograde tracer injections into the amygdala have also indicated that afferent fibers terminate in the caudal ventromedial striatum, as well as in the nucleus accumbens (Fudge, Kunishio, Walsh, Richard, & Haber, 2002; Fudge, Breitbart, & McClain, 2004; Russchen, Bakst, Amaral, & Price, 1985). Based on inputs from the amygdala and rostral agranular insula, as well as cellular and neurochemical similarities to the nucleus accumbens, we have proposed that the caudal limbic striatal region includes the lateral amygdalostriatal area, the ventromedial putamen, and medial tail of the caudate nucleus (Fudge et al., 2004).

The identification of such an anatomical ensemble, which includes elements of PFC, amygdala, and ventral striatum, may provide a unique opportunity to examine the foundations of the triadic model. In our view, the limbic striatum can be defined as that part of the striatum that receives inputs from the amygdala (Fudge et al., 2002; Fudge et al., 2004). As mentioned the amygdala projects to a broad rostrocaudal extent of the striatum, expanding the definition of the limbic striatum far beyond the nucleus accumbens. These regions receive variable inputs from prefrontal cortical areas including the anterior cingulate, medial and lateral orbital cortex, and the agranular insula (Carmichael & Price, 1996; Ferry, Ongur, An, & Price, 2000; Haber et al., 2006; Selemon & Goldman-Rakic, 1985). Determining the detailed overlap between amygdala and prefrontal cortical afferents in the striatum will help us get a grasp on how emotional inputs from amygdala may facilitate throughput from discrete prefrontal cortical regions.

Taking a step further, the resultant signal of the limbic striatum may vary along a gradient across this structure. This variation could represent different types of combination of amygdala/PFC afferents. Approach behaviors might be mediated by a unique set of afferents, while avoidance behaviors by another set of afferents. Indeed, a recent fMRI study of financial reward and loss shows that the anterior ventral striatum has relative selectivity for reward prediction, while more posterior striatum signals prediction of loss (Seymour, Daw, Dayan, Singer, & Dolan, 2007). This is consistent with appetitive/aversive ventral striatal gradients detected in rats using pharmacologic probes (Reynolds & Berridge, 2001, 2002, 2003). Such a scheme could be integrated into the triadic model by modifying the selective function of the nodes. A fractal rather than modal representation of function could be a more accurate model, that is, the triadic balance being mapped at the level of each node. Reflected in ontogeny studies, the anatomical and functional organization of afferents within each structure evolves with age. A pure fractal organization would be difficult to study using neuroimaging studies, as what is detected is the integrated neural activity within structures. However, as suggested by lesion studies (as reviewed above) and functional neuroimaging studies of development, some polarity of function seems to be attached to the triadic nodes. Thus, a combination of fractal and modular organization may be the optimal representation of the model. The study of functional connectivity may be best suited for examining the fractal aspect of the triadic model, whereas activation studies might best track their functional polarity.

Ontogeny. Most knowledge on the development of primate striatum stems from early work in nonhuman primates. In general, corticostriatal pathways develop before cortico-cortical connections (Goldman-Rakic, 1987). Cortical afferents arrive in the striatum early in the second trimester and steadily increase their innervation over the rest of gestation. The striatum undergoes a shift several weeks after corticostriatal innervation begins. The cytoarchitectural pattern changes from a homogeneous mass of densely packed cells to cellular islands of densely packed cells encapsulated by fibers and surrounded by a relatively less densely packed matrix of neurons (Goldman-Rakic, 1981). The reason for this transformation is unclear, but it is speculated that either migration of clusters of new neurons and/or the entry and retraction of afferent contacts play a role in this development. There is some indication that the dopamine innervation of the striatum plays a role in maintaining the integrity of the cellular islands, which persist throughout life (van der Kooy, 1996).

After birth, recognizable neuronal subtypes still exist in various stages of growth, as do undifferentiated cells near the ventricular wall. Rapid increases in synaptic density level off, but ultrastructural changes in synaptic modeling continue. Spine density on dendrites increases progressively over at least the next 4 months in monkeys (Brand & Rakic, 1984), and with this, the proportion of axon contacts shifts toward axospinous rather than axodendritic types. This shift is functionally significant because spines increase the overall length of the dendrite, hence its electrical resistance. The shift to axospinous contacts over axodendritic ones thus has the effect of decreasing the contribution of any individual input to the total excitatory postsynaptic potential of the cell (Gerfen, 1988; Sharpe & Tepper, 1998). Consequently, the increase in afferents arriving in the striatum during postnatal life may be balanced by the concurrent increase in spines, which may serve to attenuate the effects of any particular excitatory input to a cell. These changes concur to a refinement of striatal modulation (Gerfen, 1988; Sharpe & Tepper, 1998). The evolution of axospinous over axodendritic contacts, along with continuing degeneration of some afferent axons, suggests important alterations in information processing at least during the first months of life and perhaps well beyond.

Volumetric studies using MRI indicate that the striatum, specifically the caudate nucleus, undergoes volume loss starting on average around 10 years of age in girls and 14 years of age in boys and exhibiting a steeper volume decrease in girls than boys (Lenroot et al., 2007). Furthermore, Sowell and colleagues found that a significant volume reduction in the ventromedial putamen (an area we consider part of the limbic striatum due to its afferents from the amygdala) differed between adolescents and young adults (Sowell, Thompson, Holmes, Jernigan, & Toga, 1999). Human studies using functional neuroimaging tools are taking the lead in investigating the behavioral correlates of striatal activity tested in several laboratories (Bjork et al. 2004; Casey et al., 2008; Ernst et al., 2005; Ernst & Spear, 2008).

Dopamine, as a key mediator of striatal structures and a central component of reward function needs mention, even though it lies outside the boundaries of the present review. Thus, for completeness, we will list the dopamine models that have dominated the field of the neurobiology of reward systems (for review, Ernst & Spear, 2008). According to the *hedonic theory*, dopamine was first proposed as a translator of *hedonia* (Wise, 1980). Later, the *incentive salience theory* (Berridge, 2000) was introduced and distinguished the hedonic from the motivational attributes of reward, arguing that dopamine modulates the "wanting" rather than the "liking" of rewards. The *reward prediction error*, based on electrophysiological studies in nonhuman primates, refers to dopamine as an error signal detection that codes the difference in expected value versus actual value of received outcomes (Schultz, Dayan, & Montague, 1997). The *tonic-phasic dopamine theory* provides a mechanistic rendition of the modulation of reward processes, describing how the extrasynaptic tonic dopamine tone modulates the phasic, stimulus-bound, intrasynaptic dopamine activity (Grace, 1995). Whereas these theories have been used to explain psychopathologies, particularly addiction, none of them have integrated ontogenetic development. This is noteworthy given the wealth of data on ontogenetic changes of dopamine function across the life span, and particularly during adolescence (for review, Andersen, 2005; Laviola, Macri, Morley-Fletcher, & Adriani, 2003; Spear, 2000).

Prefrontal Cortex

Anatomy and Connectivity with Amygdala. The primate cortex in general ranges from a simple one- to two-layered primitive cortex (known as the allocortex) to a six-layered isocotex (Northcutt & Kaas, 1995). Between these extremes of differentiation are the periallocortical regions. The undifferentiated allocortical zones include the hippocampus and piriform cortex; these primitive cortices are most tightly interconnected with the amygdala. The periallocortex can show a range of transitional features, but in general it has poorly demarcated layers II and IV and a relatively rudimentary layer V. The rostral anterior cingulate (Brodmann areas 25, 32, 14) and the caudal orbital cortex (now recognized as the rostral agranular insula, or proisocortex) comprise important periallocortical regions of the prefrontal cortex. These areas are the most strongly interconnected with the amygdala (Amaral, 1986; Carmichael & Price, 1996; Ghashghaei & Barbas, 2002).

Many amygdalar subregions that send efferents to the OMPFC are the recipients of return projections (Amaral, 1986). The major amygdalar inputs to the OMPFC originate from the basal nucleus and terminate into the medial wall and the caudal orbital surface of the OMPFC. In turn, the caudal orbital surface of the OMPFC returns afferents to the intercalated neurons, modulating the output of the basal nucleus. In contrast, the medial wall of the OMPFC provides the main projections to the BLNG, that is, both basal and lateral nuclei.

Other periallocortical regions of the prefrontal cortext (PFC), while still less differentiated than isocortex, have relatively more differentiated elements than areas 25, 32, 14, and the agranular insula. These regions, including rostral areas 13, 11, and 12, receive relatively few afferents from the amygdala and project back sparingly. The isocortex forms the great majority of the primate cortex, is involved in associative and motor control functions, and is not directly interconnected with the amygdala. Nonetheless, isocortical areas, specifically those involved in working memory and planning (areas 9/46), receive inputs from the limbic cortex (Carmichael & Price, 1996; Petrides & Pandya, 1999). This organization provides an anatomical substrate for affective processing to influence mediating planning and sequencing functions via cortical–cortical interactions.

Anatomy and Connectivity with Striatum. As mentioned above, the limbic striatum can be defined by regions receiving inputs from the amygdala. Typically, these striatal regions also receive inputs from areas of the prefrontal cortex which themselves are innervated by the amygdala, creating a triangular set of inputs. It is important to remember that by this definition—as well as based on functional data—that the ventral striatum extends well beyond the nucleus accumbens. For example, the ventromedial prefrontal cortex (area 25), which is strongly interconnected with the amygdala, projects to the shell of the nucleus accumbens but also to the adjacent ventromedial caudate nucleus. More dorsal sectors of the anterior cingulate (areas 24a and b), which also receive amygdala inputs, albeit somewhat fewer, project to the head of the caudate nucleus, the central rostral putamen, and core of the nucleus accumbens (Haber et al., 2006). The posterolateral orbitofrontal cortex, again innervated by the amygdala, projects to the lateral nucleus accumbens and ventromedial putamen (Ferry et al., 2000; Fudge, Breitbart, Danish, & Pannoni, 2005). Prefrontal cortical regions that receive few amygdala inputs (such as association areas like areas 46/9,) occupy more dorsolateral regions of the striatum. However, their terminals do overlap with those from more limbic regions, such as the dorsal anterior cingulate, suggesting potential convergence of limbic and cognitive information at the level of the striatum.

Ontogeny. Similarly to the temporal lobe, including the BLNG, the prefrontal cortex is significantly expanded in higher primates compared to lower species (Gloor, 1997; Jerison, 1973). This expansion accompanies a protracted developmental period, which continues through late childhood and adolescence. A cellular explanation for this expansion, at least with respect to the prefrontal cortex, is offered by Kornack and Rakic. They have demonstrated that the duration of the cell cycle (during cell division) is up to five times longer in primates compared to rodents. At the same time, many more total rounds of division occur during the neurogenetic period in monkeys, accelerating toward the end of development (Kornack & Rakic, 1998). Together these findings provide a basis for understanding the greater size and lamination of the cortex and why its development occurs over a lengthy period postnally.

Recently, structural neuroimaging has provided information on human brain development during childhood and adolescence using relatively crude measures related to volumetric estimations of discrete brain regions. An overall increase in cortical size was reported during childhood (Durston et al., 2001; Giedd et al., 1996), which seems to co-occur with changes in dendritic density and increased myelination (Paus et al., 1999; Yakovlev et al., 2001). Between childhood and adolescence, cortical gray matter changes were found to be diffusely distributed in dorsal frontal and parietal regions, whereas between adolescence and adulthood, cortical changes seemed to be segregated within large frontal regions comprising dorsal, mesial, and orbital areas (Giedd et al., 1999; Sowell et al., 1999).

Synaptogenesis in the PFC wanes after age 2 (Huttenlocher, 1979), with synaptic pruning resulting in dendritic densities resembling adult levels by about age 16 (Huttenlocher, 1979). The rate of synaptic eliminations varies by regions, ending first in primary sensory cortices (around age 12 years) and last in the prefrontal cortex by age 16 years (Huttenlocher & Dabholkar, 1997). In addition, there is active maturation of synapse morphology, specifically of presynaptic terminals during periadolescence (Huttenlocher, 1979).

Progressive myelination changes through childhood and adolescence have also been documented in postmortem samples (Yakovlev, 1967) and more recently with magnetic resonance imaging (MRI) (Benes, Turtle, Khan, & Farol, 1994; Giedd et al., 1996; Paus et al., 1999). Significant age-related increases in white matter density (generated with 3-D masks) occurs in the arcuate fasciculus on the dominant side, and in the posterior internal capsule (Paus et al., 1999). These tracts carry axons joining the frontal and temporal speech areas (Broca's and Wernicke's areas) and cortex and brain stem (corticospinal tract), respectively. An increase in tract size is likely due to a combination of increasing axonal diameter, coupled with myelination of the tracts. The relationship between age-related changes in regional white matter density and competence in specific cognitive and motor functions remains to be explored.

In general, recent developmental functional neuroimaging studies report more diffuse activation of the prefrontal cortex during cognitive challenges in preadolescence, suggesting a less efficient or well-formed networks to carry out specific processing (Luna & Sweeney, 2004; Luna, Garver, Urban, Lazar, & Sweeney, 2004). More specifically, a shift from diffuse to focal activation has been proposed as a general developmental pattern of cortical engagement in cognitive function (Durston & Casey, 2006). During the processing of given cognitive tasks, accessory regions become less involved, whereas critical regions to the cognitive processes are recruited more readily and strongly. Hence, the narrowing of recruited regions may reflect enhanced specificity and a more efficient use of neural networks for task completion.

Conclusion: The Fractal Triadic Model and Clinicial Implications

In conclusion, this review highlights the complexity of the anatomical and functional organization of key structures to behavior and, subsequently, the many possibilities for deviation during development. This work culminates in the revised formulation of the triadic model into the *fractal triadic model*, which, although more complicated than the original description, may provide a better rendition of the various anatomical and functional elements to account for when testing specific hypotheses. Below, we extract the most salient points for the amygdala, striatum, and prefrontal cortex and close with thoughts about how such a model can help the clinician to better understand behavioral disorders in the young adults.

Three critical points dominate the review on the amygdala. *First*, lesion studies have different long-term behavioral impacts as a function of the developmental stage at which the lesion occurs. This underscores the notion of windows of vulnerability. *Second*, this differential impact does not apply indiscriminately to all behavioral responses. Innate responses, such as avoidance of snakes by monkeys, seem to be impervious to the notion of sensitive periods, whereas social behavior appears to be highly dependent on the timing of amygdala lesion. And *third*, developmental changes of the intact amygdala manifests opposite functional patterns as a function of the stimuli: challenged by threat-related stimuli, the amygdala shows greater activation in adolescents than in adults. However, challenged by receipt of losses, the amygdala shows diminished responses in adolescents relative to adults. This functional heterogeneity is consistent with the complex structure (multinuclei), connectivity of the amygdala, and anatomic evidence of immature neurons that persist throughout adolescence and into adulthood. As a result, however, it is critical to avoid overgeneralization of a given pattern of response, be it developmental or to distinct stimuli.

The striatum is larger than the amygdala and receives direct inputs, in an organized fashion, from the totality of the prefrontal cortex. The segregation of function that comprises sensory-motor, cognitive, and affective processing has been classically aligned along a dorsoventral gradient. This somatotopic organization is shown to be more complex, with the existence of a convergence of these functional paths onto distinct "patches," as well as the realization that the functional ventrodorsal gradient is present along the whole length of the rostro-caudal (antero-posterior) extent of the striatum. It is unknown whether such organization is present since birth or how it evolves across childhood and adolescence. Clearly, the few developmental histological studies suggest a refinement of striatal modulation. Similarly to the amygdala, developmental patterns of activation in humans depend on the type of stimuli/events under study. Relative to adults, adolescents show enhanced striatal activity to receipt of rewards or punishments and selection of risky choices, but reduced activity in anticipation of rewards.

Finally, the prefrontal cortex is the most complex structure with the most protracted period of maturation. It receives information from the amygdala directly and striatum indirectly (via cortico-basal ganglia loops) and, in turn, modulates both structures.

Taken together, the organization and reciprocal connectivity of these three main structures, as reviewed here, bring a "fractal" dimension to the heuristic triadic model, that is, each node (amygdala, striatum, and prefrontal cortex) is itself the seat of a triadic representation (Fig. 2-4). The next step will be to better identify the relative weight and connections among these nine subnodes (i.e., three for each main structure).

How can such a complex heuristic model of motivated behavior help the clinician interested in the young adult to better understand problems in this population? This question has two-fold answer.

First, this model arose from observations of typical changes in motivated behavior (e.g., enhanced risk taking) during the transitional period of adolescence. It was meant to provide testable neural mechanisms underlying deviant neurodevelopmental trajectories that would lead to behavioral disorders in the young adult. This highlights the critical importance of collecting information on adolescent behavior in the assessment of young adult health problems. Distinct trajectories may reflect unique dysfunctions that could be understood as specific deficits within the triadic model and provide prognostic as well as strategic information about focused therapeutic interventions. Much more work needs to be done before such a goal is attained. However, the role of clinicians in this enterprise is critical as they will supply necessary data to inform the model.

Second, while this model infers that disorders of motivated behavior can reflect dysfunction in a number of neural networks, it also suggests that there are as many possibilities for modulation and compensation to such dysfunction. In other words, the enhanced complexity adds, on the one hand, more possibilities for deficits but, on the other hand, more possibilities for plasticity. For example, if depression originates from dysfunction within the prefrontal triadic balance,

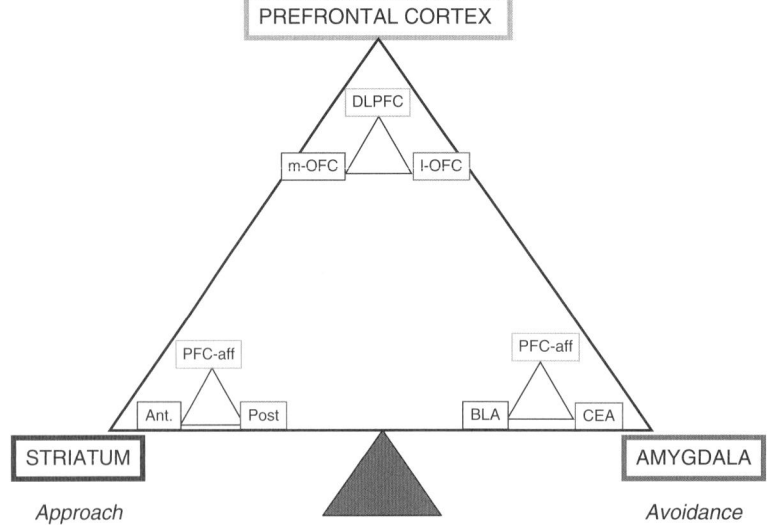

Figure 2-4. *Fractal triadic model.* In this model, each of the three representative nodes of approach, avoidance, and regulatory control is itself the seat of a triadic formation that mirrors the overall organization. Examples of regions previously identified to be associated in some studies with either appetitive or aversive responses are provided. However, similarly to the original triadic model, this representation is not over-inclusive. DLPFC, dorsolateral prefrontal cortex; m-OFC, medial orbital frontal cortex; l-OFC, lateral orbital frontal cortex; PFC-aff, prefrontal cortical afferents; Ant, anterior striatum; Post, posterior striatum; BLA, basolateral amygdala; CEA, central amygdala.

one might expect more cognitive-related alterations, and perhaps treatment could focus on the healthier nodes of the amygdala and striatum. In contrast, if the amygdala triadic balance were the primary cause of depression, then one might expect more intact cognitive function and more anxiety associated with the disorder. Here, focus might best be directed onto fostering remediation through reinforcing prefrontal and striatal balances.

At this point, although still highly speculative, such framework paves the way for focused research, helping formulate discrete questions that can be approached in studies with a priori hypotheses. A model is only valid until it is disproved by accumulation of more knowledge.

KEY POINTS

- Adolescence is characterized by biologically driven maturational changes in neural functional units that determine the characteristics of adolescent behavior (e.g., risk taking, intense emotionality).
- Therefore, extreme behaviors during adolescence are for the most part normative and serve some adaptive function in evolutionary fitness.
- The aim of understanding the neural underpinnings of this normative pattern of behavior is to help devise strategies to channel excessive behaviors into adaptive and fruitful goals.
- As a period of tremendous biological and environmental changes, adolescence is also a critical period of high vulnerability for the

development of behavioral disorders. Here, again, understanding the neural substrates of motivated behavior and their maturational trajectories across development can revolutionize treatment and particularly prevention of psychiatric disorders.

PRACTICE GUIDELINES

- Reinforce the current societal trend to protect adolescents from consequences of risky behaviors, such as substance abuse.
- Given that adolescents are more sensitive to rewards than to punishments, positive reinforcement techniques might be more powerful than negative reinforcement to help adjust behavior.
- Based on the critical importance of social acceptance by peers in the adolescent world, the judicious use of social parameters in treatment should be considered.

References

Adolphs, R. (2002). Neural systems for recognizing emotion. *Current Opinions in Neurobiology, 12,* 169–177.

Aggleton, J. P. (2000). The functional effects of amygdala lesions in humans: A comparison with findings from monkeys. The amygdala, a functional analysis (2nd ed., pp. 485–504). New York: Oxford University Press.

Alexander, G. E., & Crutcher, M. D. (1990). Functional architecture of basal ganglia circuits: Neural substrates of parallel processing. *Trends in Neuroscience, 13,* 266–271.

Alheid, G. F., & Heimer, L. (1988). New perspectives in basal forebrain organization of special relevance for neuropsychiatric disorders: The striatopallidal, amygdaloid, and corticopetal components of substantia innominata. *Neuroscience, 27,* 1–39.

Amaral, D. G. (1986). Amygdalohippocampal and amygdalocortical projections in the primate brain. In Schwarz, R. Y. A. (ed.) *Excitary amino acids and epilepsy* (pp. 3–17). New York: Plenum Publishing Company.

Andersen, S. L. (2005). Stimulants and the developing brain. *Trends in Pharmacological Sciences, 26,* 237–243.

Arnett, J. J. (1992). Reckless behavior in adolescence: A developmental perspective. *Developmental Review, 12,* 339–373.

Bauman, M. D., & Amaral, D. G. (2005). The distribution of serotonergic fibers in the macaque monkey amygdala: an immunohistochemical study using antisera to 5 hydroxytryptamine. *Neuroscience, 136,* 193–203.

Bauman, M. D., Lavenex, P., Mason, W. A., Capitanio, J. P., & Amaral, D. G. (2004). The development of mother-infant interactions after neonatal amygdala lesions in rhesus monkeys. *Journal of Neuroscience, 24,* 711–721.

Bechara, A., Tranel, D., Damasio, H., Adolphs, R., Rockland, C., & Damasio, A. R. (1995). Double dissociation of conditioning and declarative knowledge relative to the amygdala and hippocampus in humans. *Science, 269,* 1115–1118.

Benes, F. M., Turtle, M., Khan, Y., & Farol, P. (1994). Myelination of a key relay zone in the hippocampal formation occurs in the human brain during childhood, adolescence, and adulthood. *Archives of General Psychiatry, 51,* 477–484.

Bernier, P. J., Bedard, A., Vinet, J., Levesque, M., & Parent, A. (2002). Newly generated neurons in the amygdala and adjoining cortex of adult primates. *Proceedings of the National Academy of Sciences USA, 99,* 11464–11469.

Berretta, S., Pantazopoulos, H., Caldera, M., Pantazopoulos, P., & Pare, D. (2005). Infralimbic cortex activation increases c-Fos expression in intercalated neurons of the amygdala. *Neuroscience, 132,* 943–953.

Berridge, K. C. (2000). Measuring hedonic impact in animals and infants: Microstructure of affective taste reactivity patterns. *Neuroscience and Biobehavioral Reviews, 24,* 173–198.

Bjork, J. M., Knutson, B., Fong, G. W., Caggiano, D. M., Bennett, S. M., & Hommer, D.W. (2004). Incentive-elicited brain activation in adolescents: Similarities and differences from young adults. *Journal of Neuroscience, 24*, 1793–1802.

Blanchard, D. C., Canteras, N. S., Markham, C. M., Pentkowski, N. S., & Blanchard, R. J. (2005). Lesions of structures showing FOS expression to cat presentation: Effects on responsivity to a cat, cat odor, and nonpredator threat. *Neuroscience and Biobehavioral Reviews, 29*, 1243–1253.

Brand, S., & Rakic, P. (1984). Cytodifferentiation and synaptogenesis in the neostriatum of fetal and neonatal rhesus monkeys. *Anatomy and Embryology (Berlin), 169*, 21–34.

Cardinal, R. N., & Howes, N. J. (2005). Effects of lesions of the nucleus accumbens core on choice between small certain rewards and large uncertain rewards in rats. *BMC Neuroscience, 6*, 37.

Carlezon, W.A. Jr., Mague, S. D., & Andersen, S. L. (2003). Enduring behavioral effects of early exposure to methylphenidate in rats. *Biological Psychiatry, 54*, 1330–1337.

Carmichael, S. T., & Price, J. L. (1995). Limbic connections of the orbital and medial prefrontal cortex in macaque monkeys. *Journal of Comparative Neurology, 363*, 615–641.

Carmichael, S. T., & Price, J. L. (1996). Connectional networks within the orbital and medial prefrontal cortex of macaque monkeys. *Journal of Comparitive Neurology, 371*, 179–207.

Casey, B. J., Jones, R. M., & Hare, T. A. (2008). The adolescent brain. *Annals of the New York Academy of Science, 1124*, 111–126.

Chambers, R. A., Taylor, J. R., & Potenza, M. N. (2003). Developmental neurocircuitry of motivation in adolescence: A critical period of addiction vulnerability. *American Journal of Psychiatry, 160*, 1041–1052.

Costello, E. J., Pine, D. S., Hammen, C., March, J. S., Plotsky, P. M., Weissman, M. M, Biederman, J., Goldsmith, H. H., Kaufman, J, Lewinsohn, P. M., Hellander, M., Hoagwood, K., Koretz, D. S., Nelson, C. A., & Leckman, J. F. (2002). Development and natural history of mood disorders. *Biological Psychiatry, 52*, 529–542.

Crosby, E., & Humphrey, T. (1941). Studies of the vertebrate telencephalon: The nuclear pattern of the anterior olfactory nucleus, turberculum olfactorium and the amygdaloid complex in adult man. *Journal of Comparative Neurology, 74*, 309–347.

Dahl, R. E. (2004). Adolescent brain development: a period of vulnerabilities and opportunities. Keynote address. *Annals of New York Academy of Science, 1021*, 1–22.

Dorn, L., Dahl, R., Woodward, H., & Biro, F. (2006). Defining the boundaries of early adolescence: A user's guide to assessing pubertal status and pubertal timing in research with adolescence: A user's guide to assessing pubertal status and pubertal timing in research with adolecents. *Applied Developmental Science, 10*, 30–56.

Durston, S., & Casey, B. J. (2006). What have we learned about cognitive development from neuroimaging? *Neuropsychologia, 44*, 2149–2157.

Durston, S, Hulshoff Pol, H. E., Casey, B. J., Giedd, J. N., Buitelaar, J. K., & van Engeland, H. (2001). Anatomical MRI of the developing human brain: what have we learned? *Journal of the American Academy of Child and Adolescent Psychiatry, 40*, 1012–1020.

Emery, N. J., Capitanio, J. P., Mason, W. A., Machado, C. J., Mendoza, S. P., & Amaral, D. G. (2001). The effects of bilateral lesions of the amygdala on dyadic social interactions in rhesus monkeys (Macaca mulatta). *Behavioral Neuroscience, 115*, 515–544.

Ernst, M., & Spear, L. P. (in press). Reward systems. In M. de Haan & M. R. Gunnar (eds). *Handbook of developmental social neuroscience* New York: Guilford Press.

Ernst, M., Nelson, E. E., Jazbec, S., McClure, E. B., Monk, C. S., Leibenluft, E., Blair, J., & Pine, D. S. (2005). Amygdala and nucleus accumbens in responses to receipt and omission of gains in adults and adolescents. *Neuroimage, 25*, 1279–1291.

Ernst, M., Pine, D. S., & Hardin, M. (2006). Triadic model of the neurobiology of motivated behavior in adolescence. *Psychological Medicine, 36*, 299–312.

Ferry, A. T., Ongur, D., An, X., & Price, J. L. (2000). Prefrontal cortical projections to the striatum in macaque monkeys: evidence for an organization related to prefrontal networks. *Journal of Comparative Neurology, 425*, 447–470.

Fudge, J. L. (2004). Bcl-2 immunoreactive neurons are differentially distributed in subregions of the amygdala and hippocampus of the adult macaque. *Neuroscience, 127*, 539–556.

Fudge, J. L, Breitbart, M, A,, Danish, M., & Pannoni, V. (2005). Insular and gustatory inputs to the caudal ventral striatum in primates. *Journal of Comparative Neurology, 490*, 101–118.

Fudge, J. L., Breitbart, M. A., & McClain, C. (2004). Amygdaloid inputs define a caudal component of the ventral striatum in primates. *Journal of Comparative Neurology, 476*, 330–347.

Fudge, J. L., & Haber, S. N. (2000). The central nucleus of the amygdala projection to dopamine subpopulations in primates. *Neuroscience, 97*, 479–494.

Fudge, J. L., & Haber, S. N. (2002). Defining the caudal ventral striatum in primates: cellular and histochemical features. *Journal of Neuroscience, 22,* 10078-10082.

Fudge, J. L., Kunishio, K., Walsh, P., Richard, C., & Haber, S. N. (2002). Amygdaloid projections to ventromedial striatal subterritories in the primate. *Neuroscience, 110,* 257-275.

Galvan, A., Hare, T. A., Parra, C. E., Penn, J., Voss, H., Glover, G., & Casey, B. J. (2006). Earlier development of the accumbens relative to orbitofrontal cortex might underlie risk-taking behavior in adolescents. *Journal of Neuroscience, 26,* 6885-6892.

Gaspar, P., Cases, O., & Maroteaux, L. (2003). The developmental role of serotonin: news from mouse molecular genetics. *Nature Reviews Neuroscience, 4,* 1002-1012.

Gerfen, C. R. (1988). Synaptic organization of the striatum. *Journal of Electron Microscopy Technology for Medicine and Biology, 10,* 265-281.

Ghashghaei, H. T., & Barbas, H. (2002). Pathways for emotion: Interactions of prefrontal and anterior temporal pathways in the amygdala of the rhesus monkey. *Neuroscience, 115,* 1261-1279.

Giedd, J. N., Blumenthal, J., Jeffries, N. O., Castellanos, F. X., Liu, H., Zijdenbos, A., Paus, T., Evans, A. C., & Rapoport, J. L. (1999). Brain development during childhood and adolescence: A longitudinal MRI study. *Nature Neuroscience, 2,* 861-863.

Giedd, J. N., Snell, J. W., Lange, N., Rajapakse, J. C., Casey, B. J., Kozuch, P. L., Vaituzis, A. C., Vauss Y. C., Hamburger, S. D., Kaysen, D., & Rapoport, J. L. (1996). Quantitative magnetic resonance imaging of human brain development: Ages 4-18. *Cerebral Cortex, 6,* 551-560.

Gloor, P. (1997). Comparative anatomy of the temporal lobe and of the limbic system. In Pierre Gloor (ed.) *The temporal lobe and limbic system* (pp. 21-111). New York: Oxford University Press.

Gogtay, N., Giedd, J. N., Lusk, L., Hayashi, K. M., Greenstein, D., Vaituzis, A. C., Nugent, T. F. III, Herman, D. H., Clasen, L. S., Toga, A. W., Rapoport, J. L., & Thompson, P. M. (2004). Dynamic mapping of human cortical development during childhood through early adulthood. *Proceedings of the National Academy of Science USA, 101,* 8174-8179.

Goldman, P. S., & Nauta, W. J. (1977). An intricately patterned prefronto-caudate projection in the rhesus monkey. *Journal of Comparative Neurology, 72,* 369-386.

Goldman-Rakic, P. S. (1981). Prenatal formation of cortical input and development of cytoarchitectonic compartments in the neostriatum of the rhesus monkey. *Journal of Neuroscience, 1,* 721-735.

Goldman-Rakic, P. S. (1987). Development of cortical circuitry and cognitive function. *Child Development, 58,* 601-622.

Goursaud, A. P., & Bachevalier J. (2007). Social attachment in juvenile monkeys with neonatal lesion of the hippocampus, amygdala and orbital frontal cortex. *Behavioural Brain Research, 176,* 75-93.

Grace, A. A. (1995). The tonic/phasic model of dopamine system regulation: Its relevance for understanding how stimulant abuse can alter basal ganglia function. *Drug and Alcohol Dependence, 37,* 111-129.

Grace, A. A., Floresco, S. B, Goto, Y., & Lodge, D. J. (2007). Regulation of firing of dopaminergic neurons and control of goal-directed behaviors. *Trends in Neuroscience, 30,* 220-227.

Graveland, G. A., & DiFiglia, M. (1985). The frequency and distribution of medium-sized neurons with indented nuclei in the primate and rodent neostriatum. *Brain Research, 327,* 307-311.

Guyer, A.E., Monk CS, McClure-Tone EB, Nelson EE, Roberson-Nay R, Adler AD, Fromm SJ, Leibenluft E, Pine DS, Ernst M (2008). A developmental examination of amygdala response to facial expression. *Journal of Cognitive Neuroscience,* 20(9):1565-1582.

Haber, S. N., Kim, K. S., Mailly, P., & Calzavara, R. (2006). Reward-related cortical inputs define a large striatal region in primates that interface with associative cortical connections, providing a substrate for incentive-based learning. *Journal of Neuroscience, 26,* 8368-8376.

Hitchcock, J. M., & Davis, M. (1991). Efferent pathway of the amygdala involved in conditioned fear as measured with the fear-potentiated startle paradigm. *Behavioral Neuroscience, 105,* 826-842.

Holland, P. C., & Gallagher, M. (2006). Different roles for amygdala central nucleus and substantia innominata in the surprise-induced enhancement of learning. *Journal of Neuroscience, 26,* 3791-3797.

Huttenlocher, P. R. (1979). Synaptic density in human frontal cortex —developmental changes and effects of aging. *Brain Research, 163,* 195-205.

Huttenlocher, P. R., & Dabholkar, A. S. (1997). Regional differences in synaptogenesis in human cerebral cortex. *Journal of Comparative Neurology, 387,* 167-178.

Izquierdo, A., Suda, R. K., & Murray, E. A. (2005). Comparison of the effects of bilateral orbital prefrontal cortex lesions and amygdala lesions on emotional responses in rhesus monkeys. *Journal of Neuroscience, 25,* 8534-8542.

Jerison, H. (1973). *Evolution of the brain and intelligence.* New York: Academic Press.

Kalin, N. H., Shelton, S. E., Davidson, R. J., & Kelley, A. E. (2001). The primate amygdala mediates acute fear but not the behavioral and physiological components of anxious temperament. *Journal of Neuroscience*, *21*, 2067–2074.

Kemp, J. M., & Powell, T. P. (1970). The corticostriate projection in the monkey. *Brain*, *93*, 525–546.

Killcross, S., Robbins, T. W., & Everitt, B. J. (1997). Different types of fear-conditioned behaviour mediated by separate nuclei within amygdala. *Nature*, *388*, 377–380.

Killgore, W. D., & Yurgelun-Todd, D. A. (2004). Sex-related developmental differences in the lateralized activation of the prefrontal cortex and amygdala during perception of facial affect. *Perception and Motor Skills*, *99*, 371–391.

Kluver, H, & Bucy, P. C. (1997). Preliminary analysis of functions of the temporal lobes in monkeys. 1939. *Journal of Neuropsychiatry and Clinical Neuroscience*, *9*, 606–620.

Kollack-Walker, S., Watson, S. J., & Akil, H. (1997). Social stress in hamsters: Defeat activates specific neurocircuits within the brain. *Journal of Neuroscience*, *17*, 8842–8855.

Koob, G. F., Riley, S. J., Smith, S. C., & Robbins, T. W. (1978). Effects of 6-hydroxydopamine lesions of the nucleus accumbens septi and olfactory tubercle on feeding, locomotor activity, and amphetamine anorexia in the rat. *Journal of Comparative Physiology and Psychology*, *92*, 917–927.

Kordower, J. H., Piecinski, P., & Rakic, P. (1992). Neurogenesis of the amygdaloid nuclear complex in the rhesus monkey. *Brain Research Developmental Brain Research*, *68*, 9–15.

Kornack, D. R., & Rakic, P. (1998). Changes in cell-cycle kinetics during the development and evolution of primate neocortex. *Proceedings of the National Academy of Sciences USA*, *95*, 1242–1246.

LaBar, K. S., LeDoux, J. E., Spencer, D. D., & Phelps, E. A. (1995). Impaired fear conditioning following unilateral temporal lobectomy in humans. *Journal of Neuroscience*, *15*, 6846–6855.

Lapper, S. R., Smith, Y., Sadikot, A. F., Parent, A., & Bolam, J. P. (1992). Cortical input to parvalbumin-immunoreactive neurones in the putamen of the squirrel monkey. *Brain Research*, *580*, 215–224.

Laviola, G., Adriani, W., Terranova, M. L., & Gerra, G. (1999). Psychobiological risk factors for vulnerability to psychostimulants in human adolescents and animal models. *Neuroscience and Biobehavioral Reviews*, *23*, 993–1010.

Laviola, G., Macri, S., Morley-Fletcher, S., & Adriani, W. (2003). Risk-taking behavior in adolescent mice: psychobiological determinants and early epigenetic influence. *Neuroscience and Biobehavioral Reviews*, *27*, 19–31.

Lee, H. J., Groshek, F., Petrovich, G. D., Cantalini, J. P., Gallagher, M., & Holland, P. C. (2005). Role of amygdalo-nigral circuitry in conditioning of a visual stimulus paired with food. *Journal of Neuroscience*, *25*, 3881–3888.

Lee, H. J., Youn, J. M., M. J. O., Gallagher, M., Holland, P. C. (2006). Role of substantia nigra-amygdala connections in surprise-induced enhancement of attention. *Journal of Neuroscience*, *26*, 6077–6081.

Lenroot, R. K., Gogtay, N., Greenstein, D. K., Wells, E. M., Wallace, G. L., Clasen, L. S., Blumenthal, J. D., Lerch, J., Zijdenbos, A. P., Evans, A. C., Thompson, P. M., & Giedd, J. N. (2007). Sexual dimorphism of brain developmental trajectories during childhood and adolescence. *Neuroimage*, *36*, 1065–1073.

Lewis, S. J., Dove, A., Robbins, T. W., Barker, R. A., & Owen, A. M. (2003). Cognitive impairments in early Parkinson's disease are accompanied by reductions in activity in frontostriatal neural circuitry. *Journal of Neuroscience*, *23*, 6351–6356.

Luna, B., Garver, K. E., Urban, T. A., Lazar, N. A., & Sweeney, J. A. (2004). Maturation of cognitive processes from late childhood to adulthood. *Child Development*, *75*, 1357–1372.

Luna, B, & Sweeney, J. A. (2004). The emergence of collaborative brain function: FMRI studies of the development of response inhibition. *Annals of the New York Academy of Science*, *1021*, 296–309.

Macchi, G. (1951). The ontogenic development of the olfactory telencephalon in man. *Journal of Comparative Neurology*, *95*, 245–305.

Machado, C. J., & Bachevalier, J. (2006). The impact of selective amygdala, orbital frontal cortex, or hippocampal formation lesions on established social relationships in rhesus monkeys (Macaca mulatta). *Behavioral Neuroscience*, *120*, 761–786.

Masten, A. S. (2004). Regulatory processes, risk, and resilience in adolescent development. *Annals of the New York Academy of Sciences*, *1021*, 310–319.

Meunier, M., Bachevalier, J., Murray, E. A., Malkova, L., & Mishkin, M. (1999). Effects of aspiration versus neurotoxic lesions of the amygdala on emotional responses in monkeys. *European Journal of Neuroscience*, *11*, 4403–4418.

Meyer-Lindenberg, A., Hariri, A. R., Munoz, K. E., Mervis, C. B., Mattay, V. S., Morris, C. A., & Berman, K. F. (2005). Neural correlates of genetically abnormal social cognition in Williams syndrome. *Nature Neuroscience*, *8*, 991–993.

Miller, E. K. (2000). The prefrontal cortex and cognitive control. *Nature Reviews Neuroscience*, *1*, 59–65.

Millhouse, O. E. (1986). The intercalated cells of the amygdala. *Journal of Compartive Neurology, 247,* 246–271.

Monk, C. S., McClure, E. B., Nelson, E. E., Zarahn, E., Bilder, R. M., Leibenluft, E., Charney, D. S., Ernst, M., & Pine, D. S. (2003). Adolescent immaturity in attention-related brain engagement to emotional facial expressions. *Neuroimage, 20,* 420–428.

Muller, F., & O'Rahilly, R. (1990). The human brain at stages 21-23, with particular reference to the cerebral cortical plate and to the development of the cerebellum. *Anatomy and Embryology (Berlin), 182,* 375–400.

Northcutt, R. G., & Kaas, J. H. (1995). The emergence and evolution of mammalian neocortex. *Trends in Neuroscience, 18,* 373–379.

Numan, M., Numan, M. J., Marzella, S. R., & Palumbo, A. (1998). Expression of c-fos, fos B, and egr-1 in the medial preoptic area and bed nucleus of the stria terminalis during maternal behavior in rats. *Brain Research, 792,* 348–352.

O'Rourke, H., & Fudge, J. L. (2006). Distribution of serotonin transporter labeled fibers in amygdaloid subregions: implications for mood disorders. *Biological Psychiatry, 60,* 479–490.

Ohtani, N., Goto, T., Waeber, C., & Bhide, P. G. (2003). Dopamine modulates cell cycle in the lateral ganglionic eminence. *Journal of Neuroscience, 23,* 2840–2850.

Pare, D., Royer, S., Smith, Y., & Lang, E. J. (2003). Contextual inhibitory gating of impulse traffic in the intra-amygdaloid network. *Annals of New York Academy of Sciences, 985,* 78–91.

Parfitt, D. B., & Newman, S. W. (1998). Fos-immunoreactivity within the extended amygdala is correlated with the onset of sexual satiety. *Hormones and Behavior, 34,* 17–29.

Parkinson, J. A., Olmstead, M. C., Burns, L. H., Robbins, T. W., & Everitt, B. J. (1999). Dissociation in effects of lesions of the nucleus accumbens core and shell on appetitive pavlovian approach behavior and the potentiation of conditioned reinforcement and locomotor activity by D-amphetamine. *Journal of Neuroscience, 19,* 2401–2411.

Paus, T., Zijdenbos, A., Worsley, K., Collins, D. L., Blumenthal, J., Giedd, J. N., Rapoport, J. L., & Evans, A. C. (1999). Structural maturation of neural pathways in children and adolescents: in vivo study. *Science, 283,* 1908–1911.

Petrides, M., & Pandya, D. N. (1999). Dorsolateral prefrontal cortex: Comparative cytoarchitectonic analysis in the human and the macaque brain and corticocortical connection patterns. *European Journal of Neuroscience, 11,* 1011–1036.

Petrovich GD, Gallagher M. 2003. Amygdala subsystems and control of feeding behavior by learned cues. *Annals of the New York Academy of Science,* 985, 251–262

Pine, D. S., Cohen, P., Gurley, D., Brook, J., & Ma, Y. (1998). The risk for early-adulthood anxiety and depressive disorders in adolescents with anxiety and depressive disorders. *Archives of General Psychiatry, 55,* 56–64.

Pitkanen, A., & Amaral, D. G. (1998). Organization of the intrinsic connections of the monkey amygdaloid complex: Projections originating in the lateral nucleus. *Journal of Comparative Neurology, 398,* 431–458.

Prather, M. D., Lavenex, P., Mauldin-Jourdain, M. L., Mason, W. A., Capitanio, J. P., Mendoza, S. P., & Amaral, D. G. (2001). Increased social fear and decreased fear of objects in monkeys with neonatal amygdala lesions. *Neuroscience, 106,* 653–658.

Price, J. L., & Russchen, F. T. (1987). The limbic region. II. The amygdaloid complex. In B. T. Hokfelt, L. W. Swanson, & E. Amsterdam (Eds.). *Handbook of neuroanatomy* (pp 279–381).

Quirk, G. J., Likhtik, E., Pelletier, J. G., & Pare, D. (2003). Stimulation of medial prefrontal cortex decreases the responsiveness of central amygdala output neurons. *Journal of Neuroscience, 23,* 8800–8807.

Reiss, A. L., Eckert, M. A., Rose, F. E., Karchemskiy, A., Kesler, S., Chang, M., Reynolds, M. F., Kwon, H., & Galaburda, A. (2004). An experiment of nature: brain anatomy parallels cognition and behavior in Williams syndrome. *Journal of Neuroscience, 24,* 5009–5015.

Reynolds, S. M., & Berridge, K. C. (2001). Fear and feeding in the nucleus accumbens shell: Rostrocaudal segregation of GABA-elicited defensive behavior versus eating behavior. *Journal of Neuroscience, 21,* 3261–3270.

Reynolds, S. M., & Berridge, K. C. (2002). Positive and negative motivation in nucleus accumbens shell: Bivalent rostrocaudal gradients for GABA-elicited eating, taste "liking"/"disliking" reactions, place preference/avoidance, and fear. *Journal of Neuroscience, 22,* 7308–7320.

Reynolds, S. M., & Berridge, K. C. (2003). Glutamate motivational ensembles in nucleus accumbens: Rostrocaudal shell gradients of fear and feeding. *European Journal of Neuroscience, 17,* 2187–2200.

Ridderinkhof, K. R., Ullsperger, M., Crone, E. A., & Nieuwenhuis, S. (2004). The role of the medial frontal cortex in cognitive control. *Science, 306,* 443–447.

Rosene, D. L., & Van Hoesen, G. W. (1977). Hippocampal efferents reach widespread areas of cerebral cortex and amygdala in the rhesus monkey. *Science, 198*, 315–317.

Russchen, F. T., Bakst, I., Amaral, D. G., & Price, J. L. (1985). The amygdalostriatal projections in the monkey. An anterograde tracing study. *Brain Research, 329*, 241–257.

Saunders, R. C., Rosene, D. L., & Van Hoesen, G. W. (1988). Comparison of the efferents of the amygdala and the hippocampal formation in the rhesus monkey: II. Reciprocal and non-reciprocal connections. *Journal of Comparative Neurology, 271*, 185–207.

Schultz, W., Dayan, P., & Montague, P. R. (1997). A neural substrate of prediction and reward. *Science, 275*, 1593–1599.

Selemon, L. D., & Goldman-Rakic, P. S. (1985). Longitudinal topography and interdigitation of corticostriatal projections in the rhesus monkey. *Journal of Neuroscience, 5*, 776–794.

Seymour, B., Daw, N., Dayan, P., Singer, T., & Dolan, R. (2007). Differential encoding of losses and gains in the human striatum. *Journal of Neuroscience, 27*, 4826–4831.

Sharpe, N. A., & Tepper, J. M. (1998). Postnatal development of excitatory synaptic input to the rat neostriatum: An electron microscopic study. *Neuroscience, 84*, 1163–1175.

Sisk, C. L., & Foster, D. L. (2004). The neural basis of puberty and adolescence. *Nature Neuroscience, 7*, 1040–1047.

Sowell, E. R., Thompson, P. M., Holmes, C. J., Jernigan, T. L., & Toga, A. W. (1999). In vivo evidence for post-adolescent brain maturation in frontal and striatal regions. *Nature Neuroscience, 2*, 859–861.

Sowell, E. R., Trauner, D. A., Gamst, A., & Jernigan, T. L. (2002). Development of cortical and subcortical brain structures in childhood and adolescence: A structural MRI study. *Developmental Medicine and Child Neurology, 44*, 4–16.

Spear, L. P. (2000). The adolescent brain and age-related behavioral manifestations. 0*Neuroscience and Biobehavioral Reviews, 24*, 417–463.

Stefanacci, L., & Amaral, D. G. (2000). Topographic organization of cortical inputs to the lateral nucleus of the macaque monkey amygdala: a retrograde tracing study. *Journal of Comparative Neurology, 421*, 52–79.

Stefanacci, L., Clark, R. E., & Zola, S. M. (2003). Selective neurotoxic amygdala lesions in monkeys disrupt reactivity to food and object stimuli and have limited effects on memory. *Behavioral Neuroscience, 117*, 1029–1043.

Steinberg, L., & Belsky, J. (1996). A sociobiological perspective on psychopathology in adolescence. In D. Cicchetti & S. Toth (Eds.). *Rochester Symposium on Developmental Psychopathology* (pp. 93–124). Rochester, NY: University of Rochester Press.

Taylor, A. E., & Saint-Cyr, J. A. (1990). Depression in Parkinson's disease: Reconciling physiological and psychological perspectives. *Journal of Neuropsychiatry and Clinical Neuroscience, 2*, 92–98.

Thompson, C. I., & Towfighi, J. T. (1976). Social behavior of juvenile rhesus monkeys after amygdalectomy in infancy. *Physiology and Behavior, 17*, 831–836.

Turner, B. H., Mishkin, M., & Knapp, M. (1980). Organization of the amygdalopetal projections from modality-specific cortical association areas in the monkey. *Journal of Comparative Neurology, 191*, 515–543.

van der Kooy, D. (1996). Early postnatal lesions of the substantia nigra produce massive shrinkage of the rat striatum, disruption of patch neuron distribution, but no loss of patch neurons. *Brain Research Developmental Brain Research, 94*, 242–245.

Van Hoesen, G. W., Yeterian, E. H., & Lavizzo-Mourey, R. (1981). Widespread corticostriate projections from temporal cortex of the rhesus monkey. *Journal of Comparative Neurology, 199*, 205–219.

Webster, M. J., Ungerleider, L. G., & Bachevalier, J. (1991). Connections of inferior temporal areas TE and TEO with medial temporal-lobe structures in infant and adult monkeys. *Journal of Neuroscience, 11*, 1095–1116.

Whalen, P. J. (1998). Fear, vigilance, and ambiguity. *Current Directions in Psychological Science, 7*, 177–188.

Wilensky, A. E., Schafe, G. E., Kristensen, M. P., & LeDoux, J. E. (2006). Rethinking the fear circuit: the central nucleus of the amygdala is required for the acquisition, consolidation, and expression of Pavlovian fear conditioning. *Journal of Neuroscience, 26*, 12387–12396.

Wise, R. A. (1980). The dopamine synapse and the notion of "pleasure centers" in the brain. *Trends in Neuroscience, 3*, 91–95.

Yakovlev, A. G., Di, X., Movsesyan, V., Mullins, P. G., Wang, G., Boulares, H., Zhang, J., Xu, M., & Faden, A. I. (2001). Presence of DNA fragmentation and lack of neuroprotective effect in DFF45 knockout mice subjected to traumatic brain injury. *Molecular Medicine, 7*, 205–216.

Yakovlev, P. (1967). The mylogenetic cycles of regional maturation of the brain. In A. Minkowski (Ed.) *Regional development of the brain in early life.* Oxford, England: Blackwell.

Zirlinger, M., Kreiman, G., & Anderson, D. J. (2001). Amygdala-enriched genes identified by microarray technology are restricted to specific amygdaloid subnuclei. *Proceedings of the National Academy of Science USA, 98*, 5270–5275.

Zola-Morgan, S., Squire, L. R., Alvarez-Royo, P., & Clower, R. P. (1991). Independence of memory functions and emotional behavior: separate contributions of the hippocampal formation and the amygdala. *Hippocampus, 1*, 207–220.

Chapter 3

Risk-Taking Behaviors across the Transition from Adolescence to Young Adulthood

Elizabeth K. Reynolds, Jessica F. Magidson, Linda C. Mayes and Carl W. Lejuez

The transition from adolescence to adulthood (ages 18–25) can be defined as a period of exploration of identity and one's place in the world. Young adults achieve new levels of independence from their parents, adopt considerably greater responsibilities, and often make important life decisions on their own for the first time in their lives. While this is an exciting time of positive change and growth, this period of transition also is marked by a spike in the engagement in a variety of risk-taking behaviors, with the potential for very serious life-altering negative consequences. In their classic book on the topic, Jessor and Jessor (1977) defined risk taking as engagement in "behavior that is socially defined as a problem, a source of concern, or as undesirable by the norms of conventional society and the institutions of adult authority, and its occurrence usually elicits some kind of social control response" (p. 33). Focusing more on the consequences of such behavior, definitions of risk taking have also taken into consideration the possibility of positive outcomes and thus have focused on the balancing of potential for harm or danger to the individual with potential achievement or reward (Byrnes, Miller, & Schafer, 1999; Leigh, 1999). This latter view is important because it leaves room for the influence of a variety of factors that affect an emerging adult's willingness to take risks, including the potential gain from risks both in terms of positive and negative reinforcement and the corresponding opportunity costs for an unwillingness to take risks. Also relevant are developmental norms (e.g., college student drinking) that may impact the occurrence of risk behavior at one life stage and the termination of that behavior in the next life stage (Smith, Molina, & Pelham, 2002).

The goal of this chapter is to consider key risk-taking behaviors specific to emerging young adults with a focus on substance use, risky sexual activity, and delinquent behaviors (e.g., gambling, reckless driving). We begin with a sample case vignette and a review of prevalence/epidemiology, follow with etiology across various domains of biology and behavior, leading into state of the art assessment strategies for understanding, predicting, and preventing risk behavior. Finally, we conclude with a synthesis of the previous sections and relevant practice guidelines.

Case Vignette

Ty is an 18-year-old, third-generation Japanese American first diagnosed in elementary school with attention-deficit/hyperactivity disorder (ADHD) which was treated with stimulant medications. Throughout his childhood and high school years, Ty lived a regulated life at home. He was closely monitored by his parents and was required to adhere to strict rules (e.g., required to come home right after school and abide by an early curfew, and only allowed to spend the night at friends' houses on occasion). His parents provided structure with his school work, setting up time for him to do his work each day and providing close supervision and instruction. He made it through high school with average grades and only minor experimentation with alcohol and some delinquency-related behavior (e.g., physical fight with a peer, spray painting). He left for college with plans to continue a relationship with his girlfriend of 6 months who was starting her junior year in high school. Ty functioned well upon entry into college, but his impulsive and inattentive symptoms associated with ADHD made it difficult for him to make safe choices within the context of the college environment. He was faced with the challenge of succeeding academically and socially in a relatively unstructured environment while living away from home for the first time. He no longer had his parents supervising his behavior and he was presented with an array of social activities that involved opportunities for risk taking. Ty's struggle with impulse control and planning produced an unsustainable lifestyle and made successful navigation of this new environment particularly challenging. Ty began to engage in binge drinking, attending parties at which he drank heavily (i.e., over five drinks in one evening) three to four times a week. As his drinking became more frequent, he became less able to keep up with his school work and he began a dangerous pattern of procrastination that culminated in nightly Internet gambling. Further, these activities only exacerbated his fears of commitment and he began to lose touch with his girlfriend from home and instead sought more casual sexual encounters, sometimes without using any form of protection.

Throughout his first semester, his grades slipped and he ended up on academic probation. Ty felt embarrassed by his school performance and began to experience a persistent negative mood. During the next semester, more varied and frequent risk behaviors began, serving the function of helping him cope with his guilt, shame, and other negative feelings. These behaviors included marijuana use that started socially with friends but soon became more isolative as he began to use more often than his friends. As he started to miss classes, he needed to cram more heavily for exams to make up for the missed class time. This pattern of missed classes and need for cramming led to Ty increasing his dose of stimulants without supervision by his physician.

Sensing a change in their son, including a more sullen demeanor and frequent shortness during phone calls, Ty's parents became increasingly concerned. Because they were paying his college tuition, his parents continued to have some control over their son and they refused to continue paying unless he moved home for the spring semester to refocus himself and begin seeing a therapist at the University Counseling Center. Upon starting the spring semester, Ty was set up with services for his ADHD, including continued involvement with a therapist that helped him with organization techniques and a plan for studying. As Ty's negative mood decreased, he was less inclined to engage in risk-taking behavior as a coping technique. His involvement with online gambling and marijuana ceased, largely due to closer supervision from his parents at first, and diminished need over time as he began to reengage with people and activities he enjoyed prior to starting college, including reconnecting with his high school girlfriend. Soon he "grew out of" his interest in illicit drugs, and although he still drank on occasion, it was at a socially appropriate level.

Prevalence Rates/Epidemiology

Alcohol

Smith and colleagues have suggested that, in contrast to alcohol use during adolescence, alcohol use may be "normative" during young adulthood. Research consistently shows that people tend to drink the heaviest in their late teens and early to mid-twenties (Fillmore, Hartka, & Johnstone, 1991; Naimi, Brewer, & Mokdad, 2003). Specifically, young adults are especially likely to engage in binge and heavy drinking (SAMHSA, 2004). According to National Epidemiologic Survey on Alcohol and Related Conditions (NESARC) data, about 46% of young adults engaged in drinking that exceeded the recommended daily limits at least once in the past year, and 14.5% (3.9 million) had an average consumption that exceeded the recommended weekly limits (Dawson, Grant, Stinson, & Chou, 2004). This peak in heavy drinking in young adulthood is also evident in international samples (e.g., Casswell, Pledger, & Hooper, 2003). Such heavy drinking in young adulthood is associated with high-risk activities and negative consequences, such as risky sexual behavior, diminished academic performance, physical aggression, and sexual victimization (Wood, Read, Palfai, & Stevenson, 2001). Additionally, young adult drivers, ages 21–34, have the highest rates of alcohol involvement in fatal crashes (NHTSA, 2006).

Prominent attention has been given to the consequences of excessive drinking by college students (College Task Force, 2002; Weschsler et al., 2002), as 31% of undergraduate college students meet criteria for alcohol abuse according to the *Diagnostic Statistical Manual of Mental Disorders, Fourth Edition* (DSM-IV; American Psychiatric Association, 1994), and another 6% can be classified as DSM-IV alcohol-dependent (Knight et al., 2002). In 2001, 600,000 college students were unintentionally injured from alcohol-related injuries, and 696,000 were assaulted or hit by another drinking college student (Hingson, Heeren, Winter, & Wechsler, 2005). These statistics have contributed to the view that the college environment may function as a facilitator/incubator of excessive drinking, alcohol abuse, and alcohol dependence. However, it is important to clarify that although some research indicates higher rates of drinking and alcohol-related problems in college attendees (e.g., Slutske et al., 2004), other studies indicate greater likelihood of alcohol abuse and dependence among nonattendees who face many similar changes, including weakening parental control as well as a host of other challenges related to an earlier entry into adult roles (Harford, Yi, & Hilton, 2006).

Illicit Drug Use

Similar to alcohol use, during the period of emerging adulthood, illicit drug use also increases, peaks, and then declines for most young people (Arnett, 2005; Bachman et al., 2002; Bachman, Wadsworth, O'Malley, Johnston, & Schulenberg, 1997; Chen & Kandel, 1995). According to the 2002 National Survey on Drug Use and Health (NSDUH) (SAMHSA, 2003), rates of past month illicit drug use climbed steadily for youth from ages 12 to 17, peaked among 18-to 20-year-olds, and remained high for those between ages 21 and 25 before dropping for persons ages 26 through 29. In addition to continuing use, initiation of substances also occurs during this time period; for example, one-third of new marijuana users start using after age 17 as do about 70% of cocaine users (Volkow, 2004). In terms of variation in use among college attendees and non-attendees, illicit drug use has been increasing on college campuses since the mid 1990s (Mohler-Kuo, Lee, & Weschler, 2003). However, college students differ only modestly from their non-college peers in their rate of drug use and types of drugs used (Johnston, O'Malley, Bachman, & Schulenberg, 2005). The annual prevalence (i.e., use of the drug in the past year) for the use of any illicit drug among college students is 36%, compared to 39% of young adults not attending college (Johnston et al., 2005), and when considering only drugs other than marijuana rates are 19% for college students and 24% for terminal high school graduates. Thus, illicit drug use among college students does not appear to exceed rates of use in the general young adult population, and for certain drugs, rates appear to be somewhat lower in the college student population.

Cigarette Smoking

Cigarette smoking is a major public health concern in the United States, as well as internationally. In the United States, it is the leading cause of preventable death in the nation, accounting for over 440,000 premature deaths yearly (Centers for Disease Control and Prevention, 2002b). Rates of smoking in the 1990s declined in all age groups *except* ages 18–24 (Hebert, 2004), and one-third of this age group is comprised of college students (U.S. Bureau of the Census, 1997). Cigarette smoking occurs less frequently in the college student population than in the general young adult population (5.6% vs. 16%; Johnston et al., 2005). Similar rates of cigarette smoking have been found in young adult populations internationally (e.g., China; Kumra & Markoff, 2000), and young adult cigarette smoking represents a significant long-term public health issue in many countries (Peto & Lopez, 2000).

Risky Sexual Behavior

Earlier sexual maturity, later marriage, and emphasis on education have contributed to a much longer period of time between the onset of sexual maturity and marriage. The longer this period extends, the more likely it is that unmarried adolescents and young adults will become sexually active (Michael, Gagnon, Laumann, & Kolata, 1994). In terms of risky sexual behavior, those under the age of 25 are more likely than other age groups to have unprotected intercourse, to have multiple sex partners, and, particularly for young women, to choose older sex partners (Centers for Disease Control and Prevention, 2002a; Valois, Oeltmann, & Waller, 1999).

To specifically address the college population, sexual behavior among college students has been assessed in two studies utilizing national samples of college students. The first study, the National College Health Risk Behavior Survey (NCHRBS), was conducted in 1995, and the second study, the National College Health Assessment (NCHA), was conducted in 2003. While both studies surveyed the same population, they asked questions aimed at slightly different types of information and together they provide a comprehensive picture of risky sexual behavior in the college student population. According to the NCHRBS (Douglas et al., 1997), 29.6% of college students who engaged in sexual intercourse during the 3 months prior to the survey reported using a condom during their last sexual intercourse, and 79.8% reported using some form of contraception during their last sexual intercourse. Of this group, 27.9% reported using a condom most of the time or always. The NCHA (The American College Health Association, 2005) contained questions specific to negative outcomes associated with risky sex practices. In response to this survey, 26.2% of college students reported ever being tested for human immunodeficiency virus (HIV) infection, 10.1% of sexually active women reported using emergency contraception within the past school year, 2.6% of female students who had vaginal intercourse in the past year reported becoming pregnant unintentionally, and 2.0% of male students who had vaginal intercourse in the past year reported impregnating someone unintentionally. The data collected through these national surveys show that risky sex practices are evident on college campuses, and these findings extend to similar settings internationally (e.g., Bosompra, 2000; Jenkins et al., 2002). As with alcohol, it is important to note that risky sexual behavior is not limited to those attending college. In addition to unwanted pregnancy, risky sexual behavior is of great concern given its clear connection to STDs (Centers for Disease Control and Prevention, 2002a) as well as death from AIDS following infection with HIV where young adults account for the majority of cases (60% of male; 64% of female AIDS cases; Centers for Disease Control and Prevention, 2000).

Other Risk-Taking Behaviors

The emergence of young adulthood also marks the period at which many delinquent and potentially criminal behaviors peak before dropping near the end of young adulthood (Arnett, 1995). In fact, the number of violent acts committed by high school seniors has increased almost 50% over the past two decades, as have violent crime arrests, particularly for aggravated assault and robbery (U.S. Department of Health and Human Services, 2001). While not all delinquent adolescents continue such risk behaviors in young adulthood, a longitudinal study examining desistence from serious delinquency in young adulthood found that approximately 60% of delinquent adolescents continued in behaviors from reckless driving through the violent use of a weapon. Further, serious delinquency in late adolescence was identified as a risk factor for continued delinquency into young adulthood (Stouthamer-Loeber, Wei, Loeber, & Masten, 2004).

Gambling is another risk behavior that is prevalent in adolescents (Derevensky & Gupta, 2007; Jacobs, 2000) as well as young adults (Blinn-Pike, Lokken Worthy, & Jonkman, 2007; LaBrie, Shaffer, LaPlante, & Wechsler, 2003). Research indicates that approximately 15.3 million adolescents in the United States and Canada gamble and 2.2 million exhibit serious consequences from gambling (Jacobs, 2000). Similar rates of gambling in young adulthood have been found in other countries (e.g., the United Kingdom; Wardle et al., 2007). Further, problem gambling during adolescence has been shown to be a significant predictor of problem gambling during young adulthood (Winters, Stinchfield,

Botzet, & Anderson, 2002). Prevalence rates of gambling behavior are particularly high at the onset of adulthood, as the characteristics of the college setting may exacerbate gambling behavior in young adults (Winters, 2002). A meta-analysis of college student gambling studies indicates a high prevalence of lifetime problem gambling in this population (5.6%), which is almost triple the prevalence rate in older adults (Shaffer & Hall, 2001). Problem gambling on college campuses has been associated with a wide range of negative consequences and risk behaviors, including a greater likelihood to engage in risky sexual behavior and substance use, as well as experiencing more negative consequences of use (Engwall, Hunter, & Steinberg, 2004; LaBrie et al., 2003).

Gender and Race/Ethnicity Considerations

Factors such as gender, race, and socioeconomic status recently have been shown to vary in several important ways with risk behavior. The greatest amount of work has focused on gender with an interesting interaction seemingly evident (Byrnes, Miller, & Schafer, 1999). Risk behaviors are fairly equal across boys and girls in early adolescence, with girls evidencing slightly higher rates. However, through high school a reversal occurs such that risk behavior is greater in males as they enter adulthood. The Monitoring the Future Study has been tracking the substance use habits of high school students, both during high school and after graduation, since 1975 (Johnston et al., 2005). Their results show that in 12th grade, there are generally higher proportions of males than females involved in illicit drug use, especially heavy drug use (Johnston, O'Malley, Bachman, & Schulenberg, 2007). As discussed above, this study suggests that there is little gender difference in use in the lower grades. In fact, for some drugs females have slightly higher rates of annual use in 8th grade (Johnston et al., 2007).

In terms of race and ethnicity, the Monitoring the Future Study indicates that at all three grade levels (8th, 10th, and 12th) African American youth have considerably lower rates of substance use (alcohol, illicit drugs, cigarettes) than do whites (Johnston et al., 2007). By 12th grade, white students have the highest lifetime and annual prevalence-of-use rates among the three major racial/ethnic groups (white, African American, and Hispanic) for many substances (Johnston et al., 2007). In addition, while drinking among whites tends to peak around ages 19–22, heavy drinking among African Americans and Hispanics peaks later and persists longer into adulthood (Caetano & Kaskutas, 1995).

In addressing gender and race/ethnicity differences, an interesting area of disparity is among one outcome of risk behavior: sexually transmitted diseases (STDs). Research suggests that females, Hispanics, and non-Hispanic blacks are disproportionately affected by STDs (Tucker Halpern, Young, Waller, Martin, & Kupper, 2004). For example, in 2001, the gonorrhea infection rate among 15- to 19-year-old black females was almost twice as high as that for black males, and 18 times as high as the rate for white females (Centers for Disease Control and Prevention, 2002a). Black and Hispanic women account for 79% of all reported HIV infections among 13- to 19-year-old women and 75% of HIV infections among 20- to 24-year-old women in the United States, although together they represent only about 26% of U.S. women of these ages (Centers for Disease Control and Prevention, 2002a). Clearly future research is necessary to understand these dangerous disparities.

Less research is available on socioeconomic status. In the Monitoring the Future Study, socioeconomic status is indexed by parental education level. The study shows that by senior year there is little correlation of family socioeconomic status with the use of most substances. The authors suggest that this speaks to the extent of substance use across all social strata (Johnston et al., 2007); however, the potential risk factors for those in higher SES groups may differ from the documented risk factors for those in lower SES groups. It will be important for future research to examine the interactions among these variables (gender, race/ethnicity, and SES).

Etiological Factors

Genetics

Research suggests that risk behaviors, with specific relevance to substance use, have a significant genetic component (Duaux, Krebs, & Poirier, 2000). It is estimated that 40%–60% of the vulnerability to addiction can be attributed to genetic factors (Goldman, Oroszi, & Ducci, 2005; Hiroi & Agatsuma, 2005; Kreek, Nielsen, Butelman, & LaForge, 2005). Predisposition to addiction may be due to both genetic variants that are common across addictions and to those specific to a particular addiction (Kreek et al., 2005). Genetic factors may be involved in direct drug-induced effects, including alteration of a drug's effect at a receptor or a drug's absorption, distribution, metabolism, and excretion (Kreek et al., 2005).

Alcohol consumption is considered to be partially determined by genetic factors (Han, McGue, & Iacono, 1999; Heath, 1995; Heath et al., 1997; McGue, 1993, 1994), with a particularly strong genetic determination among men (Grant et al., 1999). Walters (2002) reported results from a meta-analysis of 50 family, twin, and adoption studies, in which genetic factors accounted for 20%–26% of the variability in alcohol misuse. However, Johnson, Vernon, Harris, and Jang (2004) suggest that genetic contributions to the etiology of alcoholism are not best accounted for by a simple univariate heritability estimate. For example, genetic factors may account for as much as 60% of the association between antisocial personality and alcohol dependence (Grove et al., 1990; Jang, Vernon, & Livesley, 2000; Slutske et al., 1998), and the genetic correlation between alcohol consumption and stimulus-seeking behaviors ranges from .33 and .45 (Jang et al., 2000; Mustanski, Viken, Kaprio, & Rose, 2003). Alcohol consumption has also been proposed to have a significant genotype by environment interaction. The heritability of alcohol consumption increases with age (Viken Kaprio, Koskenvuo, & Rose 1999), suggesting the reasons for alcohol consumption early in life may be more related to environmental determinants such as availability or opportunity.

A genetic basis for drug abuse has also been investigated thoroughly. For example, cannabis use is suggested to be the result of both genetic and environmental factors (Cadoret, 1992; Kendler, Karkowski, Neale, & Prescott, 2000; Kendler, Prescott, Myers, & Neale, 2003; Miles, Van den Bree, & Gupman, 2001; Tsuang et al., 1996, 1999; Van den Bree, Svikis, & Pickens, 1998). Miles et al. (2001) suggested a moderate heritability of cannabis use (.31) and a more substantial effect of the shared environment (.47). These findings support earlier findings that suggested an approximately equal distribution of variance estimates between genetic determinants, the shared environment, and unique environmental events (Tsuang et al., 1996). Tsuang et al. (1999) proposed a stage model of drug abuse that suggests a hierarchical progression toward drug abuse: exposure, initiation of use, continuation of use, regularity of use, substance abuse, and then addiction. The transition from regular use to heavy use and abuse has been demonstrated to be strongly genetic (Cadoret, 1992), with heritability ranging from 60%–80% (Kendeler, Karkowski, Neale, & Prescott, 2000).

Fisher (1958) presented the earliest evidence for a genetic determination of tobacco use, demonstrating a higher concordance rate among MZ twins than DZ twins. More current research suggests that smoking initiation and persistence demonstrates substantially greater genetic determination in men than women (Han, McGue, & Iacono, 1999; Madden et al., 1999). Li, Cheng, Ma, & Swan (2003) report that smoking initiation demonstrated a significantly higher genetic basis among women (55%) than among men (73%), while smoking persistence demonstrated a non-significantly higher genetic basis among men (57%) than among women (46%). Tobacco has also been linked to dopamine receptor polymorphisms. Research focuses on the importance of the DRD2 gene in the prediction if individuals most at risk for smoking initiation (Bierut et al., 2000; Comings et al., 1996; Wu, Hudmon, Detry, Chamberlain, & Spitz, 2000; Yoshida et al., 2001).

Numerous studies have examined the influence of genetics on the development of pathological gambling. Twin and family studies have suggested it to be hereditary, with genetic factors accounting for 35% to 54% of the risk of developing pathological gambling (Eisen et al., 1998). Genetic contribution has been shown to be stable over a 10-year period (Xian et al., 2007) and higher in men (Shah, Eisen, Xian, & Potenza, 2005; Walters, 2001; Winters & Rich, 1998). Research at the molecular level has demonstrated associations between pathological gambling and DRD1 (Sabbatini da Silva Lobo et al., 2007), as well as allele variants of the serotonin transporter gene and the monoamine-oxidase A gene, particularly in severe males (Ibañez, Blanco, Perez de Castro, Fernandez-Piqueras, & Saiz-Ruiz, 2003; Ibañez, Perez de Castro, Fernandez-Piqueras, Blanco, & Saiz-Ruiz, 2000; Perez de Castro, Ibañez, Saiz-Ruiz, & Fernandez-Piqueras, 1999). Research has also pinpointed a shared genetic vulnerability in pathological gamblers and alcohol users, with alcohol dependence accounting for 12% to 20% of the genetic variation in the risk for pathological gambling (Slutske, 2000).

It is important to stress that evidence for genetic vulnerability alone is unlikely sufficient for development of risk behaviors, and they often combine with other factors to confer risk, including gene–environment interactions and gene–gene interactions. The interaction of genes with other factors, especially environment, will be addressed in more detail below.

Neurobehavioral Contributors

A number of behavioral and cognitive changes that take place in adolescence through young adulthood may be related to maturation in the brain (Spear, 2000). Research shows that the brain continues to develop throughout adolescence and well into young adulthood. There has been a specific focus on the dopamine systems and associated mesolimbic and mesocortical brain areas. Dopamine, a neurotransmitter associated with the reward system in humans, has significant implications with regard to engagement in risk-taking behaviors. Individuals vary in their number of dopamine receptors and this variation can lead to differing levels of risky behavior (Kalat, 2004). Drugs and novel situations activate reward systems in the brain, and the mesolimbic dopamine reward pathway is a critical link that mediates drug reward (Koob, 2006). Novelty seeking and risky behaviors cause a release of dopamine in the nucleus accumbens across individuals, but there are fairly substantial differences in their "need" for novelty. Genetic differences in novelty-seeking and drug-seeking behavior may be mediated by differences in the mesolimbic dopamine systems (Bardo, Donohew & Harrington, 1996). There is some debate as to whether increases in drug-seeking behavior are related to elevations or reductions in mesolimbic DA activity. The traditional DA hypothesis of reward suggests that DA systems should be positively related to drug-seeking behavior (Spangel & Weiss, 1999). Yet others suggest that enhanced vulnerability to drug use and abuse is associated with a reward deficiency syndrome. Due to functional deficits in mesolimbic dopamine systems, individuals find reinforcing stimuli less pleasurable than others, leading them to seek out drugs and novelty as a behavioral remediation of reward deficiency. This deficiency may be due to lower than normal levels of extracellular dopamine. Another possible cause for this deficiency may be lower D_2 receptor levels caused by the expression of the A_1 allele on the D_2 receptor gene (Spear, 2000). This allele increases the probability that a person will become alcohol dependent or will engage in a variety of pleasure-seeking behaviors (Kalat, 2004). Those with an alternate form of the D_4 receptor have been shown to have novelty-seeking personalities (Donohew, Bardo, & Zimmerman, 2004). This may lead to higher levels of impulsivity, exploratory behaviors, and quick-temperedness. Studies have implicated D_4 receptors in heroin addiction and found altered distributions allelic variants of the gene encoding the D_4 receptor in alcoholics and pathological gamblers (Zuckerman & Kuhlman, 2000), although not consistently across studies.

Another factor that is linked to novelty seeking and drug use is level of monoamine oxidase (MAO). MAO is an enzyme that is involved in the catabolic degradation of the monamine neurotransmitters dopamine, serotonin, and norepinephrine. There are two forms of MAO: MAO-A and MAO-B. MAO-B is closely tied to the regulations of dopamine, while MAO-A is more involved in the regulation of serotonin and norepinephrine. MAO-B is negatively correlated with sensation seeking (low levels of MAO-B is correlated with high levels of sensation seeking). Platelet levels of MAO-B change slowly as a function of age. Levels are the lowest in adolescence and increase with age. Levels are consistently higher in women than men at all ages, corresponding with the finding that men tend to exhibit higher levels of sensation seeking. Low platelet levels of MAO-B are linked with higher levels of tobacco, drug, and alcohol use as well as higher incidence of criminal offenses (Zuckerman & Kuhlman, 2000). Low levels of MAO-B would lead to slower degradation of dopamine, ultimately increasing dopamine levels in the brain. Studies have shown that rats with high levels of novelty seeking had higher levels of dopamine activity in the nucleus accumbens both under basal conditions and during novel stimulation (Dellu, Piazza, Mayo, LeMoal, & Simon, 1996). If these findings hold true for humans, people with low platelet levels of MAO-B may be more likely to engage in novelty-seeking and drug-seeking behaviors.

The dopamine system in the brain is one of many neural systems that undergo developmental alterations in adolescence. Like many of the other systems, the dopamine system is sensitively activated by stressors. Stressors can activate dopamine projections to the prefrontal cortex as well as to the mesolimbic brain regions. Receptors for glucocorticoids (stress hormones) have been identified in the rodent brain on dopaminergic neurons in several areas of the brain, including the nucleus accumbens. Stress-induced increases in glucocorticoids may activate dopamine transmission, thus facilitating drug-taking behaviors. Stress can lead to higher activity in the mesolimbic dopamine system, which is positively related to drug-seeking behavior (Spear, 2000).

Individual Differences/Personality

Given the greater freedom that may be experienced by young adults, the impact of personality may be especially salient for this group. Sensation seeking is a personality trait defined by "the seeking of varied, novel, complex, and intense sensations and experiences, and the willingness to take physical, social, legal, and financial risks for the sake of such experience" (Zuckerman, 1979). Numerous studies have found sensation seeking to be related across multiple domains of risk-taking behaviors (Caspi et al., 1997; Lejuez et al., 2002, 2007; Zuckerman et al., 1972, 1994).

In addition to the correlations with sensation seeking, the construct of impulsivity may underlie risk-taking behaviors (e.g., Lane et al., 2003). Specifically, impulsivity has been linked to substance use vulnerability, frequency, severity including social and emotional consequences, and dependence (e.g., Allen, Moeller, Rhoades, & Cherek, 1998; Fishbein, Lozovsky, & Jaffe, 1989; King, Curtis, & Knoblich, 1991; Moeller et al., 2001; 2002; Monterosso, Ehrman, Napier, O'Brien, & Childress, 2001; Patton, Stanford, & Barratt, 1995; Petry, 2001). One difficulty in examining impulsivity and its relationship with the other key variables is the multidimensional nature of the construct (Evenden, 1999; Whiteside & Lynam, 2001). Definitions of the construct include, but are not limited to, the inability to delay gratification (Mischel, Shoda, & Rodriquez, 1989), the process of discounting a reward as a function of delay (Ainslie, 1975; Reynolds et al., 2007), and the inability to inhibit prepotent responding (Logan, 1994; Newman, Patterson, & Kosson, 1987). Several tasks and self-report instruments have been developed to measure each of these dimensions. Despite the recognized multidimensionality of impulsivity, most studies examining the construct study one dimension in isolation (for an exception, see Lane et al., 2003). Thus, it is difficult to speculate on the generalizability of the results across other dimensions of impulsivity and, more importantly, on how specific components of impulsivity are related to risk-taking behavior.

A large majority of work on personality and risk behavior has focused on individual behaviors and specific personality variables, indicating a lack of covariance across risk behaviors and the personality constructs that may underlie these behaviors (Anderson et al., 1993; Tolan & Loeber, 1993). However, more recent work has begun to focus more on the common links across these behaviors, including a higher order aspect of personality referred to as the externalizing factor (Krueger et al., 2002; Krueger, Markon, Patrick, & Iacono, 2005). Further work aimed at understanding the functional similarities across risk behaviors and the personality factors underlying them is of great importance, especially in terms of improving assessment, prevention, and treatment of individual and clusters of risk behaviors.

Developmental Precursors

Externalizing disorders such as childhood ADHD and conduct disorder (CD) have been pinpointed as developmental precursors to problematic engagement in risk-taking behavior. ADHD is characterized by developmentally inappropriate levels of inattention, hyperactivity, and impulsivity, whereas CD is characterized by a persistent pattern of disregard for rules and the rights of others (APA, 1994). Each independently has been identified as an early risk factor for the emergence of risky behavior in adolescence and adulthood, and their combination appears to pose a higher risk than either disorder alone (Flory, Milich, Lynam, Leukefeld, & Clayton, 2003; Flory, Molina, Pelham, Gnagy, & Smith, 2006; Molina, Smith, & Pelham, 1999; Thompson, Molina, Pelham, & Gnagy, 2007). Research indicates that children with ADHD report higher levels of alcohol, tobacco, and illicit drug use in adolescence compared to same-aged adolescents without a history of ADHD, and severity of ADHD symptoms in childhood also predict levels of substance use in adolescence (Molina & Pelham, 2003).

CD also has been identified as a strong predictor of early alcohol initiation and alcohol dependence (Sartor, Lynskey, Heath, Jacob, & True, 2007), as well as other substance and illicit drug use, and those with CD and ADHD demonstrate the highest levels of use (Flory et al., 2003). Research has also indicated that the link between childhood ADHD and alcohol use disorder (AUD) is only evident in older adolescents between 15 and 17 years of age (Molina, Pelham, Gnagy, Thompson, & Marshal, 2007) and continues into adulthood (Biederman et al., 2006). Additionally, childhood ADHD has been demonstrated to be a predictor of multiple risky sexual behaviors, including earlier initiation of sexual intercourse, higher rates of reported sexual partners and casual sex, and higher rates of pregnancy through early adulthood (Flory et al., 2006). Research has also linked childhood ADHD to driving-related risk behaviors, particularly when symptoms persist and CD is co-occurring (Thompson et al., 2007). Given the relationship between ADHD, CD, and a wide range of risk-taking behaviors, it is important to evaluate the presence of these disorders starting in childhood to better monitor and intervene at the onset of adolescent risk taking.

Psychopathology, Stress, and Coping

A wealth of literature suggests that affective distress is related to risk-taking behavior. There is a high comorbidity between substance use disorders and mood and anxiety disorders such as depression (Brooner, King, Kidorf, & Schmidt, 1997; Griffin, Weis, Mirin,& Lange, 1989; Weiss, Kung, & Pearson, 2003). Both cross-sectional (Clark, Lynch, Donovan, & Block, 2001) and longitudinal studies (Cooper, Wood, Orcutt, & Albino, 2003; Krueger, 1999; Wills, Sandy, & Yaeger, 2001) have demonstrated an association between trait negative affect and initiation of substance use, as well as severity of substance-related problems (e.g., Johnson & Pandina, 1993; Labouvie, Pandina, White, & Johnson, 1990). Although some evidence exists for a relationship between negative affect (e.g., depression, anxiety, anger) and sexual risk behavior, several findings have been inconclusive (Crepaz & Marks, 2001). It is hypothesized that those individuals who rely on dysfunctional styles of coping in the face of negative emotions are less able to effectively regulate their negative mood states, thus becoming vulnerable to the immediate relief promised by various risky behavioral alternatives (Westen, 1994). In turn, engagement in risky behaviors often brings relief (e.g., via distraction or euphorigenic effects of substances), thus enhancing the attractiveness of such behavior for future situations. Baker, Piper, & McCarthy (2004) provide a compelling conceptualization of these processes within the context of a negative reinforcement approach. In support of this type of conceptualization, Cooper, Agocha, and Sheldon (2000) found that drinking to cope with negative feelings was a good predictor of heavy drinking as well as drinking problems in 19- to 25-year-olds. Thus, although it is important to note that young adults are likely to engage in risk behavior that is "positive" or celebratory (e.g., Read, Wood, Kahler, Maddock, & Palfai 2003), the pressures and stresses of young adulthood increase the likelihood of risk behavior aimed at coping with stress and other forms of negative affect.

At a biological level, one's response to stress also appears to be relevant. The hypothalamic-pituitary-adrenal system (HPA axis), the anatomical structures that regulate levels of cortisol in the body in response to stress, should increase production of cortisol to mediate alarm reactions to stress, thus facilitating an adaptive phase in which alarm reactions are suppressed and the body can attempt counter-measures. Healthy regulation of the HPA axis is necessary to cope with life stressors, and low levels of cortisol in young adults with externalizing behavior may suggest HPA axis dysfunction. Further, human and animal studies have also found support for the role of HPA axis dysfunction in substance use, indicating that altered HPA axis response can lead to increased drug craving and acquisition (Brady & Sinha, 2005; Sinha, Garcia, Paliwal, Kreek, & Rounsaville, 2006). Research indicates that cortisol response may also be hereditary; non-substance-using subjects with a family history of alcoholism had lower cortisol responses than those without a family history of alcoholism, particularly when subjects had antisocial characteristics (Sorocco, Lovallo, Vincent, & Collins, 2006). Additionally, another study examining age of cannabis use initiation identified lower HPA axis activity in the early-onset group compared to subjects who had initiated cannabis use at a later age (Huizink, Ferdinand, Ormel, & Verhulst, 2006). Within the context of the various stressors associated with the transition to young adulthood outlined above, poor HPA axis functioning is likely a key factor in the development and continued use of risk behaviors, including substances to modulate the effects of stress.

Environment

Early Adversity. Data from both animal (Pryce, Bettschen, & Feldon, 2001) and human work (for review, see Fergusson, Lynskey, & Horwood, 1996) indicate that early childhood experience can have enduring consequences on the emergence and continuance of risk behavior. One specific type of adverse early experience is abuse, which has consistently been found to predict the increased likelihood of risk behaviors, including substance use and risky sexual behavior. Research linking child abuse with later risk behaviors has focused largely on childhood *sexual* abuse, with studies indicating that sexually abused individuals are at an increased risk of later engagement in risky sexual behavior (such as multiple short-term sexual encounters; exchange of sex for money, drugs, or shelter; and unprotected sex), as well as substance use (e.g., Paolucci, Genuis, & Violato, 2001). However, sexual abuse rarely occurs in the absence of a broader social context of multiple adversities, including other forms of abuse such as emotional and physical (e.g., Bornovalova, Gwadz, Kahler, Aklin, & Lejuez, 2008; Dubo, Zanarini, Lewis, & Williams, 1997). Moreover, preliminary evidence indicates that physical and emotional abuse uniquely contribute to risk behaviors (e.g., Medrano, Hatch, Zule, & Desmond, 2003). The mechanism through which childhood abuse later influences risk-taking behavior has begun to be examined, including psychosocial variables such as deficits in emotion regulation and coping (Miller & Lisak, 1999), insecure attachment (Schindler et al., 2005), disinhibition variables of risk-taking propensity and sensation seeking (Bornovalova et al., 2008), and neurocognitive changes (Weiss & Wagner, 1998), with recent movement toward integrative theories considering the interactive roles across domains.

Peer Influence. Pressure from one's peers and the desire to fit into a group greatly influence behavior (Festinger, 1950; Petraitis, Flay, & Miller, 1995). The influence of peer relationships substantially increases during adolescence. Research has suggested that many youth believe that desirable social outcomes, such as peer acceptance or peer support, will occur as a result of using substance, and they are, therefore, motivated to initiate substance use (Jenkins, 2001; Sussman et al., 1995). There is evidence that the number of friends who use illicit drugs (Jenkins & Zunguze, 1998) and smoke cigarettes (Wang et al., 1997) is positively associated with one's own illicit drug use and smoking, respectively. For example, smoking status of peers has shown differing levels of importance as a predictor of smoking behavior in adolescents across various studies. Many studies have found that a higher proportion of smoking friends predicted smoking initiation (e.g., Bauman, Carver, & Gleiter, 2001; Urberg, Degirmencioglu, & Pilgrim, 1997). Once the individual begins more frequent participation in a particular risk behavior, the individual may begin to select peers that share similar values and problem behavior, while also spending less time with less risky peers who may start to share fewer interests and who may even be disapproving of such risk behavior (Valente, Gallaher, & Mouttappa, 2004).

In addition to actual peer influence, certain behaviors may be supported by perceived behavior of others and the resulting social norms that accompany these perceptions. For example, the belief that "everyone" is drinking and drinking is acceptable is one of the strongest correlates of drinking among young adults and the subject of considerable research (e.g. Jackson, Sher, & Park, 2005). This and other types of norm misperceptions appear to contribute to problem drinking among young adults. For example, within the college setting, many students believe campus attitudes are much more permissive toward drinking than they are in reality, believe other students consume alcohol more frequently an in higher quantities than they actually do (Borsari & Carey, 2001, 2003; Perkins, 2002), and tend to misjudge the attitudes of others toward alcohol use and drunkenness (Read, Wood, Davidoff, McLacken, & Campbell, 2002). In a study conducted by Wood and colleagues (2001), social influence was cited as the strongest correlate of alcohol use and abuse. Social influence was broken down into two categories: *(1)* active: explicit invitations and *(2)* passive: perception and interpretation of drinking within a group (social modeling and misperception of peer norms).

Influence from the Virtual Environment. An interesting emerging environmental risk factor for risk-taking behavior is the Internet. The Internet can provide older adolescents with access to more risky peer groups, thereby increasing access to problem behaviors such as illicit substance use and risky sexual behavior. Gambling may be an especially great risk on the Internet because the risk behavior can occur at that moment in the virtual environment and does not require the transition to the real world as would be the case for most other risk behaviors. Research suggests that Internet gambling poses an increased risk for all ages to develop problem gambling, due to the effects of increased accessibility, use of electronic cash, as well as its solitary nature (Griffiths & Park, 2002; Wood, Griffiths, & Parke, 2007). Yet adolescent and young adult students may be most vulnerable to the effects of Internet-based problem gambling, given the lack of appropriate regulation of many Internet sites, as well as the frequency of Internet use among students (Derevensky & Gupta, 2007; Wood et al., 2007). Research examining online poker playing in a student sample ($n = 422$) found that 18% of a student sample were problem gamblers, and one-third of the students reported participation in online gambling at least twice per week (Wood et al., 2007).

Environmental Factors Specific to Emerging Adulthood. The transition to adulthood is a large contextual shift when individuals often move out of the family residence and become increasingly self-supporting (Arnett, 2005). Becoming part of the world of work and/or higher education increases the separation from the family of origin as individuals become part of new contexts. Within emerging adulthood there is cognitive development (e.g., continued brain development, the emergence of personal beliefs and values), changes in one's identity or self-definition (e.g., exploration of career roles), and affiliative transitions (e.g., shifts in relationships with parents and peers).

As an example of one common new context, a high proportion of young people, about 60%, enter college after graduating from high school (Mogelonsky, 1996). This is a higher proportion than ever before in American history. College students are faced with the challenge of succeeding academically and socially in a relatively unstructured environment, often while living away from home for the first time. They typically no longer have close parental supervision of their behavior and are presented with an array of social activities that involve opportunities for risk taking. The delayed assumption of adulthood roles, the absence of social control agents (such as parents and the high school structure), relatively easy access to alcohol (Wechsler, Lee, Kuo, & Lee, 2000), and immersion in an environment of same-age peers makes the college years a time of heightened engagement in risky behaviors (Schulenberg, O'Malley, Bachman, Wadsworth, & Johnston, 1996). Many suggest that the college campus environment itself encourages heavy drinking (Toomey & Wagenaar, 2002).

Aside from factors that enhance risk behavior, it is also important to consider factors that may reduce risk behavior. One such factor is marriage or serious committed romantic relationships. Specific to alcohol use, young married women have the greatest decreases in drinking behavior, and married men, compared with men in all other categories of living arrangements (i.e., living with parents, in a dormitory, alone, or in other arrangements) have the least robust increases (Bachman et al.,1997). Interestingly, divorce, which may occur in young adulthood, has the opposite effect, showing a relationship with increases in alcohol use (Bachman et al., 1997). Being a parent also is related to lower alcohol use for both men and women; however, during pregnancy, most women eliminate their alcohol use, although most of their husbands do not (Bachman et al., 1997). Young adults with serious alcohol problems (those who fit the diagnostic criteria for alcohol dependence) may not be as likely to choose stable roles such as marriage and parenthood, or these milestones may not affect their drinking behavior to the same extent that they affect people with less problematic drinking practices (Matzger, Delucchi, Weisner, & Ammon, 2004). Thus, although the development of a family may differ somewhat across gender, there is clear evidence of its general relationship with decreased risk behavior. With this said, it is important to acknowledge that most studies show correlation and not causation because other third variables may be influencing both greater commitment to family and reduced engagement in risk behavior.

Movement toward Integrative Models across Etiological Dimensions

In expanding the scope of risk factors, it is crucial to develop an understanding beyond the independent influence of these etiological factors, and to develop larger models that consider the interactive effects across these factors. Thus far, the greatest progress has come in the consideration of gene–environment interactions (e.g., Kaufman et al., 2007). There are a number of proposed ways in which genes and environment can interact to influence behavior including cases where *(1)* genotype increases expression of environmental risk factor, *(2)* genotype exacerbates effect of environmental risk factor, *(3)* environmental risk factor exacerbates effect of genotype, *(4)* both genotype and environmental risk factor are required, and *(5)* genotype and environmental risk factor each affects risk, creating a combined effect greater than additive (Van Duijn et al., 2005). For example, individuals who experience early life stressors are at risk for depression and anxiety. Several groups have observed an interaction between stressful life experiences and the SLC6A4 genotype in the risk for depression (Caspi, Sugden, & Moffitt, 2003). In particular, individuals homozygous for the s allele of the 5HTT gene often experience depression when environmental adversity including stress is experienced. However, these individuals do not appear to be at a substantially elevated risk in the absence of stress, and individuals with other SLC6A4 genotypes appear more resilient to stress. Stress has also been linked to substance use disorders and other risk behaviors, and neurobiological data suggest an overlap in systems underlying stress response and addiction vulnerability (Kreek et al., 2005). Few studies have directly examined gene–environment interactions in addiction (for an exception, see Kaufman et al., 2007), but several connections point to their potential relevance, including *(1)* evidence for a direct relationship between the short allele of 5HTT and addiction, *(2)* the connection of addiction with psychopathology suggesting the value of investigating similar pathways, and *(3)* the link of addiction to environmental variables, including negative life events, stress, and childhood abuse/adversity.

Moving forward, it is crucial to further develop these models to consider the manner in which gene–environment interactions may be considered together with the other etiological factors outlined above. For example, one possible model includes biological factors such as a genetic vulnerability, poor stress response due to HPA axis dysregulation, and overactivity in the mesolimbic dopamine reward pathway in the presence of stimuli associated with a risky alternative, along with with high impulsive and sensation-seeking traits, excessive stress in the adjustment to adulthood, and an environment that supports risk taking, combining to predict excessive risk behavior peaking in young adulthood. Currently, it seems reasonable to assume that the greater the number of these risk factors, the more likely the individual is to engage in problematic risk behavior, but it is necessary to develop more sophisticated interactive models and strategies to understand specifically how these factors combine to confer risk across individuals and to identify protective factors.

Assessment and Prevention

Assessment

There are several measures to assess risk taking specific to particular substances. For alcohol and substance use, the Structured Clinical Interview for DSM-IV (SCID; First, Spitzer, Gibbon, & Williams, 1995) is used to diagnose alcohol/drug abuse and dependence. Yet it is also important to take into account developmental considerations and continuous rather than dichotomous measures. The Core Alcohol and Drug Survey (Core Institute, 1994) has strong psychometric properties and is particularly relevant to the young adulthood developmental stage as well as the college context (Core Institute, 2005). Additionally, it contains items on risky behavior associated with substance use and items specific to the function underlying substance use. The Alcohol Use Disorders Identification Test (AUDIT) and the Drug Use Disorders Identification Test (DUDIT) are useful for obtaining a continuous score that takes into account the quantity and frequency of use and related consequences, which may be useful to understand the level of impairment and severity of use to distinguish from typical college drinking patterns (Saunders, Aasland, Babor, De La Fuenta, & Grant, 1993). Several specific measures are appropriate for assessment of gambling behavior, including the South Oaks Gambling Screen (Lesieur & Blume, 1987) and the Pathological Gambling Modification of the Yale-Brown Obsessive-Compulsive Scale (PG-YBOCS; Pallanti, DeCaria, Grant, Urpe, & Hollander, 2005). Additionally, standard assessments of HIV risk behaviors typically used with adult populations can also be used for HIV risk-taking behaviors in a young adult sample. For example, the AIDS Risk Assessment (ARA; Simpson, 1997) assesses drug use patterns and history as well as sexual risk behavior in 30-day and 6-month time frames.

Considering risk taking behavior more broadly, few comprehensive measures exist, particularly ones that take into account the specific characteristics of a young adult population. The Youth Risk Behavior Surveillance: National College Health Risk Behavior Survey (1997) assesses the occurrence of a variety of health risk behaviors (e.g., tobacco use, unhealthy dietary behaviors, inadequate physical activity, alcohol and other drug use, sexual behaviors that may result in HIV infection, other sexually transmitted diseases, and unintended pregnancies, behaviors that may result in unintentional injuries, such as motor vehicle crashes, and violence, including suicide); however, this assessment does not assess associated impairment or distress. Only measuring occurrence can lead to questions of impairment, and specifically, at what level of occurrence is the behavior dysfunctional. This is more apparent for some behaviors than others (e.g., condom nonuse is arguably always risky, but there is a greater debate about what number of drinks per week/night/sitting constitutes risky drinking behavior). While DSM-IV diagnoses require impairment or distress, diagnoses are not available for many risk behaviors beside alcohol/drug abuse and dependence. Relevant behavior engagement can also be gleaned from diagnoses of CD, yet this diagnosis is not developmentally appropriate. Antisocial personality disorder diagnostic information may also be useful, but it focuses heavily on criminal behaviors.

Prevention

Although great strides have been made in the prevention of a variety of risk behaviors covered above, the large majority of this work is targeted at children and early adolescents. One area for which prevention has been targeted at young adults and their unique needs is college student drinking. The National Institute of Alcohol Abuse and Alcoholism has published a comprehensive report entitled *A Call to Action: Changing the Culture of College Drinking* (NIAAA, 2002) that provides research reviews and other crucial information to assist college and university administrators and program managers in their alcohol abuse prevention efforts. In this report, individual alcohol prevention programs are designated as "Tier 1 strategies," specifying that this method has the most evidence available to support it. Following from the perspective that programs focused on skills development and attention to individual vulnerabilities are more effective than more general information-based approaches (Larimer & Cronce, 2002; NIAAA, 2002; Walters & Neighbors, 2005), these individualized interventions usually combine a motivational interviewing style with personalized feedback. This personalized feedback often includes drinking patterns and percentiles, accurate norms for alcohol use on campus, correction of myths regarding alcohol, negative drinking consequences, and protective behaviors or skills (Martens et al., 2004) that individuals can use to reduce drinking and its consequences (Dimeff, Baer, Kivlahan, & Marlatt, 1999). Thus, although all individuals are targeted, these programs are decidedly individualizing their focus.

Although there is support for individualized prevention programs, one limitation is feasibility. Several practical barriers exist, including the specialized training and ongoing supervision required of prevention staff as well as resources. Another key issue is the methodology required for identification of vulnerabilities for targeting in these individuals prevention programs. Current technologies allow for highly sophisticated identification of biological vulnerabilities, including genetics, HPA axis functioning, and neurobehavioral functioning. At the level of personality, measures of constructs such as impulsivity and sensation seeking (Zuckerman & Kuhlman, 2000) have shown the importance of personality factors in the relation to risk behavior among adolescents and young adults. Further, as discussed above, more recent efforts have moved to create dimensional higher order factors, such as the externalizing construct to consider the functional similarities across risk behavior and their personality-based determinants. Personality assessment, however, has been limited somewhat by a largely exclusive use of self-report. More recent efforts, however, have moved beyond self-report assessments to include behavioral measures to index impulsivity (Reynolds et al., 2007), risky decision making (Bechara, Damasio, Damasio, & Anderson, 1994), and risk-taking propensity (Lejuez et al., 2007). In addition to being potentially less biased than self-report measures, these tasks provide the opportunity to measure actual behavior (i.e., the participant's propensity to engage in risk on the task), which is especially useful when considering the influence of other variables that cannot be examined with a self-report measure. For example, the effect of positive or negative affect on risk taking can be examined by comparing behavior on the tasks at a baseline state and then after a mood induction. This approach could also be useful for examining the influence of substance use on subsequent risk behavior using a drug administration paradigm (e.g., will the individuals take more risks in a task under the influence of alcohol). Finally, behavioral tasks are ideally suited for studying cognitive and neurobehavioral processes as well as biological stress response changes during their administration. Although these tasks largely have been limited to research use, they are now becoming more commonly used in clinical practice for assessment and intervention planning purposes.

Key Points/Practice Guidelines

There are a number of key points that may be useful in moving forward in our understanding of adolescent risk and its emergence into adulthood. First, risk taking involves the balancing of negative and positive consequences. As such, not all risk behavior is inherently bad and some willingness to take risks in a young adult's life is crucial for discovering, developing, and consolidating his or her identity (Millstein & Igra, 1995). The line between healthy and unhealthy risk behavior, however, can sometimes blur, especially as even more hazardous behaviors may be commonplace among one's peers and the consequences of such behavior may seem distant and unlikely. Although most young adults will "grow out of" patterns of risk, some will continue in these patterns with increasing negative consequences. Second, it has become increasingly important when studying risk behavior to take a multifactorial perspective in which multiple influences are considered instead of focusing on a specific indicator or characteristic. Significant comorbidity between CD, substance use disorders, and mood disorders suggests the potential for multiple synergistic mechanisms (e.g., sensation seeking, impulsivity, poor judgment, negative affectivity) that may increase participation in a wide range of health risk behaviors (Clark & Bukstein, 1998; Zeitlin, 1999). Advancements in understanding the link between biology, environment, and behavior are crucial for moving beyond overly simplistic accounts of risk behavior, with the importance of considering unique circumstances for emerging young adults. Finally, it is useful to apply this mutlifactorial approach in understanding specific vulnerabilities among emerging young adults and developing and utilizing these advancements in clinical assessment toward implementing individualized prevention efforts. Thus, the best strategy for limiting the role of risk behavior is a more integrative biobehavioral approach that considers how all these factors come together to confer differential variability and how we might individually target these differential vulnerabilities. To date, however, efforts to integrate behavior and biology in actual practice are less common.

KEY POINTS

- Risk-taking behavior involves the balancing of negative and positive consequences, and the function of such behavior should be understood within the context of positive and negative reinforcement.
- An analysis of risk taking in young adulthood must take into account the developmental context, both in terms of the influence of normative risk-taking behavior, as well as the risk factors associated with increased levels of independence, responsibility, and autonomy.
- A multifactorial perspective is crucial in the examination of influences on young adult risk taking, rather than focusing solely on a single indicator or characteristic; specifically, multiple synergistic mechanisms (e.g., sensation seeking, impulsivity, poor judgment, negative affectivity, genetic vulnerability, adverse environment) that may increase participation in a wide range of health risk behaviors may be most relevant to consider.

PRACTICE GUIDELINES

- The distinction between healthy and unhealthy risk behaviors can sometimes blur, especially as even more hazardous behaviors may be commonplace in this population; thus, it is important for assessment approaches to consider resulting distress and functional impairments as well as potentially positive outcomes. Expressly, although risk-taking behaviors are by definition potentially harmful, it is important to take into account that behaviors may be engaged in because they also have some functional value, including some probability for desirable outcomes (e.g., social, emotional, or cognitive).
- It is important to use an integrative biobehavioral theoretical approach that considers how factors across domains come together to confer differential variability, which can further our understanding of young adult risk behavior.

- Following from this integrative approach, comprehensive risk-taking assessments tailored to the young adult population are needed. Combining self-report, behavioral, and biological/neurobehavioral assessment approaches may further enhance accuracy, comprehensiveness, and utility of assessments and their utilization in prevention and intervention efforts.

References

Ainslie, G. (1975). Specious reward: a behavioral theory of impulsiveness and impulse control. *Psychological Bulletin, 82*(4), 463–496.

Allen, T., Moeller, F., Rhoades, H., & Cherek, D. (1998). Impulsivity and history of drug dependence. *Drug and Alcohol Dependence, 50*, 137–145.

American College Health Association. (2005). American College Health Association National College Health Assessment Spring 2005 Reference Group Data Report. *Journal of American College Health, 55*, 5–16.

American Psychiatric Association. (1994). *Diagnostic and Statistical Manual of Mental Disorders* (4th ed.) Washington, DC: Author.

Anderson, E. R., Bell, N. J., Fischer, J. L., Munsch, L., Peek, C. W., & Sorell, G. T. (1993). Applying a risk-taking perspective. In N. J. Bell & R. W. Bell (Eds). *Adolescent risk taking* (pp. 165–185). Newbury Park, CA: Sage Publications.

Arnett, J. (1995). The young and the reckless: Adolescent reckless behavior. *Current Directions in Psychological Science, 4*, 67–71.

Arnett, J. J. (2005). The developmental context of substance use in emerging adulthood. *Journal of Drug Issues, 35*, 235–253.

Bachman, J. G., Wadsworth, K. N., O'Malley, P. M., Schulenberg, J., & Johnston, L.D. (1997). Marriage, divorce, and parenthood during the transition to young adulthood: Impacts on drug use and abuse. In J. Schulenberg, J. Maggs, & K. Hurrelmann (Eds.), *Health risks and developmental transitions during adolescence* (pp. 246–279). Cambridge, England: Cambridge University Press.

Bachman, J. G., O'Malley, P. M., Schulenberg, J. E., Johnston, L. D., Bryant, A. L., & Merline, A. C. (2002). *The decline of substance use in young adulthood: Changes in social activities, roles, and beliefs.* Mahwah, NJ: Lawrence Erlbaum.

Baker, T. B., Piper, M. E., & McCarthy, D. E. (2004). Addiction motivation reformulated: An affective processing model of negative reinforcement. *Psychological Review, 111*, 33–51.

Bardo, M., Donohew, R., & Harrington, N. (1996). Psychobiology of novelty seeking and drug seeking behavior. *Behavioral Brain Research, 77*, 23–43.

Bauman, K. E., Carver, K., & Gleiter, K. (2001). Trends in parent and friend influence during adolescence: The case of adolescent cigarette smoking. *Addictive Behaviors, 26*, 349–361.

Bechara, A., Damasio, A. R., Damasio, H., & Anderson, S. W. (1994). Insensitivity to future consequences following damage to human prefrontal cortex. *Cognition, 50*, 7–15.

Biederman, J., Monuteaux, M. C., Mick, E., Spencer, T., Wilens, T. E., Silva, J. M., Snyder, L. E., & Faraone, S. V. (2006). Young adult outcome of attention deficit hyperactivity disorder: A controlled 10 year follow up study. *Psychological Medicine, 36*, 167–179.

Bierut, L. J., Rice, J. P., Edenberg, H. J., Goate, A., Foroud, T., Cloninger, C. R., et al. (2000). Family-based study of the association of the dopamine D2 receptor gene (DRD2) with habitual smoking. *American Journal of Medical Genetics, 90*, 299–302.

Blinn-Pike, L., Lokken Worthy, S., & Jonkman, J. (2007). Disordered gambling among college students: A meta-analytic synthesis. *Journal of Gambling Studies, 23*, 175–183.

Bornovalova, M. A., Gwadz, M., Kahler, C. W., Aklin, W. M., & Lejuez, C. W. (2008). Sensation seeking and risk-taking propensity as mediators in the relationship between childhood abuse and HIV-related risk behavior. *Child Abuse and Neglect, 32*, 99–109.

Borsari, B., & Carey, K. B. (2001) Peer influences on college drinking: A review of the research. *Journal of Substance Abuse, 13*, 391–424.

Borsari, B., & Carey, K. B. (2003). Descriptive and injunctive norms in college drinking: A meta-analytic integration. *Journal of Studies on Alcohol, 64*, 331–341.

Bosompra, K. (2000). Determinants of condom use intentions of university students in Ghana: An application of the theory of reasoned action. *Social Science and Medicine, 52*, 1057–1069.

Brady, K. T., & Sinha, R. (2005). Co-occurring mental and substance use disorders: The neurobiological effects of chronic stress. *American Journal of Psychiatry, 162*, 1483–1493.

Brooner, R., King, V., Kidorf, M., & Schmidt, C. (1997). Psychiatric and substance use comorbidity among treatment-seeking opioid abusers. *Archives of General Psychiatry, 54,* 71–80.

Byrnes, J. P., Miller, D. C., & Schafer, W. D. (1999). Gender differences in risk taking: A meta-analysis. *Psychological Bulletin, 125,* 367–383.

Cadoret, R.J. (1992). Genetic and environmental factors in initiation of drug use and the transitions to abuse. In M. Glantz, & R. Pickens (Eds), *Vulnerability to drug abuse* (pp. 99–114). Washington, DC: American Psychological Association.

Caetano, R., & Kaskutas, L.A. (1995). Changes in drinking patterns among Whites, Blacks, and Hispanics, 1984–1992. *Journal of Studies on Alcohol, 56,* 558–565.

Caspi, A., Begg, D., Dickson, N., Harrington, H., Langley, J., Moffitt, T. E., & Silva, P. A. (1997). Personality differences predict health-risk behaviors in young adulthood: Evidence from a longitudinal study. *Journal of Personality and Social Psychology, 73,* 1052–1063.

Caspi, A., Sugden, K., & Moffitt, T. E. (2003). Influence of life stress on depression: Moderation by a polymorphism in the 5-HHT gene. *Science, 301,* 386–389.

Casswell, S., Pledger, M., & Hooper, R. (2003). Socioeconomic status and drinking patterns in young adults. *Addiction, 98,* 601–610.

Centers for Disease Control and Prevention. (2002).Youth risk behavior surveillance—United States, 2001. *Mormidity and Mortality Weekly Report, 51*(SS-4), 1–64.

Centers for Disease Control and Prevention. (2002a). *Sexually transmitted disease surveillance, 2001.* Atlanta, GA: Author.

Centers for Disease Control and Prevention. (2002b). Annual smoking-attributable mortality, years of potential life lost, and economic costs—United States, 1995–1999. (2002). *Morbidity and Mortality Weekly Report, 51,* 300–303.

Chen, K., & Kandel, D. B. (1995). The natural history of drug use from adolescence to the mid-thirties in a general population sample. *American Journal of Public Health, 85,* 41–47.

Clark, D. B., & Bukstein, O. G. (1998). Psychopathology in adolescent alcohol abuse and dependence. *Alcohol Health and Research World, 22,* 117–126.

Clark, D., Lynch, K., Donovan, J., & Block, G. (2001). Health problems for adolescents with alcohol use disorders: Self-report, liver injury, and physical examination findings and correlates. *Alcoholism: Clinical and Experimental Research, 25,* 1350–1359.

College Task Force of the National Advisory Council on Alcohol Abuse and Alcoholism. (2002). *A call to action: Changing the culture of drinking at U.S. colleges,* NIH publication no. 02-5010. Bethesda, MD: National Institute on Alcohol Abuse and Alcoholism, Department of Health and Human Services.

Comings, D. E., Ferry, L., Bradshaw-Robinson, S., Burchette, R., Shiu, C., & Muhleman, D. (1996). The dopamine D2 receptor (DRD2) gene: A genetic risk factor in smoking. *Pharmacogenetics, 6,* 73–79.

Cooper, M. L., Agocha, V. B., & Sheldon, M. S. (2000). A motivational perspective on risky behaviors: The role of personality and affect regulatory processes. *Journal of Personality, 68,* 1059–1088.

Cooper, M. L., Wood, P. K., Orcutt, H. K., & Albino, A. (2003). Personality and the predisposition to engage in risky or problem behaviors during adolescence. *Journal of Personality and Social Psychology, 84,* 390–410.

Core Institute. (1994). *Core alcohol and drug survey—Long form.* Carbondale, IL: Author, Southern Illinois University.

Core Institute. (2005). *Region Profiles of College Student Alcohol and Other Drug Use.* Carbondale, IL: Author, Southern Illinois University.

Crepaz, N., & Marks, G. (2001). Are negative affective states associated with HIV sexual risk behaviors? A meta-analytic review. *Health Psychology, 20,* 291–299.

Dawson, D. A., Grant, B. F., Stinson, F. S., & Chou, S. P. (2004). Another look at heavy episodic drinking and alcohol use disorders among college and noncollege youth. *Journal of Studies on Alcohol, 65,* 477–488.

Dellu, F., Piazza, P., Mayo, W., LeMoal, M., & Simon, H. (1996). Novelty seeking in rats and possible relationships with the sensation seeking train in humans. *Neuropsychobiology, 34,* 136–145.

Derevensky, J. L., & R. Gupta. (2007). Internet gambling among adolescents: A growing concern. *International Journal of Mental Health and Addiction, 5,* 93–101.

Dimeff, L. A., Baer, J. S., Kivlahan, D. R., & Marlatt, G. A. (1999). Brief alcohol screening and intervention for college students (BASICS): A harm reduction approach. New York: Guilford Press.

Donohew, L., Bardo, M., & Zimmerman, R. (2004). Personality and risky behavior: Communication and prevention. In R. Stelmack (Ed.), *On the psychobiology of personality: Essays in honor of Marvin Zuckerman* (pp. 223–248). Boston: Elsevier.

Douglas, K. A., Collins, J. L., Warren, C., Kann, L., Gold, R., Clayton, S., et al. (1997). Results from the 1995 National College Health Risk Behavior Survey. *Journal of American College Health, 46,* 55–66.

Duaux, E., Krebs, M. O, & Poirier, M. F. (2000). Genetic vulnerability to drug abuse. *European Psychiatry, 15*, 109–114.

Dubo, E. D., Zanarini, M. C., Lewis, R. E., & Williams, A. A. (1997). Childhood antecedents of self-destructiveness in borderline personality disorder. *Canadian Journal of Psychiatry, 42*, 63–69.

Eisen, S. A., Lin, N., Lyons, M. J., Scherrer, J. F., Griffith, K., True, W. R., Goldberg, J., & Tsuang, M. T. (1998). Familial influences on gambling behavior: an analysis of 3359 twin pairs. *Addiction, 93*, 1375–1384.

Engwall, D., Hunter, R., & Steinberg, M. (2004). Gambling and other risk behaviors on university campuses. *Journal of American College Health, 52*, 245–256.

Evenden, J. L. (1999). Varieties of impulsivity. *Psychopharmacology, 146*, 348–361.

Fergusson, D. M., Lynskey, M. T., & Horwood, L. J. (1996). Childhood sexual abuse and psychiatric disorders in young adulthood. I. Prevalence of sexual abuse and factors associated with sexual abuse. *Journal of American Academy of Child and Adolescent Psychiatry, 35*, 1355–1364.

Festinger, L. (1950). Informal social communication. *Psychological Review, 57*, 271–282.

Fillmore, K. M., Hartka, E., Johnstone, B. M. (1991). A meta-analysis of life course variation in drinking. *British Journal of Addiction, 86*, 1221–1267.

First, M. B., Spitzer, R. L., Gibbon, M. & Williams, J.B.W. (1995). The structured clinical interview for DSM-III-R personality disorders (SCID-II): I. Description. *Journal of Personality Disorders 9*(2), 83–91.

Fishbein, D., Lozovsky, D., & Jaffe, J. (1989). Impulsivity, aggression, and neuroendocrine responses to serotonergic stimulation in substance abusers. *Biological Psychiatry, 5*, 1049–1066.

Fisher, R. A. (1958). Lung cancer and cigarettes. *Nature, 182*, 108.

Flory, K., Milich, R., Lynam, D.R., Leukefeld, C., & Clayton, R. (2003). Relation between childhood disruptive behavior disorders and substance use and dependence symptoms in young adulthood: individuals with symptoms of attention-deficit/hyperactivity disorder and conduct disorder are uniquely at risk. *Psychology of Addictive Behaviors, 17*, 151–158.

Flory, K., Molina, B. S., Pelham, W. E., Gnagy, E., & Smith, B. (2006). Childhood ADHD predicts risky sexual behavior in young adulthood. *Journal of Clinical Child and Adolescent Psychology, 35*, 571–577.

Goldman, D., Oroszi, G., & Ducci, F. (2005). The genetics of addictions: Uncovering the genes. *Nature Reviews Genetics, 6*, 521–532.

Grant, J. D., Heath, A. C., Madden, P. A. F., Bucholz, K. K., Whitfield, J. B., & Martin, N. G. (1999). An assessment of the genetic relationship between alcohol metabolism and alcoholism risk in Australian twins of European ancestry. *Behavior Genetics, 29*, 463–472.

Griffin, M., Weiss, R., Mirin, S., & Lange, U. (1989). A comparison of male and female cocaine abusers. *Archives of General Psychiatry, 46*, 122–126.

Griffiths, M. D., & Parke, J. (2002). The social impact of internet gambling. *Social Science Computer Review, 20*, 312–320.

Grove, W. M., Eckert, E. D., Heston, L., Bouchard, T. J., Jr., Segal, N., & Lykken, D. T. (1990). Heritability of substance abuse and antisocial behavior: A study of monozygotic twins reared apart. *Biological Psychiatry, 27*, 1293–1304.

Han, C., McGue, M. K., & Iacono, W. G. (1999). Lifetime tobacco, alcohol and other substance use in adolescent Minnesota twins: Univariate and multivariate behavioral genetic analyses. *Addiction, 94*, 981–993.

Harford, T. C., Yi, H., & Hilton, M. E. (2006). Alcohol abuse and dependence in college and noncollege aamples: A ten-year prospective follow-up in a national survey. *Journal of Studies on Alcohol, 67*, 803–809.

Heath, A. C. (1995). Genetic influences on alcoholism risk; A review of adoption and twin studies. *Alcohol Health and Research World, 19*, 166–171.

Heath, A. C., Bucholz, K. K., Madden, P. A., Dinwiddie, S. H., Slutske, W. S., Bierut, L. J., Statham, D. J., Dunne, M. P., Whitfield, J. B., & Martin, N. G. (1997). Genetic and environmental contributions to alcohol dependence risk in a national twin sample: Consistency of findings in women and men. *Psychological Medicine, 27*, 1381–1396.

Hebert, R. (2004). What's new in Nicotine and Tobacco Research? *Nicotine and Tobacco Research, 6* Suppl 3, S279–283.

Hingson, R., Heeren, T., Winter, M., & Wechsler, H. (2005). Magnitude of alcohol-related mortality and morbidity among U.S. college students ages 18–24: Changes from 1998 to 2001. *Annual Review of Public Health, 26*, 259–279.

Hiroi, N., & Agatsuma, S. (2005). Genetic susceptibility to substance dependence. *Molecular Psychiatry, 10*, 336–344.

Huizink, A. C., Ferdinand, R. F., Ormel, J., & Verhulst, F. C. (2006). Hypothalamic-pituitary-adrenal axis activity and early onset of cannabis use. *Addiction, 101*, 1581–1588.

Ibañez, A., Blanco, C., Perez de Castro, I., Fernandez-Piqueras, J., & Saiz-Ruiz, J. (2003). Genetics of pathological gambling. *Journal of Gambling Studies, 19*, 11–22.

Ibañez, A., Perez de Castro, I., Fernandez-Piqueras, J., Blanco, C., & Saiz-Ruiz, J. (2000). Pathological gambling and DNA polymorphic markers at MAO-A and MAO-B genes. *Molecular Psychiatry*, 5, 105–109.

Jackson, K. M. Sher, K. J., & Park, A. (2005). Drinking among college students: Consumption and consequences. In Galanter, M. (Ed.), *Recent Developments in Alcoholism* (pp. 85–117). New York: Springer.

Jacobs, D. F. (2000). Juvenile gambling in North America: an analysis of long term trends and future prospects. *Journal of Gambling Studies*, 16, 119–152.

Jang, K. J., Vernon, P. A., & Livesley, W. J. (2000). Personality disorder traits, family environment, and alcohol misuse: A multivariate behavioural genetic analysis. *Addiction*, 95, 873–888.

Jenkins, J. E. (2001). Rural adolescent perceptions of alcohol and other drug resistance. *Child Study Journal*, 31, 211–224.

Jenkins, R., Manopaiboon, C., Samuel, A. P., Jeevapant, S., Carey, J. W., Kilmarx, P. H., et al. (2002). Condom use among vocational school students in Chiang Rai, Thailand. *AIDS Education and Prevention*, 14, 228–245.

Jenkins, J. E., & Zunguze, S. T. (1998). The relationship of family structure to adolescent drug use, peer affiliation, and perception of peer acceptance of drug use. *Adolescence*, 33, 811–822.

Jessor, R., & Jessor, S. L. (1977). *Problem behavior and psychological development: A longitudinal study of youth.* New York: Academic Press.

Johnston, L. D., O'Malley, P. M., Bachman, J. G., & Schulenberg, J. E. (2005). *Monitoring the future national results on adolescent drug use: Overview of key findings, 2004* (NIH publication no. 05-5726). Bethesda, MD: National Institute on Drug Abuse.

Johnston, L. D., O'Malley, P. M., Bachman, J. G., & Schulenberg, J. E. (2007). *Monitoring the future national results on adolescent drug use: Overview of key findings, 2006* (NIH publication no. 07-6202). Bethesda, MD: National Institute on Drug Abuse.

Johnson, V., & Pandina, R. (1993). Affectivity, family drinking history, and the development of problem drinking: A longitudinal analysis. *Journal of Applied Social Psychology*, 23, 2055–2073.

Johnson, A. M., Vernon, P. A., Harris, J. A., & Jang, K. L. (2004). A behavior genetic investigation of the relationship between leadership and personality. *Twin Research*, 7, 27–32.

Kalat, J. (2004). *Biological psychology* (8th ed.). Belmont, CA: Wadsworth/Thomas Learning.

Kaufman, J., Yang, B.-Z., Douglas-Palumberi, H, Crouse-Artis, M., Lipschitz, D., Krystal, J. H., & Glernter, J. G. (2007). Genetic and environmental predictors of eary alcohol use. *Biological Psychiatry*, 61, 1228–1234.

Kendler, K. S., Karkowski, L. M., Neale, M. C., & Prescott, C. A. (2000). Illicit psychoactive substance use, heavy use, abuse, and dependence in a U.S. population-based sample of male twins. *Archives of General Psychiatry*, 57, 261–269.

Kendler, K. S., Prescott, C. A., Myers, J., & Neale, M. C. (2003). The structure of genetic and environmental risk factors for common psychiatric and substance use disorders in men and women. *Archives of General Psychiatry*, 60, 929–937.

King, R., Curtis, D., & Knoblich, G. (1991). Complexity preference in substance abusers and controls: Relationships to diagnosis and personality variables. *Perceptual and Motor Skills*, 72, 35–39.

Knight, J. R., Wechsler, H., Kuo, M., Seibring, M., Weitzman, E. R., & Schuckit, M. A. (2002). Alcohol abuse and dependence among U.S. college students. *Journal of Studies on Alcohol*, 6, 263–270.

Koob, G. (2006). The neurobiology of addiction: A neuroadaptational view relevant for diagnosis. *Addiction*, 101, 23–30.

Kreek, M. J., Nielsen, D. A., Butelman, E. R., & LaForge, K. S. (2005). Genetic influences on impulsivity, risk-taking, stress responsivity and vulnerability to drug abuse and addiction. *Nature Neuroscience*, 8, 1450–1457.

Krueger, R. (1999). Personality traits in late adolescence predict mental disorders in early adulthood: A prospective-epidemiological study. *Journal of Personality*, 67, 39–65.

Krueger, R. F., Hicks, B. M., Patrick, C. J., Carlson, S. R., Lacono, W. G., & McGue, M. (2002). Etiologic connections among substance dependence, antisocial behavior, and personality: Modeling the externalizing spectrum. *Journal of Abnormal Psychology*, 111, 411–424.

Krueger, R. F., Markon, K. E., Patrick, C. P., & Iacono, W. G. (2005). Externalizing psychopathology in adulthood: A dimensional-spectrum conceptualization and its implications for *DSM–V*. *Journal of Abnormal Psychology*, 114, 537–550.

Kumra, V., Markoff, B.A. (2000). Who's smoking now? The epidemiology of tobacco use in the United States and abroad. Clinics in chest Medicine, 21(1):1–9, vii.

Labouvie, E., Pandina, R., White, H., Johnson, V. (1990). Risk factors of adolescent drug use: An affect-based interpretation. *Journal of Substance Abuse*, 2, 265–285.

LaBrie, R. A., Shaffer, H. J., LaPlante, D. A., & Wechsler, H. (2003). Correlates of college student gambling in the United States. *Journal of American College Health*, 52, 53–62.

Lane, S. D., Cherek, D. R., Rhodes, H. M., Pietras, C. J., & Tcheremissine, O. V. (2003). Relationships among laboratory and psychometric measures of impulsivity: Implications in substance abuse and dependence. *Addictive Disorders and Their Treatment, 2*, 33–40.

Larimer, M. E., & Cronce, J. M. (2002). Identification, prevention, and treatment: A review of individual-focused strategies to reduce problematic alcohol consumption by college students. *Journal of Studies on Alcohol, 114*, 148–163.

Leigh, B. C. (1999). Peril, chance, adventure: Concepts of risk, alcohol use and risky behavior in young adults. *Addiction, 94*, 371–383.

Lejuez, C. W., Aklin, W. M., Daughters, S. B., Zvolensky, M. J., Kahler, C. W., & Gwadz, M. (2007). Reliability and validity of the youth version of the balloon analogue risk task (BART-Y) in the assessment of risk-taking behavior among inner-city adolescents. *Journal of Clinical Child and Adolescent Psychology, 36*, 106–111.

Lejuez, C. W., Read, J. P., Kahler, C. W., Richards, J. B., Ramsey, S. E., Stuart, G. L., Strong, D. R., & Brown, R. A.(2002). Evaluation of a behavioral measure of risk taking: The balloon analogue risk task (BART). *Journal of Experimental Psychology: Applied, 8*, 75–84.

Lesieur, H. R., & Blume, S. B. (1987). South Oaks gambling screen (SOGS): A new instrument for the identification of pathological gamblers. *American Journal of Psychiatry, 144*, 1184–1188.

Li, M. D., Cheng, R., Ma, J. Z., & Swan, G. E. (2003). A meta-analysis of estimated genetic and environmental effects on smoking behavior in make and female adult twins. *Addiction, 98*, 23–31.

Logan, G. D. (1994). On the ability to inhibit thought and action: A users' guide to the stop signal paradigm. In T. H. Dagenbach and D. Carr (Eds.), *Inhibitory processes in attention, memory, and language* (pp. 189–239). San Diego, CA: Academic Press.

Madden, P. A. F., Health, A. C., Pedersen, N. L., Kaprio, J., Koskenvuo, M. J., & Martin, N. G. (1999). The genetics of smoking persistence in men and women: A multicultural study. *Behavior Genetics, 29*, 423–431.

Martens, M. P., Taylor, K. K, Damann, K. M., Page, J. C., Mowry, E. S., & Cimini, M. D. Protective behavioral strategies when drinking alcohol and their relationship to negative alcohol-related consequences in college students. *Psychol. Addict. Behav.* 2004 Dec; 18(4): 390–393.

Matzger, H., Delucchi, K., Weisner, C., & Ammon, L. (2004). Does marital status predict long-term drinking? Five-year observations of dependent and problem drinkers. *Journal of Studies on Alcohol, 65*, 255–265.

McGue, M. (1993). From proteins to cognitions: The behavioral genetics of alcoholism. In R. Plomin and G. McClearn (Eds.), *Nature, nurture, and psychology* (pp. 245–268). Washington, DC: American Psychological Association.

McGue, M. (1994). Genes, environment, and etiology of alcoholism. In R. Zucker, G. Boyd, & J. Howard (Eds.), *The development of alcohol problems: Exploring the biopsychosocial matrix of risk* (pp. 1–40). Rockville, MD: U.S. Department of Heath and Human Services.

Medrano, M. A., Hatch, J. P., Zule, W. A., & Desmond, D. P. (2003). Childhood trauma and adult prostitution behavior in a multiethnic heterosexual drug-using population. *American Journal of Drug and Alcohol Abuse, 29*, 463–486.

Michael, R. T., Gagnon, J. H., Laumann, E. O., & Kolata, G. (1994). *Sex in America*. Boston: Little, Brown.

Miles, D. R., Van den Bree, M. B. M., & Gupman, A. E. (2001). A twin study on sensation seeking, risk taking behavior and marijuana use. *Drug and Alcohol Dependence, 62*, 57–68.

Miller, P. M., & Lisak, D. (1999). Associations between childhood abuse and personality disorder symptoms in college males. *Journal of Interpersonal Violence, 14*, 642–656.

Millstein, S. G., & Igra, V. (1995). Theoretical models of adolescent risk-taking behavior. In J. L. Wallander & L. J. Siegel (Eds.), *Adolescent health problems* (pp. 52–71). New York: Guilford Press.

Mischel, W., Shoda, Y., & Rodriquez, M. (1989). Delay of gratification in children. *Science, 244*, 933–938.

Moeller, F. G., Dougherty, D. M., Barratt, E. S., Oderinde, V., Mathias, C. W., Harper, R. A., & Swann, A. C. (2002). Increased impulsivity in cocaine dependent subjects independent of antisocial personality disorder and aggression. *Drug and Alcohol Dependence, 68*, 105–111.

Moeller, F. G., Dougherty, D. M., Barratt, E. S., Schmitz, J. M., Swann, A. C., & Grabowski, J. (2001). The impact of impulsivity on cocaine use and retention in treatment. *Journal of Substance Abuse Treatment, 21*, 193–198.

Mogelonsky, M. (1996). The rocky road to adulthood. *American Demographics, 56*, 26–36.

Mohler-Kuo, M., Lee, J. E., & Wechsler, H. (2003). Trends in marijuana and other illicit drug use among college students: Results from four Harvard School of Public Health College Alcohol Study Surveys: 1993–2001. *Journal of American College Health, 52*, 17–24.

Molina, B. S., & Pelham, W. E. (2003). Childhood predictors of adolescent substance use in a longitudinal study of children with ADHD. *Journal of Abnormal Psychology, 112*, 497–507.

Molina, B. S., Pelham, W. E., Gnagy, E. M., Thompson, A. L., & Marshal, M. P. (2007). Attention-deficit/hyperactivity disorder risk for heavy drinking and alcohol use disorder is age specific. *Alcoholism Clinical and Experimental Research, 31*, 643–654.

Molina, B. S., Smith, B. H., & Pelham, W. E. (1999). Interactive effects of attention deficit hyperactivity disorder and conduct disorder on early adolescent substance use. *Psychology of Addictive Behaviors, 13*, 348–358.

Monterosso, J., Ehrman, R., Napier, K. L., O'Brien, C. P., Childress, A. R (2001). Three decision-making tasks in cocaine-dependent patients: do they measure the same construct? *Addiction, 96*(12), 1825–1837.

Mustanski, B. S., Viken, R. J., Kaprio, J., & Rose, R. J. (2003). Genetic influences on the association between personality risk factors and alcohol use and abuse. *Journal of Abnormal Psychology, 112*, 282–289.

Naimi, T. S., Brewer, R. D., & Mokdad, A. (2003). Binge drinking among U.S. adults. *Journal of the American Medical Association, 289*, 70–75.

National Highway Traffic Safety Administration (NHTSA). (2006). *Digest of state alcohol-highway safety-related legislation* (21st ed.). Washington, DC: Department of Transportation.

Newman, J. P., Patterson, C. M., & Kosson, D. S. (1987). Response perseveration in psychopaths. *Journal of Abnormal Psychology, 96*, 145–148.

NIAAA (2002). A call to action: Changing the culture of drinking at U.S. colleges. Retrieved May 9, 2007, from http://www.collegedrinkingprevention.gov/Reports/#task

Pallanti, S., DeCaria, C. M., Grant, J. E., Urpe, M., & Hollander, E. (2005). Reliability and validity of the pathological gambling modification of the Yale-Brown obsessive-compulsive scale (PG-YBOCS). *Journal of Gambling Studies, 21*, 431–443.

Paolucci, E. O, Genuis, M. L., & Violato C. (2001). A meta-analysis of the published research on the effects of child sexual abuse. *Journal of Psychology, 135*, 17–36.

Patton, J. H., Stanford, M. S., & Barratt E. S. (1995). Factor structure of the Barratt impulsiveness scale. *Journal of Clinical Psychology, 51*, 768–774.

Perez de Castro, I., Ibañez, A., Saiz-Ruiz, J., & Fernandez-Piqueras, J. (1999). Genetic contribution to pathological gambling: possible association between a functional DNA polymorphism at the serotonin transporter gene and affected men. *Pharmacogenetics, 9*, 397–400.

Perkins, H. W. (2002). Social norms and the prevention of alcohol misuse in collegiate contexts. *Journal of Studies on Alcohol, 14*, 164–172.

Peto, R., & Lopez, A. D. (2000). The future worldwide health effects of current smoking patterns. In C. E. Koop & C. E. Pearson (Eds.), *Global health in the 21st century*. New York: Jossey-Bass.

Petraitis, J., Flay, B. R., & Miller, T. Q. (1995). Reviewing theories of adolescent substance use: organizing pieces in the puzzle. *Psychological Bulletin, 117*, 67–86.

Petry, N. (2001). Substance abuse, pathological gambling, and impulsiveness. *Drug and Alcohol Dependence, 63*, 29–38.

Pryce, Pryce CR, Bettschen D, & Feldon J. Comparison of the effects of early handling and early deprivation on maternal care in the rat. Developmental Psychobiology. 2001 May;38(4):239–51.

Read, J., Wood, M. D., Davidoff, O. J., McLacken, X. X., & Campbell, J. F. (2002). Making the transition from high school to college: The role of alcohol-related social influence factors in students' drinking. *Substance Abuse, 23*, 53–64.

Read, J. P., Wood, M. D., Kahler, C. W., Maddock, J. E., & Palfai, T. P. (2003). Examining the role of drinking motives in college student alcohol use and problems. *Psychology of Addictive Behaviors, 17*, 13–23.

Resnick, R. J. (1997). A brief history of practice—expanded. *American Psychologist, 52*, 463–468.

Reynolds, B., Patak, M., Shroff, P., Penfold, R. B., Melanko, S., & Duhig, A. M. (2007). Laboratory and self-report assessments of impulsive behavior in adolescent daily smokers and nonsmokers. *Experimental and Clinical Psychopharmacology, 15*, 264–271.

Sabbatini da Silva Lobo, D., Vallada, H. P., Knight, J., Martins, S. S., Tavares, H., Gentil, V., & Kennedy, J. L. (2007). Dopamine genes and pathological gambling in discordant sib-pairs. *Journal of Gambling Studies, 23*, 421–433.

Sartor, C. E., Lynskey, M. T., Heath, A. C., Jacob, T. & True, W. (2007). The role of childhood risk factors in initiation of alcohol use and progress to alcohol dependence. *Addiction, 102*, 216–225.

Saunders, J., Aasland, O., Babor, T., De La Fuenta, J., & Grant, M. (1993). Development of the alcohol use disorders identification test (AUDIT): WHO collaborative project on early detection of persons with harmful alcohol consumption—II. *Addiction, 88*, 791–804.

Schindler, A., Thomasius, R., Sack, P. M., Gemeinhardt, B., Küstner U., & Eckert J. Attachment and substance use disorders: a review of the literature and a study in drug dependent adolescents. *Attachment and Human Development*. 2005 Sep;7(3):207–28

Schulenberg, J. E., O'Malley, P. M., Bachman, J. G., Wadsworth, K. N., & Johnston, L. D. (1996). Getting drunk and growing up: Trajectories of frequent binge drinking during the transition to young adulthood. *Journal of Studies on Alcohol, 57,* 289–304.

Shaffer, H. J., & Hall, M. N. (2001). Updating and refining meta-analytic prevalence estimates of disordered gambling behavior in the United States and Canada. *Canadian Journal of Public Health, 92,* 168–172.

Shah, K. R., Eisen, S. A., Xian, H., & Potenza, M. N. (2005). Genetic studies of pathological gambling: a review of methodology and analyses of data from the Vietnam Era Twin Registry. *Journal of Gambling Studies, 21,* 179–203.

Simpson, D. D. (1997). *Guidelines for the evaluation of treatment.* Invited presentation at the European Multinational Project on Evaluation of Action against Drug Abuse in Europe, Zurich, Switzerland.

Sinha, R., Garcia, M., Paliwal, P., Kreek, M. J., & Rounsaville, B. J. (2006). Stress-induced cocaine craving and hypothalamic-pituitary adrenal responses are predictive of cocaine relapse outcomes. *Archives of General Psychiatry, 63,* 324–331.

Slutske, W. S., Heath, A. C., Dinwiddie, S. H., Madden, P. A. F., Bucholz, K. K., Dunne, M. P., et al. (1998). Common genetic risk factors for conduct disorder and alcohol dependence. *Journal of Abnormal Psychology, 107,* 363–374.

Slutske, W. S., Eisen, S., True, W. R., Lyons, M. J., Goldberg, J., Tsuang, M. (2000). Common genetic vulnerability for pathological gambling and alcohol dependence in men. *Archives of General Psychiatry, 57*(7), 666–673.

Slutske, W. S., Hunt-Carter, E. E., Nabors-Oberg, R. E., Sher, K. J., Bucholz, K. K., Madden, P. A. F., Anokhin, A., & Health, A. C. (2004). Do college students drink more than their noncollege-attending peers? Evidence from a population-based longitudinal female twin study. *Journal of Abnormal Psychology, 113,* 530–540.

Smith, B. H., Molina, B. S. G., & Pelham, W. E., Jr. (2002). The clinically meaningful link between alcohol use and attention deficit hyperactivity disorder. *Alcohol Research and Health, 26,* 122–129.

Sorocco, K. H., Lovallo, W. R., Vincent, A. S., & Collins, F. L. (2006). Blunted hypothalamic-pituitary-adrenocorticol axis responsivity to stress in persons with a family history of alcoholism. *International Journal of Psychophysiology, 59,* 210–217.

Spanagel, L. P., & Weiss, F. (1999). The dopamine hypothesis of reward: past and current status. *Trends in Neuroscience, 2,* 521–527.

Spear, L. (2000). The adolescent brain and age-related behavioral manifestations. *Neuroscience and Biobehavioral Reviews, 24,* 417–463.

Stouthamer-Loeber, M., Wei, E., Loeber, R., & Masten, A. S. (2004). Desistance from persistent serious delinquency in the transition to adulthood. *Development and Psychopathology, 16,* 897–918.

Substance Abuse and Mental Health Services Administration (SAMHSA). (2003). *Results from the National Survey on Drug Use and Health: National findings.* Office of Applied Studies, NHSDA Series H-22, DHHS publication no. SMA 03-3836. Rockville, MD: Author.

Substance Abuse and Mental Health Services Administration (SAMHSA). (2004). *Results from the 2004 National Survey on Drug Use and Health: National findings.* Retrieved March 1, 2007, from http://www.oas.samhsa.gov/NSDUH/2k4NSDUH/2k4results/2k4results.htm#fig7.3.

Sussman, S., Stacy, A. W., Dent, C. W., Simon, T. R., Galaif, E. R., Moss, M. A., Craig, S., & Johnson, C. A. (1995). Continuation high schools: Youth at risk for drug abuse. *Journal of Drug Education, 25,* 191–209.

Thompson, A. L., Molina, B. S., Pelham, W., & Gnagy, E. M. (2007). Risky driving in adolescents and young adults with childhood ADHD. *Journal of Pediatric Psychology, 32,* 745–759.

Tolan, P. H., & Loeber, R. (1993). Antisocial behavior. In P. H. Tolan, B. J. Cohler (Eds). *Handbook of clinical research and practice with adolescents* (pp. 307–331). New York: Wiley.

Toomey, T. L., & Wagenaar, A. C. (2002). Environmental policies to reduce college drinking: Options and research findings. *Journal of Studies on Alcohol, 14,* 193–205.

Tsuang, M. T., Lyons, M. J., Eisen, S., Goldberg, J., True, W. R., Lin, N., Meyer, J. M., Toomey, R., & Eaves, L. J. (1996). Genetic influences on abuse of illicit drugs: a study of 3,297 twin pairs. *American Journal of Medical Genetics, 67,* 473–477.

Tsuang, M. T., Lyons, M. J., Harley, R. M., Xian, H., Eisen, S., Goldeberg, J., True, W. R., & Faraone, S. V. (1999). Genetic and environmental influence on transitions in drug use. *Behavior Genetics, 29,* 473–479.

Tucker Halpern, C., Young, M. L., Waller, M. W., Martin, S. L., & Kupper, L. L. (2004). Prevalence of partner violence in same-sex romantic and sexual relationships in a national sample of adolescents. *Journal of Adolescent Health, 35,* 124–131.

Urberg, K. A., Degirmencioglu, S. M., & Pilgrim, C. (1997). Close friend and group influence on adolescent cigarette smoking and alcohol use. *Developmental Psychology, 33,* 834–844.

U. S. Bureau of the Census. http://www.census.gov/ accessed March 7, 2009

U. S. Department of Health and Human Services, U. S. Public Health Service. (2001). *Youth violence: A report of the surgeon general.* Washington, DC: U.S. Government Printing Office.

Valente, T. W., Gallaher, P., & Mouttapa, M. (2004). Using social networks to understand and prevent substance use: A transdisciplinary perspective. *Substance Use and Misuse, 39,* 1685–1712.

Valois, R. F., Oeltmann, J. E., & Waller, J. (1999). Relationship between number of sexual intercourse partners and selected health risk behaviors among public high school adolescents. *Journal of Adolescent Health, 25,* 328–335.

Van den Bree, M. B., Svikis, D. S., & Pickens, R. W. (1998). Genetic influences in antisocial personality and drug use disorders. *Drug and Alcohol Dependence, 49,* 177–187.

Van Duijn, C. M., Clayton, D.G., Chandra, V., Fratiglioni, L., Graves, A. B., Heyman, A. et al. (2005). Interaction between genetic and environmental risk factors for Alzheimer's disease: A reanalysis of case-control studies. *Genetic Epidemiology, 11,* 6539–6551.

Viken, R. J., Kaprio, J., Koskenvuo, M., & Rose, R. J. (1999). Longitudinal analyses of the determinants of drinking and of drinking to intoxication in adolescent twins. *Behavior Genetics, 29,* 455–461.

Volkow, N. D. (2004). Exploring the why's of adolescent drug abuse. *NIDA Notes, 19,* 1–2.

Walters, G. D. (2001). Behavior genetic research on gambling and problem gambling: A preliminary meta-analysis of available data. *Journal of Gambling Studies, 17,* 255–271.

Walters, G. D. (2002). The heritability of alcohol abuse and dependence: A meta-analysis of behavior genetic research. *American Journal of Drug & Alcohol Abuse, 28,* 557–584.

Walters, S. T., & Neighbors, C. (2005). Feedback interventions for college alcohol misuse: What, why and for whom? *Addictive Behaviors, 30,* 1168–1182.

Wang, M. Q., Fitzhugh, E. C., Eddy, J. M., Fu, Q., et al. (1997). Social influences on adolescents' smoking progress: A longitudinal analysis. *American Journal of Health Behavior, 21,* 111–117.

Wardle, H., Sproston, K., Orford, J., et al. (2007). *British gambling prevalence survey.* London: UK National Centre for Social Research.

Wechsler, H., Lee, J., Kuo, M., & Lee, H. (2000). College binge drinking in the 1990s: A continuing problem—Results of the Harvard School of Public Health 1999 College Alcohol Study. *Journal of American College Health, 48,* 199–210.

Wechsler, H., Lee, J. E., Kuo, M., Seibring, M., Nelson, T. F., & Lee, H. (2002). Trends in college binge drinking during a period of increased prevention efforts. Findings from four Harvard School of Public Health College alcohol study surveys: 1933–2001. *Journal of American College Health, 50,* 203–217.

Weiss, S. R., Kung, H. C., & Pearson, J. L. (2003). Emerging issues in gender and ethnic differences in substance abuse and treatment. *Current Women, 3,* 245–253.

Weiss, M. J. S., & Wagner, S. H. (1998). What explains the negative consequences of adverse childhood experiences on adult health? Insights from cognitive and neuroscience research. *American Journal of Preventive Medicine, 14,* 356–360.

Westen, D. (1994). Toward an integrative model of affect regulation: Applications to social-psychological research. *Journal of Personality, 62,* 641–667.

White, H. R., Labouvie, E. W., & Papadaratsakis, V. (2005). Changes in substance use during the transition to adulthood: A comparison of college students and their noncollege age peers. *Journal of Drug Issues, 35,* 281–306.

Whiteside, S. P., & Lynam, D. R. (2001). The five factor model and impulsivity: Using a structural model of personality to understand impulsivity. *Personality and Individual Differences, 30,* 669–689.

Wills, T. A., Sandy, J. M., & Yaeger, A. M. (2001). Coping dimensions, life stress, and adolescent substance use: A latent growth analysis. *Journal of Abnormal Psychology, 110,* 309–323.

Winters, K. (2002). *Gambling and college students.* Retrieved August 14, 2007, from Minnesota Institute of Public Health, Gambling Problems Resource Center Web Site, http://www.miph.org/Gambling/gmb_collegestud.html

Winters, K. C., & Rich, T. (1998). A twin study of adult gambling behavior. *Journal of Gambling Studies, 14,* 213–225.

Winters, K. C., Stinchfield R. D., Botzet A., & Anderson, N. (2002). A prospective study of youth gambling behaviors. *Psychology of Addictive Behaviors, 16,* 3–9.

Wood, R. T., Griffiths, M. D., & Parke, J. (2007). Acquisition, development, and maintenance of online poker playing in a student sample. *CyberPsychology and Behavior, 10,* 354–361.

Wood, M. D., Read, J., Palfai, T., & Stevenson, J. F. (2001). Social influence processes and college student drinking: The mediation role of alcohol out come expectancies. *Journal of Studies on Alcohol, 62,* 32–43.

Wu, X., Hudmon, K. S., Detry, M. A., Chamberlain, R. M., & Spitz, M. R. (2000). D2 dopamine receptor gene polymorphisms among African-American and Mexican: A lung cancer case-control study. *Cancer Epidemiology Biomarkers and Prevention, 9,* 1021–1026.

Xian, H., Scherrer, J. F., Slutske, W. S., Shah, K. R., Volberg, R., & Eisen, S. A. (2007). Genetic and environmental contributions to pathological gambling symptoms in a 10-year follow-up. *Twin Research and Human Genetics, 10,* 174–179.

Yoshida, K., Hamajima, N., Kozaki, K., Saito, H., Maeno, K., Sugiura, T., Ookuma, K., & Takahashi, T. (2001). Assocation between the dopamine D2 receptors A2/A2 genotype and smoking behavior in the Japanese. *Cancer Epidemiology Biomarkers and Prevention, 10,* 403–405.

Youth Risk Behavior Surveillance: National College Health Risk Behavior Survey, United States, 1995. (1997). CDC surveillance summaries. *Morbidity and Mortality Weekly Report, 46*(SS-6), November 14.

Zeitlin, H. (1999). Psychiatric comorbidity with substance misuse in children and teenagers. *Drug Alcohol Dependence, 55,* 225–234.

Zuckerman, M. (1972). Personality and situational factors in the process of inferring attitudes from behavior. *Psychological Reports,* Aug 31(1), 283–9.

Zuckerman, M. (1979). *Sensation seeking: Beyond the optimal level of arousal.* Hillside, NJ: Lawrence Erlbaum.

Zuckerman, M. (1994). *Behavioral expressions and biosocial bases of sensation seeking.* New York: Cambridge University Press.

Zuckerman, M., & Kuhlman, D. (2000). Personality and risk-taking: Common biosocial factors. *Journal of Personality, 68,* 999–1029.

Chapter 4

Impact of Childhood Mental Health Problems

Leslie A. Hulvershorn, Craig A. Erickson and R. Andrew Chambers

Case 1

Tom first presented at age 5 with significant symptoms of inattention and hyperactivity. He reportedly could not sit still at school or tend to a single activity for more than 1 minute unless he was fixated on watching television. Tom's parents felt his symptoms were greatly inhibiting his ability to progress in school. With pharmacologic management of his symptoms utilizing a stimulant, Tom progressed in school with markedly reduced hyperactivity and improved attention.

After having his medication managed by his primary care physician for several years, Tom, now age 9 in 3rd grade, presented back to his psychiatrist because of increased anxiety, particularly around new people. In social settings he would look away from others, show perseveration in his thought process, and cover his face. His anxiety had become impairing in school; when anxious, he would not complete assignments. At this time, Tom continued his stimulant and began a serotonin reuptake inhibitor (SSRI) trial for treatment of anxiety. After a few months, Tom's anxiety level was significantly reduced.

Tom successfully continued his stimulants and SSRI treatment for inattention/hyperactivity and anxiety for 4 years. However, at age 13 he began to develop physical aggression to the degree that he was hitting a family member or teacher at least every other day. Given the significance of Tom's aggression, his parents agreed to an additional trial of an atypical antipsychotic. After several weeks of dose adjustment, Tom's aggressive behavior significantly decreased. Tom progressed throughout the rest of adolescence with relatively stable behavior on a consistent treatment regimen targeting inattention/hyperactivity, anxiety, and aggressive behavior.

Case 1 Commentary

Tom's diagnosis is fragile X syndrome, a unigenetic syndrome and the most common cause of inherited mental retardation. This case, involving a disorder caused by a single dysfunctional gene, is a testament to the ever-changing nature of psychopathology in childhood and adolescence—even when the genetic basis for the disorder is concretely known and relatively simple. Most psychiatric disorders of children and adolescents have far more complex pathogenesis involving the interplay of many developmentally timed genes and a great diversity of environmental influences, ranging from early perinatal events to the variable introduction and layering of psychiatric medications.

Case 2

Joe presented initially to his pediatrician at age 2 with significant language delay. Joe also exhibited poor eye contact, played only by himself, had repetitive finger-twirling movements, and lacked reciprocal social behavior. Joe was initially diagnosed with autistic disorder. After his diagnosis, Joe had regular behavior therapy, social skills training, and speech therapy throughout childhood. By age 6 he was occasionally playing with peers and developed the use of full sentences. Throughout childhood Joe continued to have difficulty developing age-appropriate peer relationships.

At age 12, Joe's parents reported that his behavior significantly changed, concurrent with outward signs of puberty. At this time, his use of speech greatly decreased. He frequently began mumbling to a friend who was not in the room. Joe began to report that the family cat was talking to him and asking him to harm others. He became aggressive toward other people and animals. He would often stare off toward the wall or ceiling. At this time, Joe's ability to care for his personal hygiene greatly decreased. He would frequently giggle and laugh to himself as if he were responding to internal stimuli.

After several trials of antipsychotic medication, Joe's attention, use of language, and self-help skills improved. His inappropriate laughter, endorsement of auditory hallucinations, and aggressive behavior all significantly decreased. After treatment, Joe's parents felt he had not returned to his prepubertal baseline but had still made significant improvement.

Case 2 Commentary

Joe is a young man who had an apparently clear-cut early-life diagnosis of autistic disorder, but he went on to develop a schizophrenia-like syndrome at the onset of puberty. Given the overlap between the negative symptoms of schizophrenia and autism, Joe's developmental psychopathology may be viewed as having both consistent and evolving features. Does he have a variant of autism that later developed psychotic features, or a very early-onset form of schizophrenia? Notably, the pathogenesis of both schizophrenia and autism are each thought to be highly complex involving multigenetic and early environmental factors. In distinction to Case 1, where a well-defined unigenetic disorder followed a quite developmentally evolving course, this case illustrates how a disorder of potentially highly variable or multigenetic etiology could also have consistent features over time yet remain elusive to diagnostic categorization.

Together, Cases 1 and 2 illustrate the mysterious nature and great complexity of the developmental progression of psychopathology from childhood into adolescence. How do we begin to tease apart the genetic and environmental contributions to these disorders? Is this nature versus nurture debate really useful? To what extent do normative developmental events contribute to psychopathological trajectories? Are diagnostic categories useful or detrimental to these considerations? In this chapter we will begin to address these and other issues related to translational research on the developmental trajectories of childhood mental health problems.

Introduction

Given a psychiatric presentation in childhood, what might caregivers predict about the longitudinal course of symptoms and later life function? This question is of particular importance given that half of all DSM-IV disorders start by age 14 (Kessler et al., 2005) and between 7% and 15% of all youth suffer from at least one mental disorder (Pihlakoski et al., 2004). Greater knowledge of the developmental trajectories of psychiatric conditions will be essential to more efficacious clinical decision making about the timing, duration, and form of treatments, producing more profound and permanently positive alterations in disease course.

Clinicians routinely observe that both within and across particular diagnoses presenting in childhood, developmental trajectories can exhibit great variability (Lewis, 1997). For example, attention-deficit/hyperactivity disorder (ADHD) diagnosed in early childhood can either persist or wane through adolescence and adulthood, or morph into a different psychopathology altogether. Yet other diagnoses, such as schizophrenia, typically emerge in early adulthood with only a subtle prodrome, although neurobiological alterations underlying this disease are likely seeded even before birth. General factors, such as gender, may also influence the trajectory of childhood illnesses into adulthood (Erickson & Chambers, 2006).

Unfortunately, our understanding of developmental trajectories of mental disorders, and hence our ability to make predictions about disease course and treatments (as interventions with long-term impact), is quite limited by a paucity of definitive empirical evidence. Many factors have contributed to this situation. For example, the types of long-term longitudinal studies needed to deepen this knowledge are immensely more expensive than cross-sectional studies and are hampered by academic or financial pressures to publish results quickly. Moreover, to define and survive in their careers, researchers often become hyperspecialized around studying a particular diagnosis of interest, or particular age group, limiting interest and efforts in characterizing a *variance* of psychiatric syndromes across developmental ages. Finally, the ever-changing nature of diagnostic categorization, the ebb and flow of popularized diagnoses, and ongoing debates about whether particular syndromes should be regarded as nested within, or independent from, others produce significant uncertainties about what exactly is being, or should be, characterized over developmental stages.

Despite these issues, interest in the therapeutic promise and potential cost-effectiveness of more permanently and advantageously altering developmental trajectories is gathering steam. An emerging field of developmental psychiatry may eventually produce what might be closer to a preventative early cure, rather than chronic palliative treatment. Fueling this field, advances in genetics and neuroscience are providing investigators with better tools for probing the age-old dilemma of nature versus nurture though a neurodevelopmental lens. Renewed interested in traditional developmental psychological theories, and their empirical validation, is in turn being driven by a need for neuroscience to be guided by overarching theoretical constructs. Emerging findings characterizing profound neurobiological changes inherent to the normal pre-adult development of the mammalian brain inspire a growing effort toward understanding the neurodevelopmental basis of psychiatric disorders.

Against this background of uncertainty, but renewed momentum toward understanding pre-adult trajectories of mental disorders, we will consider emerging themes in developmental neuroscience followed by an overview of research describing the developmental courses of differential forms of childhood mental illness. Toward defining differential developmental patterns of childhood mental illness, we propose five models (A, B, C, D, and E) that characterize the varied trajectories mental illness may take up to adulthood (Fig. 4-1). While these models are inherently imprecise given the considerable empirical uncertainty and lack of consensus regarding the relationships between syndromes, we believe they can help us begin a developmentally focused dialogue that in time will be useful in creating a predictive understanding of childhood psychopathology. Throughout the chapter we will refer to a particular model trajectory of disorders (e.g. "Model C") when research findings and/or clinical observation make the case for such characterization.

Childhood Developmental Theories

Developmental theories have long been a central topic of inquiry in psychiatry. While there has been an explosion of empirical research since the 1960s, it was theoretical formulation, based upon decades of anecdotal observation, that provided initial insights into normal and pathological child development (Kazdin et al., 1991). For Freud and many later psychoanalytic theorists such as Melanie Klein and Margaret Mahler, psychopathology had its roots in the passage between various bodily organized phases (e.g., oral, anal, oedipal, latency phases). Erik Erikson elaborated Freud's psychosexual stages from five to eight and expanded them into adulthood, incorporating concepts of developmental existential conflict resolution. Attachment theorists, starting with John Bowlby in the late 1960s, focused developmental theory on the behavioral repertoire of infants as they developed attunement to their caregivers. The study of insecure attachment and its impact on relations observed during childhood led to the development of object relations theory. In the 1950s Jean Piaget focused on the development of intellectual structures creating a continuum of stages beginning with sensorimotor and ending with formal operations. The work of self-psychologists in recent decades has placed emphasis on parental empathic failure as a predictor for psychopathology.

Impact of Childhood Mental Health Problems

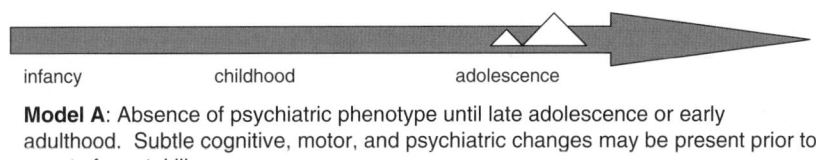

Model A: Absence of psychiatric phenotype until late adolescence or early adulthood. Subtle cognitive, motor, and psychiatric changes may be present prior to onset of mental illness.

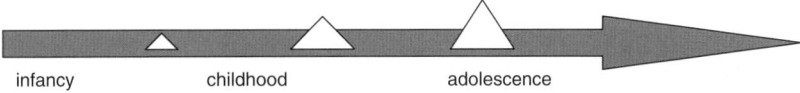

Model B: Early onset of symptoms that worsen over time but remain fairly homogeneous.

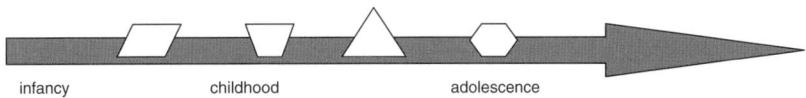

Model C: Evolution of different symptoms over time. This trajectory may be associated with considerable clinical confusion as to accuracy of prior diagnoses vs. acquisition of new diagnoses vs. presence of a single complex syndrome that evolves developmentally.

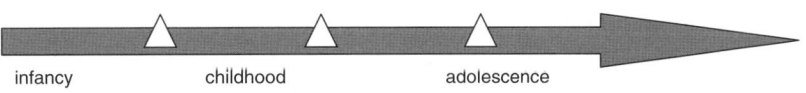

Model D: Emergence of symptoms early in life remaining fairly constant in character and severity.

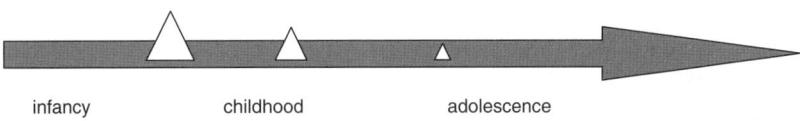

Model E: Emergence of symptoms early in life that diminish or disappear through development.

Figure 4-1. Five models of the course of mental illness from infancy to adulthood.

While the specifics and terms of developmental formulations have differed among these theorists, a general consensus pointing to the centrality of developmental change in generating adult syndromes is clear. It can be surmised that all of these theories entertain the idea that progress or outcomes of stages in developmental change depend on those that came before. The power of this idea not only relates to its intuitive clinical appeal, but the fact that it is particularly amenable to investigation from a structural/functional standpoint familiar to the physical sciences. From an engineering standpoint, the functioning of a complex structure is dependent on the functionality of its interdependent modules, and its overall design should reflect the manner or ordering in which modules were added. From a neurobiological standpoint, developmentally timed assessments of neural structures and function provide a method for understanding the physical aspects of psychological and cognitive development. Hence, a modern developmental psychopathological perspective entails the following principals: *(1)* the study of normal and pathological development are both important, and mutually informative; (2) developmental phenomena reflect dynamic changes involving multiple interacting brain systems and scales of observation ranging from the molecular to the psychological and cultural; and (3) neurobehavioral development follows a self-organizing, iterative process in which brain biology promotes interaction with the environment, which in turn changes brain biology (Cicchetti & Curtis, 2006).

Neurodevelopment of the Pre-Adult Mammalian Brain

While our understanding of how the brain changes from childhood to adolescence is itself in its earliest stages, a growing wealth of data indicates that these changes are profound and functionally meaningful, both neurobiologically and behaviorally (Romer & Walker, 2007). For example, the prefrontal cortex (PFC) undergoes significant micro- and macrostructural revision up through adolescence and early adulthood (Lewis, 1997). Local synaptic connectivity between neurons actually declines from early childhood levels, as does overall metabolic demand (Chugani, Phelps, & Mazziotta, 1987; Huttenlocher, 1979) and thickness of the cortical layer relative to the underlying white matter spaces (Giedd et al., 1996). In parallel to these changes, PFC functions of behavioral inhibition, decision making, and regulation of motivation, cognition (i.e., attention), and emotion reach new levels of efficiency and adaptability to environmental contexts (Chambers & Potenza, 2003; Spear, 2007). Meanwhile, other parts of the brain that more directly manage motivation, affect, and memory (e.g., the ventral striatum, hypothalamus, amygdala, and hippocampus, respectively) also show evidence for substantial change, whether in terms of their relative sizes, how they are innervated and modulated by specific neurotransmitters or hormones, how they interact with other brain structures, how they express specific proteins, or how they use energy to perform specific tasks (Romer & Walker, 2007).

With this neuroscientific re-invigoration of developmental psychology, exciting new translational-theoretical ideas are beginning to emerge that may soon guide more ground-breaking research into the developmental origins of psychiatric disorders as *both* genetic and environmentally dependent conditions. For example, theories that discuss the flexibililty-stability dilemma in brain development consider how and when the brain resolves two competing interests, one being the need to efficiently learn new information (favored earlier in development), and the other the need to adaptively operate based on what has been learned, usually later in development (Chambers, Potenza, Hoffman, & Miranker, 2004; Liljenstrom, 2003). Because the learning and memory attributes of specific neural networks, or even individual neurons, can be investigated biologically, physical markers of neural systems maturity can be correlated with changes in the overall adaptability of neural systems to specific stimuli (Snyder, Kee, & Wojtowicz, 2001). Over the course of postnatal development, specific genes may turn on and off over time, in a semi-predetermined way, changing the structural and functional phenotypic characteristics of individual neurons (Brumwell & Curran, 2006; Kaffman & Meaney, 2007). These structural-functional attributes in turn dictate how that neuron will respond to environmental stimuli (e.g., drugs, cognitive learning, positive or negative life experiences). Then, if stimuli are of sufficient quality, size, or duration, they in turn can alter the intracellular machinery of the neuron, such that its semi-predetermined schedule of gene activation becomes altered—either transiently or more irreversibly. In this way, neuronal phenotype, and the functionality of whole neural networks, is a reflection of the concerted impact of gene and environmental conditions, in which the developmental timing or sequencing of specific genes and environmental conditions is a critical dynamic.

Neurodevelopmental Derailment: Events in Childhood That Predispose to Mental Illness

While understanding genetic and environmental contributions are of co-equal importance to understanding the developmental progression of psychiatric disorders, the vast majority of available evidence describes neural systems function and development based on the impact of experimental environmental contingencies (e.g., pharmacological interventions, rearing conditions, stress, lesions, etc). Human genetic studies and basic science approaches that wed genetic testing and/or engineering with exposure to alternative environmental contingencies represent promising new approaches in this field. Recent investigations are beginning to examine how single genes may predispose to phenotypic components of psychiatric syndromes that may actually be shared across many different disorders (e.g., behavioral impulsivity) or how the phenotypic expression of certain genes is conditional on specific environmental events (Rende & Waldman, 2006). Yet clinical care currently extends control only over some environmental conditions that have biological impact, rather than any ability to re-engineer the genetic makeup of individual human patients. Accordingly, we limit the remainder of this section to a brief survey of how certain pre-adult environmental contingencies, abuse and neglect, may alter neurodevelopmental biology in the generation mental illness.

The potential for neurodevelopmental derailment due to abuse or neglect during early childhood has been widely supported by the maternal deprivation paradigm initially reported by H. F. Harlow and others (Sullivan et al., 2006). This model demonstrated that prolonged absence of parental caretaking and related psychological stress, even without nutritional deprivation, produce long-lasting alterations in the functioning of the hypothalamic-pituitary-adrenal (HPA) stress hormone system and persistent behavioral traits consistent with human anxiety, affective, and personality disorders (Lopez, Akil, & Watson, 1999). This work further inspired more direct investigations defining neurobiological changes associated with the induction of excess stress-related hormones or neurotransmitters in childhood. Excess corticotrophin-releasing factor, cortisol, and norepinephrine have all been variously associated with alterations in gene expression, neurotransmitter receptors, impaired neuron growth, and even neuronal death (Kaffman & Meaney, 2007; McEwen & Milner, 2007). Brain-derived neurotrophic factor (BDNF), a substance essential to neuronal growth and development, may play an important role in some of these changes, as its expression is also reduced in rats subject to maternal deprivation (Roceri, Hendriks, Racagni, Ellenbroek, & Riva, 2002). Together, some of these changes may entail lifelong and irreversible effects, such as declines in the ability of the hippocampus—a key brain area implicated in learning, memory, and multiple psychiatric disorders—to generate new neurons in adulthood (Lemaire, Lamarque, Le Moal, Piazza, & Abrous, 2006).

While neurobiological evidence is more difficult to obtain in humans, brain imaging has brought to light a number of dramatic differences in neural circuitry of children and adults affected by significant early life stress. Total corpus callosum volume was shown to be 17% smaller in abused/neglected children (mean ages, 11–12) compared to matched controls (Teicher et al., 2004). Even in adults reported free of mental illness, those who had greater than two adverse childhood events had lower anterior cingulate cortex and basal ganglia volume on MRI (Cohen et al., 2006). Maltreated, psychotropic naïve children, and adolescents with trauma-related disorders have reduced volume in many brain regions when compared to sociodemographically matched controls (De Bellis et al., 2002). Reduced cerebellar volume associated with trauma exposure has been shown to be more pronounced the earlier trauma occurs (De Bellis & Kuchibhatla, 2006).

Consistent with stress-related animal and human neuroimaging findings, early childhood neglect, abuse, and trauma have long been associated with increased risk of various forms of psychopathology. In humans, early childhood maltreatment is associated with later life elevations in affective, anxiety, personality, substance use, and posttraumatic stress disorders and is known to worsen the course of schizophrenia and bipolar disorder (Kaufman, Plotsky, Nemeroff, & Charney, 2000). Among preterm infants, greater neonatal experience of pain-related stress has been associated with reduced ability to focus at 8 months of age (Tu et al., 2007). In a sample of over 1000 socioeconomically disadvantaged high school seniors, self-reported adverse childhood events were strongly associated with adolescent depressive symptoms, drug abuse, and antisocial behavior (Schilling, Aseltine, & Gore, 2007). Early life stress and maltreatment have also been associated with increased childhood risk-taking behavior when compared to controls (Guyer et al., 2006). A dose–effect relationship of early stress was demonstrated when duration of deprivation was shown to be associated with the severity of attachment disorder in children (O'Connor & Rutter, 2000).

Precisely how the form and timing of environmental events, and their collusion with different genetic backgrounds, impact specific neural circuits and related developmental trajectories of psychiatric syndromes is not understood. A first task in approaching this problem is to begin to consider how initial clinical presentations of childhood may evolve into young adult conditions. The following sections consider how empirical evidence may point to the existence of various developmental trajectories spanning different clinical presentations in childhood.

Developmental Trajectories of Childhood Mental Illness

Anxiety Disorders

Anxiety disorders have long been thought of as amplification or persistence of early childhood temperamental features as a child ages. Kagen and colleagues followed a cohort of children from 4 months of age through early adolescence to assess the impact of early temperament on subsequent development of anxiety symptoms (Kagan & Snidman, 1999). Infants classified as "high reactive" (based upon vigorous response to stimuli) displayed significantly more distress and fear in social and nonsocial settings at 14 and 21 months of age compared to "low reactive" children who as infants demonstrated little distress when exposed to various stimuli (Kagan, 1994). By 4.5 years of age, the initially "high reactive" infants displayed fewer smiles in social settings and were generally classified as "shy and inhibited" compared to the initially "low reactive children" (Kagan, Snidman, & Arcus, 1998), and by age 7.5, those labeled as "high reactive" as infants were displaying significantly more anxiety symptoms (45%) than those initially found to be "low reactive" (15%) (Kagan, Snidman, Zentner, & Peterson, 1999). Additionally, "high reactive" infants who later appear as behaviorally inhibited during toddlerhood were predisposed to develop generalized anxiety disorder at age 12 (Schwartz, Snidman, & Kagan, 1999). In separate work, behavioral inhibition noted during early childhood was predictive of a social anxiety disorder diagnosis at a 5-year follow-up (Hirshfeld-Becker et al., 2007a, 2007b).

Among anxiety disorders, childhood posttraumatic stress disorder (PTSD) is by definition linked to early life stress exposure. As noted earlier, early stress exposure is associated with neurodevelopmental change and risk for psychopathology, including conduct, affective, and addictive disorders (Saarni & Harris, 1991). Some work has looked at what characteristics predispose certain children to developing PTSD after trauma exposure. Individuals who rated themselves as depressed or anxious as first graders, were more likely to be diagnosed with PTSD when exposed to trauma in young adulthood (Storr, Ialongo, Anthony, & Breslau, 2007). A PTSD diagnosis in children ages 20 months to 6 years followed prospectively over 2 years was predictive of subsequent functional impairment that may or may not present similar to adult cases of PTSD (Scheeringa, Zeanah, Myers, & Putnam, 2005). For those with PTSD in this cohort, re-experiencing symptoms decreased while avoidance/numbing increased over time (Scheeringa et al., 2005). Protective factors mediating against the development of PTSD have been described as previous successful coping skills, good self-esteem, strong problem-solving skills, and a positive relationship with an adult (Masten, Best, & Garmezy, 1990).

Based on these studies, we can speculate that anxiety disorders in children may have differential developmental trajectories based on whether they occur in the context of constitutional anxiety or prior traumatic stress. Overall, early infant reactivity and toddler behavioral inhibition do appear predictive of later anxiety symptoms, although many children who harbor these features do not go on to develop significant pathologic anxiety. Thus non-trauma-related anxiety in children may most typically follow various developmental courses including a path of improvement (Model E), persistence (Model D), worsening (Model B), or minor evolution among various anxiety disorders (e.g., a hybrid of Models C and D). In contrast, the development of PTSD may more often be viewed as a transition from earlier affective symptoms (Model C) that may over time morph into other affective and/or personality disorders, as significant overlap appears to exist between factors protective against and predictive of both PTSD and personality pathology. PTSD may also worsen (Model B), remain steady (Model D), or improve (Model E) with a consistent symptom set.

Unipolar Depression

While there are no nationally representative samples, unipolar depression is estimated to occur in approximately 2% of children (Kessler, Chiu, Demler, Merikangas, & Walters, 2005), with prevalence rates increasing to 6.1% by mid-adolescence through early adulthood (Blazer, Kessler, McGonagle, & Swartz, 1994). Childhood depression, while comparatively rare, does have a high rate of recurrence in adolescence and adulthood (Moffitt et al., 2007a). More severe cases predict a more protracted course and higher rate of recurrence (Sterba, Prinstein, & Cox, 2007). The course of childhood depression appears to show gender difference. In boys, recurrent early depression appears to follow significant negative life events (e.g., more of a PTSD variant), whereas in girls yearly increases in depressive symptoms occur regardless of ongoing negative life events (Silberg, Rutter, & Eaves, 2001). When diagnosed in childhood, depression may resolve completely and without recurrence in only a minority of cases (Hammen & Rudolph, 2003).

The interrelationship between depression and other aspects of childhood psychopathology has been demonstrated in several settings. Some information has pointed to symptomatic predictors of subsequent depression in youth. When controlling for conduct problems and academic skill level, inattention in first graders was significantly correlated with depressive symptoms by 3rd grade (Herman, Lambert, Ialongo, & Ostrander, 2007). Anxiety and depression in childhood have shown a strong link with anxiety predating comorbid depression in about 1 in 3 cases, depression predating anxiety in about 1 in 3 cases, and both disorders developing concurrently in the other third (Moffitt et al., 2007b). Reduced positive affect, including reduced motivation to obtain reward and reduced pleasure in experiencing reward, has been shown as a predictor of subsequent anxiety and depressive disorders (Forbes, Shaw, & Dahl, 2007).

Overall, the course of depression in childhood may follow differing pathways, including worsening symptoms over time (Model B), relative stability of illness with periodic episodes (Model D), or perhaps more rarely, improvement over time (Model E). Depression complicated by prominent anxiety, inattention, or traumatic events may also occur, leading to more heterogeneous and uncertain trajectories (Model C).

Bipolar Disorders

The diagnosis of childhood bipolar disorder remains the subject of much debate. Some have postulated that childhood bipolar disorder, as often diagnosed in the community, may actually represent a severe form of ADHD (Holtmann, Goth, Wockel, Poustka, & Bolte, 2007). Hence, ADHD has been reported as a comorbidity or possible primary diagnosis in 75%–98% of patients additionally diagnosed with youth-onset bipolar disorder (Wozniak, Biederman, & Richards, 2001). Chart review of 3- to 7-year-olds diagnosed with early-onset bipolar disorder revealed the most frequently reported clinical symptoms of mania were nonspecific and nonepisodic and included irritability, aggression, and hyperactivity (Danielyan, Pathak, Kowatch, Arszman, & Johns, 2007). In a national epidemiologic study, only 8% of adults with bipolar disorder reported childhood onset and 24% reported adolescent onset (Goldstein & Levitt, 2006). Despite the apparent rarity of adult bipolar illness originating in childhood, rates per 100,000 population of outpatient visits for childhood bipolar disorder have increased from 25 in 1994–1995 to 1003 in 2002–2003 (Moreno et al., 2007), potentially as a childhood diagnostic label that has ridden the coattails of the popular emergence of the ADHD diagnosis.

Given the uncertainty surrounding diagnosis of youth bipolar disorder, a clinical syndrome called severe mood dysregulation (SMD) has been proposed as an alternative diagnosis (Leibenluft, Charney, Towbin, Bhangoo, & Pine, 2003). SMD is characterized by "extreme, impairing, and chronic irritability, accompanied by hyperarousal symptoms" and is felt to be consistent with the broad phenotype frequently diagnosed as pediatric bipolar disorder (Brotman et al., 2006). SMD has a lifetime prevalence of 3.3% and is highly comorbid with ADHD, conduct disorder, and anxiety disorders (Brotman et al., 2006). SMD may be an appropriate surrogate diagnosis for many cases that are diagnosed as bipolar, and/or cases of ADHD complicated by robust affective symptoms, given that what is currently often labeled as childhood bipolar disorder may not often produce clear bipolar symptom development into adolescence and adulthood.

Some studies have attempted to characterize predictors of later onset bipolar disorder as assessed in genetically at-risk youth. For example, in youth with a first-degree relative with bipolar disorder, "minicycles" involving affective changes, somatic complaints, role impairment, hyper-alertness, stubbornness, anxiety, and being easily upset tended to predate full episodes of mania (Egeland et al., 2003). Notably, in this prospective report, ADHD did not predict later diagnosis of bipolar disorder. Again, severe ADHD may in some cases mimic bipolar illness and lead to a comorbid bipolar label, yet ADHD may not itself be a clear predictor of persisting or emerging bipolar illness.

Beyond debate about the proper diagnosis of youth bipolar disorder, clearly defined childhood bipolar illness, as indicated by subsequent adult bipolar illness, does appear predictive of certain clinical course features when compared to later onset illness. Childhood onset has been associated with more substance use disorders, comorbid antisocial personality, and longer periods of mood dysregulation (Goldstein & Levitt, 2006). Compared to adolescent bipolarity illness, the childhood-onset form has also been described as having a more chronic, unremitting course of illness (Masi et al., 2006).

The diagnostic controversy surrounding childhood bipolar disorder and the existence of frequent comorbidities point to Model C being a quite typical trajectory. The rarity of retrospective adult reports of the childhood onset of bipolar illness also points to Model A, implying that most cases of adult bipolar disorder may primarily entail adolescent or adult onset. More rarely, in children with first-degree relatives with bipolar illness, early symptoms of irritability, including minor mood cycling, appear predictive of later development of bipolar disorder (Model B) with symptoms worsening over time.

Disruptive Behavior Disorders

Other than the longitudinal reliability of diagnoses of mental retardation and pervasive developmental disorders (PDD), trajectories linking childhood conduct disorder (CD; and/or its minor variant, oppositional defiant disorder [ODD]) with the young adult diagnosis of antisocial personality disorder (ASPD) are perhaps the most widely recognized patterns in developmental psychiatry. However, many children with aggressive or oppositional behavior do not maintain deviance into adolescence (Petras et al., 2004), while another subset of individuals, populated with a higher percentage of females, begin antisocial behavior in adolescence (Marmorstein & Iacono, 2005).

Certain environmental factors and diagnostic complexities likely impact the extent to which CD/ODD presentations go on to ASPD. Among Finnish boys followed from age 8 to late adolescence, those with a nonintact family, low parental education, teacher complaints of hyperactivity, and parental complaints of conduct problems at age 8 independently predicted a high number of criminal offenses by age 16–20 (Sourander et al., 2006). Low parental education and early complaints of conduct problems independently predicted violence, property, traffic, and drunk-driving offenses in this cohort. These authors (Sourander et al., 2006) also found that hyperactivity in school independently predicted the majority of legal offenses.

Other studies also suggest differential developmental trajectories of disruptive behavior may be based on the presence of prominent ADHD symptoms and/or deviant peer affiliation in children aged 6–15 years (Petras et al., 2004). In one subgroup of childhood CD patients making up 11% of a clinical sample and comprised mostly of boys with severe early CD with prominent ADHD symptoms, later diagnoses consistent with ASPD were particularly reliable (Petras et al., 2004). A more common adolescent-onset trajectory (46% of the clinical sample) had members with more sophisticated social networks (comprised of friends with antisocial behavior) and a less persistent course of antisocial behavior. Other studies suggest that while early ADHD may exacerbate the likelihood of CD developing into ASPD, ADHD alone is not predictive of ASPD. For example, in a 30-year follow-up study, hyperactive boys with conduct problems had significantly more arrests, convictions, and incarcerations than controls, while hyperactive boys without conduct disorder were not at increased risk for adult criminality (Satterfield et al., 2007).

Based on these data, disruptive behavior disorders potentially follow several developmental courses. Symptom progression toward antisocial adult behavior (Model B) seems more common in boys with prominent ADHD symptoms, while the onset of new conduct problems in adolescence (Model A) may less reliably predict ASPD. Given appropriate psychosocial support, early life conduct problems are more likely to abate over time (Model E). Presentations of ADHD uncomplicated by CD are not likely to go on to ASPD traits consistent with Model C.

Addictions

Multiple lines of evidence indicate that while early childhood is typically free of substance abuse, adolescence and young adulthood is a critical period of vulnerability to acquisition and/or progression of substance use disorders into adulthood (Chambers, Taylor, & Potenza, 2003). Moreover, consistent with the broad spectrum of adult dual diagnosis presentations (i.e., substance disorder comorbidity in mental illnesses) that often transcend diagnostic categories (O'Brien et al., 2004), multiple forms of psychiatric presentations in childhood increase the risk of addictions later on. In particular, an array of externalizing disorders frequently diagnosed in boys with prominent manifestations of aggression, behavioral disinhibition, CD symptoms, and/or hyperactivity predict both earlier onset of substance use and later diagnosis of addictions (Felitti, 2003). Notably, this risk appears to be nonspecific to drug type, often involving substances that are the most frequently used and abused in the general adult population, including alcohol, marijuana, and tobacco (Chapman, Tarter, Kirisci, & Cornelius, 2007; Fite, Colder, Lochman, & Wells, 2007a, 2007b; Shelton et al., 2007).

Several studies have specifically examined risk for substance use disorders in children with ADHD and CD both as independent and comorbid presentations. As evidenced in a 25-year longitudinal birth cohort, CD symptoms in middle childhood and adolescence were generally related to later substance use disorders, even after controlling for attention problems (Fergusson, Horwood, & Ridder, 2007). ADHD diagnoses uncomplicated by CD also appear to increase the risk for subsequent acquisition of substance use disorders, while significant components of CD symptoms with the diagnosis amplify the risk (Molina, Pelham, Gnagy, Thompson, & Marshal, 2007; Tarter, Kirisci, Feske, & Vanyukov, 2007).

In summary, these data support a developmental trajectory for substance use disorders in which onset of drug addiction behavior often begins in adolescence/early adulthood (Model A). However, given the wide array of childhood psychiatric conditions that increase the risk of later onset addictions, especially those that feature ADHD and/or CD symptoms, Model C may be descriptive for a large number of cases.

Attention-Deficit/Hyperactivity Disorder

While the last decade has seen a huge increase in rates of diagnoses and treatment of ADHD in children, there remains considerable debate as to how ADHD may be considered as a pure disorder versus one that is a subsyndromal manifestation of another childhood condition (e.g., conduct disorder, affective disorders) versus a nonspecific childhood prodrome of a potentially wide variety of adult psychiatric diagnoses. Recent studies identifying behavioral features in very young children (i.e., toddlers and infants) that may predict childhood ADHD, such as high overall activity levels, anger reactivity (Auerbach, Atzaba-Poria, Berger, & Landau,

2004), and severe sleep problems (Thunstrom, 2002), may eventually help resolve aspects of this debate by identifying differential ADHD subtypes. Regardless, available evidence suggests that ADHD symptoms, whether presenting "pure" or in combination with other syndromal components (e.g., CD), frequently remain stable or decline from childhood to adolescence (Jester et al., 2005; Larsson, Larsson, & Lichtenstein, 2004; Spencer, Biederman, & Mick, 2007). Consistent with these findings, neuroimaging in ADHD children followed longitudinally through late teen years has also pointed to temporal consistency, in terms of smaller brain regions (cerebral cortex, cerebellum, total volume), although such findings are not specific to the ADHD diagnosis (Castellanos et al., 2002).

ADHD is a commonly diagnosed disorder of childhood onset with developmental patterns that can follow several models. ADHD symptoms may remit during adolescence and into adulthood, consistent with Model E, or remain stable through childhood into adulthood (Model D). However the frequent comorbidity of ADHD symptoms with other childhood disorders and eventually adult psychiatric and substance use disorders suggests Model C may capture a large portion of cases. Generally ADHD does not appear to frequently follow Model B with worsening core symptoms over time, and by definition, ADHD is a childhood-onset disorder, so Model A with adolescent or adult onset of pathology is debatable.

Psychotic Disorders

Understanding the developmental nature of childhood psychosis remains a challenge. Most children diagnosed with childhood-onset schizophrenia, even those with transient psychosis, are later found to have severe affective, psychotic, and/or behavioral disorders (Stayer et al., 2004). Conversely, the overwhelming majority of psychotic disorders have their outset during adolescence or adulthood, and numerous studies have tried to identify reliable childhood predictors of subsequent psychotic illness. For example, when retrospectively examined, adults with schizophrenia were more likely to have neurological soft signs, slowed motor development, low educational achievement, and more solitary play in childhood compared to the general population (Smith et al., 2003). Childhood histories of decreased lateralization of handedness and diminished verbal skills may represent subtle developmental impairments of lateralized cortical specializations (Leask & Crow, 2005).

Prospective neuroimaging in childhood schizophrenia has shown a pattern of change that is consistent with temporal evolution toward findings in adult-onset pathology. When imaged prospectively from ages 7–26, individuals with childhood-onset schizophrenia have significantly smaller mean cortical thickness (Greenstein et al., 2006). Cortical thickness began to normalize in parietal regions, creating a pattern more like adult-onset schizophrenia as the children aged (Greenstein et al., 2006).

While the majority of psychotic illnesses follow developmental Model A with adolescent or adult onset, the presence of prominent childhood signs point to Model B. Within the more rare set of cases of childhood-onset schizophrenia, Model C may also be applicable in which patients may later be reframed as having PDDs, schizoaffective disorders, or severe bipolar disorders. Unfortunately, psychotic illnesses in children are highly predictive of psychiatric illness of some form later on and thus do not fit well with Model E.

Summary and Conclusions

In this chapter, we have considered how neurodevelopmental research may provide new insights into understanding how and when genetic and environmental factors are integrated to generate adult psychiatric syndromes. A growing wealth of data indicating that profound changes normally occur in the brain from childhood to adolescence provide a basis for future explorations defining how psychiatric disorders can evolve clinically and neurobiologically. Toward generating a discussion about how specific childhood disorders may evolve into adulthood, we have considered how they may follow at least two of five developmental trajectories (Models A–E). Notably, this exploration is largely of an exploratory/conceptual nature. A comprehensive, quantitative view of developmental trajectories of childhood psychiatric disorders will require a number of large-scale prospective longitudinal cohort studies that are broadly inclusive of both healthy subjects and those with a wide spectrum of childhood and adult psychiatric diagnoses. Based on the available evidence presented here, and as illustrated in the introductory case vignette, the frequency with which childhood diagnoses may follow Model C (evolution of different symptoms over time), suggests the existence of considerable complexity both within and between disorders in syndromal evolution. As of yet, how variables pertaining to form and duration of treatment alter illness trajectories is also not understood. Because pharmacological treatments are known to have direct effects on brain function, studying their potentially long-term impact on developmental psychiatric trajectories is clearly of tremendous importance to both child and adult psychiatry. As exemplified by the contents of this book, the growing interest in developmental psychiatry and neuroscience aspires to correct these knowledge gaps in the coming years.

KEY POINTS

- Neurodevelopmental research is a key avenue toward understanding the integration of genetic and environmental factors in the genesis of psychiatric disorders.
- Significant changes in brain structure and function occur normally from childhood to adulthood; various perturbations in this development may lead to differential forms of adult mental illness.
- Syndromal evolution of child to adult mental disorders can be highly variable; more research is needed to understand specific environmental and genetic modifiers and the longitudinal impact of different psychiatric medications on certain presentations or trajectories.

PRACTICE GUIDELINES

- Evidence allowing accurate prognosis as to potential duration and quality of psychiatric presentations through childhood and into adulthood is not clearly defined across the broad range of psychiatric diagnoses; use caution when advising patients and families.
- Evidence pertaining to the long-term (i.e., adult) impact of psychiatric medications delivered to children is virtually nonexistent; use extreme caution when advising patients and families accordingly.
- When possible, advocate for sustained longitudinal care of child cases by a consistent treatment team over many years, not only for the sake of clinical continuity, but to enhance the anecdotal knowledge of treating clinicians about developmental trajectories.

References

Auerbach, J. G., Atzaba-Poria, N., Berger, A., & Landau, R. (2004). Emerging developmental pathways to ADHD: Possible path markers in early infancy. *Neural Plasticity, 11*(1–2), 29–43.

Blazer, D. G., Kessler, R. C., McGonagle, K. A., & Swartz, M. S. (1994). The prevalence and distribution of major depression in a national community sample: The National Comorbidity Survey. *American Journal of Psychiatry, 151*(7), 979–986.

Brotman, M. A., Schmajuk, M., Rich, B. A., Dickstein, D. P., Guyer, A. E., Costello, E. J., Egger, H. L., Angold, A., Pine, D. S., Leibenluft, E. (2006).

Prevalence, clinical correlates, and longitudinal course of severe mood dysregulation in children. *Biological Psychiatry, 60*(9), 991–997.

Brumwell, C. L., & Curran, T. (2006). Developmental mouse brain gene expression maps. *Journal of Physiology, 575*(Pt 2), 343–346.

Castellanos, F. X., Lee, P. P., Sharp, W., Jeffries, N. O., Greenstein, D. K., Clasen, L. S., Blumenthal, J. D., James, R. S., Ebens, C. L., Walter, J. M., Zijdenbos, A., Evans, A. C., Giedd, J. N., Rapoport, J. L. (2002). Developmental trajectories of brain volume abnormalities in children and adolescents with attention-deficit/hyperactivity disorder. *Journal of the American Medical Association, 288*(14), 1740–1748.

Chambers, R. A., & Potenza, M. N. (2003). Neurodevelopment, impulsivity, and adolescent gambling. *Journal of Gambling Studies, 19*(1), 53–84.

Chambers, R. A., Potenza, M. N., Hoffman, R. E., & Miranker, W. (2004). Simulated apoptosis/neurogenesis regulates learning and memory capabilities of adaptive neural networks. *Neuropsychopharmacology, 29*(4), 747–758.

Chambers, R. A., Taylor, J., & Potenza, M. (2003). Developmental neurocircuitry of motivation in adolescence: A critical period of addiction vulnerability. *American Journal of Psychiatry, 160*, 1041–1052.

Chapman, K., Tarter, R. E., Kirisci, L., & Cornelius, M. D. (2007). Childhood neurobehavior disinhibition amplifies the risk of substance use disorder: Interaction of parental history and prenatal alcohol exposure. *Journal of Developmental and Behavioral Pediatrics, 28*(3), 219–224.

Chugani, H. T., Phelps, M. E., & Mazziotta, J. C. (1987). Positron emission tomography study of human brain functional development. *Annals of Neurology, 22*(4), 487–497.

Cicchetti, D., & Curtis, W. J. (2006). The developing brain and neural plasticity: Implications for normality, psychopathology, and resistance. In D. Cicchetti & D. J. Cohen (Eds.), *Developmental Psychopathology* (2nd ed., Vol. 2, pp. 1–64). Hoboken, NJ: Wiley.

Cohen, R. A., Grieve, S., Hoth, K. F., Paul, R. H., Sweet, L., Tate, D., Gunstad, J., Stroud, L., McCaffery, J., Hitsman, B., Niaura, R., Clark, C. R., McFarlane, A., Bryant, R., Gordon, E., Williams, L. M. (2006). Early life stress and morphometry of the adult anterior cingulate cortex and caudate nuclei. *Biological Psychiatry, 59*(10), 975–982.

Danielyan, A., Pathak, S., Kowatch, R. A., Arszman, S. P., & Johns, E. S. (2007). Clinical characteristics of bipolar disorder in very young children. *Journal of Affective Disorders, 97*(1–3), 51–59.

De Bellis, M. D., Keshavan, M. S., Shifflett, H., Iyengar, S., Beers, S. R., Hall, J., Moritz, G.. (2002). Brain structures in pediatric maltreatment-related post-traumatic stress disorder: A sociodemographically matched study. *Biological Psychiatry, 52*(11), 1066–1078.

De Bellis, M. D., & Kuchibhatla, M. (2006). Cerebellar volumes in pediatric maltreatment-related post-traumatic stress disorder. *Biological Psychiatry, 60*(7), 697–703.

Egeland, J. A., Shaw, J. A., Endicott, J., Pauls, D. L., Allen, C. R., Hostetter, A. M., Sussex, J. N.. (2003). Prospective study of prodromal features for bipolarity in well Amish children. *Journal of the American Academy of Child and Adolescent Psychiatry, 42*(7), 786–796.

Erickson, C., & Chambers, R. (2006). Male adolescence: Neurodevelopment and behavioral impulsivity. In J. Grant & M. Potenza (Eds.), *Textbook of men's mental health*. Washington, DC: American Psychiatric Publishing.

Felitti, V. J. (2003). Origins of addictive behavior: Evidence from a study of stressful childhood experiences. *Prax Kinderpsychol Kinderpsychiatr, 52*(8), 547–559.

Fergusson, D. M., Horwood, L. J., & Ridder, E. M. (2007). Conduct and attentional problems in childhood and adolescence and later substance use, abuse and dependence: Results of a 25-year longitudinal study. *Drug and Alcohol Dependence, 88*(Suppl 1), S14–26.

Fite, P. J., Colder, C. R., Lochman, J. E., & Wells, K. C. (2007a). Pathways from proactive and reactive aggression to substance use. *Psychology of Addictive Behaviors, 21*(3), 355–364.

Fite, P. J., Colder, C. R., Lochman, J. E., & Wells, K. C. (2008). The Relation between childhood proactive and reactive aggression and substance use initiation. *Journal of Abnormal Child Psychology, 36*(2), 261–271.

Forbes, E. E., Shaw, D. S., & Dahl, R. E. (2007). Alterations in reward-related decision making in boys with recent and future depression. *Biological Psychiatry, 61*(5), 633–639.

Giedd, J. N., Snell, J. W., Lange, N., Rajapakse, J. C., Casey, B. J., Kozuch, P. L., Vaituzis, A. C., Vauss, Y. C., Hamburger, S. D., Kaysen, D., Rapoport, J. L. (1996). Quantitative magnetic resonance imaging of human brain development: Ages 4–18. *Cerebral Cortex, 6*(4), 551–560.

Goldstein, B. I., & Levitt, A. J. (2006). Further evidence for a developmental subtype of bipolar disorder defined by age at onset: Results from the national epidemiologic-survey on alcohol and related conditions. *American Journal of Psychiatry, 163*(9), 1633–1636.

Greenstein, D., Lerch, J., Shaw, P., Clasen, L., Giedd, J., Gochman, P., Rapoport, J., Gogtay, N.. (2006). Childhood onset schizophrenia: Cortical brain abnormalities as young adults. *Journal of Child Psychology and Psychiatry, 47*(10), 1003–1012.

Guyer, A. E., Kaufman, J., Hodgdon, H. B., Masten, C. L., Jazbec, S., Pine, D. S., Ernst, M. (2006). Behavioral alterations in reward system function: The role of childhood maltreatment and psychopathology. *Journal of the American Academy of Child and Adolescent Psychiatry, 45*(9), 1059–1067.

Hammen, C., & Rudolph, K. (2003). Childhood mood disorders. In E. Mash & R. Barkley (Eds.), *Child psychopathology* (Vol. 1, pp. 233–278). New York: Guilford Press.

Herman, K. C., Lambert, S. F., Ialongo, N. S., & Ostrander, R. (2007). Academic pathways between attention problems and depressive symptoms among urban African American children. *Journal of Abnormal Child Psychology, 35*(2), 265–274.

Hirshfeld-Becker, D. R., Biederman, J., Henin, A., Faraone, S. V., Davis, S., Harrington, K., Rosenbaum, J. F. (2007a). Behavioral inhibition in preschool children at risk is a specific predictor of middle childhood social anxiety: A five-year follow-up. *Journal of Developmental and Behavioral Pediatrics, 28*(3), 225–233.

Hirshfeld-Becker, D. R., Biederman, J., Henin, A., Faraone, S. V., Micco, J. A., van Grondelle, A., Henry, B., Rosenbaum, J. F. (2007b). Clinical outcomes of laboratory-observed preschool behavioral disinhibition at five-year follow-up. *Biological Psychiatry, 62*(6), 565–572.

Holtmann, M., Goth, K., Wockel, L., Poustka, F., & Bolte, S. (2008). CBCL-pediatric bipolar disorder phenotype: Severe ADHD or bipolar disorder? *Journal of Neural Transmission, 115*(2), 155–161.

Huttenlocher, P. R. (1979). Synaptic density in human frontal cortex—Developmental changes and effects of aging. *Brain Research, 163*(2), 195–205.

Jester, J. M., Nigg, J. T., Adams, K., Fitzgerald, H. E., Puttler, L. I., Wong, M. M., Zucker, R. A. (2005). Inattention/hyperactivity and aggression from early childhood to adolescence: Heterogeneity of trajectories and differential influence of family environment characteristics. *Development and Psychopathology, 17*(1), 99–125.

Kaffman, A., & Meaney, M. J. (2007). Neurodevelopmental sequelae of postnatal maternal care in rodents: Clinical and research implications of molecular insights. *Journal of Child Psychology and Psychiatry, 48*(3–4), 224–244.

Kagan, J. (1994). *Galen's prophecy.* New York: Basic Books.

Kagan, J., & Snidman, N. (1999). Early childhood predictors of adult anxiety disorders. *Biological Psychiatry, 46*(11), 1536–1541.

Kagan, J., Snidman, N., & Arcus, D. (1998). Childhood derivatives of high and low reactivity in infancy. *Child Development, 69*(6), 1483–1493.

Kagan, J., Snidman, N., Zentner, M., & Peterson, E. (1999). Infant temperament and anxious symptoms in school age children. *Developmental Psychopathology, 11*(2), 209–224.

Kaufman, J., Plotsky, P. M., Nemeroff, C. B., & Charney, D. S. (2000). Effects of early adverse experiences on brain structure and function: Clinical implications. *Biological Psychiatry, 48*(8), 778–790.

Kazdin, A. E., Thompson, R. A., Yates, T. T., Marans, S. R., Cohen, D. J., Chess, S., & Thomas, A. (1991). Major general theories of child and adolescent development. In M. Lewis (Ed.), *Child and adolescent psychiatry: A comprehensive textbook* (pp. 87–159). Baltimore, MD: Williams & Wilkins Co.

Kessler, R. C., Berglund, P., Demler, O., Jin, R., Merikangas, K. R., & Walters, E. E. (2005). Lifetime prevalence and age-of-onset distributions of DSM-IV disorders in the National Comorbidity Survey Replication. *Archives of General Psychiatry, 62*(6), 593–602.

Kessler, R. C., Chiu, W. T., Demler, O., Merikangas, K. R., & Walters, E. E. (2005). Prevalence, severity, and comorbidity of 12-month DSM-IV disorders in the National Comorbidity Survey Replication. *Archives of General Psychiatry, 62*(6), 617–627.

Larsson, J. O., Larsson, H., & Lichtenstein, P. (2004). Genetic and environmental contributions to stability and change of ADHD symptoms between 8 and 13 years of age: A longitudinal twin study. *Journal of the American Academy of Child and Adolescent Psychiatry, 43*(10), 1267–1275.

Leask, S. J., & Crow, T. J. (2005). Lateralization of verbal ability in pre-psychotic children. *Psychiatry Research, 136*(1), 35–42.

Leibenluft, E., Charney, D. S., Towbin, K. E., Bhangoo, R. K., & Pine, D. S. (2003). Defining clinical phenotypes of juvenile mania. *American Journal of Psychiatry, 160*(3), 430–437.

Lemaire, V., Lamarque, S., Le Moal, M., Piazza, P. V., & Abrous, D. N. (2006). Postnatal stimulation of the pups counteracts prenatal stress-induced deficits in hippocampal neurogenesis. *Biological Psychiatry, 59*(9), 786–792.

Lewis, D. A. (1997). Development of the prefrontal cortex during adolescence: Insights into vulnerable neural circuits in schizophrenia. *Neuropsychopharmacology, 16*(6), 385–398.

Liljenstrom, H. (2003). Neural stability and flexibility: A computational approach. *Neuropsychopharmacology, 28*(Suppl 1), S64–73.

Lopez, J. F., Akil, H., & Watson, S. J. (1999). Neural circuits mediating stress. *Biological Psychiatry, 46*(11), 1461–1471.

Marmorstein, N. R., & Iacono, W. G. (2005). Longitudinal follow-up of adolescents with late-onset antisocial behavior: A pathological yet overlooked group. *Journal of American Academy of Child and Adolescent Psychiatry, 44*(12), 1284–1291.

Masi, G., Perugi, G., Millepiedi, S., Mucci, M., Toni, C., Bertini, N., Pfanner, C., Berloffa, S., Pari, C. (2006). Developmental differences according to age at onset in juvenile bipolar disorder. *Journal of Child and Adolescent Psychopharmacology, 16*(6), 679–685.

Masten, A. S., Best, K., & Garmezy, N. (1990). Resilience and development: Contributions from the study of children who overcome adversity. *Developmental Psychopathology, 2,* 425–444.

McEwen, B. S., & Milner, T. A. (2007). Hippocampal formation: Shedding light on the influence of sex and stress on the brain. *Brain Research Reviews, 55*(2), 343–355.

Moffitt, T. E., Caspi, A., Harrington, H., Milne, B. J., Melchior, M., Goldberg, D., Poulton, R. (2007a). Generalized anxiety disorder and depression: Childhood risk factors in a birth cohort followed to age 32. *Psychological Medicine, 37*(3), 441–452.

Moffitt, T. E., Harrington, H., Caspi, A., Kim-Cohen, J., Goldberg, D., Gregory, A. M., Poulton, R. (2007b). Depression and generalized anxiety disorder: Cumulative and sequential comorbidity in a birth cohort followed prospectively to age 32 years. *Archives of General Psychiatry, 64*(6), 651–660.

Molina, B. S., Pelham, W. E., Gnagy, E. M., Thompson, A. L., & Marshal, M. P. (2007). Attention-deficit/hyperactivity disorder risk for heavy drinking and alcohol use disorder is age specific. *Alcoholism, Clinical and Experimental Research, 31*(4), 643–654.

Moreno, C., Laje, G., Blanco, C., Jiang, H., Schmidt, A., & Olfson, M. (2007). National trends in the outpatient diagnosis and treatment of bipolar disorder in youth. *Archives of General Psychiatry, 64*(9), 1032–1039.

O'Brien, C. P., Charney, D. S., Lewis, L., Cornish, J. W., Post, R. M., Woody, G. E., Zubieta, J. K., Anthony, J. C., Blaine, J. D., Bowden, C. L., Calabrese, J. R., Carroll, K., Kosten, T., Rounsaville, B., Childress, A. R., Oslin, D. W., Pettinati, H. M., Davis, M. A., Demartino, R., Drake, R. E., Fleming, M. F., Fricks, L., Glassman, A. H., Levin, F. R., Nunes, E. V., Johnson, R. L., Jordan, C., Kessler, R. C., Laden, S. K., Regier, D. A., Renner, J. A. Jr., Ries, R. K., Sklar-Blake, T., Weisner, C. (2004). Priority actions to improve the care of persons with co-occurring substance abuse and other mental disorders: A call to action. *Biological Psychiatry, 56*(10), 703–713.

O'Connor, T. G., & Rutter, M. (2000). Attachment disorder behavior following early severe deprivation: Extension and longitudinal follow-up. English and Romanian Adoptees Study Team. *Journal of the American Academy of Child and Adolescent Psychiatry, 39*(6), 703–712.

Petras, H., Schaeffer, C. M., Ialongo, N., Hubbard, S., Muthen, B., Lambert, S. F., Poduska, J., Kellam, S.. (2004). When the course of aggressive behavior in childhood does not predict antisocial outcomes in adolescence and young adulthood: An examination of potential explanatory variables. *Development and Psychopathology, 16*(4), 919–941.

Pihlakoski, L., Aromaa, M., Sourander, A., Rautava, P., Helenius, H., & Sillanp, A. M. (2004). Use of and need for professional help for emotional and behavioral problems among preadolescents: A prospective cohort study of 3- to 12-year-old children. *Journal of the American Academy of Child and Adolescent Psychiatry, 43*(8), 974–983.

Rende, R., & Waldman, I. (2006). Behavioral and molecular genetics and developmental psychopathology. In D. Cicchetti & D. J. Cohen (Eds.), *Developmental psychopathology* (2nd ed. Vol. 2, pp. 427–464), Hoboken, NJ: Wiley.

Roceri, M., Hendriks, W., Racagni, G., Ellenbroek, B. A., & Riva, M. A. (2002). Early maternal deprivation reduces the expression of BDNF and NMDA receptor subunits in rat hippocampus. *Molecular Psychiatry, 7*(6), 609–616.

Romer, D., & Walker, E. (2007). *Adolescent psychopathology and the developing brain* (1st ed.). New York: Oxford University Press.

Saarni, C., & Harris, P. (1991). *Children's understanding of emotion.* Cambridge, England: Cambridge University Press.

Satterfield, J. H., Faller, K. J., Crinella, F. M., Schell, A. M., Swanson, J. M., & Homer, L. D. (2007). A 30-year prospective follow-up study of hyperactive boys with conduct problems: Adult criminality. *Journal of the American Academy of Child and Adolescent Psychiatry, 46*(5), 601–610.

Scheeringa, M. S., Zeanah, C. H., Myers, L., & Putnam, F. W. (2005). Predictive validity in a prospective follow-up of PTSD in preschool children. *Journal of the American Academy of Child and Adolescent Psychiatry, 44*(9), 899–906.

Schilling, E. A., Aseltine, R. H., Jr., & Gore, S. (2007). Adverse childhood experiences and mental health in young adults: A longitudinal survey. *BMC Public Health, 7,* 30.

Schwartz, C. E., Snidman, N., & Kagan, J. (1999). Adolescent social anxiety as an outcome of inhibited temperament in childhood. *Journal of the American Academy of Child and Adolescent Psychiatry, 38*(8), 1008–1015.

Shelton, K., Lifford, K., Fowler, T., Rice, F., Neale, M., Harold, G., Thapar, A., van den Bree, M. (2007). The association between conduct problems and the initiation and progression of marijuana use during adolescence: A genetic analysis across time. *Behavior Genetics, 37*(2), 314–325.

Silberg, J. L., Rutter, M., & Eaves, L. (2001). Genetic and environmental influences on the temporal association between earlier anxiety and later depression in girls. *Biological Psychiatry, 49*(12), 1040–1049.

Smith, G. N., Lang, D. J., Kopala, L. C., Lapointe, J. S., Falkai, P., & Honer, W. G. (2003). Developmental abnormalities of the hippocampus in first-episode schizophrenia. *Biological Psychiatry, 53*(7), 555–561.

Snyder, J. S., Kee, N., & Wojtowicz, J. M. (2001). Effects of adult neurogenesis on synaptic plasticity in the rat dentate gyrus. *Journal of Neurophysiology, 85*(6), 2423–2431.

Sourander, A., Elonheimo, H., Niemela, S., Nuutila, A. M., Helenius, H., Sillanmaki, L., Piha, J., Tamminen, T., Kumpulainen, K., Moilenen, I., Almqvist, F. (2006). Childhood predictors of male criminality: A prospective population-based follow-up study from age 8 to late adolescence. *Journal of the American Academy of Child and Adolescent Psychiatry, 45*(5), 578–586.

Spear, L. (2007). The developing brain and adolescent-typical behavior patterns: An evolutionary approach. In D. Romer & E. Walker (Eds.), *Adolescent psychopathology and the developing brain* (pp. 9–30). New York: Oxford University Press.

Spencer, T. J., Biederman, J., & Mick, E. (2007). Attention-deficit/hyperactivity disorder: Diagnosis, lifespan, comorbidities, and neurobiology. *Journal of Pediatric Psychology, 32*(6), 631–642.

Stayer, C., Sporn, A., Gogtay, N., Tossell, J., Lenane, M., Gochman, P., Rapoport, J. L. (2004). Looking for childhood schizophrenia: Case series of false positives. *Journal of the American Academy of Child and Adolescent Psychiatry, 43*(8), 1026–1029.

Sterba, S. K., Prinstein, M. J., & Cox, M. J. (2007). Trajectories of internalizing problems across childhood: Heterogeneity, external validity, and gender differences. *Development and Psychopathology, 19*(2), 345–366.

Storr, C. L., Ialongo, N. S., Anthony, J. C., & Breslau, N. (2007). Childhood antecedents of exposure to traumatic events and posttraumatic stress disorder. *American Journal of Psychiatry, 164*(1), 119–125.

Sullivan, R., Wilson, D. A., Feldon, J., Yee, B. K., Meyer, U., Richter-Levin, G., Avi, A., Michael, T., Gruss, M., Bock, J., Helmeke, C., Braun, K. (2006). The International Society for Developmental Psychobiology annual meeting symposium: Impact of early life experiences on brain and behavioral development. *Developmental Psychobiology, 48*(7), 583–602.

Tarter, R. E., Kirisci, L., Feske, U., & Vanyukov, M. (2007). Modeling the pathways linking childhood hyperactivity and substance use disorder in young adulthood. *Psychology of Addictive Behavior, 21*(2), 266–271.

Teicher, M. H., Dumont, N. L., Ito, Y., Vaituzis, C., Giedd, J. N., & Andersen, S. L. (2004). Childhood neglect is associated with reduced corpus callosum area. *Biological Psychiatry, 56*(2), 80–85.

Thunstrom, M. (2002). Severe sleep problems in infancy associated with subsequent development of attention-deficit/hyperactivity disorder at 5.5 years of age. *Acta Paediatrica, 91*(5), 584–592.

Tu, M. T., Grunau, R. E., Petrie-Thomas, J., Haley, D. W., Weinberg, J., & Whitfield, M. F. (2007). Maternal stress and behavior modulate relationships between neonatal stress, attention, and basal cortisol at 8 months in preterm infants. *Developmental Psychobiology, 49*(2), 150–164.

Wozniak, J., Biederman, J., & Richards, J. A. (2001). Diagnostic and therapeutic dilemmas in the management of pediatric-onset bipolar disorder. *Journal of Clinical Psychiatry, 62*(Suppl 14), 10–15.

Chapter 5

College and Career

Jessica M. Cronce and William R. Corbin

Julie was a highly motivated student who graduated in the top 10% of her high school class. Based on the strength of her grade point average (GPA) and standardized achievement scores, Julie was admitted into her state's premier university. Julie participated in rush and was accepted into a sorority known on campus for its high degree of "sociability." At age 17, Julie moved from her parents' house into the sorority's chapter house, located off campus. Although Julie received some financial support in the form of scholarships and loans, it was not sufficient to cover all of her expenses and she had to take a part-time job working evenings as a waitress. When she was not working, Julie participated in multiple social activities, most of which involved consumption of alcohol. Her job and social activities left her with limited time to study or to sleep, and she often missed lectures. At the end of her first term, Julie's performance in her classes left her with a low GPA and she was put on academic probation. Julie had never had to cope with failure before and felt a significant amount of stress over the potential loss of her scholarship. Julie vowed to devote more time to her studies but felt significant anxiety each time she was faced with an exam or a new assignment. To cope with her anxiety, Julie engaged in even more recreational activities and attended more social events that involved drinking. Her involvement in nonacademic activities and her heavy drinking left her unable to study effectively when she devoted time to her academic projects. She also started missing shifts at her job and was subsequently fired. As her second term drew near a close and her grades had not improved, Julie began to withdraw from friends and family. She also began having difficulty sleeping and lost her appetite, which made her worry that she might have a serious medical problem. She set up an appointment in student medicine and received a referral to the counseling center. The counselor who met with Julie concluded that she was suffering from both alcohol abuse and major depressive disorder.

Unlike developmental transitions that occur in infancy and childhood, which are clearly marked by the expansion of cognitive and motor abilities, and the transition into adolescence, which is demarcated by the onset of biological changes resulting in the development of secondary sexual characteristics and the ability to reproduce, the milestones that signify the transition into young adulthood are somewhat equivocal. Within the culture of the United States, the age of 18 years holds a special significance, as it typically coincides with completion of secondary education and the assumption of rights and responsibilities associated with being an adult member of society: the right to vote in state and federal elections; full culpability for violations of the law; the ability to make medical, legal, and financial decisions without parental knowledge or consent; the capacity to live independently; the opportunity to work full time; and the freedom to engage in previously proscribed behaviors, such as gambling and tobacco use. Although this rather dramatic paradigm shift suggests that individuals may transition *out of adolescence* at 18 years of age in the United

States, this is not the same as saying that they are transitioning *into young adulthood*.

Young Adulthood versus "Emerging Adulthood"

According to qualitative research conducted by Jeffrey Arnett and his colleagues, entry into young adulthood is marked by three criteria: accepting responsibility for oneself, making independent decisions, and becoming financially independent (Arnett, 2004). These three developmental tasks often coincide with the adoption of adult role responsibilities associated with marriage, family, and long-term career stability. Based on the widening gap between the end of adolescence and the adoption of these adult role responsibilities, Arnett has posited the existence of a new developmental period bridging the transition from adolescence into young adulthood—"emerging adulthood" (Arnett, 2000). Individuals generally transverse the period of emerging adulthood between the ages of 18 to 25 years; however, much like any developmental period, emerging adulthood is not concretely tied to chronological age, but rather is marked by the completion of particular developmental tasks (Arnett, 2000). Emerging adulthood is delineated by five qualities or states experienced by the individual (Arnett, 2004). First, through a process of investigating and sampling different occupations, fields of study, and relationships, emerging adults actively engage in *identity exploration*. It is during this period that most young people make critical decisions that serve to formulate and solidify their identity in adulthood. This process of exploration exemplifies the second quality of emerging adulthood, *instability*. Emerging adults typically participate in a constellation of educational and occupational activities before settling on a particular trajectory. Similarly, over the course of emerging adulthood, individuals are normally involved in multiple romantic relationships, and they use information gleaned from these relationships to determine the qualities that they desire in a long-term romantic partner. This search for who one is and what one wants demonstrates the third quality of emerging adulthood, *self-focus*. This self-focus should not be taken to mean that emerging adults are narcissistic or selfish. In fact, many young people are acutely aware of both local and global social concerns, and they engage in philanthropic and humanitarian activities as part of the process of identity exploration. Rather, self-focus refers to the absence (or minimal presence) of routine commitments and obligations to other people, such as parents, teachers, and employers (e.g., parents no longer set curfews and determine with whom youth can associate; unlike high school teachers, college professors typically do not provide immediate negative feedback for failure to complete assignments). Emerging adults are self-focused in that they hold the principal responsibility for decisions regarding their daily activities and functioning rather than being primarily guided by outside forces. This newfound freedom of choice over major and minor life decisions in the absence of a fixed identity and stable role responsibilities tends to leave emerging adults *feeling in between*—no longer an adolescent, but not fully an adult. Emerging adults are more than an adolescent insofar as they can make independent decisions and are starting to assume responsibility for these decisions, their actions, and the resultant consequences; however, they are less than an adult insofar as they are not typically financially independent and tend to more frequently abdicate (either actively or passively) their right to make decisions, thus obviating responsibility for the outcome of those decisions. Finally, despite, or perhaps as a result of, the pervasive volatility inherent to this developmental period, emerging adulthood is marked by optimism regarding life's *possibilities*. For some individuals, it is an opportunity to escape disadvantageous home environments and/or deviant peer networks and rise above their circumstances. For others, it is an opportunity to differentiate themselves from the identities and wishes of otherwise supportive family members and friends. Although certain demographic and sociocultural features, such as socioeconomic status and teen parenthood, create a biased foundation from which to begin one's trajectory into adulthood, few doors are closed at this developmental stage; there is the hope and the potential for a bright (or better) future.

Although a literature is developing that tests hypotheses inherent to Arnett's theory, there is clearly much work that remains. Thus, in this chapter we will not attempt to resolve the ongoing debate regarding the legitimacy of emerging adulthood as a developmental period that is distinct from, and antecedent to, young adulthood. Rather, we will draw on the extant literature and attempt to elucidate the unique challenges faced by individuals in this general age range (hereafter referred to as *young adults*), specifically with respect to two major developmental tasks: participation in college and career. Furthermore, we will discuss how facing these unique challenges may impact mental health and how mental illness can impact academic and occupational performance. Finally, we will suggest methods for promoting and enhancing wellness.

The Choice between College and Career

Young adults are faced with a number of important decisions, not the least of which is whether they would be best served by primarily pursuing educational interests and goals, or whether they should devote the bulk of their time and energy to employment in the service of career objectives and financial independence. Of course, the choice to pursue college education is often in the direct service of career goal attainment and has increasingly become a prerequisite for employment in positions that offer wages and benefits that can keep pace with the rising cost of living and support a healthy lifestyle. Yet the value of practical experience cannot be underestimated, and given the rapid influx of college-educated individuals entering the job market, work experience can be the deciding factor in selection for employment and career advancement. Beyond its potential value in career attainment, working is often desirable to young adults as it can help them to begin to achieve financial independence, and employment may be necessary if auxiliary financial support from family members or social service agencies is not available. Working may also be necessary when higher education is not an option, as is the case for individuals who have not successfully completed secondary (high school) education or its equivalent (i.e., passing scores on the battery of tests necessary to earn a General Educational Development [GED] credential).

Within the United States, the event dropout rate (i.e., the percentage of students who discontinue their high school enrollment from one year to the next without receiving their diploma or its equivalent) has declined over the past few decades. In 1972, 6.1% of students enrolled in grades 10 through 12 (approximately 647,000 youth) dropped out as compared to the 3.8% of students (roughly 414,000 youth) who dropped out in 2005 (Laird, DeBell, Kienzl, & Chapman, 2007). The status dropout rate (i.e., the percentage of all individuals in a given age cohort who are not currently enrolled in school and have not received a diploma or its equivalent) has also declined over this period. Specifically, the percentage of adolescents and young adults between the ages of 16 and 24 years who prematurely ended their secondary education dropped from 14.6% in 1972 (about 4.8 million youth) to 9.4% in 2005 (constituting about 3.5 million youth; Laird et al., 2007). Among youth ages 16 to 19 years who were not enrolled in school in 2005 and had not received their diploma or GED, 35.4% participated in the labor force; that is, they reported having sought employment (either successfully or unsuccessfully) during the assessment window. Of those youth who participated in the labor force, approximately 80% were actively employed (Snyder, Dillow, & Hoffman, 2007). Almost twice as many young adults ages 20 to 24 years who had dropped out were engaged in the labor force in 2005 (about 66.2%), about 84% of whom were currently employed (Snyder et al., 2007). By comparison, 63.6% of those youth ages 16 to 19 years, and 78.4% of those young adults ages 20 to 24 who had completed high school (but were not enrolled in college) entered the workforce, 84% and 89% of whom found employment, respectively (Snyder et al., 2007).

Of course, the majority of young adults who have received their high school diploma or GED enter college. For example, 68.6% (about 1.8 million) of individuals who received a diploma or GED credential in 2004 enrolled in college the following fall (Snyder et al., 2007). In 2005, nearly 17.5 million individuals enrolled in degree-granting institutions in the United States (a 90% increase from 35 years prior [i.e., 9.2 million in 1972]), and approximately 435,000 additional individuals enrolled in non-degree-granting institutions of higher education (Snyder et al., 2007). Approximately 15 million of those students enrolled in the fall of 2005 were undergraduates, 10.1 million of whom were between the ages of 18 and 24, and nearly 8 million of whom were enrolled on a full-time basis (Snyder et al., 2007). Of the 1.6 million young adults who received their high school diploma during the 2005–2006 academic year and went on to enroll in college during the fall of 2006, 92.3% enrolled on a full-time basis (U.S. Department of Labor, Bureau of Labor Statistics, 2007a). Although these numbers are encouraging, they are a static presentation of an essentially dynamic construct. Enrollment statistics do not capture changes in enrollment status that occur between assessments. Students may opt to take a leave of absence from college (*stop out*) due to financial limitations, medical or mental health complications, or to pursue other opportunities, and then return to obtain their degree. Although longitudinal estimates of stopping out are more limited, data from the Baccalaureate and Beyond Longitudinal Study (U.S. Department of Education, 2007) tentatively suggest that rates of extended stopping out may be increasing. Among individuals receiving their first bachelor's degree during the 1992–1993 academic year, 15.9% individuals stopped out for 6 or more months (McCormick & Horn, 1996). In contrast, 30.6% of first-time bachelor's degree recipients during the 1999–2000 academic year stopped out for 6 or more months (Bradburn, Berger, Li, Peter, & Rooney, 2003). Of those youth ages 16 to 19 and 20 to 24 years who had completed some college, but were not currently enrolled in 2005, 58.2% and 70.4%, respectively, were participating in the labor force, over 90% of whom found employment (Snyder et al., 2007). Thus, cohorts of young adults that enter college now may be taking a more circuitous path en route to their degree than previous cohorts, and this path may include participation in the workforce.

Rather than stopping out to engage in work, many college students combine work with their studies (Swanson, Broadbridge & Karatzias, 2006; U.S. Department of Labor, Bureau of Labor Statistics, 2007a). As many students first enter the workforce on a part-time basis during high school (Bachman, Safron, Sy, & Schulenberg, 2003), concomitant pursuit of the immediate benefits of work (e.g., disposable income, increased independence) and the long-term benefits of education (e.g., greater earning potential, total financial independence) may be viewed as normative. Although, as previously indicated, 92.3% of recent high school graduates who enrolled in college in the fall of 2006 were full-time students, and ostensibly devoting the majority of their time to their studies, over 40% of these students also participated in the labor force, approximately 92% of whom were actively employed (U.S. Department of Labor, Bureau of Labor Statistics, 2007a). Participation in the labor force was over double (81%) among the nearly 8% of recent high school graduates enrolled in college on a part-time basis, although only 87% of these individuals were employed in the fall of 2006 (U.S. Department of Labor, Bureau of Labor Statistics, 2007a). Among all youth ages 16 to 24 years who were enrolled in college in the fall of 2006 (approximately 10.5 million individuals), nearly 50% of the full-time students and almost 86% of the part-time students participated in the labor force, over 94% of whom were actively employed (U.S. Department of Labor, Bureau of Labor Statistics, 2007a). In support of the view that work serves more than a financial function for young adults, recent data from the Current Population Survey suggest that as many as 85% of part-time workers ages 16 to 24 years are engaged in work for noneconomic reasons[a] (U.S. Department of Labor, Bureau of Labor Statistics, 2007b).

Unique Developmental Challenges and Their Mental Health Implications

A large number of studies have examined a variety of factors influencing young adults' physical and mental well-being. These studies have typically focused on traditional-age undergraduate students as opposed to their non-college counterparts. There may be multiple reasons why the focus of such studies has fixed on college

---

[a] The Bureau of Labor Statistics definition of "noneconomic reasons" for part-time work is very broad in scope, and it includes individuals who work for financial reasons but choose to not (or are unable to) work full time (Department of Labor, Bureau of Labor Statistics, 2007c). As such, this estimate must be interpreted with caution.

students; however, two of the most likely reasons relate to convenience and generalizability. The total population of undergraduate students at a given institution can typically be accessed with the assistance of the campus registrar or university directory, and thus a random sample can be readily generated. Although the outcomes of a study at a single institution may not generalize to all colleges, additional college samples can be readily obtained using the same procedures, thus increasing the external validity of the results. In addition, college students are generally circumscribed geographically, typically living on campus or within commuting distance of their institution. Thus, they are easier to assess longitudinally, especially if the research protocol is laboratory based or otherwise requires face-to-face contact with research personnel. By comparison, there is no single directory of all young adults who are *not* enrolled in college. Researchers interested in this population must attempt to obtain a representative sample through random digit dialing or mass mailing. Not only can these techniques be very expensive, but they are more likely to miss important segments of nonmatriculated youth (e.g., individuals without phone service or a place of residence, or whose phone service and/or residence is unstable; individuals who reside in penal institutions or medical care facilities), and potential factors influencing response bias cannot be readily quantified as the characteristics of those invited to participate are often unknown to the researcher. Even if all nonmatriculated youth in a given area could be identified and a random sample derived, the challenges they face and their use of various coping strategies would likely be heavily influenced by the proximal environment (e.g., local economy, including cost of living, proximity and capacity of various employers, and the accessibility of health care). Thus, nonmatriculated youth constitute a far more heterogeneous group than their college-student counterparts. This being said, some of the stressors reported by college students may reflect, to a certain extent, challenges that are universal to this developmental period (e.g., managing finances, negotiating personal relationships). Therefore, we will delineate the stressors highlighted in the available studies of college youth and discuss how these stressors may broadly apply to young adults, how they may specifically apply to individuals in college, and how they may be equated with constructs discussed in the literature on adult work stress.

Academic/Occupational Stress

As part of their 1989 cross-sectional study of Australian undergraduates, Sarros and Densten surveyed the extant literature on student stressors and noted that academic demands were consistently identified as central sources of stress. Consistent with this, 85% of the stressors identified by students in their sample rated as moderately to very stressful were related to academics, including the volume of assignments they were given to complete, receipt of poor grades on assignments, deadlines, class presentations, and unclear instructions provided by instructors. Towbes and Cohen (1996) also noted that academic factors, including overall scholastic performance, receiving poor grades, studying, and assignment overload, were reported as chronic stressors by the majority of college students in their sample. Finally, in their study examining various behavioral, health, and environmental predictors of college student stress, Dusselier, Dunn, Wang, Shelley, and Whalen (2005) included a single open-ended question asking students to identify the single factor that caused them "the greatest stress during the semester." Over half of the respondents (55%) indicated that their greatest stressor was related to their academics. Many of the specific stressors noted by students echo those found in previous studies, including exams, volume of coursework, class load, more rigorous grading practices by their professors relative to high school teachers, need for increased effort relative to high school to obtain adequate grades, and lack of time to meet academic demands. As might be expected, high levels of perceived academic stress tend to negatively impact academic performance (Akgun & Chiarrochi, 2003) and may be related to mental health outcomes including depression (Aldwin & Greenberger, 1987) and anxiety. In fact, although a host of life events and interpersonal stressors were assessed, Aldwin and Greenberger (1987) found that depression was only significantly associated with the amount of perceived stress experienced in relation to a recent academic challenge among the Caucasian students in their sample, with individuals who perceived greater academic stress endorsing more depression. Although this relation did not hold for the Korean American students in their sample, perception of a greater disparity between their own standards and their parents' standards for satisfactory school performance was positively associated with depression for this group.

Academic stress for college students finds its counterpoint in occupational stress for those engaged in a career. A number of stressors have been described within the literature, including time pressure, job complexity, and role negotiation such as work–family balance (Greenhaus & Beutell, 1985). However, unlike academic stressors and demands, which are experienced in varying degrees by college students across all institutions of higher learning, occupational stressors are less uniformly distributed across various types and places of employment. For example, individuals in jobs that routinely place them in hazardous situations (e.g., firefighters, police, military personnel) experience very different stressors than individuals with less risky positions (e.g., custodial staff, office workers, individuals in the food service industry). Several theories have been proffered as more meta-level explanations for how to predict and ameliorate job-related stress. Among the most influential has been the demand/control model (Karasek & Theorell, 1990). This model suggests that "[w]hile the psychological demands of work, along with time pressures and conflicts, are found to be significant sources of risk...work that is demanding (within limits) is not the major source of risk...[t]he primary work-related risk factor appears to be lack of control over how one meets the job's demands and how one uses one's skills" (p. 9, Karasek & Theorell, 1990). Thus, one's experience at a given job can be mapped along these two continua of *psychological demands* and relative control or *decision latitude* (Karasek & Theorell, 1990). Occupations that objectively or subjectively place a high level of psychological demands on the individual in a context of low decision latitude are termed *high-strain* and have been shown to be associated with self-reported depression and anxiety (Karasek, 1979). Individuals in high-strain jobs characterized by role ambiguity may also be more prone to burnout, "a specific type of strain that reflects a belief that the resources for coping with stressful conditions are scarce or nonexistent, leading one to experience a sense of hopelessness, fatigue, and cognitive defeat" (p. 165; Perrewé et al., 2002).

Intrapersonal/Interpersonal Stress

One feature identified as moderately stressful in the study of college students by Sarros and Densten (1989) was the students' "own expectations." Students' expectations as a source of stress may entail either an elevated baseline expectation for academic performance (e.g., perfectionism) or the disparity between expectations and subsequent objective evaluation or self-evaluation of their performance. This type of disparity may also manifest itself between students' expectations regarding their performance and the expectations of significant others (e.g., parents, professors, counselors) and may be an additional source of stress. As previously described, this type of stress has been linked to negative mental health outcomes in certain populations of students (Aldwin & Greenberger, 1987).

A large proportion of students in the study by Dusselier and colleagues (2005) identified intrapersonal and interpersonal factors when asked to indicate their greatest stressor during the past academic term. Among the chief factors reported were general adjustment to college and procrastination. Certainly, the transition to college can represent a large change for many students. For most students, college requires moving away from home and into on-campus or off-campus housing. This may embody a positive change for students coming from less than ideal home environments, or a neutral to negative change for students leaving a supportive home and peer group. Regardless, the move to independent living typically necessitates renegotiation of personal norms/preferences and interpersonal dynamics. For example, moving into a campus dormitory or a house owned by a Greek-letter organization (fraternity or sorority) generally involves adaptation to communal living, including loss of privacy, sharing resources (e.g., bathrooms, closet space), less control over eating habits (e.g., limited food selections, set serving hours in campus cafeterias), and disrupted sleeping patterns (Ross, Neibling, & Heckert, 1999). The loss of control over previously private living space can be especially disruptive to students' established behavioral patterns. Roommates in most campus dormitories are assigned randomly or based on demographic or logistical constraints (e.g., gender, year in school, space availability) rather than by some knowledge of the personalities of the parties involved. As such, a female student who prefers to start and end her day early may be paired with another female student who prefers to sleep until noon and study until the late hours of the evening or who regularly invites her boyfriend over after his late night shift. Over time, individual differences in temperament and preferred lifestyle between roommates may give rise to interpersonal conflict.

Negative interactions with other individuals in students' environment may also serve as a source of stress. Edwards, Hershberger, Russell, and Markert (2001) found a significant positive association between the frequency with which students experienced negative social interactions with adults who they felt were influential in their lives and a measure of physical health. That is, students who endorsed more frequent negative social interactions also reported more frequently experiencing symptoms of physical illness. A significant inverse association was also found between negative social interactions and a measure of mental health, suggesting that greater frequency of negative social interactions was associated with poorer psychological well-being.

Intrapersonal and interpersonal stressors associated with adjustment may also pose difficulties for young adults who engage in career activities rather than entering college. For many, entrance into the workforce coincides with departure from home and either cohabitation with one or more roommates or independent living. Nonmatriculated young adults who enter into a living arrangement with a roommate may face the same challenges as their college counterparts who engage in communal living (e.g., negotiation of shared space and resources, changes in preferred behavioral patterns); however, they may be more likely to have a prior relationship with their roommate that can serve to intensify interpersonal conflict. Rather than striking out completely on their own or moving in with strangers, young adults often seek to share an apartment with friends or romantic partners. Although the existence of this prior relationship would seemingly increase the likelihood of compatibility with respect to the personalities involved, idiosyncrasies that are accepted in a friend are frequently sources of stress in a roommate (e.g., poor personal financial responsibility, slovenliness, a tendency to freeload). Furthermore, the desire to maintain the relationship and the positive regard of the roommate may lead individuals to avoid discussions and actions that could give rise to interpersonal conflicts. Of course, short-term avoidance of interpersonal conflict often contributes to proximal intrapersonal distress and long-term negative outcomes for the relationship. Although young adults who enter into independent living situations following high school are exempt from intrapersonal and interpersonal stressors stemming from roommate relations, they are alternatively faced with intrapersonal stress related to social isolation. Transitioning to solitary living may be associated with feelings of loneliness and homesickness, especially for young adults who are forced to relocate for their job. Finally, both those career-engaged young adults who have roommates and those who opt to live alone may be faced with adjustment-related stressors associated with employment (e.g., establishing and maintaining relationships with co-workers and employers, adopting a professional persona, learning to network to obtain needed resources, negotiating role responsibilities and personal worth in the form of salary and benefits). Given that young adults entering the labor force without a college degree are likely to enter at lower-level positions, these individuals may have less control over their work environments, which, as previously indicated, has been shown to correlate with job-related stress and mental illness.

Procrastination (i.e., postponing engagement in required tasks) is another stressor common among college students as well as non-college young adults employed in the workforce. Among college students, procrastination may be prompted by a number of factors, including a belief that one does not possess the requisite skills to complete a given task (low self-efficacy), a more general belief that one lacks academic capability (low academic self-concept), general low self-esteem, fear of poor evaluation or failure, and poor time management (Farran, 2004). Of course, similar factors are likely related to procrastination on the job; however, the workplace often imposes greater structure and most of the required work takes place while in the work setting. With respect to the relation between poor time management and procrastination, research suggests that procrastination is related to disproportionate subjective weighting of short-term rewards over long-term rewards (temporal discounting; Howell, Watson, Powell, & Buro, 2006), which may in turn be related to achievement goal orientation (Howell & Watson, 2007). Specifically, college students who have a more passive orientation toward their learning goals (i.e., they simply want to avoid "failing to learn what there is to learn") are more likely to procrastinate than those who have a more active orientation (i.e., they want to learn "everything there is to learn" [p. 174; Howell & Watson, 2007]). Howell and Watson (2007) suggest that those students with the more active orientation may derive more immediate intrinsic rewards from their academic pursuits, thus promoting engagement in these tasks, and students with the more passive orientation may experience academic tasks as more aversive in the short term, thus promoting avoidance. One reason that these tasks may be experienced as aversive is lack of preparedness for task demands. Consistent with this, they found moderate negative correlations between procrastination and use of cognitive strategies, including rehearsal, elaboration, and organization, as well as use of meta-cognitive strategies, including planning, monitoring, and regulating. They also found a moderate positive association between procrastination and disorganized study habits.

Additional research on the impact of students' temporal focus has demonstrated that it may not simply be a greater focus on the nature of short-term rewards that separates procrastinators from nonprocrastinators. Although, as might be predicated based on temporal discounting, having a future orientation was negatively associated with trait procrastination, Jackson, Fritch, Nagasaka, and Pope (2003) also found that having a more negative view of the past and a fatalistic view of the present were significantly and uniquely predictive of procrastination, even after controlling for current levels of negative affect. Furthermore, students who scored high on trait procrastination also reported that their use of time was less personally meaningful and had less structure, suggesting that procrastinators are not avoiding aversive tasks (including academic and work projects) to focus on immediate rewards (Jackson et al., 2003). As might be expected, procrastination has been shown to be positively associated with levels of depression and anxiety in this population (Farran, 2004).

Financial Stress

Individuals who discontinue their secondary education before receiving their diploma (*dropout*) enter young adulthood with a large disadvantage. Relative to their peers who completed high school, individuals who dropout are less likely to obtain gainful employment, receive lower wages when employed, and are more likely to require public assistance (U.S. Department of Health and Human Services, 2003). However, college students and their high-school-educated, nonmatriculated counterparts are not immune to financial difficulties. "Lack of money" was identified as moderately stressful by the undergraduate students in the study by Sarros and Densten (1989), and financial concerns were among the frequent responses provided by students on the open-ended question in the study by Dusselier and colleagues (2005). Similarly, Ross and colleagues (1999) found that over 70% of their college student sample regarded financial struggles as a primary source of stress. Although educational expenses (e.g., tuition, educational loans, course materials) or other living expenses that are paid out of pocket (e.g., rent, food, transportation, entertainment) may contribute to financial stress, credit card debt and associated interest rates are increasingly taking their toll. Relative to other sections of the population, young adults ages 18 to 24 are the most likely to carry a credit card balance, and this phenomenon is likely related to credit card marketing targeted specifically at college students (Draut & Silva, 2004). According to data collected by the Nellie Mae

Corporation (2005), 42% of college freshmen have a credit card with a debt burden of $1,585, whereas 91% of college seniors have a credit card and owe nearly double that amount on average ($2,864). Moreover, the study revealed that over 50% of college seniors have four or more credit card accounts (as compared to only 15% of freshman), and only 21% of students pay off their balance each month (Nellie Mae Corporation, 2005). Young adults may be particularly prone to accumulating credit card debt as they are relatively less experienced in creating and maintaining a budget and may view credit cards as a means to supplement their income in order to obtain or sustain a desired lifestyle.

Combining Work with Education

Although the empirical literature is mixed with regard to the impact of concurrent work and school enrollment on the academic performance, social adjustment and overall well-being of students, from a limited-resources perspective, anything that takes time away from educational pursuits is popularly perceived as negative and a potential source of stress (Herman, 2000; Swanson et al., 2006). Even within a given study, the relation between working in combination with college and psychosocial outcomes can be unclear. For example, Swanson and colleagues (2006) found that students who were currently working reported significantly less overall satisfaction with their college experience and greater perceived stress than their nonworking counterparts; however, additional analyses examining self-reported congruence between employment, academic, long-term career, and intrapersonal/interpersonal developmental roles indicated that students typically found a balance between working and their other roles during the school year. Furthermore, greater congruence between employment and academic roles was positively associated with greater overall satisfaction with, and adjustment to, college. Greater congruence between employment and intrapersonal/interpersonal developmental roles was also positively associated with college satisfaction. Similarly, correlational data presented by Dundes and Marx (2006) suggests that college students who engage in moderate levels of work during the academic year (10 to 19 hours per week) have higher grade point averages, are more likely to spend 11 or more hours studying, and have greater efficiency relative to those students who do not work or work lesser or greater amounts; however, students who worked a moderate amount were simultaneously more likely to report increased stress level, reduced time devoted to schoolwork, and impaired attention span than those students working fewer than 10 hours. These studies suggest that how one operationalizes and measures the outcomes of interest may have important implications for the results, and future studies on this topic may benefit from using multiple measures and reporters to assess each construct.

Impact of Mental Illness on Academic and Occupational Functioning

As previously described, the unique challenges and stressors faced by college students and their nonmatriculated counterparts in the workforce are associated with various mental health problems. High rates of mental illness among college students and other young adults have important implications for the ability of these young people to succeed academically and in the workplace. In a nationally representative study in the United States, Kessler, Foster, Saunders, and Stang (1995) found that early-onset psychiatric disorders were associated with lower educational attainment, and they estimated that 3.53 million additional participants in the age range of the study would have completed high school and 4.29 million more would have completed college if these disorders were not present. Using the same sample, Kessler and Frank (1997) found that psychological disorders were associated with a greater number of work days missed or shortened. Affective disorders and comorbidity (among affective, anxiety, and substance use disorders) were most strongly associated with work impairment days. In another large sample of young adults (age 21) in New Zealand, over 97% of individuals with diagnosable psychiatric disorders reported that their symptoms interfered with work or daily activities, with percentages ranging from 72% for alcohol dependence to 100% for eating disorders and panic disorder (Newman et al., 1996).

With respect to college students, Eisenberg, Gollust, Golberstein, and Hefner (2007) found that 18.4% of undergraduates in their study reported missing academic obligations due to mental health problems, and 44.3% reported impaired academic performance resulting from mental or emotional problems. Consistent with student self-reports, a longitudinal study using academic records found that more severe depressive symptoms predicted poorer exam performance 1 year later (Andrews & Wilding, 2004). Similarly, Aertgeerts and Buntinx (2002) found that alcohol dependence during the first year of college was inversely associated with academic performance. Brackney and Karabenick (1995) identified a potential mechanism through which psychological problems contribute to academic problems, showing that students with higher levels of psychopathology reported lower self-efficacy for academic success and poorer management of resources, which, in turn, predicted academic performance.

In the workplace, the majority of research has focused on job-related stress as a potential cause of mental illness rather than focusing on poor job performance as a consequence of mental illness. Consistent with this focus, Bond and Bunce (2003) found that aspects of the workplace were predictive of mental illness, whereas mental illness did not predict aspects of the work environment. In contrast, Weisner, Vondracek, Capaldi, and Porfeli (2003) found that a history of mental illness in a sample of young adult men was associated with higher rates of unemployment. Perhaps the best model is one that includes reciprocal effects between mental illness and job performance. For example, Taris (1999) found that, although aspects of the workplace were associated with mental health, there were independent effects of mental illness on job resources, job retention, and re-employment. Regardless of the causes of mental illness, the financial costs are substantial. An analysis from a large medical database showed that only hypertension and heart disease surpassed mental illness with respect to economic burden to employers (Goetzel et al., 2004).

Stress-Management Approaches

Students in the study by Sarros and Densten (1989) were asked to rate the effectiveness of various coping strategies to manage college-related stress. Among those listed as moderately to very effective were "taking a break, putting work into perspective, exercising or physical exertion, talking with other students, socializing outside of college, support from peers, and support from tutors/lecturers." Four of these strategies ostensibly tap into social support, a putative protective factor that has been extensively examined as a moderator of the relation between stressful events and stress reactions. Exercise has also been studied as means of reducing stress, as have didactic approaches that target skills deficits related to time management. Although social support, exercise, and time management might be considered nomothetic approaches to stress management, as their utility is not circumscribed to the particular stressors described above, more idiosyncratic stress-management strategies are beyond the scope of the current chapter.

Apparent in our review, the sources of stress that impact matriculated and nonmatriculated young adults are diverse, and the source of stress most predominant in the fore at any one point in time varies across and within individuals over time. This is perhaps due to an overall limited capacity to manage stressors occurring across multiple domains. In other words, an individual who devotes the majority of his or her efforts to managing academic or work responsibilities may have less time to devote to managing interpersonal relationships or finances. Another individual or the same individual at a different time point may have pressing interpersonal or financial issues to manage and fall behind in his or her academic or work-related responsibilities. In fact, many students report that there are simply not enough hours in the day to manage all of their responsibilities. For example, in the National College Health Assessment (American College Health Association, 2006), over one-fourth (28.2%) of college students surveyed indicated that they felt "overwhelmed by all [they] had to do" on 11 or more occasions (the highest response option for the question) in the past 12 months. Given the number of responsibilities young adults must manage, learning to manage one's time effectively is a critical skill that is likely to help prevent negative mental health consequences and promote wellness.

As stated previously, the transition from adolescence to young adulthood is marked by a decrease in externally imposed structure, particularly for college students. Thus, for many young adults, it is the first time that they have been expected to take complete responsibility for structuring their own schedules. Those who feel ill-equipped to successfully manage their time may be at increased risk for negative academic and mental health outcomes. For example, Nonis, Hudson, Logan, and Ford (1998) found that perceived control over one's time was negatively correlated with perceived academic stress and positively associated with problem-solving abilities, as well as psychological and physiological health. Presumably, the development of skills to effectively manage one's time would bolster one's self-efficacy, with concomitant performance and health benefits.

Although self-help books on time management abound, the empirical research on the specific time-management skills that facilitate positive outcomes is surprisingly sparse. Although recommendations vary, monitoring of time, goal setting/prioritizing, and planning/scheduling are common to most time-management approaches. Although there does not appear to be any empirical research on the importance of time monitoring, self-monitoring of behavior is a key element of empirically supported programs focused on modifying alcohol use and maladaptive eating patterns (Fairburn, Marcus & Wilson, 1993; Sobell & Sobell, 1993). Self-monitoring is typically utilized to increase the individual's awareness of his or her behavior, as many behavioral patterns become over-rehearsed and are thus performed mindlessly. Anecdotally, use of time appears to fit this pattern as many young adults (and others outside of this age range) indicate that they are not really sure where the time goes. In addition, time monitoring would appear to be an important prerequisite to effective goal setting and planning. With respect to these latter two aspects of time management, a recent study found that both were significantly associated with academic stress (Misra & McKean, 2000). The mechanics of time management (planning/scheduling) were significantly inversely associated with three different types of academic stress (change, frustration, self-imposed), whereas setting goals and prioritizing was negatively associated with only one type of academic stress (frustration). Consistent with the previously cited study by Nonis and colleagues (1998), perceived control over time was significantly inversely associated with all five forms of academic stress assessed. In addition, perceived control was negatively associated with reactivity to stress, whereas planning and prioritizing were not reliably associated with stress reactions. The results of existing studies suggest that interventions targeting the development of time-management skills may lead to improved academic, work, and health outcomes. In fact, a recent study of a time-management intervention in the workplace showed that, for most participants, such training has a positive impact (Green & Skinner, 2005). Despite these encouraging findings, additional research on the efficacy of time-management training in college students and other young adults is sorely needed.

In addition to expediting the completion of academic and work-related responsibilities, more efficient use of time can provide greater opportunity for involvement in other activities that might promote effective management of stress. For example, social activities facilitate the development and maintenance of interpersonal relationships that provide a crucial buffering effect against stress. In the general population, social support is a well-established moderator of the relation between stress and both physical and mental health (see Cohen, 2004 for an excellent review). Social support may be particularly important during developmental transitions, including the transition from adolescence into young adulthood. In fact, a recent study by Brissette, Scheier, and Carver (2002) found that changes in social support during the first semester of college were associated with changes in stress levels. Those who reported greater increases in social support over time reported smaller increases in stress during the same time period. Another recent study showed that social support can serve as a stress buffer for college students, even in the wake of major traumatic events. Levels of stress among college students with exposure to the 9/11 terrorist attacks were associated with negative physical and mental health outcomes, but those with greater emotional and tangible social support had fewer mental health (depression) and physical health problems, respectively (MacGeorge, Samter, Feng, Gillihan, & Graves, 2004). Although specific studies of social support and work-related stress among young adults are not available, there is general support for the moderating role of social support in the work stress–health relationship. A meta-analysis evaluating the relation between various forms of social support and various health outcomes (both physical and mental) found both direct and moderating effects of social support. Better social support was associated with better physical and mental health outcomes and it moderated the effects of work-related stress on these outcomes (Viswesvaran, Sanchez, & Fisher, 1999). This research, in combination with evidence for the value of social support during important life transitions, suggests that social support is likely to play a protective role against the unique stressors faced by young adults.

Although social support has the potential to be beneficial in mitigating the effects of stress, young adults often report having too little time to engage in the myriad of social activities available to them. Exercise can also play a protective role against stress, yet competing demands associated with increased role responsibilities may keep young adults from being active. One study of a large sample of college students found that only 53% of students reported engaging in vigorous physical activity in the past month (Suminski, Petosa, Utter, & Zhang, 2002). Another recent study found that exercise decreased significantly from high school to the first 2 months of college (Bray & Born, 2004). These numbers are of concern given that studies in the general population have found that exercise (in particular, aerobic exercise) is inversely correlated with a number of negative physical and mental health outcomes, including obesity, cardiovascular disease, depression, anxiety, alcohol and tobacco use, and overall psychological well-being (Murphy, Pagano, & Marlatt, 1986; Penedo & Dahn, 2005; Petruzzello & Motl, 2006; Scully, Kremer, Meade, Graham, & Dudgeon, 1998; Ussher, Taylor, West, & McEwen, 2000). Research specifically in young adults has produced similar findings and studies have even shown that exercise can serve a long-term protective role. One study found that former college athletes relative to nonathletes were at lower risk for depression and had overall lower psychiatric distress 10 years after college (Suminski et al., 2002). Although college athletes and nonathletes may differ in important ways other than exercise level, the results are suggestive of long-term mental health benefits. Consistent with this, Bray and Born (2004) found that physical activity level in college was inversely associated with depression 25 years later. Still, such studies cannot demonstrate a causal influence of exercise on health outcomes. Thus, additional studies have examined the effects of prescribed exercise on health outcomes. Empirical studies and reviews of this literature have found reductions in anxiety, depression, and self-reported stress (Anderson, King, Stewart, Camacho, & Rejeski, 2005; North, McCullagh, & Tran, 1990; Tkachuk & Martin, 1999). Finally, much like social support, there is some evidence that exercise can serve to moderate the influence of stress. For example, Motl and Dishman (2004) found that acute exercise reduced anxiety caused by the introduction of a stressor, and Brown and Siegel (1988) found that the negative impact of stressful life events on health decreased as exercise level increased. Collectively, the literature on stress, exercise, and health provides a compelling argument for the importance of exercise for the physical and mental health of the general population and the young adult population in particular (see Petruzzello & Motl, 2006 for an excellent review of exercise and mental health in college students).

In summary, general stress-management strategies, including time management, social support, and exercise, can serve to buffer against the negative effects of stress during young adulthood. Although beyond the scope of the current chapter it is important to note that, in addition to more general stress-management strategies, specific coping skills can also serve a protective role. For example, in a sample of college students,

Largo-Wight, Peterson, and Chen (2005) found that, in addition to social support and vigorous physical activity, better problem-solving skills were associated with lower perceived stress. Other specific strategies that may serve to protect against stress include relaxation techniques and cognitive reappraisal of stressful situations. Several recent studies using interventions targeting the development of these more specific coping skills have shown promise both with college students and in the workplace (Gardner, Rose, Mason, Tyler, & Cushway, 2005; Iglesias et al., 2005; Keogh, Bond, & Flaxman, 2006).

Conclusion

In summary, young adults face a number of unique developmental challenges. Broadly, this period is marked by identity exploration, instability, self-focus, a feeling of being in between adolescence and adulthood, and optimism regarding life's possibilities (Arnett, 2004). More specifically, this period is punctuated by decisions regarding educational and occupational trajectories. For individuals who fail to complete secondary education, the choices are typically more limited, and the occupational outcomes are often less propitious. In contrast, for individuals who receive their diploma or GED, college and career opportunities are more plentiful and accessible. A college education can facilitate exploration of various fields of interest and provide basic competencies in domains inherent to all occupations, whereas employment can offer financial benefits and direct experience. College and career need not be mutually exclusive, and for a growing segment of young adults "earning and learning" in parallel has become normative (Swanson et al., 2006); however, a significant proportion of youth opt to engage in college and career in a more serial fashion, stopping out of college for extended periods of time and entering the labor force. Regardless of their chosen path, young adults engaging in these developmental tasks are faced with a myriad of unique challenges, including academic/occupational, intrapersonal/interpersonal, financial, and role-related stressors. Experiences in these domains are typically stressful because they are novel; for the first time in their lives, young adults are faced with independence and its inherent rights and responsibilities. Given the novelty of these challenges, young adults may lack the requisite skills to effectively cope and subsequently experience negative mental health outcomes, including depression and anxiety. Negative mental health outcomes may in turn impair academic and occupational functioning. Although more research is necessary to support their efficacy in mitigating or militating against the specific challenges faced by young adults engaging in college and career pursuits, nomothetic approaches to stress management, including augmenting or strengthening time-management skills, increasing/accessing social support, and engaging in physical activity, may help to increase wellness in this population.

KEY POINTS

- Young adults, regardless of whether they pursue predominantly higher education or a career, face similar challenges related to learning how to best manage time, social relationships, finances, and other aspects of living.
- College and the work place each have unique features (e.g., more or less external structure) that may present challenges and/or opportunities for young adults.
- Healthy navigation through college and career in young adulthood requires the development of skills in specific domains, including coping with stress and the appropriate management of time and resources.

> **PRACTICE GUIDELINES**
>
> - Increase awareness of behavioral patterns through self-monitoring of daily activities and provide instruction to redress specific time-management skills deficits.
> - Encourage engagement in prosocial and (non-substance-related) recreational activities that will develop and/or enhance social support.
> - Assist individuals to develop specific exercise plans that include a minimum of 30 minutes of moderate-intensity physical activity per day most days of the week. Explore and problem-solve any barriers and recommend that individuals make public commitments to adhere to their plans.

References

Aertgeerts, B., & Buntinx, F. (2002). The relation between alcohol abuse or dependence and academic performance in first-year college students. *Journal of Adolescent Health, 31*, 223–225.

Akgun, S., & Chiarrochi, J. (2003). Learned resourcefulness moderates the relationship between academic stress and academic performance. *Educational Psychology, 23*, 287–294.

Aldwin, C., & Greenberger, E. (1987). Cultural differences in the predictors of depression. *American Journal of Community Psychology, 15*, 789–813.

American College Health Association (2006). *American College Health Association-National College Health Assessment: Reference Group Data Report Fall 2005*. Baltimore, MD: Author.

Anderson, R. T., King, A., Stewart, A. L., Camacho, F., & Rejeski, W. J. (2005). Physical activity counseling in primary care and patient well-being: Do patients benefit? *Annals of Behavioral Medicine, 30*, 146–154.

Andrews, B., & Wilding, J. M. (2004). The relation of depression and anxiety to life stress and achievement in students. *British Journal of Psychology, 95*, 509–521.

Arnett, J. J. (2000). Emerging adulthood: A theory of development from the late teens through the twenties. *American Psychologist, 55*, 469–480.

Arnett, J. J. (2004). *Emerging adulthood: The winding road from the late teens through the twenties*. New York: Oxford University Press.

Bachman, J. G., Safron, D. J., Sy, S. R., & Schulenberg, J. E. (2003). Wishing to work: New perspectives on how adolescents' part-time work intensity is linked to educational disengagement, substance use, and other problem behaviors. *International Journal of Behavioral Development, 27*, 301–315.

Bond, F. W., & Bunce, D. (2003). The role of acceptance and job control in mental health, job satisfaction, and work performance. *Journal of Applied Psychology, 88*, 1057–1067.

Brackney, B. E., & Karabenick, S. A. (1995). Psychopathology and academic performance: The role of motivation and learning strategies. *Journal of Counseling Psychology, 42*, 456–465.

Bradburn, E. M., Berger, R., Li, X., Peter, K., & Rooney, K. (2003). *A descriptive summary of 1999–2000 bachelor's degree recipients 1 year later, with an analysis of time to degree* (NCES 2003–165). National Center for Education Statistics, Institute of Education Sciences, U.S. Department of Education. Washington, DC: U.S. Government Printing Office.

Bray, S. R., & Born, H. A. (2004). Transition to university and vigorous physical activity: Implications for health and psychological well-being. *Journal of American College Health, 52*, 181–188.

Brissette, I., Scheier, M. F., & Carver, C. S. (2002). The role of optimism in social network development, coping, and psychological adjustment during a life transition. *Journal of Personality and Social Psychology, 82*, 102–111.

Brown, J. D., & Siegel, J. M. (1988). Exercise as a buffer of life stress: A prospective study of adolescent health. *Health Psychology, 7*, 34–353.

Cohen, S. (2004). Social relationships and health. *American Psychologist, 59*, 676–684.

Draut, T., & Silva, J. (2004) *Generation broke: The growth of debt among young Americans*. Retrieved on September 18, 2007, from http://www.demos.org/pubs/Generation_Broke.pdf.

Dundes, L., & Marx, J. (2006). Balancing work and academics in college: Why do students working 10 to 19 hours per week excel? *Journal of College Student Retention, 8*, 107–120.

Dusselier, L., Dunn, B., Wang, Y., Shelley, M. C., II, & Whalen, D. F. (2005). Personal, health, academic, and environmental predictors of stress for residence hall students. *Journal of American College Health, 54,* 15–24.

Edwards, K. J., Hershberger, P. J., Russell, R. K., & Markert, R. J. (2001). Stress, negative social exchange, and health symptoms in university students. *Journal of American College Health, 50,* 75–79.

Eisenberg, D., Gollust, S. E., Golberstein, E., & Hefner, J. L. (2007). Prevalence and correlates of depression, anxiety, and suicidality among university students. *American Journal of Orthopsychiatry, 77,* 534–542.

Fairburn, C. G., Marcus, M. D., & Wilson, G. T. (1993). Cognitive behaviour therapy for binge eating and bulimia nervosa: A comprehensive treatment manual. In C. G. Fairburn & G. T. Wilson (Eds.). *Binge eating: Nature, assessment, and treatment* (pp. 361–404). New York: Guilford Press.

Farran, B. (2004). *Predictors of academic procrastination in college students.* Unpublished dissertation, Fordham University, New York.

Gardner, B., Rose, J., Mason, O., Tyler, P., & Cushway, D. (2005). Cognitive therapy and behavioural coping in the management of work-related stress: An intervention study. *Work and Stress, 19,* 137–152.

Goetzel, R. Z., Long, S. R., Ozminkowski, R. J., Hawkins, K., Wang, S., & Lynch, W. (2004). Health, absence, disability, and presenteeism cost estimates of certain physical and mental health conditions affecting U.S. employers. *Journal of Occupational and Environmental Medicine, 46,* 398–412.

Green, P., & Skinner, D. (2005). Does time-management training work? An evaluation. *International Journal of Training and Development, 9,* 124–139.

Greenhaus, J. H., & Beutell, N. J. (1985). Sources of conflict between work and family roles. *Academy of Management Review, 10,* 76–88.

Herman, A. M. (2000). *Report on the youth labor force.* U.S. Department of Labor, Bureau of Labor Statistics. Retrieved on September 1, 2007, from http://www.bls.gov/opub/rylf/pdf/rylf2000.pdf.

Howell, A. J., Watson, D. C., Powell, R. A., & Buro, K. (2006). Academic procrastination: The pattern and correlates of behavioural postponement. *Personality and Individual Differences, 40,* 1519–1530.

Howell, A. J., & Watson, D. C. (2007). Procrastination: Associations with achievement goal orientation and learning strategies. *Personality and Individual Differences, 43,* 167–178.

Iglesias, S. L., Azzara, S., Squillace, M., Jeifetz, M., Lores Arnais, M. R., Desimone, M. F., & Diaz, L. E. (2005). A study on the effectiveness of a stress management programme for college students. *Pharmacy Education, 5,* 27–31.

Jackson, T., Fritch, A., Nagasaka, T., & Pope, L. (2003). Procrastination and perceptions of past, present, and future. *Individual Differences Research, 1,* 17–28.

Karasek, R. A., Jr. (1979). Job demands, job decision latitude, and mental strain: Implications for job redesign. *Administrative Science Quarterly, 24,* 285–308.

Karasek, R., & Theorell, T. (1990). *Healthy work: Stress, productivity, and the reconstruction of working life.* New York: Basic Books.

Keogh, E., Bond, F. W., & Flaxman, P. E. (2006). Improving academic performance and mental health through a stress management intervention: Outcomes and mediators of change. *Behaviour Research and Therapy, 44,* 339–357.

Kessler, R. C., Foster, C. L., Saunders, W. B., & Stang, P. E. (1995). Social consequences of psychiatric disorders, I: Educational attainment. *American Journal of Psychiatry, 152,* 1026–1032.

Kessler, R. C., & Frank, R. G. (1997). The impact of psychiatric disorders on work loss days. *Psychological Medicine, 27,* 861–873.

Laird, J., DeBell, M., Kienzl, G., & Chapman, C. (2007). *Dropout rates in the United States: 2005* (NCES 2007-059). National Center for Education Statistics, Institute of Education Sciences, U.S. Department of Education. Washington, DC: National Center for Education Statistics.

Largo-Wight, E., Peterson, P. M., & Chen, W. W. (2005). Perceived problem solving, stress, and health among college students. *American Journal of Health Behavior, 29,* 360–370.

MacGeorge, E. L., Samter, W., Feng, B., Gillihan, S. J., & Graves, A. R. (2004). Stress, social support, and health among college students after September 11, 2001. *Journal of College Student Development, 45,* 655–670.

McCormick, A. C., & Horn, L. J. (1996). *A descriptive summary of 1992–1993 bachelor's degree recipients: 1 year later, with an essay on time to degree* (NCES 1996-158). National Center for Education Statistics, Institute of Education Sciences, U.S. Department of Education. Washington, DC: U.S. Government Printing Office.

Misra, R., & McKean, M. (2000). College students' academic stress and its relation to their anxiety, time management, and leisure satisfaction. *American Journal of Health Studies, 16,* 41–51.

Motl, R. W., & Dishman, R. K. (2004). Effects of acute exercise on the soleus H-reflex and self-reported anxiety after caffeine ingestion. *Physiology and Behavior, 80,* 577–585.

Murphy, T. J., Pagano, R. R., & Marlatt, G. A. (1986). Lifestyle modification with heavy alcohol drinkers: Effects of aerobic exercise and meditation. *Addictive Behaviors, 11,* 175–186.

Nellie Mae Corporation (2005). Undergraduate students and credit cards in 2004: An analysis of usage rates and trends. Retrieved on September 18, 2007, from http://www.nelliemae.com/library/research_12.html.

Newman, D. L., Moffitt, E. E., Caspi, A., Magdol, L., Silva, P. A., & Stanton, W. R. (1996). Psychiatric disorder in a birth cohort of young adults: Prevalence, comorbidity, clinical significance, and new case incidence from ages 11 to 21. *Journal of Consulting and Clinical Psychology, 64,* 552–562.

Nonis, S. A., Hudson, G. I., Logan, L. B., & Ford, C. W. (1998). Influence of perceived control over time on college students' stress and stress-related outcomes. *Research on Higher Education, 39,* 587–605.

North, T. C., McCullagh, P., & Tran, Z. V. (1990). Effect of exercise on depression. *Exercise and Sport Sciences Reviews, 18,* 379–415.

Penedo, F. J., & Dahn, J. R. (2005). Exercise and well-being: a review of mental and physical health benefits associated with physical activity. *Current Opinion in Psychiatry, 18,* 189–193.

Perrewé, P. L., Hochwarter, W. A., Rossi, A. M., Wallace, A., Maignan, I., Castro, S. L., Ralston, D. A., Westman, M., Vollmer, G., Tang, M., Wan, P., & Van Deusen, C. A. (2002). Are work stress relationships universal? A nine-region examination of role stressors, general self-efficacy, and burnout. *Journal of International Management, 8,* 163–187.

Petruzzello, S. J., & Motl, R. W. (2006). Physical activity and mental health in college students. In M. V. Landow (Ed.), *College students: Mental health and coping strategies* (pp. 41–58). New York: Nova Science.

Ross, S. E., Neibling, B. C., & Heckert, T. M. (1999). Sources of stress among college students. *College Student Journal, 33,* 312–317.

Sarros, J. C., & Densten, I. L. (1989). Undergraduate student stress and coping strategies. *Higher Education Research and Development, 8*(1), 47–57.

Scully, D., Kremer, J., Meade, M. M., Graham, R., & Dudgeon, K. (1998). Physical exercise and psychological well-being: A critical review. *British Journal of Sports Medicine, 32,* 111–120.

Snyder, T. D., Dillow, S. A., & Hoffman, C. M. (2007). *Digest of Education Statistics 2006* (NCES 2007-017). National Center for Education Statistics, Institute of Education Sciences, U.S. Department of Education. Washington, DC: U.S. Government Printing Office.

Sobell, M. B., & Sobell, L. C. (1993). *Problem drinkers: Guided self-change treatment.* New York: Guilford Press.

Suminski, R. R., Petosa, R., Utter, A. C., & Zhang, J. J. (2002). Physical activity among ethnically diverse college students. *Journal of American College Health, 51,* 75–80.

Swanson, V., Broadbridge, A., & Karatzias, A. (2006). Earning and learning: Role congruence, state/trait factors and adjustment to university life. *British Journal of Educational Psychology, 76,* 895–914.

Taris, T. W. (1999). The mutual effects between job resources and mental health: A prospective study among Dutch youth. *Genetic, Social, and General Psychology Monographs, 125,* 433–350.

Tkachuk, G. A., & Martin, G. L. (1999). Exercise therapy for patients with psychiatric disorders: Research and clinical implications. *Professional Psychology: Research and Practice, 30,* 275–282.

Towbes, L. C., & Cohen, L. H. (1996). Chronic stress in the lives of college students: Scale development and prospective prediction of distress. *Journal of Youth and Adolescence, 25,* 199–217.

U. S. Department of Education (2007). *Baccalaureate and beyond longitudinal study (B&B).* Retrieved on July 27, 2007, from http://nces.ed.gov/surveys/b&b/.

U. S. Department of Health and Human Services (2003). *Trends in the well-being of America's children and youth, 2003.* Retrieved on August 27, 2007, from http://aspe.hhs.gov/hsp/03trends/index.htm.

U. S. Department of Labor, Bureau of Labor Statistics. (2007a). *College enrollment and work activity of 2006 high school graduates* (USDL 07-0604). Retrieved on September 1, 2007, from http://www.bls.gov/news.release/pdf/hsgec.pdf.

U. S. Department of Labor, Bureau of Labor Statistics. (2007b). *Household data, annual averages: Employed and unemployed full- and part-time workers by age, sex, race, and Hispanic or Latino ethnicity.* Retrieved on September 2, 2007, from http://www.bls.gov/cps/cpsaat8.pdf.

Ussher, M. H., Taylor, A. H., West, R., & McEwen, A. (2000). Does exercise aid smoking cessation? A systematic review. *Addiction, 95,* 199–208.

Viswesvaran, C., Sanchez, J. I., & Fisher, J. (1999). The role of social support in the process of work stress: A meta-analysis. *Journal of Vocational Behavior, 54,* 314–334.

Weisner, M., Vondracek, F. W., Capaldi, D. M., & Porfeli, E. (2003). Childhood and adolescent predictors of early adult career pathways. *Journal of Vocational Behavior, 63,* 305–328.

Chapter 6

Gender Issues: Modern Models of Young Male Resilient Mental Health

William S. Pollack

While many of my colleagues in other chapters will describe the dearth of attention that both the mental health and general well-being of "young adults" has received as a group in comparison to adolescents or other adult groupings, and rightfully so (see also Arnett, 2000; Park et al., 2006), when specific categories of emotional disorders are usually delineated we tend to emphasize the most modern findings in regard to both illness and treatment in a "gender neutral" manner. When we do distinguish by gender, as in depression, eating disorders, body image difficulties, etc., the lion's share of our research has been on girls and young women (Pollack, 2006a). This is in no way meant to suggest that young adult females receive superior care or are given a greater chance of healthy adjustment within society as a whole, but only that we have too often neglected to recognize certain symptom expressions by young adult males as *distinct mental health problems*, or equally troubling, as almost "normative" dysfunctions created by a negatively synergistic effect of biology and our Western industrialized socialization patterns.

Certain disorders or experiences particularly relevant to young adult mental health are, indeed, encountered more frequently by girls and women. For example, many girls and women suffer from or are seen to be suffering from *internalizing* disorders like anxiety and depression and have experienced traumas like sexual abuse. (Child Trends, 2005; Kessler et al., 2005)

Yet in modern compilations of the greatest risks to health and mental stability during this period, almost always substance abuse, risky behavior, mortality risk (especially through suicide), and violence are most often highlighted (Arnett, 2000; Behavioral Risk Surveillance, 2005; Brown, 2004; Brown et al., 2005; Center for Substance Abuse Prevention, Substance Abuse and Mental Health Services Administration, 2005; Johnston et al., 2005; Jekielek & Brown, 2005; Park et al., 2006; Schulenberg, O'Malley, Bachman, & Johnston, 2005). Here young adult and teenage *males* are *most at risk*. So while we must remain ever vigilant to the negative aspect of young adult females' mental heath dilemmas (National Center for Statistics, 2005) perhaps not surprisingly, still, the lion's share of the victims of *externalizing* behaviors during this developmental period of usually healthy experimentation and ultimate identity cohesion (Arnett, 2000) in regard to the scourges delineated above are young *males*— often young males whose emotional predisposition to such maladies go dangerously undetected and undertreated as they attempt to, but fail to achieve a more healthy integration of self during this key stage of their life trajectories (Pollack,

2006a; Network on Transitions, 2005). For example, while we are generally knowledgeable about rising trends in single motherhood (Settersten, Furstenberg, & Raumbaut, 2005), less connection is often made between a more broad and modern diagnostic criteria for young male depression (Pollack, 1998a, 1998b, 2001c, 2001d, 2003, and below) and incredibly high rates of young male incarceration, especially for young adult males of color—with numbers as high as 11% of all black males in the United States between 20 to 24 years of age in prison (Rumbaut, 2005).

While we are generally aware that young adults (ages 18–24) have approximately twice the mortality rates than adolescents, it is perhaps a less well-known fact that *male* young adults have three times the general mortality rate than females in this age group. Unintentional injury is the leading cause for mortality in young adults, and here males again lead the pack. Homicide rates are highest as well among this age category, and here young adult males are close to *six times* more likely to die from a homicide; violent crime victimization rates for males in this age group (with the exception of being a victim of sexual assault) are much greater for males than females (Bureau of Justice Statistics, 2005a, 2005b).

So-called unintentional injury, a statistical category utilized by the Centers for Disease Control and Prevention (2005) and others, which I read as evidence of either overtly risky behavior or covert suicidal enactment (see Pollack, 2003), takes the lives of three times more young adult males than females and is often linked to motor vehicle accidents connected with substance abuse (National Center for Injury Prevention and Control, 2006).

As we move closer to the arena of normative male trauma (Pollack, 1998a, 2000a, 2000b, 2003) and more classic categories of mental heath disturbance in young adults, the need to understand our misconceptions of healthy young adult male behavior or so-called misbehavior becomes evident. Substance abuse as both a risky behavior and evidence of a continuum of mental health disorders peaks in the years we study, but, again, especially among young adult males (SAMSHA, 2004, 2005a, 2005b). Binge drinking is more likely for these males and if one can be allowed to highlight one particular mental health scourge over another, during this age period young males are up to *six times* more likely to complete a suicide than their female counterparts, yet 50% less likely (at the least) to be diagnosed as or treated for depression (see Pollack, 1998a, 1998b, 2001c, 2001d).

So why study young adult males? Because our understanding of their normative mental health has for too long gone unchallenged and the sad statistics point to a crisis in young male adult mental illness, especially in the arenas of so-called disorders of attachment, safe life skills, and depression. We must study them to rescue them from the unwitting trend toward mental health mortality, which our normative systems of development, as well as classical treatment models, have either created or maintained, or both.

The Emotional "Neighborhood" of Young Adult Males

Fred Rogers, known to generations of parents and children alike who avidly watched his public television program, "Mr. Rogers Neighborhood," meant to model healthy, mature adult functioning in a miniature virtual neighborhood—one built upon healthy connections between a diverse array of adults and the youngsters vouchsafed to their care. Fred Rogers was also an ordained minister and a quotidian philosopher of intergenerational development. He stated, "One of the greatest dignities of humankind is that each successive generation is invested in the welfare of each new generation."

Certainly, he meant this to be as true for the boys whom we were/are as a society attempting to nurture into healthy adulthood, including their young adult emotional balance and well-being, as much as their gender counterparts, the girls and young women, both of whom we aim to positively parent, mentor, teach, and, perhaps, clinically treat. Yet our normative traditional values, especially those heretofore in the arena of mental health for boys on their ways to "well-adjusted" young adulthood have in very many cases had the paradoxical effect of stunting this genuine emotional well-being as young men stumbled through their early and adolescent years, too often disconnected or disrupted in their bonds to close nurturant care from significant adult role models, as a result of our society's "boy code"(Pollack, 1998a, 1999, 2000a, 2001b, 2001c, 2006a).This is a code of masculinity that has resulted in a shame-based induced stoic denial of vulnerability in our young "men" *as a rite de passage* to adulthood, creating *a normative male-based trauma* interrupting or at least delaying the young adult male's healthy entrance to adult life. Unhappily, I will also point out in this chapter that generations of academic and clinical scientists have given the mental health imprimatur to this confusion between the absolute necessity for emotionally undisrupted bonded growth within a context of adult-to-young male emotional connection, leading to young adult masculine mental health, versus its wrong-headed impostor: the concept that psychological "separation," especially for males, was not only meant to be a normative way station to adult mental health but a necessary disidentification from their earlier female-dominated world of "coddled" succor. This now (hopefully) outdated concept of separation as the *hallmark of mental health,* especially for young males, has been one of the most salient psychological factors in impeding the mental health of our adolescent males on their way to adulthood. It has served as a capstone for the creation of a host of emotional disorders based upon this *abandonment depression* (most especially "covert depressions" and suicidal enactment) foisted upon young males, and then, supported by faulty developmental theories and clinical interventions that further crippled young males' species-specific neurobiological and psychosocial, well-adjusted urges and needs to remain emotionally connected, albeit in different capacities, throughout their formative years.

Based upon the research and clinical work of our group and others (See Pollack, 1999, 2006a), I will discuss in further detail a more modern, and indeed, practical model of young adult mental health. This model can replace our atavistic, confabulated codes of masculinity with more modern psychological concepts of "individuation" of self within a context of ongoing adult connections, jettisoning once and for all the now not only atavistic, but lingeringly harmful psychological concept of *"psychic separation"* as being necessary for our young boys to achieve emotionally balanced young adulthood, or for that matter a mentally healthy life trajectory.

Before taking us into a dismantling of these myths of pseudo-mental health for young adult males and replacing them with more positive resilient models, now founded upon an important convergence among psychoanalytically informed developmental psychology, clinical research, modern psychiatry, and new neuroscientific findings of human primate needs for "mirror" support throughout their life cycles, in both genders, perhaps a clinical vignette may be instructive. It will serve as an example of a practical intervention toward young adult mental health in one client, as well as a pragmatic metaphor for our need to modify our templates of theoretically based mental health intervention into the lives of these young adult males.

Clinical Vignette

Adam[a] was referred by his major professor in graduate school, after his expectedly brilliant career in science was becoming compromised in his pre-doctoral fellowship by increasingly and previously uncharacteristic sloppy academic work, an apparent "chip on his shoulder" as reported to the Dean by his fellow researchers, and an overt standoff with a police officer on a routine traffic stop for driving 5 miles per hour over the speed limit. Indeed, the officer was inclined to let it go with a warning, but when Adam challenged the officer's mathematical calculations, spit in his face, uttered a four-letter expletive, and appeared to be challenging him to a fight, he was held overnight in the school's security facility.

That next day Adam called my office, telling me, "I imagine everyone in my department and my girlfriend think I should see you. They say I'm too irritable these days, so I guess I'd like an appointment." Inquiries on the part of the therapist as to whether Adam had any personal interest in exploring any more specific issues were met by a sarcastic rejoinder: "I thought

---

[a] Adam is a fictitious name/merged case history used to protect privacy.

only girls and psychology majors ever *wanted* to go to therapy." After some further discussion he averred that perhaps things had not been going as well as usual and that maybe it would not hurt to have a few "talks with a shrink." I replied that I would be delighted to meet, but then the five possible suggested appointment times meant to fit with his schedule somehow were "already booked" by his "busy social schedule and studying," so it was necessary—if we were to meet at all—to listen to Adam's only two possibilities for a time and choose from those choices. I decided to schedule both, "just in case he had more important things to discuss than could be covered in one hour." With a guttural guffaw, something akin to an air of surprise admixed with disdain, he reluctantly agreed, demurring any directions to my office with the aside that his "smart phone" had GPS.

Our first meeting was somewhat of a surprise to me (and later, I discovered to Adam as well) as on first appearances he seemed and looked nothing like the air of sardonic bravado by phone had led me to imagine. Slightly shorter than average, and a bit overweight, his dress was beyond casual academic, veering into rumpled dirty, as though he had slept in his shirt; and he appeared against all evidence to the contrary in our prior phone encounter to be both anxious and somewhat "down" in his demeanor.

Before I could inform Adam of the context of this consultation and any limitations to his privacy that could ensue due to state regulations and his prior scuffle with the law, he launched into what could only be described as a "shotgun" approach of very quick staccato questions as to my training, experience, capacity to not "moralize," and what he referred to as my "scientific cure rate."

Far from being put off by this behavior, which I had been warned about by the referring professor, I found myself wondering whether I was dealing with either a severely characteralogically disordered young man or perhaps an angry young male with poor impulse control in a prodromal state of a more severe affective disorder; but, in any case, I felt neither fear, "moral disgust," nor pity. Indeed, I found myself forming an immediate impression/fantasy of a much younger boy left alone, by mistake, in a large department store while shopping with his mother, and now having what most people derisorily refer to, especially in young males, as a *tantrum*, but what I perceived to be a sullen sense of panic admixed with unexpressed sadness. It seemed almost as though he was about to cry but could find neither tears to display nor appropriate language to utter.

I decided to answer every one of Adam's questions directly, quickly, and to the point. This appeared to confuse him and I enquired as to whether there was something I had said in reply to his concerns that befuddled or bothered him. "No," he replied, his energy waning and slumping into his chair, "it's just that by this point most people walk away or the guys want to get into some kind of verbal fisticuffs." "That must be very upsetting," I responded, "as you already seem so depleted, frustrated... sad." Suddenly, he burst into tears with a strength that I believe, in retrospect, surprised us both; but Adam, clearly the most. "That's the first time I've cried since my father died," he explained, as he easily took the box of tissues I handed him. "It's very odd!" "Why odd?" I answered. "Well because I don't *feel* sad," Adam replied. "You certainly appear both sad and tired of having to fight *that* off everyday." This time he cried more softly, for several minutes.

At the end of that first session, Adam was unsure about returning, but when I assured him I would very much like to hear more about how "misunderstood" he had felt by all the others around him, he demurred and suggested an appointment for a Saturday morning: "The only day I could possibly make it."

Indeed, Adam appeared almost surprised to see me when he returned to the office that next weekend. After greeting him warmly, he noticed a sort of "puzzlement" in my eyes as he put it. "Maybe that was my response to what seemed a sense of shock on your face upon entering," I said. "I never thought you'd really be here, on your day off," Adam replied. "I'm interested in what you have to tell me about why so many other people disappoint you," I replied, and, also, "I genuinely enjoyed our last time together." I saw a beginning of a smile cross his face. I added, now with some inner trepidation, "I think if we *work together*, I might be of some help." "You mean like side by side, like, when you're trying to fix a car," he heartily responded. "Yes, that's exactly what I mean."

As this new attachment relationship developed, I learned more and more about how successful Adam had been in his younger years, taught by his parents to never rely on anyone else for success but to build up an inner "wall of strength" as he described it. "With that having given you so much success," I interpreted, "I assume, either your girlfriend or your advisor or even me asking you to take down that wall and connect more with us, wouldn't be too well received." "I'd get angry as hell," he almost shouted while making a fist. "But you'd really be scared to death, huh," I inserted, feeling our relationship had built up enough strength by then. Adam stood straight up in his chair, almost for a moment it felt to me he might lunge, then he slumped and began crying almost unconsolingly for the remainder of the hour. Before ending, I enquired if he felt good enough to leave. A different mood appeared to come over his face and he replied, "Why, just because I was acting like a baby for a while?" "Not a baby," I said, "just one of us vulnerable human beings, like your advisor or me for that matter." Again, surprised, he asked whether in the next few weeks we could get together more frequently. "Of course, I replied" and we set our course for twice-weekly meetings.

Somewhere in mid-therapy, as we were uncovering Adam's loving, but somewhat psychologically unresponsive parents, except to one aspect of his self—his intellectual prowess—I mentioned that although I had announced I would be away for several weeks and that time was soon upon us, he had hardly mentioned it. "Oh I knew you'd get into that shrink stuff one of those days." "How do you mean?" "You want me to tell you I'll miss you, that I feel abandoned like when my mother said I was too old and smart a boy to cry so much anymore and run to her for help all the time, when I got hurt on my ninth birthday! Well not this time, I'll do fine without you!"

Two days later on the last session before our 2-week-plus hiatus, he returned. "I thought you guys like to hear about dreams," Adam said somewhat sarcastically. "Sometimes, it can help get us into places that are otherwise hard to explore," I responded, adding, "but it's not just the dream, but also what it brings to your mind, when we discuss it," I said. "OK, I'm game," Adam replied as I fantasized he felt he had been challenged to a new type of chess game and was about to defeat the grandmaster. That idea I kept to myself as he began to relay his dream. "It was dark and murky out and I was lost in the woods... couldn't tell if I was a little boy or a man (Adam was 23 years old, I should add). Finally as though by magic I was finding my way to a clearing and found a road with a jeep on it, I jumped in, but it wouldn't start. Then an old man came along and helped me out and I was on my way." "What happened to the old man?" I enquired. "He wanted to get in and sit beside me, but there was only really room for one so I had to leave him behind." "So you were parted just as you took off," I remarked. "I just knew you'd say that," Adam retorted, "you think everything's about you and that damn vacation." "I don't know," I responded, "but too bad we couldn't go for a ride to Lenny's (to the local grad school lunch hangout) for a bite." "Guess you won't be there when you're on vacation," he smirked as he rose to leave this last session before our interruption.

I had assured Adam he could feel free to be in touch with me by cell phone if any issues were to arise during my absence or if he "just wanted to talk." Therefore, I was shocked and a bit worried when on our first session after my absence he arrived late and in a somewhat disheveled state. "Don't worry," he said, "I've only looked like this since yesterday. It's a weird thing, I was doing fine, better than before academically, no more weird interactions or fights and my girlfriend had said I seemed like 'a new caring man.' But about two days before I was going to see you again, I had that same dream about leaving the old man behind. This time I awoke really down and feeling alone, just like I did when my parents didn't understand I needed to cry, when I needed their support long ago." "Perhaps, there's a chance now for me to climb into the jeep," I blurted out.

Adam's whole demeanor changed and he began to laugh. After the session, I said, "Are you doing anything right now?" "Nope," Adam replied. "Then why don't we hop into my car and go down to Lenny's for a bite." Slack-jawed and open-eyed, Adam replied: "I thought you guys weren't supposed to do *real* things like that—boundaries or something." "What, I can't eat lunch with you?" I replied. Again, Adam looked shocked. "It should be separate tabs," he said. "Yes, I think that's best," I responded, "and no alcohol, just doing something positive together."

Actually, that piece of what I have referred to elsewhere as action empathy (Pollack, 1998a, 2006a) was the last actual action outside the office, as Adam began to feel a sense of, as he put it, "holding me inside" and me holding him "like a fantasy," he explained. "So now it's safe to feel," I replied. "Yep," and Adam smiled.

He continues in less intensive treatment and is about to be awarded a joint-discovery prize with his major professor for their work together, which forms the basis of his soon-to-be-defended thesis. I have little doubt that at graduation his now-steady girlfriend in an allied field will be present and that afterward they will begin making their weddings plans, now having been affianced for the last year.

Commentary

Though a complete commentary on this young adult, "male-friendly" treatment approach is not the central subject of this chapter, comments in greater detail may be found elsewhere (see Pollack, 2005). For our purposes, the underlying treatment philosophy of psychodynamic psychotherapy was modified to become male or "guy-friendly" Interconnection and understandings of inevitable mutual disconnections and their repair through both action in the present and associations to "guy code/boy code" "psychic traumas of the past" and their remediation in a "shame-free-zone" are the particular elements to highlight for the main theses of young adult, "guy" mental health upon which I will now adumbrate.

The boys and young adult males whom we treat, study, and care about (much like the young women who have been studied, even earlier, during the last decade) frequently experience intense sadness, vulnerability, and a troubling sense of isolation, disconnection, and despair within the midst of American society (Pollack, 1995a, 1995b, 1998, 2006). While many of our young males are in deep emotional pain, their suffering often remains difficult to detect, sometimes invisible. On the outside they often project a persona of bravado and pseudo-independence. But our research and clinical experience (see Pollack, 1998a, 2006a) reveal that on the inside many young men may actually feel disconnected, lonely, afraid, and desperate. However, society places at the shame-based pressure on our young "guys" to act tough, follow a strict "code of masculinity," and hide their genuine, especially any vulnerable, emotions at all costs—a process that shows itself later in young male adulthood as that "code of silence" so complained of by their female counterparts and many adults, including clinicians who find this group to be "difficult to communicate with." Consequently they lose connection with large portions of their own inner emotional selves, and we adults, who should vouchsafe their healthy growth during these periods, often lose genuine and deep emotional connections with them (Pollack et al., 2008)

As a society, a unique set of expectations is placed on boys that calls upon them to brave life's ups and downs independently (autonomously), stoically cover their pain, and above all, avoid doing anything that might *shame* either themselves or their loved ones, by not being or becoming a *real young man*. These rigid gender codes, or gender straitjackets, push many boys, especially as they move into adolescence and young adulthood to repress their yearnings for love and connection ("yearnings," which are *species*-, not gender-, specific and biologically as well as developmentally normal and necessary functions for adult emotional stability), to build an invisible, impenetrable wall of toughness around themselves, hidden by an emotional "mask" of masculine bravado or invulnerability, leaving them to experience a gamut of lonely painful problems in isolation. These problems can and do range from academic failure to drug abuse, from struggles with friends to abandonment depressions, and from attention-deficit/hyperactivity disorder to suicide and rage. Behind their masks of false invulnerability lie all their tender emotions, while in front we see the drama of action-orientation and the expression of the one full emotion they are "allowed" to express within the narrow bandwidth of developing masculinity, *anger*. Consequently it is often hard to hear young adult males' stifled but genuine voices of pain and struggle, their clamoring, their yearning for interpersonal re-connection—not only with large portions of their repressed selves within, but especially with the guiding adults who have all too often been fooled into believing that young adult males require "separation" to achieve psychological health. I have suggested this similar kind of *shame* that silences girls from expressing their voice as adolescents also takes a toll on young males (Pollack, 1998, 2000, 2006).

This classic model of boy socialization into young adulthood, which we have dubbed the "boy code" (Pollack, 1998), rests upon a premature and forced separation from the mother, all things maternal, and what in our society we have gender bifurcated as the "feminine," (i.e., all things nurturing, empathic, and bonded emotionally). This process is not only negative rather than positive in its developmental trajectory but also likely to create a premature traumatic separation, a *normative male-based developmental trauma,* leaving boys at risk for emotional maladjustment, everyday sadness, increased incidence of abandonment-like depression, and the potential for violence toward the self, suicide, as well as "commitment phobia" and rage toward others. These are all sequelae, which are the result of the profound dilemmas adolescent boys face when given that second push toward becoming a young adult male, symptomatic young adulthood that they enact before our eyes. As a result, young adult males (vs. females) engage in the lion's share of adolescent-based violence, yet the vast majority of their victims are also other young males. When added to the data on youth suicides in this age period in which males are four to six times more likely to take their own lives (National Center for Injury Prevention and Control, 2006;, Pollack, 2006a), it is not surprising that public health officials have come to see portions of the movement to young male adulthood as a major prevention challenge—which it is. Yet unlike SARS or tuberculosis, it is a challenge which we as a society, everyday, help to create: in our media images that support this code, in many of our schools, sports settings, too many of our homes, and unfortunately some of our academic training centers and consulting rooms.

What we have done to boys, even before they reach adolescence, and continue to do as they surge through young adulthood is a direct consequence of what the traditional psychological models of strength and so-called healthy development for males have emphasized. These models include the development of autonomy, separation, and individualistic coping styles, especially enforcing premature separation from nurture and an early silencing of boys' genuine expression of interdependent, humanly vulnerable self or "voice"—often beginning as early as ages 3 to 5 years (Pollack, 1995a, 1995b). Often representing core values of the dominant Caucasian Euro-American culture, this "boy code" (Pollack, 1998a, 2000a) shames young males toward extremes of self-containment, toughness, stoicism, and separation. It is a pervasive socialization system, which too often permeates traditional approaches to psychological assessments and treatment of young males. In turn, it shames our young males away from their emotional vulnerability, inter-dependence, and basic need for human connection, just when they need it most.

Through the all-too-well-known series of "boy code" admonitions to young males (especially as they enter into organized settings of growth such as schools and sports at approximately the ages of 4 to 5 years) such as: "Stand on your own two feet"; "Be a little man"; "Don't be a mamma's boy"; "Big boys don't cry!" "Don't act like a sissy"..."a wimp"..."a fag," we diminish the expression of their full biosocial emotional range. By these standards, therefore, too many boys self-critically judge themselves (and are judged) as immature, undeveloped, or deficient in intellectual/ emotional skills and failing an impossible test of masculinity. Young adult males are shamed away from exhibiting their normative characteristics of vulnerability, and they are thereby disconnected from healthy relations with each other, with potentially supportive adults, and from a full range of emotions within their own selves. And attempts to resist the "boy code" are met with cruel and endless additional shaming, a later predictor for failure to achieve mature happiness and a zest for life in young adulthood.

Unfortunately, as boys do reach beyond adolescence, even those who recognize the "box," as one young man in our studies called it, that they are locked within, they wonder about the futility of breaking out when their adult role models, especially other males, are engaging in more nuanced but equally damaging components of the same syndrome. Indeed, the young men in our research (Pollack, 1998a, 2006a) were acutely aware of how society constrains them. They particularly noticed how it holds back not just their peers but also the adult males in their midst. One young man whom I refer to here as Kevin (name concealed for confidentiality) from a working-class, predominantly Caucasian suburb of Los Angeles explained: "My father gets blocked. Like if he's upset about something at work, he can't say anything and I have no idea what he's thinking. He just sits in front of the TV, spends all his time on the Internet, or goes off on his own. He's just totally blocked." Unfortunately, when we encountered Kevin, he was in the process of beginning to use the same familiar, yet maladaptive coping mechanisms. And if we do not allow young men to express their painful emotions, even teach them how to re-connect with their sadness and to cry genuine tears, some will cry out with their fists or even bullets instead.

How then do we create more healthy, positive, and resilient visions of masculine developmental pathways? How do we promulgate and support new models for young men's developmental journeys that define what a "real boy/man" is, ones that include "mentoring," a new sense of courage, and "heroism," which is connection versus dominance or violence based? How do we find models that will allow young males to resist the demands of stereotypical and shaming homophobic gender stereotyping, bring them back into bonding with positive adult role models (of *both* genders), find true friendship with other males as well as females? How do we increase their capacity to express vulnerability and pain, without fear of being shamed, and re-connect them to the suppressed "voices" and spirituality deep within their souls?

These answers emerge from listening to the multiple pathways many young males are yearning to express and working to create them. This includes re-creating ongoing adult responsibility and bonding with younger males (recognizing what research has shown, i.e., that adult–adolescent bonding is a much more powerful force and positive vision for male youth than peer pressure will ever be) and integrating the modern findings of neurobiology into our modern psychologically based social-developmental frameworks and treatment interventions.

Let's begin first, briefly, with a new biological perspective, which emphasizes that both the males and females of the human species are "hardwired to connect" (See Pollack, 2004a). Yes, there are biological proclivities that distinguish males from females. Yes, there is evidence for young adult male neurobiological proclivity for risk taking. Yes, males engage in more rough-and-tumble activities. As academics and practitioners of all stripes, as true scientists, it behooves us to recognize these very real phenomena, which have too often been scotomas in our broader vision, or the basis of a senseless nature versus nurture argument. In so doing, however, we need not fall prey to the belief, for example, that male youth are naturally and *immutably doomed* to be more *violent* and less connected. Quite to the contrary, our most current findings suggest that biology supports both the malleability of gender difference in response to nurture contexts, as I will call them, and the species-, if not primate-specific need for bonding—the neurobiological requirement/urge to connect, which our young males need as much as the rest of us, and the fact that if this need is disrupted it may explain many young male impulsive and violent enactments which could otherwise be forestalled.

Bruce Perry (see Pollack, 1998, p.57), a premier neuroscientist in this arena has opined: "a child's capacity to think, to laugh, to love, to hate, to speak—all of it is a product of *interaction with the environment*. Sensory experiences such as touching... literally stimulate activity in the brain and the growth of neural structures" [Italics, mine]. Alan Schore places the central needs of developing children (read here as boys) within this context of emotional connection, which we adults must provide and which young males require for their health and resilience: "The idea is that we are born to form attachments, that our brains are physically wired to develop in tandem with another's, through emotional communication, before words are spoken. If things go awry, you're going to see the seeds of psychological problems, of difficulty coping, stress in human relations [emotional disturbances (... depression/ violence)] ... later on" (Schore, 2003). Schore is willing to go even further in stressing that no matter what the biological proclivities or temperamental differences, caretakers in caring support systems not only affect personality but also do so through direct impact upon neural development. Attachments formed within the matrix of a supportive adult context affect young males as people, via their developing brain structure: "the self organization of the developing brain occurs within the context of a relationship with another self, another brain. This relational context can be growth facilitating or growth inhibiting, and so it imprints into the developing ... brain either a resilience against or a vulnerability to forming later psychiatric disorders" (Schore, 2003). Dr. Ronald Dahl and others (Dahl, 2004) draw upon an extensive research corpus, which supports the hypothesis that these neurobiological developments are far from being completely mature in adolescence and that this phase of change continues at least through the period of young adult development, which in turn offers [both] special opportunities for intervention as well as distinct vulnerabilities, and forces us to re-think our social policies; and, I would add, our social responsiveness and treatment modalities as adult practitioners for our young male patients

So, therefore, if biology may underscore developmental vulnerability of the *boy code*, its findings also argue, I believe, for the potency of nurturant bonding, yes, even and, especially with male adolescents on their journey to young adulthood; as well as the significant impact adults (as well as peers) may exert upon this cohort group—including psychotherapists. Large demographic datasets do not disappoint us in supporting such hypotheses.

Here there is excellent correspondent support for the life-changing aspects of late adolescent/ young adult male bonding with nurturant adults in the larger demographic studies of Resnick and colleagues at the University of Minnesota National Longitudinal Study on Adolescent Health. I believe it is likely from their research in this arena (Resnick et al., 1997) that this chance for re-connection (especially with adult role models), and for honest emotional expression, will lead our young adult males to feel greater self-confidence, a clearer sense of positive self, diminished fear, and greater overall happiness, optimism, and personal as well as academic success. This will lead to diminished self-harm and depression, if we create for them, what our research has called "shame-free zones" (Pollack, 1998, 2003) of emotional connection within our society as well as our treatment paradigms.

Based upon a basic national survey of close to 100,000 adolescents and young adults, Resnick and his colleagues (1997) found that what affected their subjects' behaviors most were social contexts, but, again, not merely with peers but most especially the family, adults in parent-like roles, and connection to adults in school environments (who served in loco parentis) and its function of providing caring adult relationships in a sustaining context. According to the study, "parent–family connectedness" dramatically influences the level of emotional distress adolescents (and young adults suffer), their level of depression and suicidality, how much they abuse drugs and alcohol, and positive self-esteem. The study also showed other important factors that affect these behaviors, such as whether a then-adolescent boy's parents (significant attachment models) are present during key periods of the day or whether the parents have high or low expectations of his academic performance. But these factors paled in significance to the *connection factor*. Such connection, according to the study, involves "closeness to mother and/or father" and a sense of caring emanating from them, as well as "feeling loved and wanted by family members." Indeed, if one parenting (attachment) figure was positively present, these young people had two times the "protective" factors to sustain their health and well-being. If they felt "love" or affection from these parents, the protective factor rose to four times. If they felt connected to an adult who listened to their troubles in a schooling environment and felt they "fit in," again another four-time rise in protectiveness.

Now that we have re-empowered the significance of adult bonding with adolescent and young adult males as *essential*—not to unhealthy and atavistic developmental models of separation but, rather, to healthy individuation within the context of ongoing connection—we must listen to the voices of adolescent males, on the verge of young adulthood, speak for themselves.

In phases of the Listening to Boys Voices Project (see Pollack, 1998a, 1999, 2006a), we found the loneliness, isolation, depression, and bullying violence the "boy code" predicts. However, we also found the seeds of new positive young adult male developmental pathways in the yearnings, resistances, and models the subjects talked to us about, within the emotional "shame-free zones" we created for them. In particular, they talked about the sustaining qualities of genuine buddies, platonic friendships with girls/young women, and real mentors at times of need.

Modern Models of Young Male Resilient Mental Health

Indeed, a portion of our study results have allowed the young male subjects to report on those aspects of their lives that allow them to come out from behind the mask of false bravado and to re-connect with others with a full range of feelings within. The young men themselves began to report the markers of a new, genuine, *interdependent* model of male development: new rites of passage that deconstructed the boy code, resisted societal pressures of pathological independence (false, so-called self-sufficiency), and placed connection and the expression of vulnerable feelings at its center. Central components consisted of both same gender and cross-gender friendships; empathy and love as an antidote to disconnection; and adult/parent mentorship and bonding/ connection.

Though many young adult males stressed feelings of loneliness and disconnection, others emphasized the importance of having close friends, friends that "you can count on." It seems clear that—just as it seems to be true for young adult females—one's social standing as a male is very much affected by the quality and reliability of his friendships. When older subjects (ages 15 and above) were asked what advice they would give to younger boys, over and over again (100% of the sample), these young men urged the younger generation of boys to "*make special, trustworthy friends and hold onto them.*" For example:

"Make some close friends early . . . because people toss things around about you, and if you have a good friend they won't listen to that kind of thing. The friendships you have may be small in number but if they are good then they are strong."

"Don't let anyone push you around and stand up for yourself. Make a lot of friends."

"Don't waste time with people who aren't worth it. You can't be liked by everyone, so pick your friends wisely."

"Make friends and *keep them.*"

"When you're younger try to stay friends with different groups of kids. I think it's really helped me getting through . . . finding out what people are really like, not labeling."

"Don't get caught up with the wrong people. Respect your friends; they're what there is to fall back on. If you lose them you pretty much lose everything."

In addition, more than 50% of the time, their advice to these younger boys was "*be yourself,*" in other words; do not feel you need to force yourself into predetermined narrow roles, even by those you are close to. For instance:

"Go after what *you* want, don't just try to be liked by everyone."

"Explore all your options. Don't just get stuck doing the one thing everyone thinks is cool. Got to keep your options open."

A well-kept secret of adolescent males on their way to young adulthood, revealed as a consistent theme in these interviews, is that some of their most important and trusted friends are *girls and young women.* This does not appear to be pre-romantic activity (although some adults may mistake it as such) but rather solid friendship that appears to bring a sense of comfort and understanding to males. For example:

"Some of my best friends are girls. They really listen. We talk all the time . . . No sex stuff . . . more like a sister but even closer."

"With girls we do more like just talking and sharing about each other's problems. We like comfort each other."

"Over the past few years, I've developed friendships with girls. Girls give you a different point of view than a guy. They sometimes can be more sensitive with advice. When a guy gives you advice you get one half of the picture and when a girl gives you advice you get the other half of the picture. When you get advice from both sides you get the whole picture."

Young adult males were able to express a broad range of empathic, caring, and respectful feelings toward other young men, young women, and adults. For example:

> "I guess he's just always there. We always have conversations together and tell each other stuff that we don't tell other people. We're close in that way."
>
> "He knows how I feel, without asking me. Then, he'll try to cheer me up. We're real close."
>
> "When my mom is down, it hurts. Sometimes I'll try to kid her a little if her spirits are low. I owe my life to her; I want her to feel good."

Young males on their way to manhood also showed themselves to be eminently caring and loving but often likely to utilize modes of doing or "action empathy" (Pollack, 1998, 2000, 2006) other than mere words or directly expressed feelings. For example:

> "We don't say much, just [do things together], but he really understands me . . . He's there for me"
>
> "I'd do anything for him. He's my friend, That's what it's all about."
>
> "I pulled him out of the water quickly. It saved him. Why not, I love that guy—he's my best friend."

When asked who they considered to be their most important *mentors* and *heroes* (male or female) in their lives and why they look up to these individuals, over 75% of the adolescent boys on their journey to young adulthood identified mothers, fathers, grandparents, or older siblings. As one boy commented: "My mother is everything to me." Another explained: "My grandfather is my real hero. I only hope I can live up to his ideals." The consistency in these responses, of course, underscores the tremendous extent to which boys value and rely upon close relationships with adults and older supportive youth, especially young adult males (and that was a "two-way street") as attachment figures within a mental health enhancing rite of passage to adulthood.

It is my argument from our research group (see Pollack, 1999a, 2006a) and the epidemiological, psychobiological, and ethnographic data of others while the strong sway of this male developmental "guy code" may too often have been the case, it need not continue to be so. Indeed, young adult males are beginning to show us alternative, more positive visions of male development when we take the time to genuinely listen to their voices, to study and observe their behavior from the empathic perspective of coming from *within* their experience—individual and collective—rather than pre-defining it in a manner that creates what I have referred to as "gender straitjackets" for young males: inhibiting, narrowing, and psychologically suffocating models of so-called normalcy that many can only resist through actions, often not having the "voice" or language to do so, actions that too many adults later define as dysfunctional.

Given the socialization model of the boy code on the way to young adulthood, mental health for young males is achieved by providing ongoing uninterrupted connection with adult male role models who demonstrate through both action and talk a much wider breadth of healthy masculinity. "Boys no longer must be boys" who hit, hurt, or suffer silently if the definition of healthy young adult malehood eschews homophobia and separation as central to healthy adjustment.

The clinical vignette that began this chapter suggests to clinicians, especially, that of boys who have been touched by that "boy code," rather than pathologize it, one must create a haven of holding, "a shame-free zone" where long-suppressed vulnerable and sad feelings may emerge without the fear of a young male being retraumatized through shame and recognizing that true strength lies in connection not separation. To achieve this, all adults, including adult male therapists, must look within to the unconscious remnants of this code and extirpate them without either shaming themselves or their young adult patients. Then it will be a healthy connection that redefines the goal of mental health as well as mental health treatment for young adult males. Tis a consummation devoutly to be wished.

KEY POINTS

- Apparently healthy separation from adults in young adult males is actually a key factor in emotional disturbance
- Resilience for young adult males, just as for young adult females (through expressed in a different manner), comes from ongoing

connection to mentoring adult *connections* within their key environments
- Young adult males benefit substantially from psychotherapy, especially for the overt anger that covers over their attachment difficulties and covert depressions, if the treatment is modified sufficiently to deal with their socialization into the "boy code."

PRACTICE GUIDELINES

- Understand that gender differences in transitions from childhood to young adulthood exist, with girls and young women experiencing internalizing behaviors and disorders reflecting emotional lability or instability and boys and young men often projecting a more restricted emotional front.
- Recognize due to young males' "normative socialization" traumas that psychotherapy, in many cases, must shift to models of "action empathy" and recognition of our young adult male patients' need to deny their genuine dependence upon us for long periods of time.
- Realize that anger is sometimes the "emotional funnel" for a wider range of emotions in young males, most especially a male-type sense of depression/sadness resulting from premature disconnection to empathic figures in their early socialization patterns.
- Be on the lookout for "negative" and "angry" actions and wishes that may be early signs for a depressive syndrome and potential suicidal enactment (see Pollack, 2006).

References

Arnett, J. J. (2000). Emerging adulthood: A theory of development from the late teens through the twenties. *American Psychology, 44,* 469–480.

Behavioral Risk Factor Surveillance System. (2005). Prevalence data. Retrieved November 1, 2005, from http://apps.nccd.cdc.gov/brfss/

Brown, B. (2004). *Contemplating a state-level report featuring indicators of early adult well-being: Some theoretical and practical considerations.* Washington, DC: Child Trends.

Brown, B., Moore, K., & Bzostek, S. (2005). A portrait of well-being in early adulthood: A report to the William and Flora Hewlett Foundation. Retrieved November 1, 2005, from http://www.hewlett.org/Archives/Publications/portraitOfWellBeing.htm

Bureau of Justice Statistics. (2005a). Crime facts at a glance. Retrieved November 1, 2005, from http://www.ojp.usdoj.gov/bjs/glance/tables/vagetab.htm

Bureau of Justice Statistics. (2005b). Criminal victimization in the United States. 2002 statistical tables: National Crime Victimization Survey (NCJ 200561). Retrieved November 1, 2005, from http://www.ojp.usdoj.gov/bjs/pub/pdf/cvus02.pdf

Centers for Disease Control and Prevention. (2005). Youth risk behavior surveillance system. Retrieved on November 1, 2005, from http://apps.nccd.cdc.gov/yrbss

Center for Substance Abuse Prevention, Substance Abuse and Mental Health Services Administration. (2005). Alcohol and other drugs. Retrieved November 1, 2005, from http://preventionpathways.samhsa.gov/res_fact_drugs.htm

Child Trends. (2005). Original analysis of 2004 data from the American Community Survey. Requested and tabulated October 2005 [private data run]. Retrieved November 1, 2005, from http://www.census.gov/acs/www/

Dahl, R. (2004). Personal Communication.

Jekielek, S, & Brown, B. (2005). The transition to adulthood: Characteristics of young adults ages 18 to 24 in America. Retrieved November 1, 2005, from http://www.aecf.org/kidscount/pubs/transitionstoadulthood.pdf

Johnston, L. D., O'Malley, P. M., Bachman, J. G., & Schulenberg, J. E. (2005). Monitoring the future: National survey results on drug use, 1975–2004. Volume II: College students and adults ages 19–45 (NIH Publication No. 05-5728). Retrieved November 1, 2005, from http://monitoringthefuture.org/pubs/monographs/vol2_2004.pdf

Kessler, R. C., Berglund, P., & Demler O., et al. (2005). Lifetime prevalence and age-of-onset distributions of DSM-IV disorders in the National Co-Morbidity Survey replication. *Archives of General Psychiatry, 62*, 593–602.

National Center for Health Statistics. (2005). Health, United States, 2004. Retrieved November 1, 2005, from http://www.cdc.gov/nchs/hus.htm

National Center for Injury Prevention and Control. (2006). Fatal injury reports. Retrieved March 1, 2006, from http://www.cec.gov/ncipc/wisqars/

The Network on Transitions to Adulthood. (2005). The MacArthur Foundation. Retrieved November 1, 2005, from http://www.transad.pop.upenn.edu/

Park, M. J., Mulye, T. P., Adams, S. H., Brindis, C. D., & Irwin, C. E. (2006). The health of young adults in the United States. *Journal of Adolescent Health, 39*, 305–317.

Pollack, W. S. (1994). Engendered psychotherapy. Listening to the male and female voice. *Voices, The Art and Source of Psychotherapy, 30*(3), 43–47.

Pollack, W. S. (1995a). No man is an island: Toward a new psychoanalytic psychology of men. In R. Levant & W. Pollack (Eds.), *A new psychology of men* (pp. 33–67). New York: Basic Books.

Pollack, W. S. (1995b). Deconstructing disidentification: Rethinking psychoanalytic concepts of male development. *Psychoanalysis and Psychotherapy, 12*(1), 30–45.

Pollack, W. S. (1998a). *Real boys: Rescuing our sons from the myths of boyhood.* New York: Random House.

Pollack, W. S. (1998b). Mourning, melancholia, and masculinity: Recognizing and treating depression in men. In W. S. Pollack & R. F. Levant (Eds.). *New psychotherapy for men* (pp. 147–166). New York: Wiley.

Pollack, W. S. (1998c, August 30). Back to school: The hidden suffering of boys in the classroom [editorial]. *San Jose Mercury News,* Perspectives page.

Pollack, W. S. (1998d, September 6). How US schools are stifling male students [editorial]. *Sacramento Bee,* Forum page.

Pollack, W. S. (1999). The sacrifice of Isaac: A new psychology of boys and men. *SPSMM Bulletin, 4*, 7–14.

Pollack, W. S. (2000a). *Real boys' voices.* New York: Random House.

Pollack, W. S. (2000b). The Columbine syndrome: Boys and the fear of violence. *The National Forum, 80*(4), 39–42.

Pollack, W. S. (2001a). Preventing violence through family connection. *The Brown Child and Adolescent University Behavior Letter, 12,* 1–4.

Pollack, W. S. (2001b). *Real boys workbook.* New York: Random House.

Pollack, W. S. (2001c). New psychoanalytically treatment models for adult and young adult men. In G. R. Brooks & G. E. Good (Eds.), *The new handbook of psychotherapy and counseling with men* (pp. 527–543). San Francisco: Jossey Bass.

Pollack, W. S. (2001d). Suicide among adolescents [Foreword]. In J. Portner (Ed.) *One in thirteen* (pp. vii–xii). Beltsville, MD: Robins Lane Press.

Pollack, W. S. (2002). Suicide prevention in conjunction with ShowTime Presentation: Bang Bang You're Dead [video].

Pollack, W. S. (2003). Relational psychoanalytic treatment for young adult males. *Journal of Clinical Psychology, 59*(11), 1205–1213.

Pollack, W. S. (2004a). Parent–child connections: The essential component for positive youth development and mental health, safe communities, and academic achievement. *New Directions for Youth Development, 103*(Fall), 17–30.

Pollack, W. S. (2004b). "Real boys, "real" girls, "real" parents: Preventing violence through family connection. In R. H. Rozensky, N. G. Johnson, C. D. Goodheart, & W. R. Hammond (Eds.), *Psychology builds a healthy world* (pp. 35–47). Washington, DC: American Psychological Press.

Pollack, W. S. (2005). Sustaining and reframing vulnerability and connection: Creating genuine resilience in boys and young males. In S. G. Goldstein & R. Brooks (Eds.). *Handbook of resilience* (pp. 65–77). New York: Plenum.

Pollack, W. S. (2006a). The war for boys: Hearing their voices, healing their pain. *Professional Psychology: Research and Practice, 37*(2), 190–195.

Pollack, W. S. (with Gary Cohen) (2006b). *Real boys* (revised final 3rd ed.) [video]. New York: Halcyon Productions.

Pollack, W. S., & Levant, R. F. (Eds.) (1998). *New psychotherapy for men.* New York: Wiley.

Pollack, W. S., Modzeleski, W., & Rooney, G. (2008). *Prior knowledge of potential school based violence: Information students learn may prevent a targeted attack.* Washington, DC: United States Department of Education and United States Secret Service.

Resnick, M. D., Bearman, P. S., Blum, R. W., Bauman, K. E., Harris, K. M., Jones, J., Tabor, J., Beuhring, T., Sieving, R. E., Shew, M., Ireland, M., Bearinger, L. H., & Udry, J. R. (1997). Protecting adolescents from harm. *Journal of the American Medical Association, 278*(10), 823–832.

Rumbaut, R. G. (2005). Young adults in the United States: A profile. Philadelphia: The network on transitions to adulthood. Research Network Working Paper, No. 4, funded by the MacArthur Foundation. Retrieved March 1, 2005, from http://www.transad.pop.upenn.edu/news/wp.htm

Schore, A. N. (2003). *Affect dysregulation and the self.* New York: W.W Norton & Co.

Schulenberg, J., O'Malley, P. M., Bachman, J. G., & Johnston, L. (2005). Early adult transitions and their relations to well-being and substance use. In R. A. Settersten, F. F. Furstenburg, & R. G. Rumbaut (Eds.), *On the frontier of adulthood: Theory, research and public policy.* Chicago: University of Chicago Press.

Settersten, R. A, Furstenburg, F. F., & Raumbaut, R. G. (Eds.). (2005). *On the frontier of adulthood: Theory, research and public policy.* Chicago: University of Chicago Press.

Substance Abuse and Mental Health Services Administration (SAMHSA). (2004). Gender differences in substance dependence and abuse. The NSDUH report. Retrieved on October 29, 2004, from http://www.drugabusestatistics.samhsa.gov/2k4/genderDependence/genderDependence.cfm

Substance Abuse and Mental Health Services Administration (SAMHSA). (2005a). Results from the 2003 National Survey on Drug Use and Health: National findings (DHHS Publication No. SMA 04-3964). Retrieved November 1, 2005, from http://www.drugabusestatistics.samhsa.gov/nsduh.htm

Substance Abuse and Mental Health Services Administration (SAMHSA). (2005b). Substance use tables. Retrieved November 1, 2005, from http://www.icpsr.umich.edu/

Chapter 7

Cultural and Ethnic Considerations in Young Adult Mental Health

Declan T. Barry and Mark Beitel

Jiro,[a] a single Japanese immigrant male, was 23 years old when he presented at a Northwest Ohio university-based psychology clinic because of "difficulty concentrating...and slipping grades." At intake, he was formally attired in shirt and tie; his answers were brief and he maintained little eye contact. He came to the clinic upon the recommendation of his faculty advisor. Despite being an honors student in school and college in Japan and maintaining a perfect GPA in his first year of graduate school in the United States, he had experienced difficultly concentrating, especially while studying, during his second year in the United States and had failed a class in each of the previous two semesters. After graduating college in Japan 2 years previously, Jiro had moved to the United States to pursue a master's program in business and marketing; he sometimes felt lonely: he had no family members in the United States, except for a distant cousin on the East Coast, whom he had visited once since his arrival in the United States, and had no close friends. His family in Japan had not been informed about Jiro's academic problems because he did not wish to "burden" them. The clinician recommended a course of psychological testing to rule out cognitive and/or physiological deficits. Subsequently, the client was administered intellectual, achievement, and neuropsychological tests that indicated an IQ of 117 ("Superior range") and the absence of a learning disorder and neuropsychological impairment. Jiro was informed that his testing scores did not explain his difficulty concentrating; his clinician suggested that further psychological assessment focusing on Jiro's feelings and characteristic way of interacting with people might illuminate the reason(s) for his difficulty concentrating. After the clinician reviewed that people's psychological functioning may influence their ease or difficulty in concentrating and studying, Jiro agreed to further testing and was administered semi-structured clinical interviews for diagnosing Axis-I and Axis-II DSM-IV (American Psychiatric Association, 1994) psychiatric disorders. He was subsequently diagnosed with generalized anxiety disorder, mood disorder, not otherwise specified, and avoidant personality disorder features. Jiro was informed of the diagnosis; the clinician explained that his anxiety, mood, and characteristic style of interacting with people might, in part, explain his difficulty concentrating and studying. The clinician recommended that Jiro begin a course of psychotherapy so that he could learn additional skills to regulate his anxiety and mood, which would improve his ability to concentrate and study. Jiro agreed to initially participate in five sessions and then reconsider if he wished to proceed. Jiro completed a trial of 25 weekly

---

[a] The client's identifying information has been altered to protect his confidentiality. The first author of this chapter was Jiro's clinician. The cultural formulation presented in this vignette is based on the authors' research and may be useful in assessment and treatment. Components of this cultural assessment, which are often omitted from standard case formulations, will be discussed in this chapter.

sessions of individual psychotherapy, which largely comprised cognitive-behavioral and humanistic/experiential therapy interventions. In early sessions, Jiro exhibited a "marginalization" mode of acculturation (i.e., he largely avoided socializing and communicating with Americans and with Asian ethnic peers), a strong interdependent self-construal (i.e., self-concept is viewed as flexible, variable, and guided by external factors, such as roles, status, and relationships) accompanied by a weak independent self-construal (i.e., the self is viewed as a separate, stable, autonomous, and bounded entity), an attenuated Japanese/Asian ethnic identity (he reported shame concerning his ethnic background, attenuated sense of ethnic belonging, and an absence of ethnic pride), and concerns about intimacy (although Jiro had dated in college in Japan, he had not done so since his arrival in the United States). During treatment, Jiro began making friends with American, Japanese, and international students. The focus of earlier sessions involved prescribing assignments related to socializing and communication, and discussions regarding the patient's performance on these tasks. For example, Jiro was assigned a stepwise set of socialization/communication tasks; he tracked his thoughts and feelings before, during, and following each assignment. Examples of initial tasks were comprised of his asking one question in a particular class on a specific day and greeting one person at class on a particular day. Jiro was also instructed to limit the amount of time he spent in the library and studying (prior to attending therapy, he routinely spent more than 6 hours each weeknight studying and more than 8 hours per day on both Saturday and Sunday). The focus in later sessions was on identifying cognitions that appeared to influence Jiro's anxiety, mood, and style of interaction with others, including his initial strong traditional sex role identification (e.g., "A man should never show any weakness"), harsh self-criticism (e.g., "I am a failure, I have disgraced my family by failing in the United States"), perceived harsh criticism of others (e.g., "Americans just see me as a burned-out Asian geek"), and reduced empathy for others (e.g., "Chinese people are dirty, I keep away from them"), and involved examining the relative advantages/disadvantages of his assumptions and prescribing "homework" to test his cognitions/assumptions. The clinician continued to explain the rationale for therapy assignments and in-session interventions and focused on drawing the client's attention to his pre-existing strengths and then assisting him to harness and ameliorate them. Treatment ended with the mutual agreement of the patient and clinician. Jiro reported that he had received A's on all of his classes since beginning treatment, had experienced decreased difficulty studying, attenuated anxiety, improved mood, and increased enjoyment interacting with others. He started attending Asian and international student campus organizations and joined the softball team associated with his graduate program. He started dating a Japanese woman whom he had met in one of his classes. By the end of treatment, Jiro exhibited an integrated mode of acculturation (i.e., he socialized and communicated with Japanese and American individuals with comparable ease) and salient independent (i.e., self is viewed as a separate, stable, autonomous, and bounded entity) and interdependent self-construals (but weaker in comparison to treatment initiation). In comparison to pre-treatment, Jiro exhibited a stronger Japanese ethnic identity, specifically increased ethnic pride and sense of belonging, a stronger egalitarian sex-role ideology, and increased desire for and less anxiety concerning intimacy.

Introduction

Humans have a proclivity for classifying and grouping information (Bartlett, 1932; Fiske, 1993). Mental health professionals often group information about patients based on age. For example, psychiatrists and clinical psychologists often specialize in treating patients belonging to particular age groups, including childhood, adolescence, adulthood, and late adulthood. This is not surprising given that members of certain age groups may face unique developmental tasks (e.g., autonomy in childhood) and may be more prone to exhibit specific psychiatric disorders (e.g., depression in adulthood). Some researchers have drawn attention to specific age periods because of their putative role in subsequent human development and mental health; for example, childhood has been conceptualized as a "critical" or "sensitive" developmental period (e.g., Bowlby, 1988; Freud, 1923/1960). One of the purposes of the current volume is to draw attention to mental health issues pertaining to "young adulthood" (i.e., the period between 18 and 29 years).

Lodged between adolescence with its focus on identity development and older adulthood with its focus on generativity, young adulthood has received relatively little attention as a developmental stage. As a stage, young adulthood was outlined by Erikson (1950/1963). He saw the major challenges of this stage in terms of overcoming *isolation* in favor of *intimacy* with friends and romantic partners. The newly consolidated identity, forged in adolescence, must find a way to connect with others in healthy and sustainable ways. The action, therefore, in young adulthood centers around *affiliation* with others: One's social circle widens and one has more control than ever before over the type and frequency of social contacts. Certainly, in the United States, one's potential network widens tremendously as the legally autonomous young adult typically goes off to college, to work, and/or to military service. Young adulthood, then, provides the necessary training and social contacts to prepare one for life's next developmental crisis—generativity versus stagnation in later adulthood.

From an Eriksonian perspective, the developmental task of young adulthood is to achieve *intimacy* with the people one meets. If all goes well, then the psychosocial crisis is resolved favorably and the virtue of *love* develops. Healthy rituals in this stage involve parties with friends as well as dating and, subsequently, marriage. The pathology of this stage has to do with *elitism* and *exclusivity*, forming rigid and unhealthy attachments with a select few. Should things go poorly, and the developmental milestones are not met, isolation is likely to occur.

In recent years, mental health professionals have increasingly recognized the role of cultural factors in the diagnosis and treatment of mental disorders (Lewis-Fernandez & Kleinman, 1995). The Diagnostic and Statistical Manual (DSM-IV-TR; American Psychiatric Association, 2000)—the predominant U.S. psychiatric classification system—now includes sections related to capturing patients' cultural contexts, including a general introductory cultural statement, information concerning cultural considerations for the use of diagnostic categories and criteria, a listing of culture-bound syndromes and idioms of distress, and a suggested outline for a cultural formulation. In 2001, the U.S. Department of Health and Human Services (DHHS) issued a supplement to the Surgeon General's report on mental health that underscored the role of ethnicity and race in accounting for several disparities in mental health care in the United States, including limited access to effective mental health services for Americans of ethnic and racial minority descent compared with those of European descent. Researchers have also highlighted the importance of attending to gender differences nested within cultural variables (Barry & Grilo, 2002; Johnson & Glassman, 1998) and patients' gender when attempting to individualize treatment for ethnic/racial minority individuals (U. S. Department of Health and Human Services, 2001). This chapter discusses issues related to cultural and ethnic considerations pertaining to young adult mental health and offers practice recommendations for clinicians who work with young adult patients of ethnic/racial minority descent.

Ethnicity, Race, and Mental Health Research

Young adults, similar to humans of all ages, function within a specific cultural milieu and thus, depending on their geographic location, are exposed to cultural norms that differ from their counterparts in other parts of the world (Hofstede & Bond, 1984; Wan, Chiu, Peng, & Tam, 2007). Furthermore, in any multicultural society, young adults from different ethnic/racial groups may be exposed to varying cultural norms regarding parameters of appropriate behavior, including help-seeking behaviors (Cauce et al., 2002). However, considerable debate exists concerning the key ingredients of culture and the extent to which it affects human behavior (Brislin, 1993; Greenfield, Keller, Fuligni, & Maynard, 2003; Segall, Lonner, & Berry, 1998). Culture has been defined as "the man-made part of the environment" that is comprised of accepted behaviors, beliefs, and institutions that exhibit great variability but which make sense to its members (Herskovits, 1948). Individuals use culture as a lens to filter information and to make sense of the world, other people, and themselves (Barry & Bullock, 2001). Culture may also act as a buffer to minimize human awareness of vulnerability (Solomon, Greenberg, & Pyszcynski, 1991) and may satiate our basic human need to belong (Baumeister & Leary, 1995). Although many authors draw attention to the importance of culture, its usefulness as an explanatory concept in examining psychological phenomena resides in the investigator's ability to "unpackage" or deconstruct it (Poortinga, van de Vijver, Joe, & Koppel, 1989; Whiting, 1976). Mental health researchers have traditionally deconstructed culture by using two categorical variables: ethnicity and race.

Ethnicity is a sociodemographic designation that is commonly used by mental health professionals to classify young adults and other individuals. Betancourt and Lopez (1993) note that ethnicity is typically used to assign group membership based on cultural, nationality, or linguistic factors. Race was initially viewed as a biological classification based on shared, fixed, immutable inborn traits (e.g., skin color) that could predictably categorize individuals into mutually exclusive groups. It is important to consider the history and origin of the construct of race when discussing possible racial differences in mental health outcomes (Smedley & Smedley, 2005). Many scientists in the 1800s and 1900s employed an essentialist approach to argue that traits, such as morality and intelligence, could be hierarchically arranged by racial group membership with Caucasians comprising the apex (e.g., Porteus, 1926). This position was used to justify government-sanctioned discrimination of racial minority group members, including young adults (Davenport, 1923). Increased public criticism of race-based research, especially in the civil rights era, coupled with researchers' inability to identify putative biological markers of race resulted in its decreased use (Owens & King, 1999); instead of race differences, researchers increasingly examined constructs such as socioeconomic status (Takeuchi & Gage, 2003). However, in recent years, the human genome investigation has revitalized interest in the genetic foundations of race (Collins, 2004; Henig, 2004). Decisions about the inclusion/exclusion criteria of ethnicity and race occur within a sociopolitical context and are as much based on domestic and foreign policy concerns of their day as they are on scientific or anthropological data (Takeuchi & Gage, 2003; Yanow, 2003).

In the 1970s, the U.S. Federal Government issued a directive to standardize census data collection efforts that were, in part, required by the Voting Rights Act and affirmative action (U.S. Office of Management and Budget [OMB], 1978). Revisions by the OMB in 1997 resulted in the inclusion of six racial categories in the Census 2000: American Indian or Alaska Native (AIAN), Asian, Native Hawaiian and Other Pacific Islander, black or African American, white, and "Some Other Race." Census 2000 also employed two categories for ethnicity: Hispanic or Latino and Not Hispanic or Latino, with the stipulation that Hispanics or Latinos may be of any race. The existence of such ethnic and racial group categories facilitates intergroup comparison on different indicators, including mental health and mental illness, and has been instrumental in documenting mental health disparities among young adults (see Mays, Ponce, Washington, & Cochran, 2003).

Ethnicity, Race, and Mental Health Disparities

Beginning in the 1970s, Stanley Sue and colleagues (1974, 1978) began documenting that extant mental health systems in the United States were not adequately serving the needs of ethnic and racial minority groups. The landmark 1985 DHHS report of the Secretary's Task Force on Black and Minority Health documented a disparity in a variety of health indicators (e.g., hospital admissions, physician visits) among ethnic and racial minority groups. Epidemiological findings concerning significant differences in morbidity and mortality between ethnic and racial groups focused attention on health disparities (Hummer, Benjamins & Rogers, 2004); this area has become a major priority for federal health research funding (National Institutes of Health, 2002), and the eradication of ethnic/race health disparities is one of the cardinal goals of the Department of Health and human Service's Healthy People 2010 initiative (U. S. Department of Health and Human Services, 2000). Differences in access to effective mental health services across ethnic and racial groups (i.e., mental health disparities) have also garnered increased research attention. In particular, two issues have shaped the debate surrounding mental health disparities: comparative prevalence rates of psychiatric disorders and comparative rates of mental health service utilization. We now address these issues as they pertain to young adults from ethnic/racial minority backgrounds.

In the 2000 U.S. Census, 4.1 million Americans (1.5%) identified themselves as American Indian or Alaska Native (AIAN) solely or in combination with one or more ethnic/racial categories; 755,680 were young adults (U.S. Census Bureau, 2002). Similar to African Americans, AIAN young adults are disproportionately represented in at-risk populations, including those with low socioeconomic status and those with low education level (U. S. Department of Health and Human Services, 2001). Although large epidemiological and randomized controlled trials have advanced the field of mental health, information regarding AIAN status has traditionally not been measured, or has been measured in such small numbers to obviate relevant statistical analyses (Manson, 2003). In order to address such gaps in the literature, the American Indian Service Utilization, Psychiatric Epidemiology, Risk and Protective Factors Project (AI-SUPERPFP) was conducted on two American Indian reservation populations (Southwest and Northern Plains tribes). The lifetime prevalence of having any DSM-IV (American Psychiatric Association, 1994) psychiatric disorder was approximately 42% for both tribes. In comparison to those older than 44 years, participants aged 15 to 24 years were at higher risk for substance use disorders compared with no disorder [odds ratio (OR) 1.5, $p < .001$)] and depressive and/or anxiety disorders (OR 2.1, $p < .01$) (Beals et al., 2005). In comparison to other population-based psychiatric epidemiology studies, alcohol use disorders and PTSD were more common in the two American Indian populations. Alcohol use disorders in both tribes were significantly associated with increased likelihood of liver problems/pancreatitis, head injuries, hearing problems, and vision problems (Shore et al., 2006). Members of both tribes exhibited a style of drinking, characterized as high quantity, low frequency (O'Connell et al., 2006). Furthermore, lifetime exposure to at least one trauma (62.4%–67.2% among men and 66.2%–69.8% among women) was common; in comparison to results of the National Comorbidity Survey, men and women from both tribes were more likely to report that they witnessed trauma, including trauma to loved ones, and they were often victims of physical attacks (Manson, Beals, Klein, & Croy, 2005). Whereas trauma in the general population has been found to peak between the ages of 16 and 20 years (Breslau et al., 1998), no age difference emerged until the 45 to 54 year age range, when lifetime prevalence of trauma declined among members of the Southwest tribe (Manson et al., 2005). In addition to alcohol use disorders and posttraumatic stress disorder, American Indians appear to have elevated rates of suicide and suicide attempts. Suicide is the second and third leading causes of death among AIAN groups aged 15 to 24 years and 25 to 44 years, respectively (Centers for Disease Control and Prevention, 2003; Indian Health Service, 2000–2001).

In the 2000 U. S. Census, 10.2 million (3.6%) of the population identified themselves as Asian and approximately 400,000 (0.1%) identified themselves as Native Hawaiian and Other Pacific Islander (U.S. Census Bureau, 2002). Of these respective groups, 2,119,653 and 89,732 were young adults. While Census 2000 distinguished Asian and Native Hawaiian and Other Pacific Islander, most of the relevant mental health research on these populations has used the term "Asian American and Pacific Islander" (AAPI). In contrast to other ethnic/racial minority groups, AAPI have traditionally been characterized as "a model minority" who rarely use mental health services because of purported low rates of psychopathology (Hu, Snowden, Jerrell, & Nguyen, 1991). More recently, the "myth of the model minority" has been disputed (Association of Asian Pacific Community Health Organizations, 1995). One of the few epidemiologic studies to examine prevalence rates of psychiatric disorders among AAPI found that lifetime prevalence rates for major depression (6.9%) and dysthymia (5.2%) among Chinese Americans in Los Angeles were much lower than those reported for whites in the National Comorbidity Survey (Kessler et al., 1994; Takeuchi et al., 1998). Young adults were significantly less likely to have experienced a mood disorder than those aged 50 to 65 years. Studies to date indicate that AAPI are less likely than whites to use mental health services (Matsuoka, Breaux, & Ryujin, 1997; Zhang, Snowden, & Sue, 1998). A study of Chinese, Japanese, and Korean immigrants in the United States, the majority of whom were young adults, found that men were significantly less willing than women to use psychological services or to recommend such services to distressed friends (Barry & Grilo, 2002). Findings from the National Latino and Asian American Study (NLAAS; Alegria et al., 2004; Heeringa, 2004) indicate that foreign-born Asian Americans are significantly less likely to seek mental health services than their U.S.-born counterparts (Abe-Kim et al., 2007). The prevalence of psychiatric disorders among Asian Americans is associated with higher rates of perceived discrimination (Gee, Spencer, Chen, Yip, & Takeuchi, 2007). Assessment of psychiatric problems in AAPI young adults is further complicated because DSM-IV (American Psychiatric Association, 1994) diagnostic categories and AAPI indigenous labels of subjective distress may not correspond well. Unlike Western medicine, some Asian cultures have not traditionally dichotomized body and mind; this characteristic, coupled with reticence regarding emotional expression, may result in exclusive reporting of somatic symptoms (Lin & Cheung, 1999). However, the finding that Asian Americans may have difficulty identifying psychological symptoms is not unequivocal (Chun, Enomoto, & Sue, 1996). Conclusions about prevalence rates of psychiatric disorders and mental health utilization rates in young AAPI adults are difficult to make given the relative paucity of relevant large-scale epidemiological studies.

In the 2000 U.S. Census, 34.7 million Americans (12.3%) identified themselves as black or African American; 6.4 million were young adults (U.S. Census Bureau, 2002). While the prevalence rates of psychiatric disorders for African Americans who live in the community parallel those of European Americans, many more African American young adults belong to at-risk groups (e.g., homeless, incarcerated) that typically have higher rates of psychopathology (U. S. Department of Health and Human Services, 2001). In comparison to Caucasian and Hispanic individuals aged 18 to 23, African Americans are more likely to report having been shot or shot at or knowing someone who was killed (Turner & Lloyd, 2004). One area of clinical concern is the escalating suicide rate among young African Americans, especially males (ages 15 to 19), which according to one estimate increased 70% between 1979 and 1997 (Joe & Kaplan, 2001).

Two national surveys—The National Ambulatory Medical Care Survey (NAMCS) and The National Hospital Ambulatory Medical Care Survey (NHAMCS)—have played a pivotal role in documenting health care disparities in the United States. Both surveys were designed to collect information about the provision and use of ambulatory medical care services—one in primary care settings (NAMCS), the other in hospital emergency and outpatient departments (NHAMCS). Snowden and Pingitore (2002), using data from the 1997 NAMCS data, found that African Americans were more likely to seek mental health care from primary care physicians than psychiatrists and were less likely to receive psychotropic medications from primary care providers. Among those aged 15–24 (data was not provided on young adults), the rates of visits for a mental health reason to a primary care physician and a psychiatrist were 10% and 5% for African Americans and 6% and 8% for Caucasians, respectively. In a separate analysis of NAMCS and NHAMCS databases regarding prescription of atypical antipsychotic medications from 1992 through 2000, Daumit et al. (2003) found that whereas African Americans and Hispanics were significantly less likely than whites to receive an atypical antipsychotic medication in the early 1990s, by the end of the decade, there was no disparity between Hispanics and whites across psychiatric diagnoses; however, the adjusted odds of African Americans receiving these medications in visits specified for psychotic disorders was still 25% lower than whites. Atypical antipsychotic medications (e.g., olanzapine, risperidone) appear to be more effective than traditional antipsychotic medications for negative symptoms of psychosis and carry fewer serious adverse side effects (Kapur & Remington, 2000). Richardson, Anderson, Flaherty, & Bell (2003) examined racial differences in psychosocial and pharmacotherapy interventions from the 1997 NHAMCS and found that after controlling for diagnosis and other factors, African Americans were more likely to receive pharmacotherapy and less likely to receive psychotherapy than were whites. A higher proportion of African Americans in the 16–29 age range made visits to a hospital for depression-related reasons than among their white counterparts.

According to the U.S. Census Bureau (2003), the Hispanic population rose from approximately 22 million (9.1%) in 1990 to 39 million (13.4%) in 2003 and now outnumbers the African American population. In the 2000 Census, 8.1 million Hispanics were young adults. Mexican Americans, many of whom are immigrants, comprise the largest Hispanic subgroup in the United States. Two large-scale epidemiological studies have examined the mental health status of Mexican Americans: Los Angeles, California, site of the Epidemiologic Catchment Area (LAECA; Burnam, Hough, Karno, Escobar, & Telles, 1987) and the Mexican American Prevalence and Services Survey (MAPSS; Vega et al., 1998). Both studies found higher rates of anxiety, mood, and substance use disorders among U.S.-born relative to foreign-born Mexican Americans. More recently, Grant and co-workers (2004), using data from the National Epidemiologic Survey on Alcohol and Related Conditions (NESARC; Grant, Moore, Shephard, & Kaplan, 2003), found that Mexican Americans were at significantly lower risk than U.S.-born non-Hispanic whites of psychiatric morbidity; foreign-born Mexican Americans and foreign-born non-Hispanic whites were at significantly lower risk of DSM-IV mood, anxiety, and substance use disorders than their U.S.-born counterparts. Lifetime rates of major depressive disorder (MDD) were lower among young adults in comparison to those aged 45–64 (Hasin, Goodwin, Stinson, & Grant, 2005). Hispanic, Asian, and African American racial/ethnic group membership was associated with decreased risk of MDD, whereas Native American racial group membership was associated with increased risk.

Another nationally representative survey National Latino and Asian American Study (NLAAS; Alegria et al., 2004; Heeringa, 2004) examined prevalence rates of psychiatric disorders and mental health utilization among four Hispanic ethnic subgroups: "Cuban," "Mexican," "Puerto Rican," and "Other Latino." The prevalence of depressive, anxiety, and substance use disorders and mental health service use among Puerto Ricans was significantly higher ($p < .05$) than among the other Latino ethnic subgroups (Alegria et al., 2007a, 2007b). The prevalence of past year psychiatric disorders did not differ significantly among those aged 18–34 (16.5%), 35–49 (14.3%), 50–64 (14.2%), and 65 or higher (14.2%). Higher rates of psychiatric disorder and mental health service use were observed for U.S.-born third-generation Latino Americans in comparison to immigrants.

The National Epidemiologic Survey on Alcohol and Related Conditions (NESARC; Grant et al., 2004), sponsored by the National Institute on Alcohol Abuse and Alcoholism (NIAAA), is perhaps the most comprehensive epidemiologic study that has examined the prevalence rates of *Diagnostic and Statistical Manual*, fourth edition (DSM-IV; APA, 1994) psychiatric disorders among African American, Asian, Caucasian, Hispanic, and Native American respondents aged 18 and older. The NESARC, conducted between 2001 and 2002, comprised a nationally representative face-to-face survey of 43,093 civilian noninstitutionalized adult respondents. Overall, American Indians reported the highest rate of each psychiatric disorder and Asian Americans, the lowest (Huang et al., 2006). The respective rates of mood disorder, anxiety disorder, and personality disorder for American Indians (15.3%, 15.3%, 24.1%) were significantly higher than those among African Americans (8.8%, 10.4%, 16.6%), Asians (7.4%, 6.9%, 10.1%), Caucasians (9.4%, 11.7%, 14.6%), and Hispanics (8.0%, 8.8%, 14.0%).

In addition to examining prevalence rates, it may also be important to consider the strength of the association between different psychiatric disorders for different ethnic/racial groups when considering potential ethnicity/race-based disparities. For example, Huang et al. (2006) found noticeable disparities in the co-occurrence of psychiatric disorders among specific race/ethnic subgroups in the NESARC; whereas the association between alcohol use disorder and mood disorder among African Americans (OR = 3.5) was significantly stronger than that among Caucasians (OR = 2.0), the association between alcohol use disorder and personality disorder among Asians (OR = 5.0) was significantly greater than among African Americans (OR = 2.5), Caucasians (OR = 1.9), and Native Americans (OR = 1.7). A different examination of the NESARC revealed that alcohol dependence was significantly associated with most anxiety disorders among African Americans, Asians, and Caucasians, but not among American Indians (Smith et al., 2006). A greater understanding of potentially different patterns of psychiatric comorbidities among young adult members of ethnic/racial groups may help mental health specialists target their clinical interventions.

Research on health care disparities has also highlighted potential differences in delays in treatment seeking and in the quality of care received by members of ethnic/racial minority groups. The NSC-R examined delays in treatment seeking and odds of ever making treatment contacts among African Americans, Caucasians, and Hispanics. In comparison to Caucasians, African Americans and Hispanics reported significantly longer delays and lower odds of ever making treatment contact (Wang et al., 2005). Among those who received mental health treatment in the prior year, African American status was negatively associated with service use. In the National Survey of American Life, which included information on 3,570 African Americans, young adults were less likely to obtain services in response to mental health problems than those aged 30–60 and women were more likely to seek mental health services than men (Neighbors et al., 2007). In the Community Tracking Study, a nationally representative survey of 1,636 civilian, non-institutionalized adults conducted during 1997 and 1998, the minority (30.4%) of those with a probable depressive or anxiety disorder received at least 1 appropriate treatment for their disorder. Of the different age groups examined, those between 18 and 29 years old were least likely to have received appropriate care (standardized prediction was 20%). The standardized prediction of appropriate care was higher for Caucasians (34%) than for African Americans (17%) and Hispanics (24%) (Young et al., 2001). More detailed information regarding delays in onset of treatment for specific disorders across ethnic/racial groups might facilitate the development of more targeted mental health treatments and public health interventions. The relatively short delays in treatment seeking found for respondents with mood disorders in the NSC-R may be, in part, attributable to educational programs and quality improvement programs in primary care settings (Wang et al., 2005).

Substance Use Disorders in Young Adulthood

Substance use disorders deserve special attention in any discussion of cultural considerations pertaining to psychiatric disorders in young adulthood. Data from the 2005 National Survey on Drug Use and Health (NSDUH, 2005; Substance Abuse and Mental Health Services Administration, 2006) suggest that young adulthood is associated with the highest rates of illicit drug use in the past month. The rates of current drug use for adults aged 18–20, 21–25, and 26–29 were 22.3%, 18.7%, and 12.9%, respectively. The rate of heavy alcohol use (i.e., five or more alcoholic beverages on the same occasion on each of 5 or more days in the last 30 days) was 15.3% for individuals aged 18 to 25. Furthermore, the rate of driving under the influence of alcohol was highest among adults aged 21–25 (27.9%), followed by those aged 26–29 (22.6%) and 18–20 (19.8%), respectively. In the NESARC, the prevalence of alcohol use and dependence for men and women was highest among adults aged 18 to 29 (i.e., young adults). Among young adults who self-identified as African American, Asian, Caucasian, Hispanic, and Native American, respective prevalence rates of alcohol abuse were 6.9%, 4.8%, 10.2%, 9.1%, and 15.3% among men and 2.1%, 3.9%, 5.6%, 3.0%, and 6.7% for women (Grant et al.,

2004). Drawing on the 1995 and 2000 NIAAA-sponsored National Alcohol Survey, which oversampled African Americans (n = 1,341) and Hispanics (n = 869), Schmidt, Greenfield, and Bond (2007) found that compared with Caucasians, African Americans and Hispanics with more severe alcohol problems were significantly less likely to have received alcohol treatment. Among those with an alcohol use disorder, young adults were about half as likely as those aged 30 or higher to have used alcohol services, and African Americans and Hispanics were less likely than Caucasians to have utilized such services. In particular, Hispanics as compared to Caucasians were less likely to have received professional substance abuse treatment. Hispanics cited financial and logistical barriers to services, including lack of knowledge about how to locate services, lack of financial resources, and inability to obtain child care. The increase in racial/ethnic minority young adults attending college may have exposed them to binge and heavy drinking, which appear to be common among college students in the United States (National Center for Education Statistics, 2005; Wechsler et al., 2002).

Three-Factor Approach

Whereas ethnicity and race-based categories have been useful in drawing attention to mental health care disparities in the overall American population (Mays et al., 2003), the degree to which these categories are useful to mental health practitioners is debatable. Not only is there controversy over whether ethnicity and race may be social constructs that do not accurately capture the differences between Americans (Williams, 1994, 1997), the common practice of attributing putative cultural, biological, or social etiologies to reported ethnicity/race-based differences on psychosocial functioning measures is flawed; rather than inferring such causation, it is incumbent on mental health researchers to measure putative causal variables directly (Barry & Garner, 2001). To illustrate this point, consider the categorization of Asian American and Pacific Islander (AAPI)—a term used by many mental health professionals—whose members comprise 43 ethnic groups and speak over 100 languages. The extent of shared heritage, values, rituals, and traditions between individuals of Filipino and Pakistani descent, for example, is debatable, as is any assumption that differences on psychosocial functioning found between men from these two groups can (without testing) be attributed to cultural, biological, or social causation (see Foster & Sharp, 2002; Lee, Mountain & Koenig, 2001; Shields et al., 2005). Problems with solely relying on categorical measures of culture, such as ethnicity and race, have prompted researchers to recommend that (similar to the notion of culture itself) the constructs of ethnicity and race should be deconstructed. Phinney (1996) outlined three dimensions of ethnicity/race: cultural values and norms; salience and meaning of ethnic or racial identity; and experiences associated with ethnic/racial minority status. Barry and colleagues (Barry & Beitel, 2006; Barry, Bernard, & Beitel, 2006; Barry, Elliott, & Evans, 2000; Barry & Garner, 2001) have outlined a three-factor model to better assist mental health clinicians and researchers in deconstructing the concept of culture. The three factors—acculturation, self-construal, and ethnic identity—are cultural variables that have been shown to be related to human psychosocial functioning among individuals of ethnic/racial minority status (Berry, 1980; Markus & Kitayama, 1991; Phinney, 1996; Singelis, Bond, Sharkey, & Li, 1999).

Acculturation, self-construal, and *ethnic identity* provide mental health professionals who work with young adults from diverse ethnic/racial backgrounds a dimensional approach to examining culture. This approach acknowledges that culture is not static but rather dynamic and complex, and it may provide a more differentiated measure of culture than such categorical variables as race and ethnicity (Barry & Garner, 2001; Barry & Grilo, 2002). These three factors allow researchers and clinicians to directly measure issues related to culture rather than inferring them in a post-hoc fashion based on findings related to ethnicity/race differences (Barry & Garner, 2001; Barry & Grilo, 2003). A brief overview of the three components follows.

Acculturation encompasses social interaction and communication styles that individuals adopt when interacting with individuals and groups from another culture (Barry & Garner, 2001). It comprises competence and ease/comfort in communicating with both ethnic/racial group peers and out-group members. Communication difficulty resulting from cultural differences between ethnic/racial minority patients and their providers has been associated with underutilization of and unwillingness to use health care services (Barry & Grilo, 2002; Ma, 1999). The process and outcome of acculturation may also influence how symptoms are expressed and, in turn, subsequent entry into or use of the mental health system (Aponte & Barnes, 1995). Berry's (1980) scheme may be used to classify socialization and communication patterns: *assimilation* for socialization and communication primarily with individuals from the majority culture, *separation* for socialization and communication primarily with ethnic/racial peers, *integration* for socialization and communication with members of both minority and majority cultural groups, and *marginalization* for absence of socialization and communication with ethnic/racial minority peers or majority culture members.

Acculturation is a central feature of "being with others" for ethnic minorities in any culture and presents an added complication of psychosocial development with which majority members simply do not have to contend. Many cultural minority members deal with physical and emotional *isolation* on a daily basis. Partly as a consequence of their physical relocation and entrance into another culture, immigrants are at high risk for isolation and may present for treatment with this issue—much as Jiro did (described in the clinical vignette). Cultural minority members make choices, and have choices imposed upon them, about the nature and extent of social contact with majority and minority group members. For minority members, this state of affairs adds to the complexity of establishing *intimacy* with others. In general, one's cultural minority status confers a variety of advantages and disadvantages in the quest for psychosocial development. With respect to the core psychosocial task of young adulthood, a likely consequence is that the psychosocial work of *affiliation* may be compromised, thereby increasing the risk for developmental problems. An added complication may be the degree of discord between majority and minority rituals of affiliation. For example, the minority culture may have strong guidelines for in-group/out-group relationships (e.g., dating/marriage) and/or the majority culture may harbor stereotypes and prohibitions against minority affiliations. One potential outcome is that the psychosocial virtue of *love* may be more difficult to attain. The pathology of *elitism* may be chosen, or fallen back upon as a default stance, and/or may be foisted upon the cultural minority member. Unfortunately, elitism and/or isolation will limit one's abilities to thrive in the next stage of adult generativity.

Self-construal refers to two types of self-concept, independent and interdependent, which appear to be linked to the degree to which one's culture makes a distinction between the individual and the group (Markus & Kitayama, 1991). Variations in self-construal may influence recognition and reporting of psychiatric symptoms, communication styles, and use of mental health services (Lin & Cheung, 1999; Oetzel, 1998; Yeh, 1999). Independent self-construal refers to a self that is viewed as a separate, stable, autonomous, and bounded entity, whereas interdependent self-construal is described as flexible, variable, and guided by external factors such as roles, status, and relationships. Americans of ethnic/racial minority status may differ from those of European descent in terms of the salience of their self-construals. For example, Asian Americans, unlike Americans of European descent, tend to have more salient interdependent rather than independent self-construals (Chung, 1992).

The psychosocial construct of self-construal is also intimately linked with the psychosocial tasks and perils of young adulthood. Self-construal itself may be viewed as an identity development process, the bulk of whose work gets done in the previous psychosocial stage of adolescence. However, its attainment may promote or inhibit the work of young adulthood. For example, a strong sense of interdependence may facilitate *affiliation* and reduce *isolation* within one's circle of like-minded group members. It may be a more complicating factor when relating to out-group members with strong independent self-construal orientations. Cultural minority members espousing interdependent self-construal models may find that they are required to do *identity* work as they acculturate in addition to the difficult psychodevelopmental work of *intimacy* attainment.

The third factor—*ethnic identity*—may be a more useful psychological construct than ethnicity (Phinney, 1996). Ethnic identity may be viewed as the ethnic component of social identity, defined by Tajfel (1981) as: "that part of an individual's self-concept which derives from his knowledge of his membership of a social group (or groups) together with the value and emotional significance attached to that membership" (p. 255). Ethnic identity has been identified as an important cultural variable in examining psychosocial functioning and health care utilization among ethnic/racial minority young adults (Brinson & Kottler, 1995; Pillay, 2005).

Ethnic identity is certainly a vital part of general *identity* development, and much work in this area gets done in adolescence. Ethnic identity commitments guide the nature and extent of intimate contacts and affiliations, as well as their attendant ritual manifestations, for example, dating/marriage. While a strong and consolidated ethnic identity confers many advantages, it is easy to generate a list of potential drawbacks. To begin with, the psychosocial virtue of *love* may be *pathologically* ascribed to one's ethnic group, leading to the pathologies of *elitism* and *exclusivity*, which are likely to cause development difficulties as well as larger societal problems, for example, racism, nationalism, etc.

Models of Mental Illness

Attending to patients' cultural norms is an important component of diagnosing mental health disorders. Kleinman, among others, has highlighted the importance of examining explanatory models (i.e., patients' perception of the etiology and nature of their presenting symptoms and disorders) in arriving at valid diagnoses and in developing optimal treatment recommendations (Kleinman & Benson, 2006). Culture-based attributions regarding mental illness may influence help-seeking behaviors of young adults and their family members. For example, among family members of patients with schizophrenia attending a teaching hospital in India, those who reported that mental illness was a function of spirits typically viewed traditional healers as the providers of choice (Banerjee & Roy, 1998). Thus, when making treatment recommendation to patients from different cultural groups, clinicians might benefit from attending to their patients' models of mental illness and to the perceived credibility of their proposed interventions.

Conclusions

Ethnic/racial minority young adults are an important clinical group whose psychological functioning and mental health needs are not well understood. Findings from recent epidemiological studies suggest that young adults from ethnic/racial minority groups have higher rates of specific psychiatric disorders than do their Caucasian counterparts. Evidence-based treatments for ethnic/racial minority young adults are scarce. Further research on psychologically meaningful dimensions of culture, gender, and development may inform the development of such treatments for this population.

KEY POINTS

- In multicultural societies, cultural minority young adults compared to their cultural majority counterparts appear to be at higher risk for specific psychiatric disorders.
- Although ethnicity and race are commonly used constructs in the United States, their meaning may differ across cultures, and their usefulness in understanding clinically relevant facets of culture is limited.

- Developing effective psychological treatments for ethnic/racial minority young adults will likely involve increased understanding of the complex and dynamic relationships between culture, gender, and developmental variables.
- Culture-based models of mental illness and mental health may influence patients' help-seeking behaviors and decision making about treatments.

PRACTICE GUIDELINES

- Empirically test culture-related assumptions in a clinically meaningful manner.
- Assess multiple psychologically meaningful dimensions of culture, gender, and development.
- Consider framing clinical interventions to emphasize strengths and/or building skills and avoid focusing on weaknesses. Provide a concrete, convincing rationale for culturally informed, clinical interventions.

References

Abe-Kim, J., Takeuchi, D. T., Hong, S., Zane, N., Sue, S., Spencer, M. S., Appel, H., Nicdao, E., & Alegría, M. (2007). Use of mental health-related services among immigrant and U.S.-born Asian Americans: Results from the National Latino and Asian American Study. *American Journal of Public Health, 97,* 91–98.

Alegría, M., Mulvaney-Day, N., Torres, M., Polo, A., Cao, Z., & Canino, G. (2007a). Prevalence of psychiatric disorders across Latino subgroups in the United States. *American Journal of Public Health, 97,* 68–75.

Alegría, M., Mulvaney-Day, N., Woo, M.., Torres, M., Gao, S., & Ordo, V. (2007b). Correlates of past-year mental health service use among Latinos: Results from the National Latino and Asian American Study. *American Journal of Public Health, 97,* 76–83.

Alegría, M., Takeuchi, D., Canino, G., Naihua, D., Shrout, P., Meng, X. L.,Vega, W., Zane, N., Vila, D., Woo, M., Vera, M., Guarnaccia, P., Aguilar-Gaxiola, S., Sue, S., Escobar, J., Lin, K.M., & Gong, F. (2004). Considering context, place, and culture: The National Latino and Asian American Study. *International Journal of Methods in Psychiatric Research, 13,* 208–220.

American Psychiatric Association. (1994). *Diagnostic and statistical manual of mental disorders* (4th ed.). Washington, DC: Author.

American Psychiatric Association. (2000). *Diagnostic and statistical manual of mental disorders* (4th ed. Text revision). Washington, DC: Author.

Aponte, J. F., & Barnes, J. M. (1995). Impact of acculturation and moderator variables on the intervention and treatment of ethnic groups. In J. F. Aponte, R. Y. Rivers, & J. Wohl (Eds.), *Psychological interventions and cultural diversity* (pp. 19–39). Boston: Allyn and Bacon.

Association of Asian Pacific Community Health Organizations. (1995). *Taking action: Improving access to health care for Asians and Pacific Islanders.* Oakland, CA: Association of Asian Pacific Community Health Organizations.

Banerjee, G., & Roy, S. (1998). Determinants of help-seeking behaviour of families of schizophrenic patients attending a teaching hospital in India: An indigenous explanatory model. *International Journal of Social Psychiatry, 44*(3), 199.

Barry, D. T., & Beitel, M. (2006). Sex role ideology among East Asian immigrants in the United States. *American Journal of Orthopsychiatry, 76,* 512–517.

Barry, D. T., Bernard, M. J., & Beitel, M. (2006). Gender, sex role ideology, and self-esteem among East Asian immigrants in the U. S. *Journal of Nervous and Mental Disease, 194,* 708–711.

Barry, D. T., & Bullock, W. A. (2001). Culturally creative psychotherapy with a Latino couple by an Anglo therapist. *Journal of Family Psychotherapy, 12,* 15–30.

Barry, D. T., Elliot, R., & Evans, E. M. (2000). Foreigners in a strange land: Ethnic identity and self-construal in male Arab immigrants. *Journal of Immigrant Health, 2,* 133–144.

Barry, D. T., & Garner, D. M. (2001). Eating concerns in East Asian immigrants. *Journal of Eating and Weight Disorders, 6,* 90–98.

Barry, D. T., & Grilo, C. M. (2002). Cultural, psychological, and demographic correlates of willingness to use psychological services among East Asian Immigrants. *Journal of Nervous and Mental Diseases, 190,* 32–39.

Barry, D. T., & Grilo, C. M. (2003). Cultural, self-esteem, and demographic correlates of perception of personal and group discrimination among East Asian immigrants. *American Journal of Orthopsychiatry, 73,* 223–229.

Bartlett, F. C. (1932). *Remembering.* Cambridge, England: Cambridge University Press.

Baumeister, R. G., & Leary, M. R. (1995). The need to belong: Desire for interpersonal attachments as a fundamental human motivation. *Psychological Bulletin, 117,* 479–529.

Beals, J., Manson, S. M., Whitesell, N. R., Spicer, P., Novins, D. K., Mitchell, C. M. (2005). Prevalence of DSM-IV disorders and attendant help-seeking in two American Indian reservation populations. *Archives of General Psychiatry, 62,* 99–108.

Berry, J. W. (1980). Acculturation as varieties of adaptation. In A. Padilla (Ed.), *Acculturation: Theory, models and some new findings* (pp. 9–25). Boulder, CO: Westview.

Betancourt, H., & Lopez, S. R. (1993). The study of culture, ethnicity, and race in American psychology. *The American Psychologist, 48,* 629–637.

Breslau, N., Kessler, R. C., Chilcoat, H. D., Schultz, L. R., Davis, G. C., & Andreski, P. (1998). Trauma and posttraumatic stress disorder in the community. *Archives of General Psychiatry, 55,* 626–632.

Brislin, R. W. (1993). *Understanding culture's influence on behavior.* Orlando, FL: Holt, Rinehart & Wilson.

Bowlby, J. (1988). *A secure base: Parent–child attachment and healthy human development.* New York: Basic Books.

Brinson, J. A., & Kottler, J. A. (1995). Minorities' underutilization of counseling centers' mental health services: A case for outreach and consultation. *Journal of Mental Health Counseling, 17,* 371–385.

Burnam, M. A., Hough, R. L., Karno, M., Escobar, J. I., & Telles, C. A. (1987). Acculturation and lifetime prevalence of psychiatric disorders among Mexican Americans in Los Angeles. *Journal of Health and Social Behavior, 28,* 89–102.

Cauce, A. M., Domenech-Rodriguez, M., Paradise, M., Cochran, B. N., Shea, J. M., Srebnik, D., & Baydar, N. (2002). Cultural and contextual influences in mental health help-seeking: A focus on ethnic minority youth. *Journal of Consulting and Counseling Psychology, 70,* 44–55.

Centers for Disease Control and Prevention. (2003). Injury mortality among American Indian and Alaska Native children and youth. *Morbidity and Mortality Weekly Report, 52,* 697–701.

Chun, C. A., Enomoto, K., & Sue, S. (1996). Health care issues among Asian Americans: implications of somatization. In P. M. Kato & T. Mann (Eds.), *Handbook of diversity in health psychology.* New York: Plenum.

Chung, D. (1992). Asian cultural commonalities: A comparison with mainstream American culture. In S. Furuto, R. Biswas, D. Chung, & F. Ross-Sheriff (Eds.), *Social work practice with Asian Americans* (pp. 27–44). Newbury Park, CA: Sage.

Collins, F. S. (2004). What we do and don't know about race, ethnicity, genetics, and health at the dawn of the genome era. *Nature Genetics, 36,* 1–3.

Daumit, G. L., Crum, R. M., Guallar, E., Powe, N. R., Primm, A. B., Steinwachs, D. M., & Ford D. E. (2003). Outpatient prescriptions for atypical antipsychotics for African Americans, Hispanics, and Whites in the United States. *Archives of General Psychiatry, 60,* 121–128.

Davenport, C. B. (1923). Eugenics in race and state. *Scientific Papers of the Second International Conference of Eugenics: Vol. 2.* Baltimore: Williams & Wilkins.

Erikson, E. H. (1963). *Childhood and society.* New York: Norton. (Original work published 1950).

Fiske, S. T. (1993). Social cognition and social perception. *Annual Review of Psychology, 44,* 155–194.

Foster, M. W., & Sharp, R. R. (2002). Race, ethnicity, and genomics: Social classifications as proxies of biological heterogeneity. *Genome Research, 12,* 844–850.

Freud, S. (1960). The ego and the id. (J. Riviere, Trans.). New York: W. W. Norton. (Original work published 1923).

Gee, G. C., Spencer, M., Chen, J., Yip, T., & Takeuchi, D. T. (2007). The association between self-reported racial discrimination and 12-month DSM-IV mental disorders among Asian Americans nationwide. *Social Science & Medicine, 64,* 1984–1996.

Grant, B. F., Moore, T. C., Shepard, J., & Kaplan, K. (2003). Source and accuracy statement, Wave 1 National Epidemiological Survey on Alcohol and Related Conditions (NESARC). Bethesda, MD: National Institute on Alcohol Abuse and Alcoholism.

Grant, B. F., Stinson, F. S., Hasin, D. S., Dawson, D. A., Chou, S. P., & Anderson, K. (2004). Immigration and lifetime prevalence of DSM-IV psychiatric disorders among Mexican Americans and non-Hispanic Whites in the United States: Results from the National Epidemiological Survey on Alcohol and Related Conditions. *Archives of General Psychiatry, 61,* 1226–1233.

Greenfield, P. M., Keller, H., Fuligni, A., & Maynard, A. (2003). Cultural pathways through universal development. *Annual Review of Psychology, 54,* 461–490.

Hasin, D. S., Goodwin, R. D., Stinson, F. S., & Grant, B. F. (2005). Epidemiology of major depressive disorder. *Archives of General Psychiatry, 62,* 1097–1106.

Heeringa, S. G. (2004). Technical sample design documentation 2002–2003 National Latino and Asian American Study (NLAAS). Ann Arbor, MI: Institute for Social Research, University of Michigan.

Henig, R. M. (2004, October 10). The genome in black and white (and gray). *The New York Times Magazine,* pp. 47–51.

Herskovits, M. J. (1948). *Man and his works.* New York: Knopf.

Hofstede, G., & Bond, M. (1984). Hofstede's culture dimensions: An independent validation using Rokeach's value survey. *Journal of Cross-Cultural Psychology, 15,* 417–433.

Hu, T., Snowden, L. R., Jerrell, J. M., & Nguyen, T. D. (1991). Ethnic populations in public mental health services: Choices and level of use. *American Journal of Public Health, 81,* 1429–1434.

Huang, B., Dawson, D. A., Stinson, F. S., Hasin, D. S., Ruan, W. J., Saha, T. D., Smith, S. M., Goldstein, R. B., & Grant, B. F. (2006). Prevalence, correlates, and comorbidity of nonmedical prescription drug use and drug use disorders in the United States: Results of the National Epidemiologic Survey on Alcohol and Related Conditions. *Journal of Clinical Psychiatry, 67,* 1062–1073.

Hummer, R. A., Benjamins, M. R., & Rogers, R. G. (2004). Racial and ethnic disparities in health and mortality among the U.S. elderly population. In N. Anderson, R. Bulatao, & B. Cohen (Eds.), *Critical perspectives on racial and ethnic differences in health in late life* (pp. 53–94). Washington, DC: National Academies Press.

Indian Health Service. (2000–2001). Trends in Indian health. Rockville, MD: Public Health Service, U.S. Department of Health and Human Services.

Joe, S., & Kaplan, M. S. (2001). Suicide among African American men. *Suicide and Life-Threatening Behavior, 31,* 106–121.

Johnson, P. B., & Glassman, M. (1998). The relationship between ethnicity, gender and alcohol consumption: A strategy for testing competing models. *Addiction, 93,* 583–588.

Kapur, S., & Remington, G. (2000). Atypical antipsychotics. *British Medical Journal, 321,* 1360–1361.

Kessler, R. C., McGonagle, K. A., Zhao, S., Nelson, C. B., Eshleman, S., Wittchen, H. U., & Kendler, K. S. (1994). Lifetime and 12-month prevalence of DSM-III-R psychiatric disorders in the United States: Results from the National Comorbidity Study. *Archives of General Psychiatry, 51,* 8–19.

Kleinman, A., & Benson, P. (2006). Anthropology in the clinic: The problem of cultural competency and how to fix it. *Public Library of Science Medicine, 3*(10), e294.

Lee, S., Mountain, J., & Koenig, B. A. (2001). The meanings of "race" in the new genomics: implications for health disparities research. *Yale Journal of Health Policy, Law, and Ethics, 1,* 33–75.

Lewis-Fernandez, R., & Kleinman, A. (1995). Cultural psychiatry: Theoretical, clinical, and research issues. *Psychiatric Clinics of North America, 18,* 433–448.

Lin, K.-M., & Cheung, F. (1999). Mental health issues for Asian Americans. *Psychiatric Services, 50,* 774–780.

Ma, G. X. (1999). Access to health care by Asian Americans. In G. X. Ma & G. Henderson (Eds.), *Ethnicity and health care: A sociocultural approach* (pp. 99–121). Springfield, IL: Charles C. Thomas.

Manson, S. M. (2003). Extending the boundaries, bridging the gaps: Crafting mental health: Culture, race, and ethnicity, a supplement to the Surgeon General's report on mental health. *Culture, Medicine, and Psychiatry, 27,* 395–408.

Manson, S. M., Beals, J., Klein, S. A., & Croy, C. D. (2005). Social epidemiology of trauma among two American Indian reservation populations. *American Journal of Public Health, 95,* 851–859.

Markus, H. R., & Kitayama, S. (1991). Culture and the self: Implications for cognition, emotion, and motivation. *Psychological Review, 98,* 224–253.

Matsuoka, J. K., Breaux, C., & Ryujin, D. J. (1997). National utilization of mental health services by Asian Americans/Pacific Islanders. *Journal of Community Psychology, 25,* 141–145.

Mays, V. M., Ponce, N. A, Washington, D. L., & Cochran, S. D. (2003). Classification of race and ethnicity: Implications for public health. *Annual Review of Public Health, 24,* 83–110.

National Center for Education Statistics. (2005). *Postsecondary participation rates by sex and race/ethnicity, 1974–2003* (NCES 2005–028). Washington, DC: Government Printing Office.

National Institutes of Health. (2002). *Strategic research plan and budget to reduce and ultimately eliminate health disparities, Vol 1*. Washington, DC: U.S. Department of Health and Human Services.

Neighbors, H. W., Caldwell, C., Williams, D. R., Nesse, R., Taylor, R. J., Bullard, K M., Torres, M., & Jackson, J. S. (2007). Race, ethnicity, and the use of services for mental disorders. *Archives of General Psychiatry, 64*, 485–494.

O'Connell, J., Novins, D. K., Beals, J., Croy, C., Baron, A. E., Spicer, P., Buchwald, D., & American Indian Service Utilization, Psychiatric Epidemiology, Risk and Protective Factors Project Team. (2006). The relationship between patterns of alcohol use and mental and physical health disorders in two American Indian populations. *Addiction, 101*, 69–83.

Oetzel, J. G. (1998). The effects of self-construals and ethnicity on self-reported conflict styles. *Communication Reports, 11*, 133–144.

Owens, K., & King, M. C. (1999). Genomic views of human history. *Science, 286*, 451–453.

Phinney, J. S. (1996). When we talk about American ethnic groups, what do we mean? *American Psychologist, 51*, 918–927.

Pillay, Y. (2005). Racial identity as a predictor of the psychological health of African American students at a predominantly White university. *Journal of Black Psychology, 31*, 46–66.

Poortinga, Y. H., van de Vijver, F., Joe, R., & Koppel, J. M. H. (1989). Peeling the onion called culture: A synopsis. In C. Kagitcibasi (Ed.), *Growth and progress in cross-cultural psychology* (pp. 22–34). Berwyn, PA: Swets North American.

Porteus, S. D. (1926). *Temperament and race*. Boston: Richard G. Badger.

Richardson, J., Anderson, T., Flaherty, J., & Bell, C. (2003). The quality of mental health care for African Americans. *Culture, Medicine, and Psychiatry, 27*, 487–498.

Schmidt, L. A., Ye, Y., Greenfield, T. K., & Bond, J. (2007). Ethnic disparities in clinical severity and services for alcohol problems: Results from the National Alcohol Survey. *Alcoholism: Clinical and Experimental Research, 31*(1), 48–56.

Segall, M. H., Lonner, W. J., & Berry, J. W. (1998). Cross-cultural psychology as a scholarly discipline: On the flowering of culture in behavioral research. *American Psychologist, 53*, 1101–1110.

Shields, A. E., Fortun, M., Hammonds, E. M., King, P. A., Lerman, C., Rapp, R., & Sullivan, P. F. (2005). The use of race variables in genetic studies of complex traits and the goal of reducing health disparities: A transdisciplinary perspective. *American Psychologist, 60*, 77–103.

Shore, J. H., Beals, J., Orton, H., Buchwald, D., & AI-SUPERPFP Team. (2006). Comorbidity of alcohol abuse and dependence with medical conditions in two American Indian reservation communities. *Alcoholism: Clinical and Experimental Research, 30*, 649–655.

Singelis, T. M., Bond, M. H., Sharkey, W. F., & Li, C. S. Y. (1999). Unpackaging culture's influence on self-esteem and embarrassability. *Journal of Cross-Cultural Psychology, 30*, 315–341.

Smedley, A., & Smedley, B. D. (2005). Race as biology is fiction, racism as a social problem is real: anthropological and historical perspectives on the social construction of race. *American Psychologist, 60*, 16–26.

Smith, S. M., Stinson, F. S., Dawson, D. A., Goldstein, R., Huang, G., & Grant, B. F. (2006). Race/ethnic differences in the prevalence and co-occurrence of substance use disorders and independent mood and anxiety disorders: results from the National Epidemiologic Survey on Alcohol and Related Conditions. *Psychological Medicine, 26*, 987–998.

Snowden, L. R., & Pingitore, D. (2002). Frequency and scope of mental health service delivery to African Americans in primary care. *Mental Health Services Research, 4*, 123–130.

Solomon, S., Greenberg, J., & Pyszcynski, T. (1991). A terror management theory of social behavior: the psychological functions of self-esteem and cultural world-views. *Advances in Experimental Social Psychology, 24*, 93–159.

Substance Abuse and Mental Health Services Administration. (2006). Results from the 2005 National Survey on Drug Use and Health: National findings (Office of Applied Studies, NSDUH Series H-30, DHHS Publication No. SMA 06-4194). Rockville, MD.

Sue, S., Allen, D. B., & Conaway, L. (1978). The responsiveness and equality of mental health care to Chicanos and Native Americans. *American Journal of Community Psychology, 6*, 137–146.

Sue, S., McKinney, H., Allen, D., & Hall, J. (1974). Delivery of community mental health services to black and white clients. *Journal of Consulting and Clinical Psychology, 42*, 794–801.

Tajfel, H. (1981). *Human groups and social categories*. Cambridge, England: Cambridge University Press.

Takeuchi, D., Chung, R. C-Y., Lin, K-M., Shen, H., Kurasaki, K., Chun, C. A., & Sue, S. (1998). Lifetime and twelve-month prevalence rates of major depressive episodes and dysthymia among Chinese Americans in Los Angeles. *American Journal of Psychiatry, 155*, 1407–1414.

Takeuchi, D. T., & Gage, S-J., L. (2003). What to do with race? Changing notions of race in the social sciences. *Culture, Medicine, and Psychiatry, 27,* 435–445.

Turner, R. J., & Lloyd, D. A. (2004). Stress burden and the lifetime incidence of psychiatric disorder in young adults. *Archives of General Psychiatry, 61,* 481–488.

U.S. Census Bureau. (2002). *American Indian and Alaska Native population: 2000.* Retrieved November 22, 2005, from http://www.cdc.gov/omh/Populations/ AIAN/AIAN.htm.

U.S. Census Bureau. (2003). *Annual resident population estimates of the United States by age, race, and Hispanic or Latino origin: April 1, 2000 to July 1, 2003.*

U.S. Department of Health and Human Services. (2000). Healthy People 2010. 2nd ed. Vol 1. *Understanding and improving health and objectives for improving health.* Washington, DC: Author.

U.S. Department of Health and Human Services. (2001). *Mental health: Culture, race, and ethnicity: A supplement to mental health: A report of the Surgeon General.* Washington, DC: Author.

U.S. Office of Management and Budget. (1978). *Directive No. 15: Race and ethnic standards for federal statistics and administrative reporting.* Washington, DC.: Author.

Vega, W. A., Kolody, B., Anguilar-Gaxiola, S., Alderete, E., Catalano, R., & Caraveo-Anduaga, J. (1998). Lifetime prevalence of DSM-III-R psychiatric disorders among urban and rural Mexican Americans in California. *Archives of General Psychiatry, 55,* 771–778.

Wan, C., Chiu, C. Y., Peng, S., & Tam, K. P. (2007). Measuring cultures through intersubjective cultural norms: Implications for predicting relative identification with two or more cultures. *Journal of Cross-Cultural Psychology, 38,* 213–226.

Wang, P. S., Lane, M., Olfson, M., Pincus, H. A., Wells, K. B., & Kessler, R. C. (2005). Twelve-month use of mental health services in the United States. *Archives of General Psychiatry, 62,* 629–640.

Weschler, H., Lee, J. E., Kuo, M., Seibring, M., Nelson, T. F., & Lee, H. (2002). Trends in college binge drinking during a period of increased prevention efforts. Findings from four Harvard School of Public Health College Alcohol Study surveys: 1993–2001. *Journal of American College Health, 50,* 203–217.

Whiting, B. B. (1976). The problem of the packaged variable. In K. F. Riegel & J. A. Meecham (Eds.), *The developing individual in a changing world* (pp. 303–309). New York: Hawthorne.

Williams, D. R. (1994). The concept of race in Health Services Research: 1966 to 1990. *Health Services Research, 29,* 261–274.

Williams, D. R. (1997). Race and health: Basic questions, emerging directions. *Annals of Epidemiology, 7,* 322–333.

Yanow, D. (2003). *Constructing "race" and "ethnicity" in America: Category-making in public policy and administration.* Armonk, NY: M. E. Sharpe.

Yeh, C. J. (1999). Invisibility and self-construal in African American men: Implications for training and practice. *The Counseling Psychologist, 27,* 810–819.

Young, A. S., Klap, R., Sherbourne, C. D., & Wells, K. B. (2001). The quality of care for depression and anxiety disorders in united states. *Archives of General Psychiatry, 58*(1), 55–61.

Zhang, A. Y., Snowden, L., & Sue, S. (1998). Differences between Asian and White Americans' help seeking and utilization patterns in the Los Angeles area. *Journal of Community Psychology, 26,* 317–326.

Chapter 8

Body Image

Jennifer L. Greenberg, Sherrie S. Delinsky, Hannah E. Reese, Ulrike Buhlmann and Sabine Wilhelm

Alex was brought in by his parents for treatment of body dysmorphic disorder (BDD). Alex was 16 years old and a junior in high school. Because he had missed so many days of school he was in danger of repeating a grade. When he did attend school, he was generally tardy and would spend most of the day going back and forth between the guidance counselor's office and the bathroom. Growing up, Alex prided himself on being a loyal son and friend, grade A student, and avid soccer player. However, at 12, around the time of puberty, Alex developed mild acne. Alex began picking at his skin for 10–15 minutes every morning in an effort to fix his blemishes or to prevent new ones from forming. He bought over-the-counter creams to try to reduce outbreaks and subsequent redness. Over the next few years, Alex found it increasingly difficult to be around his friends at school or in social situations, for fear they would make fun of him or not like him based on his "terrible skin." At age 14, he begged his mother to take him to the dermatologist, who prescribed a new regimen of topical creams and washes. His morning routine grew to consist of repeated washing, skin picking, and application of topical creams and concealer, and occupied 1–2 hours each morning. If Alex was interrupted, for example by his mother trying to coax him out of the house for school, he became upset, agitated, and, at times, physically aggressive. He made up excuses to avoid spending time with friends.

He started spending at least 1 hour per day lifting weights in addition to his prerequisite soccer workouts so that he could achieve the lean, muscular abdomen and biceps with which he had now become preoccupied. At 15, over a course of 6 months, Alex dropped 40 pounds. He restricted the amount and types of food he ate, eating only 1–2 meals per day and excluding most fats and carbohydrates. Because he was never satisfied with his progress toward this end, Alex refused to wear anything other than long-sleeved shirts, including to soccer and to the gym. Alex could not concentrate in class because of his concerns that others were staring at his face or body. Alex spent most of his time alone and spent hours each day worried about and trying to enhance his appearance; he became so depressed he contemplated suicide.

Body image is the subjective view of one's physical appearance derived from both perceptual (evaluation of body size) and affective/cognitive (attitudes toward one's body) components. Because of the strong influence of thoughts and feelings on body image, actual appearance often has little bearing on sense of attractiveness. Living amidst ubiquitous sociocultural messages of the beauty "ideal," children and adults learn to measure themselves and others against impossible standards. Thus, discrepancies may develop between the way young adults view their bodies and what they view to be the ideal, resulting in body-image dissatisfaction. Negative body image is a precursor to future pathology, and by early adolescence it can already predict the development of eating disorders and depression.

In this brief review, we explicate factors contributing to the development of body image, body-image dissatisfaction, and disturbance. We also explore the role of gender and culture, as they may potentially moderate the pathways for body-image development and disturbances. Lastly, we discuss the current status of empirically supported programs for the prevention and treatment of body-image disturbance and make suggestions for future research directions.

Significance of Body Image

In recent years, pervasive body-image concerns among young women have led to increasing empirical and clinical attention to body image (Cash, Morrow, Hrabosky, & Perry, 2004; Thompson, Heinberg, Altabe, & Tantleff-Dunn, 1999). Whereas body dissatisfaction used to be more prevalent among young Caucasian females, rates of body dissatisfaction appear to be on the rise in men and across ethnic minorities (Roberts, Cash, Feingold, & Johnson, 2006). In addition, the rapid increase in overweight and obesity among American children and adolescents over the last 30 years has contributed to increased body dissatisfaction, negative psychological sequelae, and the addition of health-related consequences, such as high blood pressure, high cholesterol, and pediatric diabetes. However, body image may be linked only weakly to actual appearance.

Body image is a multidimensional construct comprised of self-perceptions and attitudes regarding one's physical appearance. Attitudes involve two dimensions: body satisfaction and importance of appearance (Cash, 2002). In order to assess body satisfaction, some people rely on overall appearance, while others judge themselves based on specific physical characteristics, including body weight/shape or specific body parts (e.g., hair, nose, skin). Because body image has been closely related to self-esteem, individuals for whom appearance is highly important in determining sense of self may be more vulnerable to fluctuations in self-esteem and negative body image (Rudiger, Cash, Roehrig, & Thompson, 2007).

Body image is more influential in determining self- or body-esteem than actual body shape/size. For example, perceived weight, when compared to actual weight, is consistently more highly associated with psychological sequelae (e.g., body-image dissatisfaction, poor self-esteem; see Pesa, Syre & Jones, 2000). In other words, perceptions and attitudes adolescents have about their bodies are better determinants of their body image and self-esteem than their actual bodies.

Various aspects of body-image concerns have been implicated as precursors for future pathology. Importantly, whereas body-image disturbance is a risk factor and the hallmark feature of body image and eating disorders, it is not uncommon. Body-image dissatisfaction and disturbance appear on a continuum and at staggering rates throughout the U.S. population, a phenomenon dubbed "normative discontent" by Rodin, Silberstein, & Striegel-Moore (1984). Data from large community samples have also suggested high rates of disordered eating and attempts to control weight among U.S. women (Forman-Hoffman, 2004), adolescents (McVey, Tweed, & Blackmore, 2004), and middle-aged women (McLaren & Kuth, 2004). Recent data have implicated a worsening trend for body-image disturbances across gender, age, and culture (Becker, Gilman, & Burwell, 2005; Cash et al., 2004; Shaw, Ramirez, Trost, Randall, & Stice, 2004). The negative impact of body-image dissatisfaction on self-esteem, mood, sexual functioning, quality of life, and eating behaviors (Cash & Fleming, 2002a, 2002b; Cash et al., 2004; Johnson & Wardle, 2005; Stice, 2002; Wiederman, 2002) underscores the need for early identification of body-image concerns and efforts to support development of positive body image.

Whereas people with higher levels of investment (i.e., derive their self-esteem or concept largely from appearance) are more prone to fluctuating and negative body image, a positive body image has been associated with positive psychological and physical sequelae, including a self-worth less driven by appearance, less body-image disturbance, fewer body-image cognitive distortions, less disturbed eating attitude, and lower body mass index ([BMI]; Rudiger et al., 2007). Positive body image has also been associated with higher quality of life, self-esteem, optimism, and social support among males and females and lower levels of disordered eating among females (e.g., Rudiger et al., 2007).

Developmental Course

Body Image in Adolescence

Adolescence is characterized by significant physical, psychological, emotional, and social changes. A growing body of data suggests a worsening of body dissatisfaction and eating disorder symptoms over adolescence. Increased levels of body dissatisfaction and disordered eating between the ages of 11 and 16 years have been reported in American, Australian, and Scottish girls (e.g., Hoare & Hoare, 1998; Striegel-Moore et al., 2000). During this time, physical and hormonal changes occur as a result of puberty, which have long been implicated in the development of body-image concerns in both sexes. Girls tend to report increased body dissatisfaction following puberty, due in part to increased body fat. Boys, on the other hand, tend to be generally satisfied with shape and weight, or they desire increased muscularity. Concurrently, adolescents are growing increasingly dependent on peer groups for identification and approval.

As girls get older they are more likely to report higher levels of appearance-related social comparisons, body dissatisfaction, and eating disturbances (see Halliwell & Harvey, 2006). The role of peer-based social comparisons in mediating sociocultural ideals and internalization may help to explain the increase in body dissatisfaction that occurs during adolescence. However, in a sample of 507 U.K. boys and girls, Halliwell & Harvey (2006) recently found that body dissatisfaction and internalization of sociocultural attitudes remained relatively consistent between ages 11 and 16. Therefore, an increase in body-image concerns is not universal in adolescence. Adolescent girls, particularly those with high levels of peer comparison and internalization, may be more vulnerable to body dissatisfaction and its consequences. Furthermore, it is likely that these predisposing factors are in place before adolescence.

Body Image in Childhood

Perceptions and attitudes about our bodies (i.e., body image) are typically in place by adolescence, and they tend to remain relatively stable over time if left untreated. Ubiquitous social pressures from an early age (e.g., sociocultural messages from the television, parental influences) may contribute to early development of body image. In fact, children as young as 6-years-old have reported body-image dissatisfaction, including expressions of wanting to be thinner and a fear of being fat (Gardner, Friedman, & Jackson, 1999; Smolak and Levine, 2001a). This effect was particularly salient among females, although gender differences only manifested around age 9 (Gardner et al., 1999). The early onset of body-image dissatisfaction is particularly disconcerting given the high propensity for dieters to progress to pathological eating and clinically diagnosable eating disorders.

In spite of continued media messages promoting youth and the thin ideal, some recent data suggest that young college women's body images may be improving despite a significantly heavier average body weight (e.g., Cash et al., 2004). This encouraging trend begs for greater examination of the factors mediating the relationships between direct and indirect influences on body dissatisfaction. For example, increased public awareness of body image, obesity, and eating disorders and efforts to enhance media literacy may serve a protective role against body-image dissatisfaction and its deleterious effects (Cash et al., 2004; Levine & Piran, 2004; Levine & Smolak, 2001, 2002; Stice, 2002).

Gender Differences

Gender differences consistently emerge when comparing body image in adolescent girls and boys, with young girls typically experiencing higher levels of body image and related concerns (e.g., Varnado-Sullivan, Horton, & Savoy, 2006). A closer examination of levels of perceived pressures, social comparison, and internalization may help to explicate some of the variance in body-image dissatisfaction and disturbance between and within sexes.

Most girls wish to be thinner than their perceived size and overestimate the extent to which males find thinner figures attractive. To a lesser extent, boys may be dissatisfied with their perceived shape/weight; however, boys typically desire greater muscularity and overestimate the extent to which girls prefer larger, muscular shapes. Discrepancies between actual and ideal body images result in body-image disturbance, lower self-esteem, and maladaptive behaviors. These consequences can be dangerous.

In boys the muscular ideal can lead to disordered eating, steroid use, and repeated attempts at cosmetic correction. Cafri, van den Berg, & Thompson (2006) examined risky behaviors (e.g., use of substances, such as anabolic steroids or prohormones, and dieting to gain weight) in the pursuit of weight control and muscularity in adolescent boys (n = 269). They found that boys who endorsed symptoms of muscle dysmorphia (MD) were more likely to use substances, and that body dissatisfaction and BMI were significant predictors of dieting to gain weight. Higher exercise frequency and participation in sports have also been associated with increased body-image concerns and eating pathology in young males, although exercise frequency has also been linked to higher self-esteem in boys (Cafri et al., 2006; Varnado-Sullivan et al., 2006).

Relative to boys, girls perceive more pressure to control their weight (McCabe & Ricciardelli, 2001; Polce-Lynch, Myers, Kliewer, & Kilmartin, 2001). Perceived pressure to be thin is associated with internalization of sociocultural ideals and is a risk factor for the development of body-image dissatisfaction and disordered eating in adolescent girls and boys. Perceived pressure may come from media, family, or peer sources. For all adolescents, social comparisons (i.e., peer comparisons) appear to at least partially moderate the relationship between perceived pressure to control weight and internalization of sociocultural messages (Halliwell & Harvey, 2006). However, the pathway by which internalization affects body-image concerns and disturbances differs for boys and girls.

It may be that girls are more likely than boys to notice, internalize, and make peer comparisons based on sociocultural ideal media messages; subsequently, girls report more body dissatisfaction and eating pathology than their male counterparts. In other words, girls are more likely to be aware of and internalize sociocultural messages regarding appearance (from the media and from peers), feel badly about their own appearance as it compares to the ideal and to others', and feel pressured to lose or control their weight. Interestingly, even without reporting body dissatisfaction, girls who internalize sociocultural messages are more vulnerable to disordered eating (Halliwell & Harvey, 2006). However, in boys the relationship between internalization and disordered eating is fully mediated by body dissatisfaction.

While most studies on gender differences in body image have examined shape and weight, other appearance-related concerns have received less attention. Phillips and colleagues (1997, 2006) examined gender differences in the clinical features of adolescents and adults with body dysmorphic disorder (BDD). She found gender differences similar to those found in the general population. Regardless of gender, most adolescents and adults were concerned with skin, hair, stomach, weight, and teeth. Females were more likely to be preoccupied with their hips and their weight, pick their skin, and use makeup to camouflage "imperfections." Men were more likely to be preoccupied with body build (e.g., muscularity), genitals, and hair thinning and to use a hat for camouflage. Interestingly, Phillips found that men were as likely as women to seek nonpsychiatric medical and surgical treatment, although women were more likely to receive such treatment with the exception of cosmetic surgery, which men and women were equally likely to receive.

Sociocultural Factors

Media Influences

The media, primarily consisting of television, movies, and magazines, sends a clear message that beauty and thinness are important, desirable, and within every person's reach. Given the pervasiveness of these media messages, it is not surprising that there is now a substantial literature examining the impact of the mass media and its images of beauty on the body image and satisfaction of young adults.

Although not without exceptions, the evidence largely supports a consistent, moderate negative effect of the media. Correlational work supports an association between viewing images of thin models or idealized images of beauty and body dissatisfaction (for review, see Thompson et al., 1999). Additionally, prospective studies have found media exposure to predict and temporally precede the development of weight concerns and appearance dissatisfaction (Dohnt & Tiggeman, 2006; Field et al., 2001). Perhaps most importantly, however, experimental work has demonstrated a clear effect of media images of beauty on body dissatisfaction. A recent meta-analysis conducted on 25 studies that randomly assigned women to view images of thin models versus normal or plus-size models or inanimate objects found a medium negative overall effect (d = −.31) on body satisfaction (Groesz, Levine, & Murnen, 2002).

Recent research in this area has focused on identifying the moderators and mediators of this effect of the media on body image. In other words, which individuals are particularly affected by these messages and why? Clearly, most young adults are exposed to images of beauty and thinness in the media and only a fraction develop body-image concerns. Several studies have identified high internalization of the thin ideal as rendering individuals particularly vulnerable to media messages (Brown & Dittmar, 2005; Dittmar & Howard, 2004; Stice & Shaw, 2004; Yamamiya, Cash, Melnyk, Posavec, & Posavec, 2005). Those individuals who readily endorse and agree with the sociocultural standards of beauty are more likely to be less satisfied with their own bodies after viewing appearance-related images in the media. The tendency to make social comparisons has also been found to affect the degree to which the media affects one's body image and satisfaction (Dittmar & Howard, 2004; Engeln-Maddox, 2005). A very recent series of studies (Trampe, Stapel, & Siero, 2007) revealed that baseline level of body dissatisfaction moderated the effect of images of thin models on body image such that only those women who were dissatisfied with their bodies initially were negatively affected by viewing pictures of thin models. This effect appeared to be mediated by the degree to which the body-dissatisfied women made social comparisons. The body-dissatisfied women compared themselves to others more frequently and also compared themselves indiscriminately with models, non-models, and neutral objects (e.g., vases), while the body-satisfied women only engaged in social comparison with other non-models.

Peers and Teasing

Peers may play a particularly important role in the body-image development of young adults. As adolescents transition from the home to college or independent living, they may become increasingly more reliant on peers for emotional support and information about norms and values. Research suggests that peers may influence body image through both direct and indirect means.

Perhaps the most direct form of influence is teasing. Indeed, a substantial literature including both longitudinal studies and experimental work suggests that appearance-related teasing is related to negative body image and disturbed eating behavior (for review, see chapter 5 of Thompson et al., 1999).

Researchers have also proposed that peers may play a powerful indirect role in shaping an individual's body image and disordered eating by fostering a climate in which appearance and thinness are highly valued and creating norms around eating and dieting behaviors. The primary evidence for this hypothesis comes from studies demonstrating greater similarity on measures of body image and eating behavior within social peer groups than between peer groups. For example, an early and influential study demonstrated that members of a sorority demonstrated high levels of similarity in levels of binge eating (Crandall, 1988). Perhaps, most importantly, these women were not similar when they joined the sorority, but their eating behaviors converged over a period of 7 months, suggesting that the social climate of the sorority may have reinforced this behavior. Additional, cross-sectional work examining similarities in body-image concerns and disordered eating in adolescent cliques has also demonstrated considerable similarity within peer groups when compared to peers outside the peer group (Hutchinson & Rapee, 2007; Paxton, Schutz,

Wertheim, & Muir, 1999). Much of the work in this area, however, does not allow us to disentangle two primary pathways that may be causing this within-group similarity. While it is entirely possible that peers are in fact influencing each other through the process of socialization, it is also possible that individuals select peers who are already similar to themselves on these attitudes and behaviors. A recent study by Zalta and Keel (2006) attempted to clarify this issue in a study examining bulimic symptomatology in college women. Because of the unique living arrangements in their college sample, they were able to tease apart the two influences and found evidence for both selection and socialization. Specifically, individuals selected peers who were similar to themselves in certain personality traits (e.g., perfectionism), which rendered them more likely to developing disordered eating. Subsequent to this selection, it appeared that socialization of bulimic symptomatology only operated among peer groups who were at a similar high risk for developing disordered eating. Thus, it appears that socialization may be a powerful force in influencing disordered eating but only among individuals with pre-existing vulnerabilities.

Cultural Differences

Stereotypical depictions of an eating disorder patient have focused on young, affluent Caucasian women. However, recent epidemiologic data show a growing incidence of body-image disorders across ethnically and socioeconomically diverse populations. It is unclear whether these data reflect a true rise in body-image dissatisfaction or whether this is at least partially an artifact of previously underrecognized or untreated symptomatology.

Most studies have examined cultural differences in body image within Western countries and suggest that ethnic minorities within these countries have less body dissatisfaction and lower risk for associated pathology. This may be due in part to the level of acculturation within the mainstream culture, assuming an inverse relationship between level of acculturation and body dissatisfaction (e.g., Altabe & O'Garo, 2002; Kawamura, 2002). In other words, the more one adopts the values, attitudes, and sociocultural standards of the mainstream culture as their own, the more vulnerable they are to developing negative body image. However, recent data (e.g., Roberts et al., 2006; Shaw et al., 2004) have emerged to suggest a convergence of body-image dissatisfaction across ethnicities. In other words, the gap in ethnic differences in body dissatisfaction may be growing smaller as sociocultural pressures for thinness become increasingly widespread.

Black, Latina, and Asian females tend to be more satisfied with their overall shape/weight and specific body parts than white females (e.g., Altabe, 2001; Celio, Zabinski, & Wilfley, 2002; Mayville, Katz, Gipson, & Cabral, 1999; Shaw et al., 2004; Soh, Touyz, & Surgenor, 2006). Moreover, blacks and Latinos report less internalization of the thin ideal and less perceived pressure to control weight when compared to Asians or whites. Nonetheless, these differences seem to be fading. Shaw et al. (2004) found no ethnic differences among adolescent and adult females in risk factors for body-image disorders (e.g., perceived pressure to be thin, body dissatisfaction, negative affect, and self-esteem) or eating disorder symptomatology (e.g., fear of fat, weight and shape concerns, compensatory behaviors). If sociocultural factors impact ethnic groups equally, currently successful prevention and treatment efforts might be equally effective for ethnic minority and white individuals (Shaw et al., 2004). The generalization of current prevention and treatment approaches is particularly salient in light of the global rise of body dissatisfaction. To this end, the tripartite model, which implicates the influence of direct (peer, parental, and media) and mediating factors (internalization of media images/ideals) in the development of body dissatisfaction and eating disturbances in the United States (Keery, van den Berg, & Thompson, 2004; Shroff & Thompson, 2006), was recently replicated in a sample of Japanese undergraduate women (Yamamiya, Shroff, & Thompson, 2008), suggesting an overlap in the sociocultural variables found to influence body image and eating disturbances in Japan and the United States.

Sociocultural theorists have implicated the rapid spread of Western cultural values (e.g., the thin ideal, individualism, competition) in the etiology and growing prevalence of body-image dissatisfaction and disorders (e.g., Warren, Gleaves, Cepeda-Benito, del Carmen Fernandez, & Rodriguez-Ruiz, 2005). For example, a cross-sectional study of women living in a traditional Fijian village found significantly higher prevalence of overweight, obesity, and body-image concerns from 1989 to 1998, a period of social change and changing attitudes toward body shape in Fiji (Becker et al., 2005). Similar findings have been reported among Chinese and Polynesian women who became increasingly dissatisfied with their bodies after increased exposure to Western culture (Yang, Gray, & Pope, 2005).

Notably, variants of body-image dissatisfaction have been identified in Western and non-Western countries for centuries, including in the United States, United Kingdom, Australia, Singapore, Taiwan, Kenya, Iran, South Africa, Egypt, Greece, Italy, Saudi Arabia, Curaçao, Hong Kong, and Japan (for review, see Soh et al., 2006). For example, *Fushokubyo* ("non-eating illness") has been recognized in Japanese literature since the seventeenth and eighteenth centuries. *Shubo-kyofu* (a variant of *Taijin kyofusho*) is a Japanese phobia of having a deformed body that bears striking resemblance to body dysmorphic disorder (Suzuki, Takei, Kawai, Minabe, & Mori, 2003). Traditional cultural values are not necessarily protective against body dissatisfaction. In a study of Taiwanese women in Taiwan and the United States, those who identified more strongly with Taiwanese culture reported higher levels of body dissatisfaction and disordered eating (Tsai, Curbow, & Heinberg, 2003). Thus, sociocultural factors may have differential effects on body-image concerns; degree of acculturation, socioeconomic status, peer, family, and media should be addressed as important sociocultural influences.

Cross-cultural differences have been long noted in the core symptomatology of body image and related disorders (e.g., fear of fatness in anorexia nervosa). Clinicians need to be able understand differential presentation and culturally specific meanings of body-image concerns across diverse populations and be sensitive to the various pathways by which sociocultural factors may influence body-image concerns. Although numerous studies have examined cultural differences, disparities in access to health care and methodological limitations have made it difficult to accurately measure prevalence and symptoms across cultures (Franko, Becker, Thomas, & Herzog, 2007). In addition, examining stages of acculturation (e.g., such as time spent in residence, socioeconomic status, ethnic group identification and relatedness, and language) may be beneficial in helping to establish culturally sensitive classification systems as well as in developing appropriate targets for prevention and treatment efforts.

Body-Image Disturbance

Many people dislike some aspect of their appearance. However, some individuals become so distressed about how they look that it interferes with their daily life. Body-image disturbance is both a risk factor and core feature of eating and other body-image disorders.

Neurobiology of Body-Image Disturbance

The exact pathophysiology of body-image disorders is not well known. However, in addition to the sociocultural and psychological factors already discussed, emerging data from neuropsychological, neuroimaging, and pharmacological studies suggest an aberrant neurobiological system involving multiple networks. Emotions and body image are regulated largely via the right hemisphere, and newly acquired body-image disorders subsequent to right hemispheric regions are well documented involving the parietal cortex (see Kaye, 2008) and fronto-temporal regions (Gabbay et al., 2003; see Feusner, Yaryura-Tobias, & Saxena, 2008). Increased left hemispheric activation (involving the prefrontal and lateral temporal regions), associated with visual biases, has been found in patients with body-image disorders (Feusner, Yaryura-Tobias, & Saxena, 2008; Kaye, 2008). Neuropsychological studies of patients with BDD (e.g., Deckersbach et al., 2000) and anorexia nervosa (AN; e.g., Lopez et al., 2007; Sherman et al., 2006) found that patients selectively attend to small details in an attempt to organize information, in lieu of a more global processing approach. In other words, these individuals tend to get caught up in the details and have trouble seeing the big picture. Preliminary neuroimaging studies also implicate executive dysfunction (frontal-striatal dysfunction) and potential biases in visual and visual-spatial processing (e.g., Carey, Seedat, Warwick, van Heerden, & Stein, 2004; Feusner, Townsend, Bystritsky, & Bookheimer, 2007). For example, a recent fMRI study of BDD patients found left hemispheric activation (i.e., local processing of information) compared to controls, specifically in the lateral prefrontal cortex (associated with behavior and decision making), lateral temporal lobe regions (associated with visual memory), and dorsal anterior cingulate (associated with cognitive and motor control; Feusner et al., 2007). Similarly, higher medial prefrontal and anterior cingulate cortex activation has been found for individuals with AN (ill and recovered) compared to controls (see Kaye, 2008). Lastly, psychopharmacologic treatment and challenge studies in BDD (Phillips, Albertini, & Rasmussen, 2002), AN, and BN (see Kaye, 2008) have implicated 5-HT (serotonin) and DA (dopamine) dysregulation. Serotonin plays a role in modulating constructs such as mood, aggression, and appetite, while dopamine is involved in modulating motivation, reward, learning, and decision making; dysregulation of these neurotransmitters may contribute to the selective attention (obsessionality) and dysregulated mood states (e.g., anxiety, depression) and inhibition observed in individuals with body-image disorders (Feusner, Yaryura-Tobias, & Saxena, 2008; Kaye, 2008; Saxena & Feusner, 2006; Wagner et al., 2007). For example, it has been suggested that overactive D2/D3 receptors in the antero-ventral striatum (a region associated with reward and reinforcement) may account in part for the difficulty of AN patients to discriminate or respond appropriately to salient stimuli, such as food and other hedonic pleasures (Frank et al., 2005). Greater activation of this region in recovered AN patients may also support neuropsychological findings (e.g., Lopez et al., 2007; Sherman et al., 2006) that indicate use of more local, detailed (rather than global or hedonic) strategies in this population. In addition, dorsal caudate dopamine D2/D3 receptor binding in the striatal region has been positively correlated with anxiety and harm avoidance (Frank et al., 2005); rather than responding to stimuli—positive or negative—based on associated rewards, individuals with increased DA receptor binding in this region may be more likely to behave based on anxiety or harm avoidance.

Body Dysmorphic Disorder

Classified as a somatoform disorder in DSM-IV, BDD is defined as a preoccupation with an imagined or slight defect in appearance; if a slight physical anomaly is present, the concern must be excessive (APA, 2000). Moreover, the concerns must cause clinically significant distress or impairment in social, occupational, or other important areas of functioning, and it cannot be better accounted for by another mental disorder (e.g., dissatisfaction with body shape and size in anorexia nervosa).

Preoccupations commonly focus on the face or head (e.g., skin, hair, or nose), but any other body part may also be the focus of concern (APA, 2000). As noted, among individuals with *muscle dysmorphia,* which may occur more commonly among males, the primary preoccupation focuses on muscle size and shape. Individuals with BDD experience significant distress about their perceived defect that often compels them to think about it for many hours a day. Consequently, suffering and impairment in everyday functioning occur. Avoidance of everyday activities may lead to substantial social isolation, including being housebound for years and suicide attempts (e.g., Phillips, McElroy, Keck, Pope, & Hudson, 1993). Frequent checking in (or avoidance of) mirrors and other reflective surfaces (e.g., store windows), excessive grooming behaviors (e.g., hair combing, makeup application, or skin picking), and frequent request for reassurance about the perceived defect are common; however, these provide only temporary relief. Furthermore, individuals with BDD frequently compare their body parts with others and are often concerned that other people might take special notice of their perceived defect. Camouflaging the "defect" (e.g., wearing a hat to hide perceived hair loss) is also very common. Like social phobia, BDD is characterized by a strong fear of negative evaluation by others (e.g., Hollander, Neville, Frenkel, Josephson, & Liebowitz, 1992). Individuals with BDD may also experience ideas of reference related to their appearance (APA, 2000). That is, they often believe that others take special notice of the perceived defect and talk about it or mock it. In other words, delusional BDD patients are convinced about the existence of the defect and are not able to consider that the flaw or defect might only exist in their imagination. Those patients may qualify for a diagnosis of delusional disorder, somatic subtype. However, Phillips and colleagues suggested that both delusional and nondelusional forms of BDD reflect one single disorder with different degrees of insight (Phillips, McElroy, Keck, Hudson, & Pope, 1994).

BDD usually begins in adolescence and its course tends to be chronic if left untreated. Several studies have investigated the prevalence of BDD, and studies using clinician-administered interviews have found rates of 0.7% to 3% (e.g., Bienvenu et al., 2000; Otto, Wilhelm, Cohen, & Harlow, 2001), indicating that BDD is a common mental disorder. Prevalence rates in dermatology and reconstructive surgery settings are even higher (e.g., Phillips, Dufresne, Wilkel, & Vittorio, 2000; Sarwer, Wadden, Pertschuk, & Whitaker, 1998). These prevalence rates are consistent with observations that individuals with BDD often do not seek psychological help, but they consult dermatologists, plastic surgeons, or dentists (Phillips et al., 1993) because they are too ashamed and embarrassed to seek professional help (McElroy, Phillips, & Keck, 1994).

Over the past decade both psychological and pharmacological treatments for BDD have received increased attention. Whereas medication studies mostly examined selective serotonin reuptake inhibitors (SSRIs; e.g., Hollander et al., 1999; Phillips, Albertini, & Rasmussen, 2002; Phillips & Najjar, 2003), psychological treatments mainly focused on behavior therapy or cognitive-behavioral therapy (e.g., McKay et al., 1997; Rosen, Reiter, & Orosan, 1995; Wilhelm, Otto, Lohr, & Deckersbach, 1999). Specifically, cognitive-behavioral therapy involves gradual exposure to anxiety-provoking situations or stimuli (e.g., social situations) and prevention of any avoidance behaviors (e.g., not making eye contact) or rituals performed to decrease the anxiety or distress associated with the situation or stimuli (e.g., mental review of the situation). The patient is asked to do the exposure until the accompanying anxiety or discomfort decreases (i.e., habituation). Further, maladaptive appearance-related interpretations are identified and modified to more accurate, healthier beliefs. Whereas both medication and psychological treatment studies have obtained promising results (Williams, Hadjistavropoulos, & Sharpe, 2006), future research needs to further develop effective treatment strategies for BDD.

Eating Disorders

Body-image disturbances form the core of eating disorders. In addition to shape/weight concern, eating disorders are characterized by attempts to control body weight by restriction of food intake and other compensatory strategies (APA, 2000). Anorexia nervosa (AN) and bulimia nervosa (BN) are the best characterized eating disorders; however, those who do not meet criteria for either AN or BN may be diagnosed within a third category, eating disorder not otherwise specified (ED-NOS). Binge eating disorder has been the most widely studied disorder within this NOS category.

Anorexia nervosa typically begins during adolescence and has a prevalence of 0.3% in young girls and women (Hoek & van Hoeken, 2003). AN is defined by a refusal to maintain normal body weight (e.g., resulting $< 85\%$ of expected weight or a BMI < 17.5 kg/m^2), an intense fear of losing control or gaining weight despite objective underweight, overinvestment in body shape/weight, and in postmenarcheal females, absence of menses (amenorrhea) for at least 3 consecutive months. Some AN patients rely exclusively on severe caloric restriction (restricting type) in order to control weight, while others also engage in regular binge episodes or purging behavior (e.g., vomiting or laxative use; binge eating/purging type). Extreme dietary restriction is difficult to uphold and can lead to binge eating, depression, social withdrawal, intense preoccupation with food, altered hormone secretion, and decreased metabolic rate (Wilson, Grilo, & Vitousek, 2007). Treatment outcome data are limited by the relative rarity and medical complications associated with AN; however, psychological treatments, including family therapy, have received empirical support.

The Maudsley model (see Lock, le Grange, Agras, & Dare, 2001) is the best-studied and most widely available treatment for AN. In a series of randomized controlled trials and case series, it has been shown to be highly effective, particularly with younger individuals with a recent onset, as a means of preventing posthospitalization weight loss in AN patients (e.g., Russell, Szmukler, Dare, & Eisler, 1987; see Wilson et al., 2007). The intervention typically involves 10–20 family-based sessions in which parents are coached in taking over their child's eating and weight behaviors until the child is compliant with the prescribed eating and weight strategies. The child's rights are made contingent upon resolution of the eating disorder. Of the individual treatments for AN, cognitive-behavioral therapy, described by Garner and Vitousek, is the most frequently studied. There is currently no empirical basis for the use of antidepressants with this population.

Bulimia nervosa is characterized by recurrent episodes of binge eating (uncontrolled consumption of an objectively large amount of food), regular compensatory behaviors designed to influence shape/weight (e.g., self-induced vomiting, misuse of laxatives, diuretics, enemas, fasting, excessive exercise), and overconcern with shape/weight. People with BN are usually within a normal or low body weight range, although BN can occur in overweight individuals (Wilson et al., 2007). Similar to AN, BN affects mostly young females; the prevalence has been estimated at 1%–2% in community samples (Hoek & van Hoeken, 2003). BN is chronic with symptoms waxing and waning over time, and relapse or morphing of BN into ED-NOS is not uncommon (Milos, Spindler, Schnyder, & Fairburn, 2005).

CBT (Fairburn, Marcus, & Wilson, 1993) for BN has received the most extensive examination and support. Treatment consists of 16–20 sessions that seek to enhance motivation for change, replace dysfunctional dieting with a regular pattern of eating, decrease concern with shape/weight and prevent relapse. Although many patients improve, CBT for BN typically eliminates binge eating and purging in 30%–50% of cases (Wilson et al., 2007). There is also evidence for the efficacy of interpersonal psychotherapy (IPT), originally developed as a short-term treatment for depression, which was adapted for BN by Fairburn. IPT helps patients identify and change current interpersonal problems likely maintaining the eating disorder. Adaptations of CBT treatments for use with adolescents have been described (see Lock, 2005; Wilson & Sysko, 2006) and family treatments are being evaluated. This is promising in light of the early onset of symptoms and the well-established role of BN and eating pathology as risk factors for future psychopathology. Although treatments for eating disorders, particularly BN, fare well, there is room for improvement. More direct and efficacious interventions targeting body-image disturbance are needed, particularly for adolescents.

Treatment and Prevention of Body-Image Disturbance

Treatment Programs

Cognitive-behavioral treatments have been among the most widely used and effective therapies for the treatment of body-image disturbances. As treatments for body image related to eating and body dysmorphic pathology have already been discussed, the present section will be limited to the discussion of empirically supported treatments for body image in the normative population.

The majority of empirically supported therapies designed to treat body-image disturbance combine cognitive and behavioral techniques (Cash, 1995; Rosen, 1997; Stice, Trost, & Chase, 2003; for a review, see Farrell, Shafran & Lee, 2006). Techniques address disturbances in cognition, affect, and behavior thought to maintain body-image disturbance and include cognitive restructuring (challenging the accuracy of maladaptive thinking), behavioral experiments (behavioral tasks designed to test predictions based on maladaptive thinking), and perceptual retraining.

Mirror retraining, which involves a systematic, nonjudgmental exposure to body image, can be used to reduce body image–related anxiety and avoidance and as a form of perceptual retraining (e.g., Delinsky & Wilson, 2006; Rosen, 1997). Mirror retraining encourages mindfulness of present emotional experiences and has been shown to be effective in improving body-image behaviors (checking, avoidance), cognitions (weight/shape concerns, body dissatisfaction, thin ideal internalization, dysfunctional beliefs about appearance), dieting, mood, and self-esteem (Delinsky & Wilson, 2006).

Cash's (1995) and Rosen's (1997) cognitive-behavioral treatment programs have been the most extensively studied. Both programs address perceptual, cognitive, affective, and behavioral components of body image. A review of the outcome literature suggests that while Rosen and Cash's programs have been helpful in reducing body-image disturbance, the effects may be nonspecific. CBT has been reported to be more effective than no treatment or nonspecific treatments; however, these studies have not been replicated reliably. In addition, while CBT has been compared to nonspecific treatments, such as exercise therapy or reflective therapy, and to waitlist or no treatment controls, studies comparing CBT to active treatments are scarce. In addition, studies that manipulated the format and delivery of CBT provide evidence to suggest that current treatments could be more parsimonious. For example, condensed versions of Cash's treatment (e.g., three sessions, eight weekly 20-minute sessions, self-help with 5–10 minute weekly therapist telephone contact) demonstrated comparable results to the full course of therapy.

Prevention Programs

The potential negative impact of exposure to the sociocultural thin ideal on young adults has been well documented; however, not all youth exposed to sociocultural pressures develop poor body image nor subsequent poor self-esteem, low mood, or body-image or eating disturbances. Further investigation of the possible moderators of this effect will help to elucidate the most effective targets for prevention efforts. Personal factors (negative body image, low self-esteem), socioenvironmental factors (internalization), and behavioral factors (dieting and binge eating) have already been identified as risk factors (e.g., Irving & Neumark-Sztainer, 2002; Levine & Piran, 2004; Sherwood & Neumark-Sztainer, 2001). Furthermore, because elementary school (ages 6–11) seems to be a critical period in the development of negative body image and eating disorders, many programs have targeted efforts toward this group (Levine & Smolak, 2001, 2002; Sherwood & Neumark-Sztainer, 2001). Extant prevention programs emphasize three key areas: knowledge, attitudes, and behavior, and they typically include a combination of health education, media literacy, and dissonance induction strategies.

Health education programs provide information on healthy weight control behaviors, body image, eating disorders, and social pressure resistance skills, and they have been effective in reducing risk for disordered eating and increasing health care utilization (e.g., Stice, Shaw, Burton, & Wade, 2006).

Media literacy is used to attenuate the effects of idealized media messages. Individuals are taught to critically analyze and deconstruct information from various media sources. While these strategies have been associated with reduced body dissatisfaction and eating pathology, the overall data on media literacy have been mixed (Stice & Shaw, 2004). The biggest limitation of media literacy programs has been their effectiveness in increasing awareness of sociocultural pressures without influencing internalization of such ideals. Because internalization of these ideals has been strongly linked to body dissatisfaction and its accompanying pathology, the addition of strategies that could reduce internalization might prove more effective.

Dissonance induction, grounded in cognitive dissonance theory (Festinger, 1957), includes verbal, written, and behavioral exercises by which individuals learn to critique and counterargue against sociocultural ideals. Young adults are encouraged to challenge idealized messages of beauty and may be asked to question the validity of a message or propose alternatives to proposed messages (see Engeln-Maddox, 2005). According to dissonance theory, engaging in activities that contradict the internalized sociocultural ideal should result in inconsistent thoughts (i.e., mixed messages), thereby creating psychological discomfort that motivates people to modify their beliefs and attitudes in order to restore consistency (e.g., Stice, et al., 2006).

Many existing prevention programs are school based with a focus on education and empowerment, and most have been effective in reducing negative self-talk, internalization of cultural thin ideals, unhealthy weight management strategies, and in promoting positive self-esteem in girls and boys (Grave, De Luca, & Campello, 2001; Levine & Smolak, 2002; Smolak & Levine, 2001b). Unfortunately, prevention approaches have not been consistently effective and existing programs have been criticized for lacking ecological validity. A recent review of 21 school-based prevention programs found the most effective programs were interactive, involved parents, increased self-esteem, and provided media literacy (O'Dea, 2005). A brief (two-session) school-based prevention program developed for adolescent boys was effective in improving area-specific body image (i.e., musculature), self-esteem, and affect, but not other areas of body satisfaction (Stanford & McCabe, 2005), which may suggest the importance of taking into account specific areas of concern (e.g., muscles in males). However, additional studies are needed to determine the necessary and effective parts of these programs and their long-term impact.

KEY POINTS

- Body-image concerns and related disturbances have become increasingly pervasive among young adults of both sexes and cross-culturally.
- Body-image disturbance puts youth at risk for developing body-image disorders; therefore, early identification and treatment of body-image concerns are key.
- Body-image disorders are more than a matter of vanity; they can be severely debilitating and, if left untreated, are associated with the development of additional medical and psycho-pathology and morbidity.
- The interplay of biological, social, and cultural factors in the development, presentation, and treatment of body image and body-image disturbance underscores the need for more comprehensive intervention and prevention approaches.

PRACTICE GUIDELINES

- Providers need to specifically query youth about potential body-image concerns.
- Youth commonly experience appearance-related concerns; providers need to assess concerns with regard to time, distress, and avoidance to determine when concerns become pathological.
- Prevention and intervention efforts should provide education and skills to buffer against the internalization of unrealistic sociocultural standards of beauty and the accompanying pressures adolescents and young adults face in trying to attain this ideal.

References

Altabe, M. N. (2001). Issues in the assessment and treatment of body image disturbance in culturally diverse populations. In J. K. Thompson (Ed.), *Body image, eating disorders, and obesity: An integrative guide for assessment and treatment* (pp. 129–147). Washington, DC: American Psychological Association.

Altabe, M., & O'Garo, K. N. (2002). Hispanic body images. In T. F. Cash & T. Pruzinsky (Eds.), *Body image: A handbook of theory, research and clinical practice* (pp. 250–256). New York: Guilford Press.

American Psychiatric Association (APA). (2000). *Diagnostic and statistical manual of mental disorders* (4th ed., Text revision). Washington, DC: Author.

Becker, A. E., Gilman, S. E., & Burwell, R. A. (2005). Changes in prevalence of overweight and in body image among Fijian women between 1989 and 1998. *Obesity Research, 13*(1), 110–117.

Bienvenu, O. J., Samuels, J. F., Riddle, M. A., Hoehn-Saric, R., Liang, K.-Y., Cullen, B. A. M., Grados, M. A., & Nestadt, G. (2000). The relationship of obsessive–compulsive disorder to possible spectrum disorders: Results from a family study. *Biological Psychiatry, 48*, 287–293.

Brown, A., & Dittmar, H. (2005). Think "thin" and feel bad: The role of appearance schema activation, attention level, and thin-ideal internalization for young women's responses to ultra-thin media ideals. *Journal of Social & Clinical Psychology, 24*, 1088–1113.

Cafri, G., van den Berg, P., & Thompson, J. K. (2006). Pursuit of muscularity in adolescent boys: Relations among biopsychosocial variables and clinical outcomes. *Journal of Clinical Child & Adolescent Psychology, 35*(2), 283–291.

Carey, P., Seedat, S., Warwick J., van Heerden, B., & Stein, D. J. (2004). SPECT imaging of body dysmorphic disorder. *Journal of Neuropsychiatry and Clinical Neurosciences, 16*(3), 357–359.

Cash, T. F. (1995). *What do you see when you look in the mirror? Helping yourself to a positive body image.* New York: Bantam Books.

Cash, T. F. (2002). Cognitive behavioral perspectives on body image. In T. F. Cash & T. Pruzinsky (Eds.), *Body image: A handbook of theory, research, and clinical practice* (pp. 38–46). New York: Guilford Press.

Cash, T. F., & Fleming, E. C. (2002a). Body image and social relations. In T. F. Cash & T. Pruzinsky (Eds.), *Body image: A handbook of theory, research, and clinical practice* (pp. 277–286). New York: Guilford Press.

Cash, T. F., & Fleming, E. C. (2002b). The impact of body-image experiences: Development of the Body Image Quality of Life Inventory. *International Journal of Eating Disorders, 31*, 455–460.

Cash, T. F., Morrow, J. A., Hrabosky, J. I., & Perry, A. A. (2004). How has body image changed? A cross-sectional investigation of college women and men from 1983 to 2001. *Journal of Consulting and Clinical Psychology, 72*, 1081–1089.

Celio, A. A., Zabinski, M. F., & Wilfley, D. E. (2002). African American body images. In T. F. Cash & T. Pruzinsky (Eds.). *Body image: A handbook of theory, research and clinical practice* (pp. 234–242). New York: Guilford Press.

Crandall, C. S. (1988). Social contagion of binge-eating. *Journal of Personality and Social Psychology, 55*, 588–598.

Deckersbach, T., Savage, C. R., Phillips, K. A., Wilhelm, S., Buhlmann, U., Rauch, S. L., Baer, L., & Jenike, M. A. (2000). Characteristics of memory dysfunction in body dysmorphic disorder. *Journal of the International Neuropsychological Society, 6*, 673–681.

Delinsky, S. S., & Wilson, G. T. (2006). Mirror exposure for the treatment of body image disturbance. *International Journal of Eating Disorders, 39*(2), 108–116.

Dittmar, H., & Howard, S. (2004). Thin-ideal internalization and social comparison tendency as moderators of media models' impact on women's body-focused anxiety. *Journal of Social & Clinical Psychology, 23*, 768–791.

Dohnt, H., & Tiggemann, M. (2006). The contribution of peer and media influences to the development of body satisfaction and self-esteem in young girls: A prospective study. *Developmental Psychology, 42*, 929–936.

Engeln-Maddox, R. (2005). Cognitive responses to idealized media images of women: The relationship of social comparison and critical processing to body image disturbance in college women. *Journal of Social & Clinical Psychology, 24*, 1114–1138.

Fairburn, C. G., Marcus, M. D., & Wilson, G. T. (2003). Cognitive-behaviour therapy for binge eating and bulimia nervosa: A comprehensive treatment manual. In C. G. Fairburn & G. T. Wilson (Eds.), *Binge eating: Nature, assessment, and treatment* (pp. 361–404). New York: Guilford Press.

Farrell, C., Shafran, R., & Lee, M. (2006). Empirically evaluated treatments for body image disturbance: A review. *European Eating Disorders Review, 14*, 289–300.

Festinger, L. (1957). *A theory of cognitive dissonance.* Evanston, IL: Row, Peterson.

Feusner, J. D., Townsend, J., Bystritsky, A., & Bookheimer, S. (2007). Visual information processing of faces in body dysmorphic disorder. *Archives of General Psychiatry, 64*(12), 1417–1425.

Feusner, J. D., Yaryura-Tobias, J., & Saxena, S. (2008). The pathophysiology of body dysmorphic disorder. *Body Image, 5,* 3–12.

Field, A. E., Camargo, C. A., Taylor, C. B., Berkey, C. S., Roberts, S. B., & Colditz, G. A. (2001). Peer, parent, and media influences on the development of weight concerns and frequent dieting among preadolescent and adolescent girls and boys. *Pediatrics, 107,* 54–60.

Forman-Hoffman, V. L. (2004). High prevalence of abnormal eating and weight control practices among U.S. high-school students. *Eating Behaviour, 5,* 325–336.

Frank, G., Bailer, U., Henry, S., Drevets, W., Meltzer, C., Price, J., Mathis, C., Wagner, Hoge, J., Ziolko, S., Barbarich-Marsteller, N., Weissfeld, L., & Kaye, W. H. (2005). Increased dopamine D2/D3 receptor binding after recovery from anorexia nervosa measured by positron emission tomography and [11C]raclopride. *Biological Psychiatry, 58*(11), 908–912.

Franko, D. L., Becker, A. E., Thomas, J. J., & Herzog, D. B. (2007). Cross-ethnic differences in eating disorder symptoms and related distress. *International Journal of Eating Disorders, 40*(2), 156–164.

Gabbay, V., Asnis, G. M., Bello, J. A., Alonso, C. M., Serras, S. J., & O'Dowd, M. A. (2003). New onset of body dysmorphic disorder following frontotemporal lesion. *Neurology, 61*(1), 123–125.

Gardner, R. M., Friedman, B. N., & Jackson, N. A. (1999). Body size estimation, body dissatisfaction, and ideal size preference in children six through thirteen. *Journal of Youth and Adolescence, 28*(5), 603–618.

Grave, R. D., De Luca, L., & Campello, G. (2001). Middle school primary prevention program for eating disorders: A controlled study with a twelve-month follow-up. *Eating Disorders: The Journal of Treatment & Prevention, 9*(4), 327–337.

Groesz, L. M., Levine, M. P., & Murnen, S. K. (2002). The effect of experimental presentation of thin media images on body satisfaction: A meta-analytic review. *International Journal of Eating Disorders, 31,* 1–16.

Halliwell, E., & Harvey, M. (2006). Examination of a sociocultural model of disordered eating among male and female adolescents. *British Journal of Health Psychology, 211,* 235–248.

Hoare, P., & Hoare, L. (1998). Eating habits, body-esteem and self-esteem in Scottish children and adolescents. *Journal of Psychosomatic Research, 45,* 425–431.

Hoek, H.W., & van Hoeken, D. (2003). Review of the prevalence and incidence of eating disorders. *International Journal of Eating Disorders, 34,* 383–396.

Hollander, E., Allen, A., Kwon, J., Aronowitz, B., Schmeidler, J., Wong, C., & Simeon, D. (1999). Clomipramine vs. desipramine crossover trial in body dysmorphic disorder: Selective efficacy of a serotonin reuptake inhibitor in imagined ugliness. *Archives of General Psychiatry, 56,* 1033–1042.

Hollander, E., Neville, D., Frenkel, M., Josephson, S., & Liebowitz, M. R. (1992). BDD diagnostic issues and related disorders. *Psychosomatics, 33,* 156–165.

Hutchinson, D. M., & Rapee, R. M. (2007). Do friends share similar body image and eating problems? The role of social networks and peer influence in early adolescence. *Behaviour Research and Therapy, 45,* 1557–1577.

Irving, L. M., and Neumark-Sztainer, D. (2002) Integrating the prevention of eating disorders and obesity: Feasible or futile? *Preventive Medicine, 34,* 299–309.

Johnson, F., & Wardle, J. (2005). Dietary restraint, body dissatisfaction, and psychological distress: A prospective analysis. *Journal of Abnormal Psychology, 114,* 119–125.

Kaye, W. (2008). Neurobiology of anorexia nervosa and bulimia nervosa. *Physiol Behav, 94*(1), 121–135.

Kawamura, K. Y. (2002). Asian American body images. In T. F. Cash & T. Pruzinsky (Eds.), *Body image: A handbook of theory, research and clinical practice* (pp. 243–249). New York: Guilford Press.

Keery, H., van den Berg, P., & Thompson, J. K. (2004). A test of the tripartite influence model of body image and eating disturbance in adolescent girls. *Body Image, 1,* 237–251.

Levine, M. P., & Piran, N. (2004). The role of body image in the prevention of eating disorders. *Body Image, 1*(1), 57–70.

Levine, M. P., & Smolak, L. (2001). Primary prevention of body image disturbances and disordered eating in childhood and early adolescence. In J. K. Thompson & L. Smolak (Eds.), *Body image, eating disorders, and obesity in youth: Assessment, prevention, and treatment* (pp. 237–260). Washington, DC: American Psychological Association.

Levine, M. P., & Smolak, L. (2002). Ecological and activism approaches to the prevention of body image problems. In T. F. Cash & T. Pruzinsky (Eds.), *Body image: A handbook of theory, research, and clinical practice* (pp. 497–505). New York: Guilford Press.

Lock, J. (2005). Adjusting cognitive behavior therapy for adolescents with bulimia nervosa. *American Journal of Psychotherapy, 59,* 267–281.

Lock, J., le Grange, D., Agras, W. S., & Dare, C. (2001). *Treatment manual for anorexia nervosa: A family-based approach.* New York: Guilford Press.

Lopez, C., Tchanturia, K., Stahl, D., Booth, R., Holliday, J., & Treasure, J. (2008). An examination of the concept of central coherence in women with anorexia nervosa. *International Journal of Eating Disorders, 41*(2), 143–152.

Mayville, S., Katz, R., Gipson, M., & Cabral, K. (1999). Assessing the prevalence of body dysmorphic disorder in an ethnically diverse group of adolescents. *Journal of Child and Family Studies, 8*(3), 357–362.

McCabe, M. P., & Ricciardelli L. A. (2001). The development of the perceived sociocultural influence on body image and body change questionnaire. *International Journal of Behavioural Medicine, 8*, 20–41.

McElroy, S. L., Phillips, K. A., & Keck, P. E. (1994). Obsessive-compulsive spectrum disorders. *Journal of Clinical Psychiatry, 55*, 33–51.

McKay, D., Todaro, J., Campisi, T., Moritz, E. K., Neziroglu, F., & Yaryura-Tobias, J. A. (1997). Body dysmorphic disorder: A preliminary evaluation of treatment and maintenance using exposure with response prevention. *Behaviour Research and Therapy, 35*, 67–70.

McLaren, L., & Kuh, D. (2004). Body dissatisfaction in midlife women. *Journal of Women and Aging, 16*, 35–54.

McVey, G., Tweed, S., & Blackmore, E. (2004). Dieting among preadolescent and young adolescent females. *Canadian Medical Association Journal, 170*, 1559–1561.

Milos, G., Spindler, A., Schnyder, U., & Fairburn, C. G. (2005). Instability of eating disorder diagnoses: Prospective study. *British Journal of Psychiatry, 187*, 573–578.

O'Dea, J. (2005). School-based health education strategies for the improvement of body image and prevention of eating problems: An overview of safe and successful interventions. *Health Education, 105*(1), 11–33.

Otto, M. W., Wilhelm, S., Cohen, L. S., & Harlow, B. L. (2001). Prevalence of body dysmorphic disorder in a community sample of women. *American Journal of Psychiatry, 158*, 2061–2063.

Paxton, S. J., Schutz, H. K., Wertheim, E. H., & Muir, S. L. (1999). Friendship clique and peer influences on body I age concerns, dietary restraint, extreme weight-loss behaviors, and binge-eating in adolescent girls. *Journal of Abnormal Psychology, 108*, 255–266.

Pesa, J. A., Syre, T. R., & Jones, E. (2000). Psychosocial differences associated with body weight among female adolescents: The importance of body image. *Journal of Adolescent Health, 26*(5), 330–337.

Phillips, K. A., Albertini, R. S., & Rasmussen, S. A. (2002). A randomized placebo-controlled trial of fluoxetine in body dysmorphic disorder. *Archives of General Psychiatry, 59*, 381–388.

Phillips, K. A., & Diaz, S. F. (1997). Gender differences in body dysmorphic disorder. *Journal of Nervous and Mental Disorders, 185*(9), 570–577.

Phillips, K. A., Didie, E. R., Menard, W., Pagano, M. E., Fay, C., & Weisberg, R. B. (2006). Clinical features of body dysmorphic disorder in adolescents and adults. *Psychiatry Research, 141*(3), 305–314.

Phillips, K. A., Dufresne, R. G. Jr., Wilkel, C., & Vittorio, C. (2000). Rate of body dysmorphic disorder in dermatology patients. *Journal of the American Academy of Dermatology, 42*, 436–441.

Phillips, K. A., McElroy, S. L., Keck, P. E. Jr., Hudson, J. I., & Pope, H. G. (1994). A comparison of delusional and nondelusional body dysmorphic disorder in 100 cases. *Psychopharmacology Bulletin, 30*, 179–186.

Phillips, K. A., McElroy, S. L., Keck, P. E. Jr., Pope, H. G., & Hudson, J. I. (1993). Body dysmorphic disorder: 30 cases of imagined ugliness. *American Journal of Psychiatry, 150*, 302–308.

Phillips, K. A., & Najjar, F. (2003). An open-label study of citalopram in body dysmorphic disorder. *Journal of Clinical Psychiatry, 64*, 715–720.

Polce-Lynch, M., Myers, B. J., Kliever, W., & Kilmartin, C. (2001). Adolescent self-esteem and gender: Exploring relations to sexual harassment, body image, media influence and emotional expression. *Journal of Youth and Adolescence, 30*, 225–244.

Roberts, A., Cash, T. F., Feingold, A., & Johnson, B. T. (2006). Are black-white differences in females' body dissatisfaction decreasing? A meta-analytic review. *Journal of Consulting and Clinical Psychology, 74*(6), 1121–1131.

Rodin, J. Silberstein, L., & Striegel-Moore, R. (1984). Women and weight: A normative discontent. Nebraska Symposium on Motivation. *Nebraska Symposium on Motivation, 32*, 267–307.

Rosen, J. C. (1997). Cognitive-behavioral body image therapy. In D. M. Garner, & P. E. Garfinkel (Eds.), *Handbook of treatment for eating disorders* (2nd ed.). New York: Guilford Press.

Rosen, L. C., Reiter, J., & Orosan, P. (1995). Cognitive-behavioural body image therapy for body dysmorphic disorder. *Journal of Consulting and Clinical Psychology, 63*, 263–269.

Rudiger, J. A., Cash, T. F., Roehrig, M., & Thompson, J. K. (2007). Day-to-day body image states: Prospective predictors of intra-individual level and variability. *Body Image, 4*(1), 1–9.

Russell, G. F. M., Szmukler, G. I., Dare, C., & Eisler, I. (1987). An evaluation of family therapy in anorexia nervosa and bulimia nervosa. *Archives of General Psychiatry, 44,* 1047–1056.

Sarwer, D. B., Wadden, T. A., Pertschuk, M. J., & Whitaker, L. A. (1998). The psychology of cosmetic surgery: A review and reconceptualization. *Clinical Psychology Review, 18,* 1–22.

Saxena, S., & Feusner, J. (2006). Toward a neurobiology of body dysmorphic disorder. *Primary Psychiatry, 13(7),* 41–48.

Shaw, H., Ramirez, L., Trost, A., Randall, & Stice, E. (2004). Body image and eating disturbances across ethnic groups: More similarities than differences. *Psychology of Addictive Behaviors, 18,* 12–18.

Sherman, B. J., Savage, C. R., Eddy, K. T., Blais, M. A., Deckersbach, T., Jackson, S. C., Franko, D. L., Rauch, S. L., Herzog, D. B. (2006). Strategic memory in adults with anorexia nervosa: Are there similarities to obsessive-compulsive spectrum disorders? *International Journal of Eating Disorders, 39,* 468–476.

Sherwood, N. E., & Neumark-Sztainer, D. (2001). Internalization of the sociocultural ideal: Weight-related attitudes and dieting behaviors among young adolescent girls. *American Journal of Health Promotion, 15(4),* 228–231.

Shroff, H., & Thompson, J. K. (2006). The tripartite influence model of body image and eating disturbance: A replication with adolescent girls. *Body Image, 3(1),* 17–23.

Smolak, L., & Levine, M. P. (2001a). Body image in children. In J. K. Thompson & L. Smolak (Eds.), *Body image, eating disorders, and obesity in youth: Theory, assessment, treatment, and prevention* (pp. 41–66). Washington, DC: American Psychological Association.

Smolak, L., & Levine, M. P. (2001b). Two-year follow-up of a primary prevention program for negative body image and unhealthy weight regulation. *Eating Disorders: Journal of Treatment and Prevention, 9(4),* 313–325.

Soh, N. L., Touyz, S. W., & Surgenor, L. J. (2006). Eating and image disturbances across cultures: A review. *European Eating Disorders Review, 14,* 54–65.

Stanford, J. N., & McCabe, M. P. (2005). Evaluation of a body image prevention programme for adolescent boys. *European Eating Disorders Review, 13,* 360–370.

Stice, E. (2002). Risk and maintenance factors for eating pathology: A meta-analytic review. *Psychological Bulletin, 128,* 825–848.

Stice, E., & Shaw, H. (2004). Eating disorder prevention programs: A meta-analytic review. *Psychological Bulletin, 130,* 206–227.

Stice, E., Shaw, H., Burton, E., & Wade, E. (2006). Dissonance and healthy weight eating disorder prevention programs: A randomized efficacy trial. *Journal of Consulting and Clinical Psychology, 74(2),* 263–275.

Stice, E., Trost, A., & Chase, A. (2003). Healthy weight control and dissonance-based eating disorder prevention programs: Results from a controlled trial. *International Journal of Eating Disorders, 33,* 10–21.

Striegel-Moore, R. H., Schreiber, G. B., Lo, A., Crawford, P., Obarzanek, E., & Rodin, J. (2000). Eating disorder symptoms in a cohort of 11 to 16-year-old black and white girls: The NHLBI growth and health study. *International Journal of Eating Disorders, 27(1),* 49–66.

Suzuki, K., Takei, N., Kawai, M., Minabe, Y., & Mori, N. (2003). Is *Taijin Kyofusho* a culture-bound syndrome? *American Journal of Psychiatry, 160(7),* 1358.

Thompson, J. K., Heinberg, L. J., Altabe, M., & Tantleff–Dunn, S. (1999). *Exacting beauty: Theory, assessment and treatment of body image disturbance.* Washington, DC: American Psychological Association.

Trampe, D., Stapel, D. A., & Siero, F. W. (2007). On models and vases: Body dissatisfaction and proneness to social comparison effects. *Journal of Personality and Social Psychology, 92,* 106–118.

Tsai, G., Curbow, B., & Heinberg, L. (2003). Sociocultural and developmental influences on body dissatisfaction and disordered eating attitudes and behaviors of Asian women. *Journal of Nervous and Mental Disease, 191,* 309–318.

Varnado-Sullivan, P. J., Horton, R., & Savoy, S. (2006). Differences for gender, weight and exercise in body image disturbance and eating disorder symptoms. *Eating and Weight Disorders, 11(3),* 118–125.

Wagner, A., Aizenstein, H., Venkatraman, V. K., Fudge, J., May, J. C., Mazurkewicz, L., Frank, G. K., Bailer, U. F., Fischer, L., Nguyen, V., Carter, C., Putnam, K., & Kaye, W. H. (2007). Altered reward processing in women recovered from anorexia nervosa. *American Journal of Psychiatry, 164(12),* 1842–1849.

Warren, C. S., Gleaves, D. H., Cepeda-Benito, A., del Carmen Fernandez, M., & Rodriguez-Ruiz, S. (2005). Ethnicity as a protective factor against internalization of a thin ideal and body dissatisfaction. *International Journal of Eating Disorders, 37(3),* 241–249.

Wiederman, M. W. (2002). Body image and sexual functioning. In T. F. Cash & T. Pruzinsky (Eds.), *Body image: A handbook of theory, research, and clinical practice* (pp. 287–294). New York: Guilford Press.

Wilhelm, S., Otto, M. W., Lohr, B., & Deckersbach, T. (1999). Cognitive behavior group therapy for body dysmorphic disorder: A case series. *Behaviour Research and Therapy, 37,* 71–75.

Williams, J., Hadjistavropoulos, T., & Sharpe, D. (2006). A meta-analysis of psychological and pharmacological treatments for body dysmorphic disorder. *Behaviour Research and Therapy, 44,* 99–111.

Wilson, G. T., Grilo, C. M., & Vitousek, K. M. (2007). Psychological treatment of eating disorders. *American Psychologist, 62*(3), 199–216.

Wilson, G. T., & Sysko, R. (2006). Cognitive-behavioral therapy for adolescents with bulimia Nervosa. *European Eating Disorders Review, 14,* 8–16.

Yamamiya, Y., Cash, T., Melnyk, S. E., Posavec, H. D., & Posavec, S. S. (2005). Women's exposure to thin and beautiful media images: Body image effects of media-ideal internalization and impact-reduction interventions. *Body Image, 2*(1), 74–80.

Yamamiya, Y., Shroff, H., & Thompson, J. K. (2008). The tripartite influence model of body image and eating disturbance: A replication with a Japanese sample. *International Journal of Eating Disorders, 41*(1), 88–91.

Yang, C. F., Gray, P., & Pope, H. G. Jr. (2005). Male body image in Taiwan versus the West: Yanggang Zhiqi meets the Adonis complex. *American Journal of Psychiatry, 162*(2), 263–269.

Zalta, A. K., & Keel, P. K. (2006). Peer influence on bulimic symptoms in college students. *Journal of Abnormal Psychology, 115,* 185–189.

Chapter 9

Coping with Stress and Trauma in Young Adulthood

Scott M. Hyman, Steven N. Gold and Rajita Sinha

In today's industrialized society, the transition to young adulthood has taken on more meaning than simply turning 18, getting married, having children, or settling into a career. Rather, self-sufficiency, financial independence, independent decision making, and the ability to accept full responsibility for one's choices and actions mark the passage to adulthood (Arnett, 2000, 2004). Many individuals in their early to mid twenties do not feel that they have become full adults, and it is only when the aforementioned qualities are attained, typically by age 30, that they feel they have clearly reached young adulthood (Arnett, 2000, 2004).

Some authors define young adulthood as the years spanning the ages of 18 and 25 (e.g., Park, Mulye, Adams, Brindis, & Irwin, Jr., 2006; Szajnberg & Massie, 2003), whereas others distinguish between emerging adulthood (ages 18–25) and young adulthood (the late twenties through the thirties) as distinct developmental periods (Arnett, 2000, 2004). According to the latter conceptualization, changes in the timing of marriage and parenthood in the past few decades has created a distinct and prolonged developmental period where possible life avenues are explored before finally settling into adult roles (Arnett, 2000, 2004). This extended exploratory period, characterized by demographic diversity, instability, and change, has been termed emerging adulthood (Arnett, 2000, 2004). For the purpose of this chapter, we will discuss stress, trauma, and coping as they pertain to the developmental period spanning Arnett's (2000, 2004) conceptualization of both emerging and young adulthood (ages 18 through the thirties).

Case Vignette I

Richard, a 25-year-old Caucasian male, entered a Masters in Business Administration program directly out of college and started a job at a large brokerage firm soon after graduating. Richard had been a full-time student prior to taking the job and had little real-world work experience other than a few part-time jobs (e.g., waiting tables) that carried little responsibility. Although he had some difficulty with a few college and Master's level courses, he did not worry much about failing exams since other people were not affected by his grade, and he was always able to make up courses or earn extra credit in other ways. Richard drank socially throughout his academic career and only suffered minor consequences, such as having to miss a few early classes because of a hangover.

After securing a well-paying job at a reputable firm, Richard was under constant pressure to earn money for his clients, and he soon became terribly concerned that any mistake would have tremendous negative ramifications for him, the firm, and for those to whom he provided consultation. Richard stayed at work very late, and he obsessed over every decision. He was losing sleep because of work pressures, and he felt panicky upon waking. He dreaded going into work out of fear that he would slip up and ruin a client's finances and the reputation of the company. He was constantly tired, and he felt angry and sad that his entire existence seemed to revolve around worrying about work.

Over time, he made some friends at the office and began going out to bars with co-workers in order to help him relax after a stressful day. He found the effects of alcohol soothing, and he eventually began drinking in the mornings prior to going into work to relieve anxiety. One day, a co-worker commented that he smelled of alcohol. Richard became extremely concerned that this information would be relayed to his supervisor and a heightened level of anxiety ensued. He worried that he would lose his job and never be employed in this business again. With fear of impending job loss and humiliation, he sought help for work-related stress.

Case Vignette 2

Wayne, a 36-year-old African American male, sought out therapy for trauma 18 years after having been repeatedly verbally demeaned, physically beaten, and in general "literally tortured" by his openly racist dorm roommate during his freshman year in college. As is often the situation in cases of severe interpersonal trauma, he was in many ways even more disturbed by the failure of his parents and other "authority figures" to believe his reports of being assaulted or to come to his aid than by the attacks themselves. He was especially disturbed that his parents had repeatedly told him to "stop fooling around" and to "get down to work" at school because they were convinced that his complaints were merely a ruse he was employing in an attempt to get out of going to college.

Throughout his childhood his parents had ridden him hard to achieve at both academics and athletics, droning into him that "a black man has to work twice as hard as anybody else to get anywhere in this world." Wayne explained to his therapist that (apparently in response to this indoctrination) he had in fact always put much more effort than anyone else he knew into athletics, school, and work. He bitterly complained that despite this he was stuck in a job well below his capabilities, his income was considerably below that of his friends, and he had never been able to sustain a romantic relationship.

His chief complaint at admission was that in the intervening years since being victimized by his college roommate he had devoted an inordinate amount of time almost every day ruminating about the assault and that he was consumed with rage that no one had put credence in or responded to his pleas for help. He also was disturbed by his lack of progress in his career and his failure to establish a stable primary relationship.

Entering into emerging/young adulthood can be a prized achievement and an exciting time full of new freedoms and possibilities. However, it can also be a period of considerable life stress as new roles and responsibilities are embraced and greater self-reliance is required to navigate difficult life situations (Arnett, 2004). In this sense, the emerging/young adult years can be a particularly vulnerable period where stress can contribute to the manifestation or consolidation of psychiatric and/or substance use disorders (Schulenberg, Sameroff, & Cicchetti, 2004). Indeed, cigarette use, binge drinking, heavy alcohol consumption, and illicit drug use peaks during the early twenties (Park et al., 2006). Rates of substance abuse and dependence are highest between the ages of 18 and 25 and then show a decline (Park et al., 2006). Moreover, adults aged 18 to 24 are at three-times greater risk of suicide than adolescents between ages 12 and 17, and 75% of all lifetime cases of diagnosable mental disorders begin by age 24 (Park et al., 2006).

The heightened manifestation of psychiatric and substance use problems during the early twenties may partially reflect inexperience adapting to the responsibilities of this period, problems entering into and maintaining intimate relationships, and failures in coping with sudden, unforeseen stressors. In fact, cigarette companies have historically counted on the transitional stress of young adulthood to market their cigarettes to young men and women (Ling & Glantz, 2002). Furthermore, stress has been associated with substance misuse and suicidal behavior (Mitchell & Dennis, 2006; Sinha, 2005; van Praag, 2004), both of which may represent maladaptive attempts to escape from problems and/or regulate affect. As such, emerging/young adults at greatest risk of developing mental health problems may be those who experience the most intense and prolonged life stress (particularly traumatic stress), who are most sensitive to stress, and who are most lacking in coping skills and social supports necessary to tolerate and overcome life's many disappointments and frustrations.

In this chapter, we will discuss some of the role transitions that can make emerging/young adulthood a particularly stressful developmental period, and the risk and resilience factors that may account for differences in adjustment. Regarding risk factors, we place particular emphasis on traumatic stress, since trauma can severely derail adult development and interfere with the establishment of a stable life structure. Left untreated, trauma can interfere on a long-term basis with the establishment of a stable career trajectory and the formation of healthy, long-term relationships. We will also discuss how difficulties coping with disappointments and setbacks related to the major developmental tasks of this period (establishment of work roles and intimate relationships) can lead to increased life stress and psychosocial impairment. Finally, we will discuss how treatment can address transitional life stress and traumatic stress in emerging/young adults.

"Welcome to the Real World": New Roles and Responsibilities of Emerging/Young Adults

It is not uncommon for family, friends, and co-workers to condescendingly welcome a newly transitioned adult to the real world upon hearing them complain that they had to work another late night or pay another bill, and it may be at this precise moment that reality sets in and the once paramount concerns of the past become comparatively trivial.

Whichever road one chooses following completion or discontinuation of secondary education, whether it is higher education, military service, entry into the workforce, or becoming a stay-at-home parent, new roles and responsibilities will be undertaken, and new stressors will abound. It is expected that young men and women will leave their parents' homes and cope effectively with the new demands of adult life (Scharf, Mayseless, & Kivenson-Baron, 2004). Those with the most mature life skills (e.g., financial responsibility, problem-solving and decision-making skills, ability to regulate emotions, social competence, ability to seek social support), who attend to their physical health, who are psychologically well adjusted, who behave ethically, who have healthy relationships, who are educated, who are engaged in productive pursuits, who "give back" to the community, and who are less threatened by their new roles and responsibilities are expected to cope best with this transition and meet with the most success (Benson, Scales, Hawkins, Oesterle, & Hill, 2004; Scharf et al., 2004). Of course, the types of stressors faced by emerging/young adults will vary according to their vocational and educational choices and sociocultural context. For instance, in the United States, most young men and women (over 60%) will enter higher education following completion of high school (Bianchi & Spain, 1996 as cited in Arnett, 2000), whereas in Israel, the majority of young Jewish men and women will leave home for mandatory service in the armed forces, where they will be responsible for others' lives and expensive military equipment (Scharf et al., 2004). A career in law enforcement will certainly convey different stressors than life in the business world, and manual labor will differ from office work in relation to stress exposure. Whatever the case, how well these young men and women cope with the stressors inherent to their new environments will likely impact their sense of self-efficacy and determine their overall level of adjustment throughout adult life.

Stress in Tackling the Developmental Tasks of Emerging/Young Adulthood

In Western cultures, two major developmental goals of emerging/young adulthood are that of establishing vocational identities and intimate relationships (Roisman, Masten, Coatsworth, & Tellegen, 2004). Accomplishing these goals requires sufficient labor/educational skills and interpersonal and conflict resolution skills necessary to maintain employment and establish/maintain intimate social relationships. Failure to gain competence in these domains and difficulties coping with problems related to them can cause considerable occupational and relationship stress.

As was portrayed in the first case vignette, the transition from full-time student to full-time employment can be one of the most difficult challenges of emerging/young adulthood. In the school setting, failure to perform typically affects only the individual, with no real consequences for other students or the educational institution. In the work setting, however, the employee carries a greater responsibility to others (e.g., co-workers, clients, patients) and to their particular business/health organization as a whole. Wrong decisions can have large ramifications for many parties, with much more being at stake than just receiving a failing grade (e.g., money; jobs; heath; survival of a business). Indeed, entering the workforce can open oneself up to a variety of stressors for which emerging/young adults may not be fully prepared, and difficulties regulating negative affect associated with work stress may lead to the development of psychopathology. Support for this contention comes from a recent longitudinal study that found that work stress precipitated the onset of major depression and generalized anxiety disorder in previously healthy young adult men and women (Melchior et al., 2007). In addition, a recent prospective epidemiologic study found that work environments characterized by high job strain (low control and high demands) increased the likelihood of developing drug dependence in young adulthood (Reed, Storr, & Anthony, 2006).

The need to develop intimacy in friendships and romantic partnerships also becomes paramount during these years (Roisman et al., 2004). Failure to establish intimate relationships can result in a lack of social support and social isolation, which serve as stressors by increasing negative affect, feelings of alienation, and loneliness (Cohen, 2004). Supportive relationships, in addition to reducing isolation, can help to diminish or eliminate the effects of stress by assisting with coping and by promoting less threatening interpretations of negative life events (Cohen, 2004; Ozbay et al., 2007). On the other hand, unsupportive social relationships can increase stress (Cohen, 2004), and negative relationship transitions, such as marital separation or divorce, can lead to feelings of distress (Lee & Gramotnev, 2007). Thus, an emerging/young adult's ability to enter into and maintain healthy intimate relationships by implementing adaptive communication, conflict resolution, and problem-solving skills may define his or her competency in this domain and partially determine quality of life and overall level of stress.

Vulnerability Factors

Emerging/young adulthood can be particularly taxing for individuals who have unsuccessful marriages, become parents too soon, who do not complete school, who fail to find work, or who get involved with drugs or crime (Jekielek & Brown, 2005; Osgood, Foster, Flanagan, & Ruth, 2005). All of these factors can hinder their ability to achieve financial stability and/or establish fulfilling relationships (Jekielek & Brown, 2005; Osgood et al., 2005). Having limited physical, social, and educational resources can be particularly detrimental and stress provoking. Specifically, individuals involved with mental health, juvenile and foster care systems, those who have reentered society from the criminal justice system, those who are in special education, those who have disabilities and chronic illnesses, and runaway/homeless youth are at greatest risk for having difficulties with the transition to adulthood (Osgood et al., 2005). Consequently, these individuals may be at high risk of experiencing additional stress-related problems during adulthood. For instance, having a criminal history can restrict employment and educational opportunities, which can lead to further criminal involvement (Uggen & Wakefield, 2005) and a greater likelihood of experiencing subsequent life stress (e.g., arrest; incarceration). Individuals with emotional disturbances may be shunned from social interactions that form the basis of healthy friendships and romantic relationships (Levine & Wagner, 2005), and individuals with chronic physical conditions may face constant social stigma and experience greater social isolation than their healthy peers (Blum, 2005). Moreover, runaway and homeless youth may struggle to find affordable housing during their transition, since they cannot rely on their families for support, and individuals with physical disabilities may have the added stress of having to arrange for medical services or devices to assist them with daily living (Osgood et al., 2005). Finally, as coping styles in adolescence predict how an individual will tend to cope with stress in young adulthood (Hussong & Chassin, 2004), youth who failed to develop adaptive coping will continue to be at a disadvantage when facing stress as young adults.

Indeed, navigating emerging/young adulthood can be stressful enough for individuals who start out with sufficient educational and social resources and no physical, intellectual, and coping deficiencies. However, the transition may be much more difficult and stress-provoking for the vulnerable populations described above. Not only do they face more problems, setbacks, and inconveniences, but they are also more limited in resources and supports needed to help them through the many challenges and stresses of adult life.

Traumatic Stress and the Derailment of Adult Development

Trauma represents the most extreme form of adverse life event, and there is evidence that traumatic stress, especially in response to repeated trauma that occurs early in life, can have large ramifications on development, psychosocial functioning, psychological adjustment, and even physical health (Anda et al., 2006; van der Kolk, 2005). Childhood maltreatment and other forms of trauma may alter brain-stress responding (Bugental, 2004; DeBellis, 2002) and sensitize individuals to the effects of subsequent life stressors (Glaser, Os, Portegijs, & Myin-Germeys, 2006; Harkness, Bruce, & Lumley, 2006). With the development of post-traumatic stress disorder (PTSD), the combination of chronically elevated levels of arousal, often in the form of more or less constant anxiety, intrusive and disturbing recollections of traumatic events that distract from focused attention on the present and have a disorganizing effect on behavior, and an avoidance of situations associated with traumatic experiences that is subject to stimulus generalization (American Psychiatric Association, 2000) can interfere appreciably with routine daily functioning.

Traumatic stress, especially when it results from protracted child abuse, may disrupt the maturation of self-regulatory systems that enable a person to modulate and tolerate aversive affective states (Cicchetti & Toth, 2005; Hein, Cohen, & Campbell, 2005). Markedly reduced resiliency to stress, a proclivity to be emotionally overwhelmed, and a tendency to disorganized behavior in the form of rage reactions and impulsive behavior are common. These trends make it exceedingly difficult, and in some instances impossible, for young adults affected by trauma to establish effective interpersonal relationships and stable career patterns.

The combination of chronic arousal (i.e., sleep difficulty, irritability, difficulty concentrating, hypervigilence, and exaggerated startle), intrusive re-experiencing of trauma (i.e., through distressing recollections of the event, disturbing dreams, and flashbacks), and persistent behavioral avoidance of people and situations that arouse recollections of the trauma and which can result in diminished participation in social activities and estrangement from others are also likely to intensely compromise coping abilities. In a desperate attempt to obtain even momentary relief from prolonged periods of elevated distress, trauma survivors are at markedly increased risk to develop reliance on maladaptive forms of coping such as substance abuse (Dube et al., 2002, 2003; Edwards, Dunham, Ries, & Barnett, 2006; Felitti, 2003), nonchemical patterns of addictive behavior such as pathological gambling (Kausch, Loreen, & Rowland, 2006; Petry & Steinberg, 2005) and sexual compulsivity (Carnes & Delmonico, 1996), vulnerability to dissociative responses to stress (Argargun et al., 2003; Van den Bosch, Herheul, Langeland, & Van den Brink, 2003), and self-injurious behavior (Yates, 2004). Treatment for PTSD therefore often requires balancing targeting traumatic stress symptoms with treating addictive and compulsive behavior patterns (Ford & Russo, 2006).

In treating young adults with trauma-related difficulties stemming from extensive histories of child abuse, it is especially important to take into account the impact of family of origin background. A dysfunctional family environment commonly associated with childhood maltreatment trauma is characterized by a lack of consistent affection, structure, and guidance that results in deficits in basic living and coping skills necessary to care for oneself, make sound decisions and overcome problems, and alleviate feelings of distress (Gold, 2000). This type of family environment has repeatedly been found to be marked by low levels of adaptation, cohesion, expressiveness, and encouragement of independence and elevated degrees of conflict and control (Gold, Hyman, & Andres-Hyman, 2004). This pattern is not limited to maltreating families; families of children who are abused by nonfamilial perpetrators exhibit the same constellation of traits (Gold et al., 2004; Ray & Jackson, 1994). Moreover, these family characteristics have been shown to contribute to maladjustment in adulthood independent of the impact of abuse trauma (Higgins & McCabe, 2003). It is therefore crucial in working with young adults with trauma-related difficulties to assess for developmental gaps and deficits in adaptive capacities that require remediation in order to assist them in successfully navigating the developmental tasks of young adulthood; exclusively trauma-focused intervention cannot be expected to effectively address these areas (Gold, 2008).

Indeed, the second case vignette illustrates several key points about traumatic stress in response to an incident occurring in young adulthood: *(1)* Without appropriate treatment, posttraumatic stress disorder (PTSD) can continue indefinitely and may even worsen in severity over time (Flannery, 1999; Goenjian et al., 2005). *(2)* When trauma occurs in young adulthood and is not resolved, major developmental tasks from this period, especially the establishment of the elements of a stable adult life structure such as progressing in career and forming an enduring romantic partnership, are at high risk of being derailed (Gold, 2008). *(3)* Trauma in young adulthood can interfere with the consolidation of identity, especially the process of resolving apparent inconsistencies between the roles imposed on the individual when she or he was growing up and current self-perceptions that are inconsistent with them. *(4)* In addition to disrupting current developmental tasks, trauma is most likely to be debilitating to individuals who were reared in a family environment that did not adequately meet their developmental needs in their formative years (Finzi-Dottan & Karu, 2006; Gold, 2008; Gold, Hyman, & Andres-Hyman, 2004; Higgins & McCabe, 2000).

Stress and Substance Use in Emerging/Young Adulthood

In recent years, there has been a rise in illicit drug use among college students, in most student subgroups, and across students enrolled in all types of colleges (Gledhill-Hoyt, Lee, Strote, & Wechsler, 2000). Furthermore, there has been an increase in prescription drug abuse among 12–17 year olds (Under the Counter, 2005). These are just some examples of the growing drug problem afflicting young people. Considering these increases and the fact that substance use and misuse peaks during the early twenties (Park et al., 2006), it is important to consider how stress can lead to substance use and how engaging in maladaptive drug-use behaviors can sensitize individuals to the effects of stress and facilitate poor coping, both of which can interfere with a successful adult transition.

Stress Increases Risk of Substance Use

There is substantial evidence that stress can increase an individual's vulnerability to substance use, particularly when life stress is high and coping resources are impoverished (Sinha, 2005; Wills, 1990; Wills & Hirky, 1996). As demonstrated in the first case vignette, the transitional stress and newfound responsibilities of emerging/young adulthood (e.g., new work roles) may be related to the increases in substance use seen during this period, and the risk of developing substance use disorders may be particularly high for those who are most deficient in coping ability (e.g., individuals raised in abusive families). Some support for this contention comes from a recent prospective epidemiologic study that found that work environments characterized by high job strain (low control and high demands) increased the likelihood of developing drug dependence in young adulthood (Reed, Storr, & Anthony, 2006) and literature indicating that greater use of maladaptive avoidance coping strategies are related to a greater likelihood of drug use initiation and higher levels of ongoing use (Wills & Hirky,

1996). As such, stress should be considered as an etiological factor in the initiation and/or escalation of substance use during this period and should be a primary target when considering prevention strategies and clinical intervention.

Substance Use Alters Stress and Reward Pathways

In addition to stress influencing drug abuse in vulnerable individuals, there is emerging evidence that brain stress systems are activated by drugs of abuse, and chronic use results in neuroadaptations that enhance stress sensitivity, increase craving and wanting of drugs, and also enhance the salience of drugs, thereby promoting continued drug use (Fox, Hong, Siedlarz, & Sinha, 2007; Sinha, 2005). Thus, secondary and college-aged students who become involved with substances, either through social or coping motives, may be placing themselves at risk of experiencing greater stress during emerging/young adulthood. The brain changes that can result from continual and chronic substance use can cause greater stress sensitivity and an overreliance on substance use as a fast-acting, yet maladaptive, coping strategy. While coping through substance use may provide immediate, yet temporary, relief from problems and associated distress, coping in this manner prevents goal-directed problem solving that can potentially result in further difficulties (e.g., using drugs to cope with relationship stress rather than working through the problem can lead to a breakup). Moreover, with increasing drug use, greater legal, social, and occupational problems may arise, thereby increasing life stress and interfering with adult functioning. Finally, alterations in brain-stress and reward pathways can increase drug craving and compulsive drug seeking (Sinha, 2005), thereby perpetuating substance use disorders and severely derailing successful emerging/young adult development. It is, therefore, important when working with emerging/young adults to assess for substance use and to develop a conceptualization of how substance use may be contributing to stress and hindering the development of a more adaptive coping repertoire. Interventions focused on reducing or eliminating substance use and on teaching adaptive modes of coping will likely have an effect on reducing stress during emerging/young adulthood.

Tailoring Stress-Coping Interventions to Emerging/Young Adults

Emerging/young adults must begin to develop optimal ways of coping with stress as they adapt to their new environments and take on their new adult roles and responsibilities. How skillfully they employ various coping strategies will partially determine their level of adjustment (Hussong & Chassin, 2004). Excessive reliance on parents and/or maladaptive coping strategies (e.g., drug abuse, avoidance) to solve problems and/or regulate affect could lead to greater stress while hindering the development of a more adaptive stress-coping repertoire. Trying various coping strategies and observing their effectiveness may be a process by which emerging/young adults build upon previously developed strategies and streamline their ability to cope with stress as they move through adulthood.

Coping factors associated with resilience to stress and stress-induced psychiatric disorders include feeling positive emotions (e.g., optimism and humor); the ability to reappraise, reframe, or find meaning in a stressful situation or event; acceptance of stressful circumstances; finding spirituality/religion; seeking social support; actively approaching problems (and not avoiding them); and regular exercise (Southwick, Vythilingam, & Charney, 2005). Importantly, increasing any one or combination of resiliency factors will likely have beneficial effects on other ones (Southwick et al., 2005). For instance, becoming more optimistic may facilitate social support seeking and vice versa. As such, cognitive-behavioral, pharmacological, and social support interventions focused on bolstering any of these resiliency factors will likely have beneficial effects in reducing stress and improving mental health. Importantly, interventions may meet with the most success if specifically tailored to the developmental stage of the treated individual.

Indeed, evidence suggests that younger adults differ from older adults with respect to the types of stressors they face, their emotional reactions to stress, the ways in which they characteristically cope with stress, and their overall effectiveness in coping with stress. For example, one study found that younger adults were more likely to describe anger in response to interpersonal problems than older adults, and they also reported more intense negative reactions to interpersonal stress (Birditt & Fingerman, 2003). Another study found that thinking optimistically to manage negative affect was greater among middle-aged adults than younger adults (Chapman & Hayslip Jr., 2006). Other researchers found that a higher percentage of college seniors report directly facing problems, whereas younger students take a more passive approach to dealing with stress (Jackson & Finney, 2002). Moreover, a recent review indicated that younger adults are less adept at solving problems and regulating affect than older adults who are better able to use their experiences in social and emotional situations to choose diverse and appropriate emotion regulation and instrumental coping strategies to solve problems effectively (Blanchard-Fields, 2007). Indeed, coping seems to mature with age. As such, stress-focused interventions tailored toward facilitating the development and/or reorganization of adaptive coping strategies and the elimination or minimization of maladaptive coping strategies may be beneficial to the well-being and mental health of emerging/young adults, and particularly for those who are severely deficient in coping ability.

Stress Prevention through Proactive Coping

Probably the best way to manage stress is to proactively cope with it, or prevent it from happening in the first place. Indeed, stress can often be thwarted by thinking ahead to what might be needed in a given situation and taking the effort to prepare for possible adversity (Greenglass, 2003). Emerging/young adults, who have less experience than older adults in addressing stressful situations on their own, may benefit from education regarding what stressors to expect in certain situations and how to plan accordingly. For instance, a new employee may be able to prevent or minimize work-related stress by discussing with a more experienced co-worker the types of problems that have arisen at the workplace and how the experienced co-worker handled problems in the past. Steps can then be taken to prepare should a similar problem arise. A student who is planning to work in addition to taking a full class load may not have the time and energy to consistently keep up with class readings, and cramming for exams may be his/her only recourse. Yet, for this student, taking a lighter class load at the start of the semester may help reduce academic stress. In addition to seeking information from more experienced adults, therapists working with emerging/young adults may self-disclose how they prevented stressful situations from happening in their own lives in order to model effective ways of proactively coping with life stress. Indeed, education and counseling related to proactive coping may help individuals prevent many of the stressors that make emerging/young adulthood so difficult.

Actively Facing Stressors

Even if proactive coping is implemented flawlessly, it is unlikely that one would be able to avert all stressors, and there must eventually be a shift to coping strategies needed to deal with unforeseen stressful situations (e.g., illness; layoff; break-up with a significant other) as they arise. Once harm, threat, or challenge is identified, one must evaluate the coping strategies that will meet with the most success in managing the stressful situation (Lazarus & Folkman, 1984). The best choice of coping strategies may depend on the particular stressor at hand. In instances when a solution is possible and immediate action could solve the problem, it is best to actively approach the problem and not avoid it (i.e., by procrastinating on an assignment; through drinking or drug use), since avoidance does nothing to solve the problem and can even lead to increased stress (e.g., procrastinating on a work assignment can lead to high stress when rushing to make a deadline). Training in effective ways to solve problems and resolve interpersonal conflicts may help emerging/young adults identify and cope with stressful situations without feeling overwhelmed, helpless, or out of control.

In instances when nothing can be done to fix a problem (e.g., when dealing with the death of a loved one), or when trying to solve a problem may make a situation worse (e.g., arguing a ticket with a police officer), a shift in focus must be made to regulate one's emotional stress response in order to be able to think more rationally, reduce impulsiveness, and meet with a more positive or less damaging outcome. Indeed, a primary focus of emotion regulation is on keeping a stressful situation from becoming worse by overreacting to it or reacting in a negative manner that can lead to increased stress (e.g., acting out in anger at one's boss could result in job loss; squeezing a girlfriend's arm to make her accept an apology can lead to greater conflict). Emotion regulation skills can also be implemented to enhance problem solving and conflict-resolution efforts by reducing emotional reactions that can interfere with rational thought and prosocial behavior.

Therapeutic Interventions

Various cognitive-behavioral and mindfulness/ acceptance-based techniques have been developed to teach individuals ways to alter problems and regulate emotional stress responses to problems. Cognitive restructuring, which involves learning to think critically in order to modify appraisals of stressful situations and alter erroneous cognitions that maintain stress (e.g., finding meaning in a stressful situation; viewing a stressor as a challenge; challenging the accuracy of one's thoughts; thought stopping), and behavioral coping skills training, which involves learning specific behavioral skills to prevent or manage stressful situations (e.g., social skills training, problem-solving training, relaxation training, time management training, and organizational skills training), can be employed to teach individuals ways to reduce emotional stress reactions, enlist social support (coping assistance), and overcome or prevent stress (Gardner, Rose, Mason, Tyler, & Cushway, 2005; Lazarus & Folkman, 1984). Indeed, cognitive- behavioral interventions have proven effective in the treatment of mood, anxiety, and substance use disorders (Butler, Chapman, Forman, & Beck, 2006; Carroll, 1996; Leichsenring, Hiller, Weissberg, & Leibing, 2006; Norton & Price, 2007). Some popular therapies that incorporate cognitive and behavioral techniques include cognitive therapy (e.g., Beck & Emery, 1985), rational emotive behavior therapy (Ellis & Dryden, 2007), and stress inoculation training (Meichenbaum, 1985).

Mindfulness-based stress reduction (MBSR) was developed by Jon Kabat-Zinn (1990) and involves directing attention to what is happening in the moment and suspending the impulse to judge what one is experiencing in an effort to build up a resistance to stress and respond adaptively to problematic situations. It has been shown to have an effect on reducing stress, improving mood, enhancing positive coping strategies, and decreasing negative coping strategies (Chang et al., 2004; Proulx, 2003; Walach et al., 2007) and can be applied to young adults as they attempt to cope with the stressors of adulthood. Mindfulness/acceptance-based techniques have been incorporated into structured therapies such as dialectical behavior therapy (DBT) to address affect dysregulation in patients with borderline personality disorder (Linehan, 1993), acceptance and commitment therapy (Hayes, Strosahl, & Wilson, 1999), and mindfulness-based cognitive therapy for depression (Segal, Williams, & Teasdale, 2002).

For individuals diagnosed with simple PTSD, prolonged exposure therapy has the best empirical support (Foa, 2000; Foa & Meadows, 1997). However, this form of treatment can be emotionally taxing because it requires confronting the traumatic event or events that engendered the client's difficulties to begin with. Therefore, exposure-based interventions require sufficient coping capacities to productively process traumatic material without becoming overwhelmed by it. Since young adults may react more intensely to certain stressors than older adults (Birditt & Fingerman, 2003) and because they may not be as adept at coping as older adults (Blanchard-Fields, 2007), some level of training in coping strategies may be crucial before exposure-based intervention is initiated. The three categories of skills training discussed above: stress reduction training, mindfulness training, and training in judgment and reasoning can be extremely valuable in optimizing the success of exposure therapy. Mastery of stress reduction greatly reduces the likelihood that the client will become overwhelmed by the traumatic material. Training in mindfulness helps diminish the probability that during exposure the client will be inundated with vivid flashbacks by supporting the ability to stay grounded in the present while reviewing recollections of past trauma. The development of strong judgment and reasoning skills assists the client in developing a more rational appraisal of the traumatic situation and its impact.

Encouraging Stress Reducing Activities Outside of Therapy

Two already popular activities among emerging/young adults that have stress-reducing effects are exercise and yoga (Michalsen et al., 2005). The growing popularity of fitness clubs and yoga studios may have something to do with the beneficial effects exercise has on mood and cognitive functioning and its ability to reduce an individual's sensitivity to stress (Southwick et al., 2005; Tsatsoulis & Fountoulakis, 2006). Yoga, which appears to be more popular among women than men, is an ancient Indian practice that combines muscle relaxation with stretching, meditation, and exercise and which has stress-reducing benefits comparable to cognitive-behavioral therapy (Granath, Ingvarsson, von Thiele, & Lundberg, 2006; Michalsen et al., 2005; Smith, Hancock, Blake-Mortimer, & Eckert, 2007). Additionally, researchers have found it to have other stress-related benefits such as pain relief (Michalsen et al., 2005). Moreover, exercise and yoga can improve one's body image, enhance self-confidence, and thereby reduce stress in social, dating, and/or sexual situations. Indeed, yoga and exercise should be encouraged among emerging/young adults as a nonstigmatizing and social mean of reducing life stress and preventing mental health problems.

Spirituality, whether through organized religion or a personal belief in a higher power, has also been found to enhance coping and protect against illness possibly by providing a framework for understanding and making sense of adversity (Southwick et al., 2005). Support for this contention comes from a recent meta-analysis of 49 studies which found that individuals who used positive religious coping strategies (benevolent religious reappraisals, seeking spiritual support, collaborative religious coping, etc.) experienced greater positive adjustment to stress than individuals who did not utilize these strategies (Ano & Vasconcelles, 2005). Indeed, spirituality can be harnessed as a means of coping with life stress and may be encouraged among emerging/young adults who are open to it. Attendance at social support focused community functions with a spiritual component (e.g., organized religion, Alcoholics Anonymous) may also be encouraged as a means of enhancing resilience to stress and stress-induced psychiatric disorders (Southwick et al., 2005).

Conclusion

Emerging/young adulthood can be a stressful developmental period that can convey an increased risk for the development of psychiatric and substance use disorders. The types of stressors emerging/young adults face will vary according to their culture, choices, and circumstances. How well they cope with the stressors inherent to their new environments will impact their level of adjustment throughout adult life. Two major developmental tasks of this period are to establish vocational identities and intimate relationships, and failure to gain competence and success in these domains can cause considerable occupational and relationship stress. Emerging/young adulthood may be most difficult for individuals with physical, intellectual, and coping deficiencies and poor educational and social resources. Exposure to traumatic stress can be particularly detrimental as it can severely derail young adult development and interfere with a stable career trajectory and the formation of healthy, intimate relationships. Moreover, stress can lead to substance use in vulnerable individuals, and chronic substance abuse can further increase stress sensitivity, disrupt adaptive coping, and interfere with a successful adult transition.

Stress-coping focused interventions must be specifically tailored to emerging/young adults who are less experienced than older adults at solving problems and regulating affect through the use of diverse and appropriate coping strategies. Interventions geared toward the development and reorganization of adaptive strategies (e.g., planning; seeking social support) and the elimination or minimization of maladaptive coping strategies (e.g., avoidance, addiction) may benefit emerging/young adults and particularly traumatized individuals and those who are otherwise deficient in coping ability.

Interventions administered within the therapeutic environment (e.g., cognitive-behavioral therapy; mindfulness-based stress reduction) and self-administered outside of therapy (e.g., exercise and yoga) are effective and should be strongly encouraged.

KEY POINTS

- Entering into emerging/young adulthood can be a stressful developmental period, particularly for vulnerable individuals (e.g., intellectually and socially disadvantaged), that can convey an increased risk for the development of psychiatric and substance use disorders. How well they cope with the stressors inherent to their new environments will impact their level of adjustment throughout adult life.
- Traumatic stress can be particularly detrimental as it can severely derail young adult development and interfere with a stable career trajectory and the formation of healthy, intimate relationships, which are two major developmental tasks of this period.
- Stress, and particularly traumatic stress, can lead to maladaptive coping through substance abuse, which can further increase stress sensitivity, disrupt adaptive coping, and interfere with a successful adult transition.
- Emerging/young adults may react more intensely to stress than older adults and may be less experienced than older adults at solving problems and regulating negative affect through the use of diverse and appropriate coping strategies.

PRACTICE GUIDELINES

- Careful clinical assessment of current life stressors, traumatic stress, and the maladaptive stress reactions associated with them (e.g., substance abuse, PTSD, depression) is necessary for effective treatment planning with emerging/young adults who may be having difficulty adjusting to their new adult roles and responsibilities. Stress-coping focused interventions, especially traumatic stress–focused interventions (exposure therapy) should be specifically tailored to emerging/young adults who are less experienced than older adults at coping with stress. Bolstering coping skills and any combination of resiliency factors (e.g., social support, spirituality) may reduce reliance upon maladaptive methods of coping, facilitate a successful adult transition, and increase the likelihood that trauma-focused interventions will be successful.
- Stress should be considered an etiological factor in the initiation and perpetuation of substance use disorders during this period and should be a primary target for intervention. Clinicians should also be mindful of the effects of substance abuse on brain-stress and reward systems, which can sensitize individuals to the effects of stress, facilitate poor coping, and interfere with a successful transition to young adulthood.

(Practice Guidelines continued)

- Cognitive-behavioral and mindfulness/acceptance-based interventions administered within the therapeutic environment and stress-reducing social activities undertaken outside of therapy (e.g., exercise, yoga) are effective and should be strongly encouraged.

References

American Psychiatric Association. (2000). *Diagnostic and statistical manual of mental disorders* (4th ed., Text revision). Washington, DC.

Anda, R. F., Felitti, V. J., Bremner, J. D., Walker, J. D., Whitfield, C., Perry, B. D., Dube, S. R., & Giles, W. H. (2006). The enduring effects of abuse and related adverse experiences in childhood: A convergence of evidence from neurobiology and epidemiology. *European Archives of Psychiatry and Clinical Neuroscience, 256*(3), 174–186.

Ano, G. G., & Vasconcelles, E. B. (2005). Religious coping and psychological adjustment to stress: A meta-analysis. *Journal of Clinical Psychology, 61*(4), 461–480.

Argargun, M. Y., Kara, H., Oezer, O. A., Selvi, Y., Kiran, U., & Kiran, S. (2003). Nightmares and dissociative experiences: The key role of childhood traumatic events. *Psychiatry & Clinical Neurosciences, 67*(2), 139–145.

Arnett, J. J. (2000). Emerging adulthood: A theory of development from the late teens through the twenties. *American Psychologist, 55*(5), 469–480.

Arnett, J. J. (2004). *Emerging adulthood: The winding road from the late teens through the twenties.* New York: Oxford University Press.

Beck, A. T., & Emery, G. (1985). *Anxiety disorders and phobias: A cognitive perspective.* USA: Basic Books.

Benson, P. L., Scales, P. C., Hawkins, J. D., Oesterle, S., & Hill, K. G. (2004). *Executive summary: Successful young adult development.* A report submitted to the Bill & Melinda Gates Foundation.

Birditt, K. S., & Fingerman, K. L. (2003). Age and gender differences in adults' descriptions of emotional reactions to interpersonal problems. *Journal of Gerontology, 58B*(4), 237–245.

Blanchard-Fields, F. (2007). Everyday problem solving and emotion: An adult developmental perspective. *Current Directions in Psychological Science, 16*(1), 26–31.

Blum, R. W. M. (2005). Adolescents with disabilities in transition to adulthood. In D. W. Osgood, E. M. Foster, C. Flanagan & C. R. Ruth (Eds.), *On your own without a net: The transition to adulthood for vulnerable populations* (pp. 1–26). Chicago: The University of Chicago Press.

Bugental, D. B. (2004). Thriving in the face of early adversity. *Journal of Social Issues, 60*(1), 219–235.

Butler, A. C., Chapman, J. E., Forman, E. M., & Beck, A. T. (2006). The empirical status of cognitive-behavioral therapy: A review of meta-analyses. *Clinical Psychology Review, 26,* 17–31.

Carnes, P. J., & Delmonico, D. L. (1996). Childhood abuse and sexual addictions: Research findings in a sample of self-identified sexual addicts. *Sexual Addiction & Compulsivity, 3*(3), 258–268.

Carroll, K. M. (1996). Relapse prevention as a psychosocial treatment: A review of controlled clinical trials. *Experimental and Clinical Psychopharmacology, 4*(1), 46–54.

Chang, V. Y., Palesh, O., Caldwell, R., Glasgow, N., Abramson, M., Luskin, F., Gill, M., Burke, A., & Koopman, C. (2004). The effects of a mindfulness-based stress reduction program on stress, mindfulness self-efficacy, and positive states of mind. *Stress and Health, 20,* 141–147.

Chapman, B. P., & Hayslip Jr., B. (2006). Emotional intelligence in young and middle adulthood: Cross-sectional analysis of latent structure and means. *Psychology and Aging, 21*(2), 411–418.

Cicchetti, D., & Toth, S. L. (2005). Child maltreatment. *Annual Review of Clinical Psychology, 1,* 409–438.

Cohen, S. (2004). Social relationships and health. *American Psychologist, 59*(8), 676–684.

DeBellis, M. D. (2002). Developmental traumatology: A contributory mechanism for alcohol and substance use disorders. *Psychoneuroendocrinology, 27,* 155–170.

Dube, S. R., Anda, R. F., Felitti, V. J., Edwards, V. J., & Croft, J. B. (2002). Adverse childhood experiences and personal alcohol abuse as an adult. *Addictive Behaviors, 27,* 713–725.

Dube, S. R., Felitti, V. J., Dong, M., Chapman, D. P., Giles, W. H., & Anda, R. F. (2003). Childhood abuse, neglect, and household dysfunction and the risk of illicit drug use: The adverse childhood experiences study. *Pediatrics, 111,* 564–572.

Edwards, C., Dunham, D. N., Ries, A., & Barnett, J. (2006). Symptoms of traumatic stress and substance use in a non-clinical sample of young adults. *Addictive Behaviors, 31*(11), 2094–2104.

Ellis, A., & Dryden, W. (2007). *The practice of rational emotive behavior therapy* (2nd ed.). New York: Springer.

Felitti, V. J. (2003). Ursprünge des Suchtverhaltens—Evidenzen aus einer Studie zu belastenden Kindheitfahrungen [Origins of addictive behavior: Evidence from a study of stressful childhood experiences], *Praxis der Kinderpsychologie und Kinderpsychiatrie, 52*(8), 547–559.

Finzi-Dottan, R., & Karu, T. (2006). From emotional abuse in childhood to psychopathology in adulthood: A path mediated by immature defense mechanisms and self-esteem. *Journal of Nervous and Mental Disease, 194*(8), 616–621.

Flannery, R. B. (1999). Psychological trauma and posttraumatic stress disorder: A review. *International Journal of Emergency Mental Health, 1*(2), 135–140.

Foa, E. B. (2000). Psychosocial treatment of posttraumatic stress disorder. *Journal of Clinical Psychiatry, 61*(5), S49–S51.

Foa, E. B., & Meadows, E. A. (1997). Psychosocial treatments for posttraumatic stress disorder: A critical review. *Annual Review of Psychology, 48,* 449–480.

Ford, J. D., & Russo, E. (2006). Trauma-focused, present-centered, emotional self-regulation approach to integrated treatment for posttraumatic stress and addiction: Trauma adaptive recovery group education and therapy (TARGET). *American Journal of Psychotherapy, 60*(4), 335–355.

Fox, H. C., Hong, K. A., Siedlarz, K., & Sinha, R. (2007). Enhanced sensitivity to stress and drug/alcohol craving in abstinent cocaine dependent individuals compared to social drinkers. *Neuropsychopharmacology, 33*(4), 796–805.

Gardner, B., Rose, J., Mason, O., Tyler, P., & Cushway, D. (2005). Cognitive therapy and behavioral coping in the management of work-related stress: An intervention study. *Work & Stress, 19*(2), 137–152.

Glaser, J., Os, J. V., Portegijs, P. J. M., & Myin-Germeys, I. (2006). Childhood trauma and emotional reactivity to daily life stress in adult frequent attenders of general practitioners. *Journal of Psychosomatic Research, 61,* 229–236.

Gledhill-Hoyt, J., Lee, H., Strote, J., & Wechsler, H. (2000). Increased use of marijuana and other illicit drugs at US colleges in the 1990s: results of three national surveys. *Addiction, 95*(11), 1655–1667.

Goenjian, A. K., Walling, D., Steinberg, A. M., Karayan, I., Najarian, L. M., & Pynoos, R. (2005). A prospective study of posttraumatic stress and depressive reactions among treated and untreated adolescents 5 years after a catastrophic disaster. *American Journal of Psychiatry, 162*(12), 2302–2308.

Gold, S. N. (2000). *Not trauma alone: Therapy for child abuse survivors in family and social context.* Lillington, NC: Taylor & Francis.

Gold, S. N. (2008). Benefits of a contextual approach to understanding and treating complex trauma. *Journal of Trauma & Dissociation, 9*(2), 269–292.

Gold, S. N., Hyman, S. M., & Andres-Hyman, R. C. (2004). Family of origin environments in two clinical samples of survivors of intra-familial, extra-familial, and both types of sexual abuse. *Child Abuse & Neglect, 28,* 1199–1212.

Granath, J., Ingvarsson, S., von Thiele, U., & Lundberg, U. (2006). Stress management: A randomized study of cognitive behavioral therapy and yoga. *Cognitive Behaviour Therapy, 35*(1), 3–10.

Greenglass, E. R. (2003). Proactive coping and quality of life management. In E. Frydenberg, (Ed.), *Beyond coping: Meeting goals, visions, and challenges* (pp. 37–62). Oxford, England: Oxford University Press.

Harkness, K. L., Bruce, A. E., & Lumley, M. N. (2006). The role of childhood abuse and neglect in the sensitization to stressful life events in adolescent depression. *Journal of Abnormal Psychology, 115*(4), 730–741.

Hayes, S. C., Strosahl, K. D., & Wilson, K. G. (1999). *Acceptance and commitment therapy: An experiential approach to behavior change.* New York: Guilford Press.

Hein, D., Cohen, L., & Campbell, A. (2005). Is traumatic stress a vulnerability factor for women with substance use disorders? *Clinical Psychology Review, 25,* 813–823.

Higgins, D. J., & McCabe, M. P. (2000). Multi-type maltreatment and the long-term maladjustment of adults. *Child Abuse Review, 9,* 6–18.

Higgins, D. J., & McCabe, M. P. (2003). Maltreatment and family dysfunction in childhood and the subsequent adjustment of children and adults. *Journal of Family Violence, 18*(2), 107–120.

Hussong, A. M., & Chassin, L. (2004). Stress and coping among children of alcoholic parents through the young adult transition. *Development and Psychopathology, 16,* 985–1006.

Jackson, P. B., & Finney, M. (2002). Negative life events and psychological distress among young adults. *Social Psychology Quarterly, 65*(2), 186–201.

Jekielek, S., & Brown, B. (2005). *The transition to adulthood: Characteristics of young adults ages 18 to 24 in America.* A Kids Count/PRB/Child Trends Report on Census 2000. The Annie E. Casey Foundation.

Kabat-Zinn, J. (1990). *Full catastrophe living: Using the wisdom of your body and mind to face stress, pain, and illness.* New York: Delacorte.

Kausch, O., Loreen, R., & Rowland, D. Y. (2006). Lifetime histories of trauma among pathological gamblers. *The American Journal on Addictions, 15*(1), 35–43.

Lazarus, R. S., & Folkman, S. (1984). *Stress, appraisal and coping*. New York: Springer.

Lee, C., & Gramotnev, H. (2007). Life transitions and mental health in a national cohort of young austrailian women. *Developmental Psychology, 43*(4), 877–888.

Leichsenring, F., Hiller, W., Weissberg, M., & Leibing, E. (2006). Cognitive-behavioral therapy and psychodynamic psychotherapy: Techniques, efficacy, and indications. *American Journal of Psychotherapy, 60*(3), 233–259.

Levine, P., & Wagner, M. (2005). Transition for young adults who received special education services as adolescents: A time for challenge and change. In D. W. Osgood, E. M. Foster, C. Flanagan, & C. R. Ruth (Eds.), *On your own without a net: The transition to adulthood for vulnerable populations* (pp. 1–26). Chicago: The University of Chicago Press.

Linehan, M. M. (1993). *Cognitive behavioral therapy of borderline personality disorder*. New York:Guilford Press.

Ling, P. M., & Glantz, S. A. (2002). Why and how the tobacco industry sells cigarettes to young adults: Evidence from industry documents. *American Journal of Public Health, 92*(6), 908–916.

Meichenbaum, D. (1985). *Stress inoculation training*. New York: Pergamon Press.

Melchior, M., Caspi, A., Milne, B. J., Danese, A., Poulton, R., & Moffitt, T. E. (2007). Work stress precipitates depression and anxiety in young, working women and men. *Psychological Medicine, 37*(8), 1119–1129.

Michalsen, A., Grossman, P., Scil, A., Langhorst, J., Ludtke, R., Esch, T., Stefano, G. B., & Dobos, G. J. (2005). Rapid stress reduction and anxiolysis among distressed women as a consequence of a three-month intensive yoga program. *Medical Science Monitor, 11*(12), CR555–561.

Mitchell, A. J., & Dennis, M. (2006). Self harm and attempted suicide in adults: 10 practical questions and answers for emergency department staff. *Emergency Medicine Journal, 23,* 251–255.

Norton, P. J., & Price, E. C. (2007). A meta-analytic review of adult cognitive-behavioral treatment outcome across the anxiety disorders. *The Journal of Nervous and Mental Disease, 195*(6), 521–531.

Ozbay, F., Johnson, D. C., Dimoulas, E., Morgan III., C. A., Charney, D., & Southwick, S. (2007). Social support and resilience to stress: From neurobiology to clinical practice. *Psychiatry, 4*(5), 35–40.

Osgood, D. W., Foster, E. M., Flanagan, C., & Ruth, C. R. (2005). Introduction: Why focus on the transition to adulthood for vulnerable populations? In D. W. Osgood, E. M. Foster, C. Flanagan, & C. R. Ruth (Eds.), *On your own without a net: The transition to adulthood for vulnerable populations* (pp. 1–26). Chicago: The University of Chicago Press.

Park, M. J., Mulye, T. P., Adams, S. H., Brindis, C. D., & Irwin, Jr., C. E. (2006). The health status of young adults in the United States. *Journal of Adolescent Health, 39,* 305–317.

Petry, N. M., & Steinberg, K. L. (2005). Childhood maltreatment in male and female treatment-seeking pathological gamblers. *Psychology of Addictive Behaviors, 19*(2), 226–229.

Proulx, K. (2003). Integrating mindfulness-based stress reduction. *Holistic Nursing Practice, 17*(4), 201–208.

Ray, K. C., & Jackson, J. L. (1994). Childhood sexual abuse: An examination of family functioning. *Journal of Interpersonal Violence, 9*(2), 270–277.

Reed, P. L., Storr, C. L., & Anthony, J. C. (2006). Drug dependence enviromics: Job strain in the work environment and risk of becoming drug-dependent. *American Journal of Epidemiology, 163*(5), 404–411.

Roisman, G. I., Masten, A. S., Coatsworth, J. D., & Tellegen, A. (2004). Salient and emerging developmental tasks in the transition to adulthood. *Child Development, 75*(1), 123–133.

Scharf, M., Mayseless, O., & Kivenson-Baron, I. (2004). Adolescents' attachment representations and developmental tasks in emerging adulthood. *Developmental Psychology, 40*(3), 430–444.

Schulenberg, J. E., Sameroff, A. J., & Cicchetti, D. (2004). The transition to adulthood as a critical juncture in the course of psychopathology and mental health. *Development and Psychopathology, 16,* 799–806.

Segal, Z. V., Williams, J. M. G., & Teasdale, J. D. (2002). *Mindfulness-based cognitive therapy for depression: A new approach to preventing relapse.* New York: Guilford Press.

Sinha, R. (2005). Stress and drug abuse. In N. H. K. T. Steckler & J. M. H. M. Reul (Eds.), *Handbook of stress and the brain. Part 2. Stress: Integrative and clinical aspects* (Vol. 15, pp. 333–356). Amsterdam: Elsevier.

Smith, C., Hancock, H., Blake-Mortimer, J., & Eckert, K. (2007). A randomized comparative trial of yoga and relaxation to reduce stress and anxiety. *Complementary Therapies in Medicine, 15,* 77–83.

Southwick, S. M., Vythilingam, M., & Charney, D. S. (2005). The psychobiology of depression and resilience to stress: Implications for prevention and treatment. *Annual Review of Clinical Psychology, 1,* 255–291.

Szajnberg, N. M., & Massie, H. (2003). Transition to young adulthood: A prospective study. *International Journal of Psychoanalysis, 84,* 1569–1586.

The National Center on Addiction and Substance Abuse at Columbia University. Under the Counter: The Diversion and Abuse of Controlled Prescription Drugs in the U. S. CASA, New York 2005.

Tsatsoulis, A., & Fountoulakis, S. (2006). The protective role of exercise on stress system dysregulation and comorbidities. *Annals of the New York Academy of Science, 1083,* 196–213.

Uggen, C., & Wakefield, S. (2005). Young adults reentering the community from the criminal justice system: The challenge of becoming and adult. In D. W. Osgood, E. M. Foster, C. Flanagan, & C. R. Ruth (Eds.), *On your own without a net: The transition to adulthood for vulnerable populations* (pp. 1–26). Chicago: The University of Chicago Press.

Van den Bosch, L. M. C., Herheul, E., Langeland, W., & Van den Brink, W. (2003). Trauma, dissociation, and posttraumatic stress disorder in female borderline patients with and without substance abuse problems. *Australian & New Zealand Journal of Psychiatry, 37,* 549–555.

van der Kolk, B. A. (2005). Developmental trauma disorder: Toward a rational diagnosis for children with complex trauma histories. *Psychiatric Annals, 35*(5), 401–408.

Van Praag, H. M. (2004). Stress and suicide: Are we well-equipped to study this issue? *Crisis,25*(2), 80–85.

Walach, H., Nord, E. Zier, C., Dietz-Waschkowski, B., Kersig, S., & Schupbach, H. (2007). Mindfulness-based stress reduction as a method for personnel development: A pilot evaluation. *International Journal of Stress Management, 14*(2), 188–198.

Wills, T. A. (1990). Stress and coping factors in the epidemiology of substance use. In Kozlowski et al. (Eds.), *Research advances in alcohol and drug problems* (Vol. 10), 215–250. New York: Plenum Press.

Wills, T. A., & Hirky, A. E. (1996). Coping and substance abuse: A theoretical model and review of the evidence. In M. Zeichnec & N. S. Eudler (Eds.), *Handbook of coping: Theory, research, and applications* (pp. 279–302). New York: Wiley.

Yates, T. M. (2004). The developmental psychopathology of self-injurious behavior: Compensatory regulation in posttraumatic adaptation. *Clinical Psychology Review, 24*(1), 35–74.

Chapter 10

Intimate Romantic Relationships in Young Adulthood: A Biodevelopmental Perspective

Beth A. Auslander and Susan L. Rosenthal

Roman is a 21-year-old male who grew up in a family characterized by much conflict and instability. His parents were alcoholics and while drinking they engaged in domestic violence. When not drinking, his parents were very attentive and caring toward him and were involved in his life. His parents separated several times before finally divorcing when he was 13 years of age. Roman has not had many close friendships over the years. He acknowledges that he has difficulty maintaining friends in part because he loses his temper easily. He also notes that he has trouble sustaining romantic relationships. He relates that he enters relationships with much enthusiasm, often sharing intimate details extremely early on in relationships, perhaps too early. He gets jealous easily and fears that the relationship will end. He has trouble managing conflicts with partners and notes that he has had physical altercations with partners.

Introduction

A major goal of adolescence and young adulthood is to develop a healthy sense of sexuality. According to the National Commission on Adolescent Health, this means appreciating one's body, delaying sexual behavior until cognitively, emotionally, and physically mature, and engaging in responsible relationships that are consensual, mutually respecting, nonexploitive, pleasurable, and protective against pregnancy and sexually transmitted infections (STIs) (Haffner, 1995). Implicit in this definition is that an individual both feel an appreciation or respect for oneself and also one's romantic partner.

In the present chapter, we describe young adult relationships within a biological and developmental framework. We begin this chapter by discussing the biological underpinnings of social behavior. Next, we review developmental theories on attachment and intimacy that suggest that early relationships between parent and child and peer relationships provide the basis for later romantic relationships. We end this chapter with a discussion of young adult romantic and sexual relationships by reviewing the data on sexual behavior, sexually transmitted infections, and relationship quality and conflict within romantic relationships among this population.

Theoretical Understanding of the Development of Intimacy

Neurobiological Basis of Pair Bonding and Romantic Attachment

An animal model that has been widely used to help understand biology's role in social behavior is the prairie vole (Insel & Young, 2001), a mammal that forms monogamous pair bonds (Williams, Insel, Harbaugh, & Carter, 1994). Oxytocin has been implicated in pair bonding for female prairie voles (Insel & Hulihan, 1995; Williams et al., 1994), and vasopressin has been implicated in pair bonding for male prairie voles (Insel & Hulihan, 1995; Winslow, Hastings,

Carter, & Insel, 1993). That is, when oxytocin was administered to nonmating prairie voles, partner preference developed for females but not for males. In contrast, infusion of vasopressin in nonmating prairie voles resulted in partner preference for males but not females. When oxytocin was blocked by antagonists in mating prairie voles, pair bonding in females was prevented and when vasopressin was blocked by antagonists, pair bonding in males was prevented (Insel & Hulihan, 1995).

In humans, oxytocin and vasopressin increase during sexual arousal, orgasm, and self-stimulation (Carmichael et al., 1987; Carmichael, Warburton, Dixen, & Davidson, 1994; Murphy, Seckl, Burton, Checkley, & Lightman, 1987). Other research has found an association between the release of oxytocin and affiliation cues toward a romantic partner (Gonzaga, Turner, Keltner, & Campos, 2006). Further research (Bartels & Zeki, 2004) has indicated that certain regions of the brain's reward system that have an increased number of oxytocin and vasopressin receptors become activated when individuals view pictures of their romantic partners, while other regions of the brain that have been implicated as playing a role in negative emotions, such as judgment, become deactivated. Interestingly, some of the same regions activated for romantic love were activated for maternal love. Insel and Young (2001) have suggested that "for attachment to occur, these neuropeptides must link social stimuli to dopamine pathways associated with reinforcement" (p. 135).

Attachment Theory

Early interactions with parents can lay the foundation for later romantic relationships, and thus, it is important to have insight into these formative relationships. Bowlby (1969) proposed that an attachment between parent and child develops based on parental responsiveness to infant needs. Ainsworth (1979) further noted that varying levels of parent responsiveness can result in different attachment styles. If a caregiver consistently responds to a child's needs and distress, the child develops a "secure" attachment. Such children are able to explore their environment and cope with distress, knowing that their mother is nearby to help if needed. If a caregiver overreacts or inconsistently responds to a child's needs, then an "ambivalent/anxious" attachment can result. These children may respond ambivalently to their mothers; at times, they may cling to them and at other times they may display anger toward them. If a caregiver does not respond at all or is rejecting of a child's needs, then an "avoidant" attachment style can develop. Children with an avoidant attachment style often will appear detached from their mother and may not respond to their mother upon her return. Through the parent–child attachment, the child learns whether he or she can count on the parent to be there and whether he or she can turn to the parent during periods of distress. According to Bowlby (1973), these early interactions between parent and infant create what he referred to as "internal mental models" or blueprints for relationships. They tell individuals what to expect in a relationship, how to interpret different experiences within a relationship, and how to respond in relationships.

Support for the relationship of attachment to romantic relationships has been found; for example, perceiving parents as being supportive was found to be associated with perceiving romantic partners as supportive (Furman, Simon, Shaffer, & Bouchey, 2002). In another study, inappropriate physical or intimate contact and role-reversal behaviors (e.g., child nurturing the parent or acting in a caretaking role) by the parent during early adolescence were related to higher levels of physical perpetration and victimization within young adult romantic relationships (Linder & Collins, 2005). It could be that when individuals experience such negative interactions with their parents they do not learn how to regulate their emotions and deal with conflict in their romantic relationships (Linder & Collins, 2005).

Adult relationships and attachment styles can be characterized in much the same way as those between the parent and child (Hazan & Shaver, 1987). Young adults with *secure attachment* styles tend to have positive relationships. That is, they are more likely than those in the other attachment groups to value and experience intimacy within a relationship (Mikulincer & Erev, 1991; Monteoliva & Garcia-Martinez, 2005). They tend to experience more satisfaction and happiness and less loneliness in their romantic relationships (Hazan & Shaver, 1987; Monteoliva & Garcia-Martinez, 2005; Moore & Leung, 2002). Compared to those with other attachment styles, those with secure attachment styles perceive themselves more positively in terms of attractiveness (Bogaert & Sadava, 2002) and tend to be more comfortable communicating and expressing emotions and concerns within the romantic relationship (Furman & Simon, 2006). Given all this, it is not surprising that they experience more stability within the relationship and perceive the relationship as likely to endure (Hazan & Shaver, 1987; Monteoliva & Garcia-Martinez, 2005).

Individuals with *anxious attachment* styles seek and strongly desire intimacy but have difficulty achieving it (Hazan & Shaver, 1987). It could be that ambivalent persons interact with partners in a way that distances them from their partner or it could be that they choose partners who have little interest or ability to develop an intimate relationship. They tend to be dependent and jealous (Hazan & Shaver, 1987) and to fear abandonment (Bogaert & Sadava, 2002). Attachment anxiety is associated with increased sexual risk. Those with greater attachment anxiety compared to those with lower attachment anxiety have less confidence in using condoms and more negative beliefs about condoms, such as: "using condoms means they do not trust their partner" and "a partner would be upset if they used condoms" (Kershaw et al., 2007). In terms of sexual behavior, higher attachment anxiety is related to an earlier age of first intercourse, more lifetime sexual partners, more infidelity, less frequent communication with partners about contraception and HIV/AIDS, decreased use of condoms, and a greater likelihood of having unprotected sex with a risky partner (Bogaert & Sadava, 2002; Feeney, Peterson, Gallois, & Terry, 2000; Kershaw et al., 2007).

It has been thought that those with *avoidant styles* may be less interested than those with other attachment styles in developing close, committed sexual relationships. They are less likely to report qualities consistent with a well-functioning (e.g., satisfying) relationship, and they are more likely to fear intimacy and closeness (Hazan & Shaver, 1987), minimize or avoid discussing concerns in the relationship (Furman & Simon, 2006), and foresee the relationship as ending (Hazan & Shaver, 1987; Monteoliva & Garcia-Martinez, 2005). These findings are consistent with a more accepting view of casual sex (Feeney, Noller, & Patty, 1993) and to be more likely to engage in sex for manipulative reasons than those with secure or anxious attachment styles (Davis, Shaver, & Vernon, 2004).

Hence, these results suggest that in order to foster healthy sexuality, one most also foster the development of secure emotional attachments in early childhood. In addition, understanding individuals' attachment styles may be useful when intervening therapeutically.

Social Cognitive Theory

According to social cognitive theory, individuals can develop skills and behaviors by observing or attending to models in their environment, storing the information learned, and then enacting on behaviors based on certain expected outcomes (Bandura, 1989). This theory would suggest that parents could play an influential role in their offspring's development of romantic relationships through their modeling of behaviors in their own romantic relationships. Children observe parents interacting in their romantic relationship and learn to imitate these behaviors later on in their adult romantic relationships.

Research examining the relationship between family structure (i.e., married versus divorced) and young adult children's romantic relationships found that those from married families tended to fare better in their romantic relationships than those from divorced families. For instance, young adult children from married/intact families were more likely than those from divorced families to experience intimacy (Ensighn, Scherman, & Clark, 1998) and a secure attachment with their romantic partners (Summers, Forehand, Armistead, & Tannenbaum, 1998) and less likely to have negative perceptions of marriage (e.g., fears of relationship ending) (Wallerstein & Lewis, 2004). Maternal remarriage is also associated with positive outcomes; young adult children of mothers who remarry compared to young adult children of mothers who do not remarry reported increased intimacy and passion and fewer problems in romantic relationships (Shulman, Scharf, Lumer, & Maurer, 2001).

More recent research suggests that it may not be the family structure per se that is important but rather the specific attitudes and behaviors children witness in their parents' romantic relationships. For instance, Cunningham and Thornton (2006) found a relationship between parents and young adult children's attitudes toward premarital sex, cohabitation, and being single, especially when parents' marital quality was high. In terms of behaviors, cross-sectional studies have found that interparental conflict was related to less intimacy in young adults' romantic relationships (Ensighn et al., 1998) and more accepting attitudes of aggression in romantic relationships, including verbal and physical aggression toward romantic partners (Kinsfogel & Grych, 2004). In a longitudinal study, parental marital discord at age 13 predicted marital discord at age 30 years. This study further found that specific negative behaviors, such as jealousy, proneness to anger, and moodiness, were associated with poorer adult marriages (Amato & Booth, 2001). These findings taken together support social cognitive theory and suggest that parents need to be mindful of the behaviors they display and model in their romantic relationships.

Sullivan, Erikson, and Gilligan: Theories of Intimacy

Sullivan (1953) noted that preadolescence marks an important period with regard to the development of intimate relationships as it is during this time that individuals begin forming relationships with same-sex peers. He argued that although qualities necessary for romantic relationships, such as intimacy and closeness, are founded in parental relationships, the growth and enhancement of such qualities take place through friendships. For the first time, individuals learn to become sensitive to the needs of others and to develop and pursue common goals. Sullivan further proposed that after an individual develops same-sex relationships in preadolescence and opposite sex relationships in early adolescence, he or she can concentrate on developing a sense of self in late adolescence.

Recent research lends support to Sullivan's theory of intimacy. Early friendships appear to serve as a practice ground for individuals to experiment with skills or competencies, such as reciprocity and cooperation. Relationships with best friends have been shown to have a direct effect on the capacity for closeness and commitment in romantic relationships (Scharf & Mayseless, 2001). Further, perceptions of support and negative interactions in current friendships are associated with perceptions in current romantic relationships (Connolly, Furman, & Konarski, 2000). Having better quality friendships also appears to serve as a protective factor against perpetration and victimization in later romantic relationships. It could be that individuals with positive experiences in friendships expect to have the same types of interactions in their romantic relationships or it could be that those with positive friendships possess the necessary skills (e.g., conflict resolution) to negotiate relationships effectively (Linder & Collins, 2005).

In keeping with Sullivan's theory, research also has demonstrated that friendships mediate the connection between parent relationships and romantic relationships (Furman et al., 2002; Scharf & Mayseless, 2001). Similarities between friendships and romantic relationships, such as the contemporary nature of friendships with romantic relationships and the equal status associated with each, may help explain why friendships seem to play a more influential role. Also it is often through peer networks that romantic relationships emerge; hence, romantic relationships developing out of these peer networks are likely to be similar to the friendships existing within them (Connolly et al., 2000).

Erikson (1968) proposed that individuals develop through eight life stages that build on each other. At each stage, there is a psychosocial crisis to be addressed that includes both positive and negative poles. Erikson believed that during adolescence, the psychosocial crisis is "identity versus identity confusion" and that during young adulthood the psychosocial crisis is "intimacy versus isolation." In order to develop an identity, Erikson noted that the adolescent "must make a series of ever-narrowing selections of personal, occupational, sexual, and ideological commitments" (1968, p. 245). According to him, a true sense of identity consists of "a feeling of being at home in one's body, a sense of knowing where one is going, and an inner assuredness of anticipated recognition from those who count" (1968, p. 165). Given that he believed that each stage builds upon the other, Erikson theorized that identity must be fully formed in order for there to be real intimacy, which he described as a "counterpointing as well as a fusing of identities" (1968, p. 135). For Erikson, if a strong sense of identity is not established, one's identity could get lost in the relationship.

Sullivan and Erikson's theories of intimacy can seem contradictory. As noted above, Sullivan's theory proposed that intimacy develops before identity and Erikson's theory suggests the opposite—that identity must be present before intimacy develops. Researchers have examined the timing of identity and the timing of intimacy to help resolve this debate. According to a review of studies, there is some support for identity needing to be intact before intimacy can give rise, but this seems to be more true for men than for women (Orlofsky, 1993). This leads to another interesting point as to whether men and women differ with respect to identity and intimacy development. Carol Gilligan has argued that Erikson's theory of identity development was male biased as it did not take into account the female perspective. According to Gilligan, identity may precede intimacy for males, but for women identity and intimacy develop simultaneously. She believed that women come to define themselves within the context of their relationships (Gilligan, 1979). When considering these differing views, it may be better not to conclude that one (i.e., identity or intimacy) precedes the other but rather to conclude that identity and intimacy are forever intertwined. That is, the more one develops a sense of self, the more able one is to seek out relationships and experience closeness, and the more one establishes intimacy in a relationship, the more one learns about oneself and is able to develop a stronger sense of self.

The Intimacy Process Model

Reiss and Patrick (1996) proposed an intimacy process model illustrating intimacy as a complex, continual process through which a series of interactions between two partners take place over time. In their model, each partner influences the other through his/her thoughts, feelings, and behavior. Communication of emotions is a central part of the intimacy process model as well as the response to the emotion. According to the model, the "self-disclosing person" either verbally or nonverbally expresses a thought or feeling to the "responsive listener." Typically, individual factors (e.g., needs, values) as well as situational factors (e.g., goals of the relationship) influence what is expressed by the self-discloser. The responsive listener perceives the self-expression within his or her own framework of individual and situational factors and responds according to these. The response is interpreted within the self-disclosing person's framework of individual and situational factors which thereby determines how the self-disclosing person feels about the response. If the self-disclosing person experiences the response as supportive, validating, and caring, then the interaction could be experienced as intimate. If the response is viewed by the self-discloser as distancing or rejecting, the interaction would not be experienced as intimate. The responsive listener then has a reaction to the self-discloser's reaction. If the responsive listener's response to the self-disclosing person is viewed in a positive manner, then the responsive listener will feel appreciated and valued. The more each person in the interaction feels validated or appreciated, the more likely intimate interactions are to occur in the future.

Reiss and Patrick (1996) further noted that attachment and intimacy have many commonalties. For instance, attachment and intimacy both involve a bond between two people, require individuals to regulate and express emotions, involve responsiveness to the other individual, and are associated with positive health outcomes.

Romantic and Sexual Relationships

Romantic relationships begin to evolve over the adolescent period, giving rise to young adult relationships. Although many *young* adolescents may show interest in dating, few report being in a current romantic relationship (Connolly, Craig, Goldberg, & Pepler, 1999; Feiring, 1996). If they are in a relationship, it is typically brief

(Feiring, 1996), and it may be nonexclusive (Short et al., 2003). By *late* adolescence, romantic relationships are longer in duration as the dyad begins to take precedence over the peer group. Qualities, such as reciprocity and commitment, become more important in romantic relationships at this stage (Connolly & Goldberg, 1999).

During adolescence and young adulthood, individuals form their sexual identity, the label (e.g., heterosexual, homosexual) used by a person to define his or her sexual attractions, thoughts, and behaviors (Diamond, 2003). Previously, homosexual-committed relationships were thought to be pathological and inferior to heterosexual relationships (Roisman, Clausell, Holland, Fortuna, & Elieff, 2008). However, recent studies have not found this to be the case. Individuals in same- and opposite-sex committed relationships have been found to report similar levels of satisfaction and to perform similarly on observed measures of relationship quality (Roisman et al., 2008). Further, variables that predict relationship satisfaction and stability in heterosexual relationships also have been shown to predict relationship satisfaction and stability in homosexual relationships (Kurdek, 2004). Therefore, committed relationships appear to function the same way regardless of whether the relationship is same sex or opposite sex.

According to the *National Survey of Adolescent and Young Adults: Sexual Health Knowledge, Attitudes, and Experiences*, 11% of young adult males and 29% of young adult females reported that they were currently married, living as married, or had been married (Kaiser Family Foundation, 2003). Many young adults have a series of monogamous steady relationships. Within these relationships, a majority of young adults said that they feel that it is an expectation that they will have sex. In addition, they believe that it is expected that by a certain age they will be sexually experienced. This might help explain why 61% of the young adults surveyed believed that it is good idea to wait to have sex but at the same time acknowledged that most people do not wait (Kaiser Family Foundation, 2003). While most individuals believe that sex should occur within steady relationships, not all sexual encounters occur in a steady relationship. In the literature, such encounters have been referred to in a variety of ways, such as casual sex, hookups, one-night stands, and anonymous sex (Cubbins & Tanfer, 2000; Grello, Welsh, & Harper, 2006; Paul, McManus, & Hayes, 2000). Among a sample of undergraduate students, 53% reported having had sex with someone whom they were not romantically involved (Grello et al., 2006). One-third of these were with persons the individual did not know very well; the remainder was with friends. The latter has led to the term "friends with benefits." These are relationships that are often emotionally intimate, involve occasional sex, but for some reason are not labeled as "boyfriend/girlfriend" relationships. Gender differences exist with regard to the frequency and impact of casual relationships. First, more males than females reported having engaged in a casual coital relationship (Grello et al., 2006; Paul et al., 2000). Second, while both genders reported entering relationships being aware that it was casual, more females than males believed that it could possibly evolve into a romantic relationship. Finally, although males who have had casual sex tend to have the fewest depressive symptoms, females who have had casual sex tend to have the most depressive symptoms (Grello et al., 2006).

Results from the national survey and other studies with young adult and college populations have indicated that by this age, most have engaged in some sexual behavior. For example, 80% of the young adults (18 to 24 years) in the *National Survey of Adolescent and Young Adults: Sexual Health Knowledge, Attitudes, and Experiences* (Kaiser Family Foundation, 2003) reported that they have had sexual intercourse. Almost one-fourth (24%) of the young adult virgins in this survey noted that they had engaged in "intimate" behavior with a partner and 12% said that they had experienced oral sex. While some individuals initiate intercourse during their early adolescent years, one in four stated that their first experience occurred in young adulthood (Kaiser Family Foundation, 2003). Most young adults with vaginal sex experience have had more than one sexual partner, with approximately 40% of the young adults in the national survey reporting having had between 2 to 5 lifetime sexual partners. Of concern is that 14% of them have had 10 or more lifetime sexual partners (Kaiser Family Foundation, 2003). Sexually experienced young adults engage in a variety of sexual behaviors; for example, 84% reported having had oral sex as well (Kaiser Family Foundation, 2003). The rates of heterosexual anal intercourse among nonvirgin college populations range between 20% to 32% (Baldwin & Baldwin, 2000; Civic, 2000; Flannery, Ellingson, Votaw, & Schaefer, 2003).

Gender and race/ethnic differences are apparent in sexual history/behavior of young adults. Young adult males have had more lifetime partners than females and report initiating intercourse at an earlier age. White adolescents/young adults are more likely to have engaged in oral sex than African American and Latino adolescents/young adults; however, African American and Latino adolescent/young adults initiate sexual intercourse at earlier ages than white adolescents/young adults. African Americans also report having more partners. Asian American adolescents/young adults report the lowest rates of sexual activity (Kaiser Family Foundation, 2003).

Research has found that adolescents and young adults report that the most common reasons for engaging in sex are for sexual pleasure and intimacy-related purposes. Other reasons include coping with negative emotions, self-affirmation, partner approval, and peer approval. Motives for having sex have been found to differ by gender. Males tend to report a greater range of motives for having sex than women. Having sex for intimacy-related purposes appears to be protective against sexual risk-taking behavior. This could be because sexual behavior is more likely to occur within a monogamous, steady relationship (Cooper, Shapiro, & Powers, 1998).

Sexually Transmitted Infections

Over half of the 18.9 million sexually transmitted infections (STIs) diagnosed every year are among young people ages 15 to 24 (Weinstock, Berman, & Cates, 2004). For example, Chlamydia is more prevalent among the 15- to 19-year old and 20- to 24-year-old age groups than any other age groups (Centers for Disease Control and Prevention, 2006) and the highest prevalence rate among women for the human papillomavirus is in the 20- to 24-year-old age group (Dunne et al., 2007). Sexually transmitted infections are not just found among those with multiple partners. Approximately 50% of those infected with an STI had only one partner within the last year (Ford, Jaccard, Millstein, Bardsley, & Miller, 2004). Women experience the burden of STIs, as they and their offspring can suffer serious long-term complications, including pelvic inflammatory disease, cervical cancer, pregnancy complications, infertility, neonatal complications, and even death (Aral, 2001; Boonstra, 2000; Hutto, 1987; Nahmias et al., 1971; Stagno & Whitley, 1999).

Despite the high prevalence rates of STIs among this age group, the majority of young adults do not perceive themselves to be at risk for STI infection (Ford et al., 2004), and many are not protecting themselves against STIs. For example, a study involving a national sample of young adults found that 55% percent reported using condoms "regularly" (Kaiser Family Foundation, 2003). Other studies with college students and military recruits suggest that inconsistent condom use can range from 64% to 71% (Civic, 2000; Hwang, Shafer, Pollack, Chang, & Boyer, 2007; Roberts & Kennedy, 2006). Even if condoms are used, they are often used ineffectively; one study with young adult women found that in the 3 months prior, 44% delayed condom use and 19% experienced condom slippage/breakage (Civic et al., 2002). A recent literature review suggested that young people do not use condoms for the following reasons: lack of knowledge about STIs, low perceived risk, inaccurate assumption that oral contraceptives protect against STIs, male resistance to condoms, difficulties negotiating condom use (especially for women), and implication that condoms convey mistrust (East, Jackson, O'Briaen, & Peters, 2007).

Relationship Quality and Conflict

Previous research has indicated that the majority of late adolescent/young adults reported feeling satisfied in their romantic relationships (Auslander et al., 2007; Cramer, 2004). Support seems to play an influential role in relationship satisfaction with those reporting higher levels of support also reporting higher degrees of relationship satisfaction (Cramer, 2004). Over time, differences in opinion occur, and how individuals handle these differences also seems to be important with regard to relationship satisfaction. Among a college population, a negative conflict style (e.g., becoming irritated, avoiding discussion) was found to be associated with lower relationship satisfaction (Cramer, 2000).

Unfortunately, dating violence is not an uncommon event in young adulthood. According to a review of the literature conducted by Lewis and Fremouw (2001), the prevalence rates of physical violence within a romantic relationship typically fall between 21% and 45%. These rates are much higher when dating violence is defined more broadly to include both psychological and sexual victimization. In fact, in a longitudinal study following women through college, 88% of them reported that they had been verbally threatened, physically assaulted, or sexually assaulted by a romantic partner (Smith, White, & Holland, 2003). While one often thinks of dating violence as being one way, it can often be bidirectional. Among a sample of female college students, 28% reported both perpetrating violence and being victimized within dating relationship (Orcutt, Garcia, & Pickett, 2005). There are gender differences with regard to dating violence. Women tend to report at least equal but sometimes higher rates of perpetrating violence than men, while men tend to report higher rates of victimization than women. However, women tend to experience more consequences or injury from dating violence than do men (Orcutt et al., 2005). Longitudinal studies have indicated that previous exposure to violence, whether it be child physical abuse, witness to domestic violence as a child, or assault during adolescence, predicts dating violence in young adulthood (Linder & Collins, 2005; Smith et al., 2003).

Conclusion

Major developmental tasks of young adulthood include achieving intimacy and developing a healthy sense of sexuality. We are beginning to develop a better understanding of the role neurobiology plays in romantic attachments. A young adult's ability to form satisfying, lasting, and healthy relationships appears to be largely influenced by his or her early relationships with parents and friends. It is easy to focus on the adverse outcomes of sexual relationships such as STIs; however, it is important to remember that sexuality is a natural part of these intimate relationships, can provide pleasure, and represents an important way to express closeness and intimacy.

KEY POINTS

- Neuropeptides (oxytocin and vasopressin) have been implicated in the development of pair bonds in animals and romantic attachments in humans.
- The parent–child and parental romantic relationships can lay the foundation for young adult romantic relationships, and friendships can serve as a practice ground for skills to be used in romantic relationships.
- Most young adults have engaged in vaginal sex or some type of intimate sexual behavior. Sexual behavior among adults appears to differ across gender and race ethnicity. Compared to other age groups, adolescents/young adults are at the highest risk group for sexually transmitted infections.
- Most young adults report feeling satisfied in their romantic relationships. However, dating violence is not uncommon.

> **PRACTICE GUIDELINES**
>
> - Interventions that foster secure attachments between parent and child should be encouraged as this could later impact young adult relationships. Parents should be taught how to respond to their children's needs and how best to take an active role in their life.
> - Practitioners are encouraged to ask parents about how their romantic relationships are going and provide guidance or appropriate referral if there is discord or violence.
> - Practitioners are encouraged to be specific when asking young adults questions about their romantic relationships and sexual behavior, so that appropriate guidance, treatment, and/or referral can be made.

References

Ainsworth, M. D. (1979). Infant–mother attachment. *American Psychologist, 34,* 932–937.

Amato, P. R., & Booth, A. (2001). The legacy of parents' marital discord: Consequences for children's marital quality. *Journal of Personality and Social Psychology, 81,* 627–638.

Aral, S. O. (2001). Sexually transmitted diseases: Magnitude, determinants and consequences. *International Journal of STD and AIDS, 12,* 211–215.

Auslander, B. A., Rosenthal, S. L., Fortenberry, D., Biro, F. M., Bernstein, D. I., & Zimet, G. D. (2007). Predictors of sexual satisfaction in an adolescent and college population. *Journal of Pediatric and Adolescent Gynecology, 20,* 25–28.

Baldwin, J. I., & Baldwin, J. D. (2000). Heterosexual anal intercourse: An understudied, high-risk sexual behavior. *Archives of Sexual Behavior, 29,* 357–373.

Bandura, A. (1989). Social cognitive theory. *Annals of Child Development, 6,* 1–60.

Bartels, A., & Zeki, S. (2004). The neural correlates of maternal and romantic love. *NeuroImage, 21,* 1155–1166.

Bogaert, A. F., & Sadava, S. (2002). Adult attachment and sexual behavior. *Personal Relationships, 9,* 191–204.

Boonstra, H. (2000). Campaign to accelerate microbicide development for STD prevention gets under way. *The Guttmacher Report on Public Policy, 3,* 3–5.

Bowlby, J. (1969). *Attachment and Loss: Vol. 1. Attachment.* New York: Basic Books.

Bowlby, J. (1973). *Attachment and Loss. Vol 2. Separation: Anxiety and Anger.* New York: Basic Books.

Carmichael, M. S., Humbert, R., Dixen, J., Palmisano, G., Greenleaf, W., & Davidson, J. M. (1987). Plasma oxytocin increases in the human sexual response. *Journal of Clinical Endocrinology and Metabolism, 64,* 27–31.

Carmichael, M. S., Warburton, V. L., Dixen, J., & Davidson, J. M. (1994). Relationships among cardiovascular, muscular, and oxytocin responses during human sexual activity. *Archives of Sexual Behavior, 23,* 59–79.

Centers for Disease Control and Prevention. (2006). *Trends in reportable sexually transmitted diseases in the United States, 2005: National surveillance data for chlamydia, gonorrhea, and syphilis.* Atlanta, GA: Author.

Civic, D. (2000). College students' reasons for nonuse of condoms within dating relationships. *Journal of Sex and Marital Therapy, 26,* 95–105.

Civic, D., Scholes, D., Ichikawa, L., Gorotahaus, L., McBride, C. M., Yarnall, K. S. H., & Fish, L. (2002). Ineffective use of condoms among young women in managed care. *AIDS Care, 14,* 779–788.

Connolly, J., Craig, W., Goldberg, A., & Pepler, D. (1999). Conceptions of cross-sex friendships and romantic relationships in early adolescence. *Journal of Youth and Adolescence, 28,* 481–494.

Connolly, J., Furman, W., & Konarski, R. (2000). The role of peers in the emergence of heterosexual romantic relationships in adolescence. *Child Development, 71,* 1395–1408.

Connolly, J., & Goldberg, A. (1999). Romantic relationships in adolescence: The role of friends and peers in the emergence and development. In W. Furman, B. B. Brown, & C. Feiring (Eds.), *The development of romantic relationships in adolescence* (pp. 266–290). New York: Cambridge University Press.

Cooper, M. L., Shapiro, C. M., & Powers, A. M. (1998). Motivations for sex and risky sexual behavior among adolescents and young adults: A functional perspective. *Journal of Personality and Social Psychology, 75,* 1528–1558.

Cramer, D. (2000). Relationship satisfaction and conflict style in romantic relationships. *Journal of Psychology, 134,* 337-341.

Cramer, D. (2004). Satisfaction with a romantic relationship, depression, support and conflict. *Psychology Psychotherapy, 77,* 449-461.

Cubbins, L. A., & Tanfer, K. (2000). The influence of gender on sex: A study of men's and women's self-reported high-risk sex behavior. *Archives of Sexual Behavior, 29,* 229-257.

Cunningham, M., & Thorton, A. (2006). The influence of parents' marital quality on adult children's attitudes toward marriage and its alternatives: Main and moderating effects. *Demography, 43,* 659-672.

Davis, D., Shaver, P. R., & Vernon, M. L. (2004). Attachment style and subjective motivations for sex. *Personality and Social Psychology Bulletin, 30,* 1076-1090.

Diamond, L. M. (2003). New paradigms for research on heterosexual and sexual-minority development. *Journal of Clinical Child and Adolescent Psychology, 32,* 490-498.

Dunne, E. F., Unger, E. R., Sternberg, M., McQuillan, G., Swan, D. C., Patel, S. S., & Markowitz, L. E. (2007). Prevalence of HPV infection among females in the United States. *Journal of the American Medical Association, 297,* 813-819.

East, L., Jackson, D., O'Briaen, L., & Peters, K. (2007). Use of the male condom by heterosexual adolescents and young people: Literature review. *Journal of Advanced Nursing, 59,* 103-110.

Ensighn, J., Scherman, A., & Clark, J. J. (1998). The relationship of family structure and conflict to levels of intimacy and parental attachment in college students. *Adolescence, 33,* 575-582.

Erikson, E. H. (1968). *Identity youth and crisis.* New York: W.W. Norton.

Feeney, J. A., Noller, P., & Patty, J. (1993). Adolescents' interactions with the opposite sex: Influence of attachment style and gender. *Journal of Adolescence, 16,* 169-186.

Feeney, J. A., Peterson, C. B., Gallois, C., & Terry, D. J. (2000). Attachment style as a predictor of sexual attitudes and behavior in late adolescence. *Psychology and Health, 14,* 1105-1122.

Feiring, C. (1996). Concepts of romance in 15-year-old adolescents. *Journal of Research on Adolescence, 6,* 181-200.

Flannery, D., Ellingson, L., Votaw, K. S., & Schaefer, E. A. (2003). Anal intercourse and sexual risk factors among college women, 1993-2000. *American Journal of Health Behavior, 27,* 228-234.

Ford, C. A., Jaccard, J., Millstein, S. G., Bardsley, P. E., & Miller, W. C. (2004). Perceived risk of Chlamydial and Gonococcal infection among sexually experienced young adults in the United States. *Perspectives on Sexual and Reproductive Health, 36,* 258-264.

Furman, W., & Simon, V. A. (2006). Actor and partner effects of adolescents' romantic working models and styles on interaction with romantic partners. *Child Development, 77,* 588-604.

Furman, W., Simon, V. A., Shaffer, L., & Bouchey, H. A. (2002). Adolescents' working models and styles for relationships with parents, friends, and romantic partners. *Child Development, 73,* 241-255.

Gilligan, C. (1979). Woman's place in man's life cycle. *Harvard Educational Review, 49,* 431-446.

Gonzaga, G. C., Turner, R. A., Keltner, D., & Campos, B. (2006). Romantic love and sexual desire in close relationships. *Emotion, 6,* 163-179.

Grello, C. M., Welsh, D. P., & Harper, M. S. (2006). No strings attached: The nature of casual sex in college students. *Journal of Sex Research, 43,* 255-267.

Haffner, D. W. (1995). Facing facts: Sexual health for America's adolescents. *Journal of Adolescent Health,* Volume 22, Number 6, June 1998, pp. 453-4597.

Hazan, C., & Shaver, P. (1987). Romantic love conceptualized as an attachment process. *Journal of Personality and Social Psychology, 52,* 511-524.

Hutto, C. (1987). Intrauterine herpes simplex virus infections. *Journal of Pediatrics, 110,* 97-101.

Hwang, L. Y., Shafer, M. B., Pollack, L. M., Chang, Y. J., & Boyer, C. B. (2007). Sexual behaviors after universal screening of sexually transmitted infections in healthy young women. *Obstetrics and Gynecology, 109,* 105-113.

Insel, T. R., & Hulihan, T. J. (1995). A gender-specific mechanism for pair bonding: Oxytocin and partner preference formation in monogamous voles. *Behavioral Neuroscience, 109,* 782-789.

Insel, T. R., & Young, L. J. (2001). The neurobiology of attachment. *National Reviews. Neuroscience, 2,* 129-136.

Kaiser Family Foundation. (2003). *National survey of adolescents and young adults: Sexual health, knowledge, attitudes, and experiences.* Henry J. Kaiser Family Foundation. Retrieved January 1, 2007, from http://www.kff.org

Kershaw, T. S., Milan, S., Westdahl, C., Lewis, J., Rising, S. S., Fletcher, R., & Ickovics, J. (2007). Avoidance, anxiety, and sex: The influence of romantic attachment on HIV-risk among pregnant women. *AIDS Behavior, 11,* 299-311.

Kinsfogel, K. M., & Grych, J. H. (2004). Interparental conflict and adolescent dating relationships: Integrating cognitive, emotional, and peer influences. *Journal of Family Psychology, 18,* 505-515.

Kurdek, L. A. (2004). Are gay and lesbian cohabiting couples really different from heterosexual married couples? *Journal of Marriage and the Family, 66,* 880–900.

Lewis, S. F., & Fremouw, W. (2001). Dating violence: A critical review of the literature. *Clinical Psychology Review, 21,* 105–127.

Linder, J. R., & Collins, W. A. (2005). Parent and peer predictors of physical aggression and conflict management in romantic relationships in early adulthood. *Journal of Family Psychology, 19,* 252–262.

Mikulincer, M., & Erev, I. (1991). Attachment style and the structure of romantic love. *British Journal of Social Psychology, 30,* 273–291.

Monteoliva, A., & Garcia-Martinez, J. M. (2005). Adult attachment style and its effect on the quality of romantic relaitonships in Spanish students. *Journal of Social Psychology,145,* 745–747.

Moore, S., & Leung, C. (2002). Young people's romantic attachment styles and their associations with well-being. *Journal of Adolescence, 25,* 243–255.

Murphy, M. R., Seckl, J. R., Burton, S., Checkley, S. A., & Lightman, S. L. (1987). Changes in oxytocin and vasopressin secretion during sexual activity in men. *Journal of Clinical Endocrinology and Metabolism, 65,* 738–741.

Nahmias, A. J., Josey, W. E., Naib, Z. M., Freeman, M. G., Fernandez, R. J., & Wheeler, J. (1971). Perinatal risk associated with maternal genital herpes simplex virus infection. *American Journal of Obstetrics and Gynecology, 110,* 825–837.

Orcutt, H. K., Garcia, M., & Pickett, S. M. (2005). Female-perpetrated intimate partner violence and romantic attachment style in a college student sample. *Violence and Victims, 20,* 287–302.

Orlofsky, J. L. (1993). Intimacy status: Theory and research. In J. E. Marcia (Ed.), *Ego identity: A handbook for psychosocial research* (pp. 111–133). New York: Springer-Verlag.

Paul, E. L., McManus, B., & Hayes, A. (2000). "Hookups": Characteristics and correlates of college students' spontaneous and anonymous sexual experiences. *Journal of Sex Research, 37,* 76–88.

Reiss, H. T., & Patrick, B. C. (1996). Attachment and intimacy: Component processes. In E. T. Higgins & W. W. Kruglanski (Eds.), *Social psychology: Handbook of basic principles* (pp. 523–563). New York: Guilford Press.

Roberts, S. T., & Kennedy, B. L. (2006). Why are young college women not using condoms? Their perceived risk, drug use, and developmental vulnerability may provide important clues to sexual risk. *Archives of Psychiatric Nursing, 20,* 32–40.

Roisman, G. I., Clausell, E., Holland, A., Fortuna, K., & Elieff, C. (2008). Adult romantic relationships as contexts of human development: A multi-method comparison of same-sex couples with opposite-sex dating, engaged, and married dyads. *Developmental Psychology, 44,* 91–101.

Scharf, M., & Mayseless, O. (2001). The capacity for romantic intimacy: Exploring the contribution of best friend and marital and parental relationships. *Journal of Adolescence, 24,* 379–399.

Short, M. B., Succop, P. A., Mills, L., Stanberry, L. R., Biro, F. M., & Rosenthal, S. L. (2003). Non-exclusivity in adolescent girls' romantic relationships. *Sexually Transmitted Diseases, 30,* 752 – 755.

Shulman, S., Scharf, M., Lumer, D., & Maurer, O. (2001). Parental divorce and young adult children's romantic relationships: Resolution of the divorce experience. *American Journal of Orthopsychiatry, 71,* 473–478.

Smith, P. H., White, J. W., & Holland, L. J. (2003). A longitudinal perspective on dating violence among adolescent and college-age women. *American Journal of Public Health, 93,* 1104–1109.

Stagno, S., & Whitley, R. J. (1999). Herpesvirus infections in neonates and children: Cytomegalovirus and herpes simplex virus. In K. K. Holmes, P. F. Sparling, P. M. Mardh, S. M. Lemon, W. E. Stamm, P. Piot, & J. N. Wasserheit (Eds.), *Sexually transmitted diseases* (3rd ed., pp. 1191–1212). New York: McGraw-Hill.

Sullivan, H. S. (1953). *The interpersonal theory of psychiatry.* New York: W.W. Norton.

Summers, P., Forehand, R., Armistead, L., & Tannenbaum, L. (1998). Parental divorce during early adolescence in Caucasian families: The role of family process variables in predicting the long-term consequences for early adult psychosocial adjustment. *Journal of Consulting and Clinical Psychology, 66,* 327–336.

Wallerstein, J. S., & Lewis, J. M. (2004). The unexpected legacy of divorce: Report of a 25-year study. *Psychoanalytic Psychology, 21,* 353–370.

Weinstock, H., Berman, S., & Cates, W. (2004). Sexually transmitted diseases among American youth: Incidence and prevalence estimates, 2000. *Perspectives on Sexual and Reproductive Health, 36,* 6–10.

Williams, J. R., Insel, T. R., Harbaugh, C. R., & Carter, C. S. (1994). Oxytocin administered centrally facilitates formation of a partner preference in female prairie voles (*Microtus ochrogaster*). *Journal of Neuroendocrinology, 6,* 247–250.

Winslow, J. T., Hastings, N., Carter, C. S., & Insel, T. R. (1993). A role for central vasopressin in pair bonding in monogamous prairie voles. *Nature, 365,* 545–548.

Chapter 11

Marriage in Young Adulthood

Hui Liu, Sinikka Elliott and Debra J. Umberson

Young adulthood is a typical life course stage during which most people establish their first significant intimate relationships, and many of these relationships evolve into what is arguably the most significant love relationship, marriage. This chapter focuses on the predictors and consequences of marriage in young adulthood, defined as the period from age 18 to 30. We conclude with a review of some contemporary debates and important directions for research on the topic of marriage in young adulthood.

Recent Changes to Marriage

The United States witnessed remarkable changes in marriage during the last few decades. Average age at first marriage increased; the proportion of never married (especially for African Americans) increased; and cohabitation and marital dissolution rose dramatically (Casper & Bianchi, 2001). All of these changes in marriage are most striking among young adults.

Delay of Marriage

One of the most notable changes in the institution of marriage in the United States is the delay of first marriage. Although fewer Americans marry now than in past decades, the long-term view indicates that Americans are simply delaying marriage rather than avoiding marriage altogether (see Oppenheimer, 1997). Age at first marriage began to increase in the 1950s. Figure 11-1 shows that the age at first marriage decreased modestly before 1950 in the United States and then increased stably for both men and women. Despite the increase in age at first marriage, Figure 11-1 shows that young adulthood (roughly between ages 18 and 30) continues to be the life period when Americans, on average, experience their first marriage.

At all time periods, the average age of marriage has been older for men than for women. In addition, African Americans and those with higher education tend to marry at older ages than whites and those with lower education. According to the U.S. Census Bureau, between 2000 and 2002, the median age at first marriage was 26.4 for white men and 24.7 for white women, compared to 28.6 for black men and 28.1 for black women. For high school graduates, the median age at first marriage was 26.8 for men and 25.2 for women, whereas for those without any diploma it was 25.8 for men and 22.7 for women (Simmons & Dye, 2004).

Cohabitation and Same-Sex Unions

Delaying marriage increases young adults' exposure to nonmarital relationships. Indeed, most unmarried young Americans are involved in other types of intimate relationships. According to a report from the National Center for Health Statistics, more than 85% of young adults aged 20–24 report having had at least one same-sex or opposite-sex intimate partner during the previous year, although only 16% of men and 28% of women in this age group have ever been married (Mosher, Chandra, & Jones, 2005). This rapidly growing living arrangement

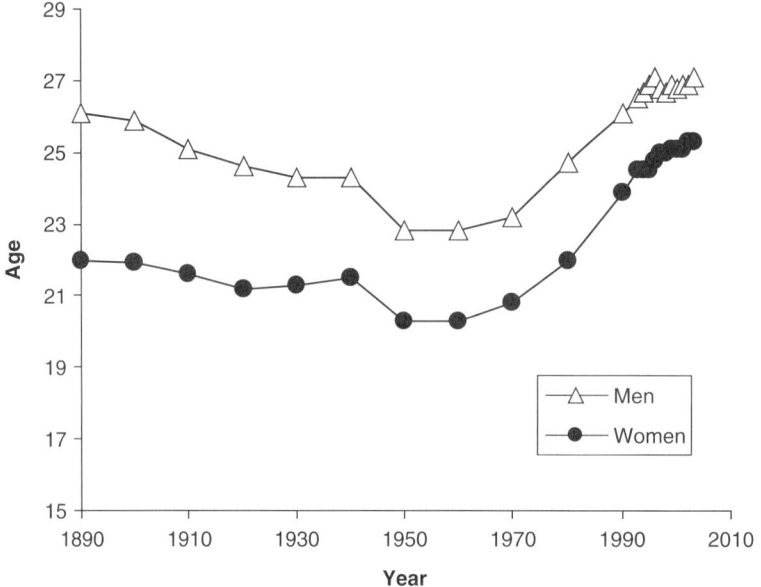

Figure 11-1. U. S. median age at first marriage, 1890–2003 (*Source*: U.S. Bureau of the Census, Information Please Database, Copyright © 2006 Pearson Education, Inc.).

in the United States is most prevalent in young adulthood, and it is even more prevalent among African Americans and individuals with less education (Teachman, Tedrow, & Kyle, 2000). Among cohabiting couples, about 11% are gay or lesbian (U.S. Census Bureau, 2001). To date, although a few states have some form of domestic partnership or civil union rights for gay and lesbian couples, Massachusetts and Connecticut are the only states to allow gays and lesbians the right to legally marry (Hull, 2006).

Is cohabitation an alternative to marriage in modern America? Although cohabitation is more likely to replace marriage for African Americans and for young adults with less education, it is not a substitute for marriage for most Americans (Smock, 2000). On the one hand, cohabiting couples share some similarities to married couples, such as sharing a home and engaging in emotional and sexual intimacy (Musick & Bumpass, 2006). On the other hand, cohabitors do not appear to reap the same benefits as the married. For example, compared to married couples, cohabiting couples are more likely to separate their income (Brines & Joyner, 1999), engage in more risky health behaviors (Horwitz & White, 1998),

report strain in their relationships (Skinner, Bahr, Crane, & Call, 2002), experience psychological distress (Brown, 2000), and eventually divorce (Heaton, 2002). At present, cohabitation represents an uninstitutionalized unit in the American marriage system (Smock, 2000), and some sociologists argue that institutional legitimacy is responsible for many of the benefits of legal marriage for individual well-being (Waite & Gallagher, 2000). Due to the lack of national data on gay and lesbian relationships, research on the links between same-sex unions and health and well-being remain largely "speculative" (Elliott & Umberson, 2004, p. 38).

Marital Dissolution

Today, half of all first marriages in America end in divorce and, until the 1980s, the divorce rate rose steadily. Figure 11-2 illustrates changes in the divorce rate in America from 1900 to 2005. America has witnessed a modest decline in the divorce rate since 1980, but this trend does not apply to those not having completed high school, for whom the divorce rate has continued to increase (Raley & Bumpass, 2003).

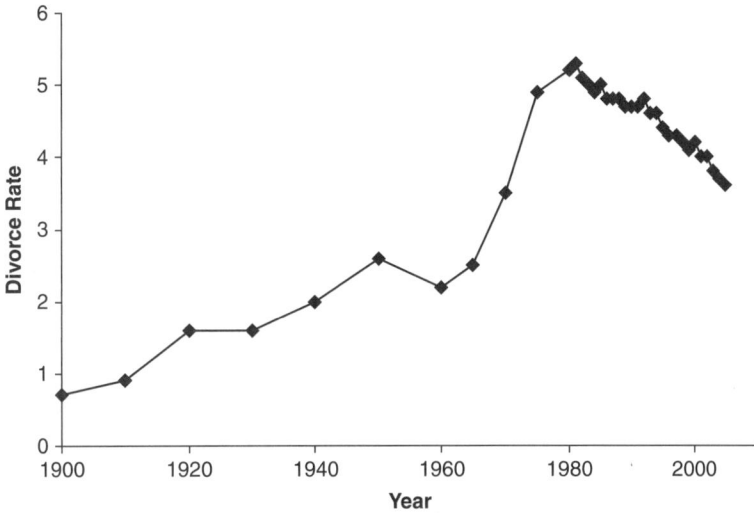

Figure 11-2. U. S. divorce rate per 1,000 population, 1900–2005 (*Source*: U.S. Dept. of Health and Human Services, National Center for Health Statistics. Information Please Database, Copyright © 2006 Pearson Education, Inc.).

Divorce is more likely when people marry at a younger age (Heaton, 2002). The risk of divorce is especially high for those who marry in their teen years. A national survey shows that nearly half of women who marry before 18 divorce within 10 years, compared to a quarter of those married at the age of 25 or older (Bramlett & Mosher, 2002). Along with marrying at an early age, other factors associated with higher risk of marital dissolution include the following: African American status (Raley & Bumpass, 2003), lower levels of education (Raley & Bumpass, 2003), having been married previously (Goldstein, 1999), premarital cohabitation (Smock, 2000), having parents who divorced (Feng, Giarrusso, Bengston, & Frye, 1999), poor health status (Joung, Van de Mheen, Stronks, Van Poppel, & Mackenbach, 1998), and engaging in risky health behaviors (Ostermann, Sloan, & Taylor, 2005).

Consequences of Marriage for Young Adults

While most family scholars agree that the meanings and implications of marriage for today's young adults are different from those of their parents' and grandparents' generations, scholars and politicians continue to emphasize the value of marriage for individuals' well-being (Waite & Gallagher, 2000). Most of the arguments in favor of marriage are premised on a research literature showing that marriage is associated with favorable consequences for both mental and physical health.

Mental Health

The relationship between marriage and mental health is well established and, until recently, the association between being married and better mental health was an unchallenged social fact. This association, however, depends on a number of factors. The mental health advantage of the married is most apparent when comparing the married with the previously married—the divorced, separated, and widowed (Umberson & Williams, 1999). As alternatives to marriage, in the form of cohabitation and gay and lesbian unions, become more common and acceptable among young adults, the mental health advantage of the married young adults relative to their never-married counterparts may diminish (Marks, 1996). In fact, the never-married and married are very similar for certain measures of mental health (Marks, 1996). A great deal of research focuses on explaining why the married are presumably in better mental health than the unmarried. The two primary categories of explanation fall within either a social causation framework or a social selection framework.

Causation Perspective. According to the causation perspective, the married have better mental health than the unmarried because *(1)* resources provided by marriage contribute to mental health (Waite & Gallagher, 2000) or *(2)* the stress associated with marital dissolution (through divorce or widowhood) undermines mental health (Williams & Umberson, 2004).

The Marital Resource Model. The marital resource model suggests that marriage provides social, psychological, and economic resources that promote mental health. Marriage may expand one's social connections with others and these connections may further benefit mental health (House, Landis & Umberson, 1988). Marriage may provide a sense of belonging, meaning, and purpose in ways that enhance well-being (Umberson & William, 1999). Moreover, emotional support from a spouse is particularly important to mental health in the face of stress. The influence of marriage on access to emotional support varies by gender, with women more likely to provide emotional support to a spouse and men more likely to receive support from a spouse (Erickson, 2005). However, as a result of women's increasing labor force participation and changing gender norms, young wives may have less time and be less inclined to provide emotional/social/health support to their husbands than in the past. Yet research reveals that wives continue to be overwhelmingly responsible for domestic work and young couples establish a fairly traditional domestic division of labor after the birth of a child (Walzer, 1998).

Marriage may also promote mental health by increasing available economic resources through specialization, economies of scale, and the pooling of wealth (Waite & Gallagher, 2000), and, on average, women receive more of an economic benefit from marriage than do men (Ross, Mirowsky & Goldsteen, 1990). Economic hardship contributes to psychological distress (Mirowsky & Ross, 2003). Increased economic resources through marriage may lead to enhanced psychological well-being, not only by reducing the chances of distress from economic hardship but also by providing financial means for psychological treatment in the case of mental illness (Ross, Mirowsky, & Goldsteen, 1990). However, women's economic benefits from marriage may not be as significant among recent younger cohorts because of increases in young women's gains from education and employment (see a review in Oppenheimer, 1997). In turn, marriage has become less valued as a source of economic stability among young adults (Teachman, Tedrow, & Kyle, 2000).

Stress Model. In contrast to the marital resource model, which attributes mental health benefits to the positive effects of marriage, the stress or "crisis" model suggests that the strain of marital dissolution undermines the mental health of the divorced, separated, and widowed, which, in turn, leads to marital status differences in mental health (Williams & Umberson, 2004). According to the stress model, the benefits of marriage for mental health are not as great as the costs of marital dissolution for mental health. Recent research adds growing empirical support for the stress model. Williams (2003) finds that transitions to divorce/separation/widowhood are associated with increases in depression and declines in life satisfaction. A more recent study by Strohschein, McDonough, Monette, & Shao (2005) suggests that losing a spouse brings more distress than gaining one brings well-being. These findings are more consistent with a stress model than a resource model in explaining marital differences in psychological well-being. Young adults lack expertise in handling stressful life events and suffer more from marital dissolution in terms of declines in psychological well-being in comparison to midlife adults (Marks & Lambert, 1998).

Selection Perspective. While the causation framework argues that marriage leads to better mental health, the social selection framework suggests that the main reason for the better mental health of the married relative to the unmarried is the favorable characteristics of individuals who get and stay married. Marriage selection works through two stages. First, individuals in better mental health or with more favorable characteristics are more likely to get married. Second, those in poorer mental health or with fewer favorable characteristics are more likely to divorce.

A national study by Forthofer, Kessler, Story, & Gotlib (1996) found that those with psychiatric disorders are more likely to get married prior to age 19—and teen marriage is strongly related to marital disruption—but less likely to get married later. Adolescents with psychiatric disorders may marry early to escape stressful environments during childhood, but they are less attractive in the marriage market when they get older (Forthofer et al., 1996). Individuals in poor physical health are also more likely to get divorced and thus selected out of marriage (Joung et al., 1998). Poorer economic prospects—which are in turn associated with decreased psychological well-being—lower the probability of young adults getting married (Oppenheimer, 1997) and boost the probability of divorce (Raley & Bumpass, 2003). This effect of economic prospects on marriage becomes more salient among younger cohorts, especially for women (Sweeney, 2002).

As a whole, the research evidence suggests that both causation and selection influence the link between marriage and mental health (see Wade & Pevalin, 2004). The key question is whether selection or causation predominates in explaining the relationship between marriage and mental health. Most social science research on marriage and mental health emphasizes causation over selection (Waite & Gallagher, 2000). The influence of selection and protection factors that matter most in young adulthood may be different from those factors that matter most later in life. This is an empirical question that researchers have not yet adequately addressed.

Social Factors Influencing the Mental Health Benefits of Marriage. Although, on average, it appears that young married adults enjoy better mental health than those who are unmarried (at least in comparison to the previously married), some individuals appear to benefit more from marriage than others. The social factors that have received the most research attention in this regard are gender, marital quality, and parental status.

Gender. One of the most frequently cited findings in sociological research on marriage is that marriage benefits young men's mental health more than young women's (Umberson & Williams, 1999). Moreover, the adverse effects of divorce on mental health seem to be greater for young men than for young women (Williams & Umberson, 2004). Nevertheless, the argument that marriage benefits men more than women has been, and continues to be, challenged and contested.

The debates over gender differences in marital benefits began in the 1970s, when Jesse Bernard (1972) and Walter Gove (Gove & Tudor, 1973) argued that men benefit more than women from marriage because women are more depressed than men due to their less rewarding/more demanding roles within marriage and the family. Since the 1970s, dozens of studies support this claim (see a review in Williams & Umberson, 2004). A recent study by Joyner and Udry (2000) suggests that gender difference in the mental health benefits of intimate relationships begins very early in the life course. Female adolescents are more depressed than male adolescents, partly as a consequence, Joyner and Udry argue, of the different benefits they derive from romantic involvement.

In response to Gove and Bernard's early work, Bruce Dohrenwend (Dohrenwend & Dohrenwend, 1976) argued that women are not more distressed than men when dimensions of psychological well-being other than depression are considered. In this view, men only appear to benefit more from marriage because most research uses depression (psychological distress) as a measure of mental health (Horwitz, White, & Howell-White, 1996b). This may bias results because men and women express psychological upset in different ways. Externalizing expressions of distress, such as alcohol consumption, are more common among men, while internalizing expressions of distress, such as depression, are more common among women (Rosenfield, 1999). This gendered expression of psychological distress emerges in early adolescence (Price & Lavercombe, 2000). Hence, focusing on depression as the sole or primary measure of mental health more likely captures women's psychological distress, but it may not fully reflect men's levels of distress. When both female and male prevalent measures of mental health (e.g., depression and alcohol consumption) are used, studies suggest that both young men and young women may benefit from marriage (Horwitz, White, & Howell-White, 1996b).

However, empirical evidence of gendered expressions of distress is not exclusive. Horwitz and colleagues (1996a) analyze longitudinal data and focus on young adulthood and mental health. They find that, although divorce increases depression more for young women than for young men, divorce does not increase alcohol problems more for young men than for young women. This suggests that the use of a gendered mental health measure cannot eliminate, although it may reduce, gender differences in young adults' response to marital dissolution.

In sum, gender differences in the mental health benefits of marriage remain a controversial topic. The empirical evidence generally suggests that marriage benefits men's and women's mental health in *different* ways. Women benefit more from increased economic resources through marriage, whereas men benefit more from social support and network connections offered by marriage (Ross, Mirowsky, & Goldsteen, 1990). However, corresponding to social change in the meanings and implications of gender and marriage, the previously observed gender differences in marital benefits may have diminished among young generations (Simon, 2002; Williams, 2003), especially if we compare the married to the never-married.

Marital quality. Although marriage is generally associated with positive mental health, not all marriages are equally beneficial to mental health. Marital quality plays a key role. A marriage characterized by high levels of marital satisfaction and low levels of conflict is beneficial to mental health (Horwitz, Mclaughlin, & White, 1997). Some studies suggest that marital quality has a greater impact on the mental health of young women than young men (Horwitz, Mclaughlin, & White, 1997), but studies that consider a wider age range of adults find that marital quality affects the mental health of men and women in similar ways (Umberson, Chen, House, Hopkins, & Slaten, 1996; Williams, 2003).

For several decades, social scientists argued that marital quality was highest early in marriage, dipped with the arrival of children, and then rose again in later life. However, recent research using more sophisticated statistical techniques shows that marital quality is at its highest very early in marriages and that marital quality tends to diminish over time, with no upturn later in the life course (VanLaningham, Johnson, & Amato, 2001). Since marital quality is highest early in marriage, young adults who marry are likely to enjoy the benefits of high marital quality. However, the marital quality of young couples tends to decline over time (Umberson, Williams, Powers, & Chen, 2005).

While marital quality is highest very early in marriage, some adults begin their marriage with better marital quality than others. Of particular concern for young adults, getting married prior to the age of 19 is associated with lower marital quality (Forthofer et al., 1996). Other factors associated with reduced marital quality include physical illness (Wickrama, Lorenz, & Conger, 1997), premarital cohabitation (Skinner et al., 2002), poor marital quality of parents (Feng et al., 1999), and lower levels of locus of control (Myers & Booth, 1999).

Children. While many couples believe that having a child will bring them closer, research suggests that having children imposes stress on relationships—especially in terms of financial strain, time constraints, and strain around childcare and the division of domestic labor (Bird, 1997). This negative impact of having a child on relationship quality is more salient for younger than for older parents because younger parents have fewer available resources to ease the strains of parenting young children (Umberson et al., 2005). In comparison to childless couples, young couples with minor children at home experience declines in marital quality—and lower marital quality is, in turn, detrimental to mental health (Umberson et al., 2005). Although a few studies find that parenting experiences increase psychological distress for both men and women, these effects are generally found to be stronger for women than for men because of women's greater involvement in raising children (Bird, 1997).

Evidence suggests that having young children lowers marital quality and thus adds to stress levels and psychological distress; however, some longitudinal studies of newlyweds suggest that marital quality declines in the early years of marriage regardless of whether one has a child (McHale & Huston, 1985). It is also notable that, in comparison to the childless, parents report feeling a greater sense of meaning and purpose in life (Umberson & Williams, 1999). Moreover, while having children in young adulthood may be stressful in a number of ways, having independent adult children in later life may actually contribute to marital quality and psychological well-being (Umberson et al., 2005).

Health Behavior

Young adulthood is a period of life in which numerous health behaviors are at their worst. Research shows that early adolescence and the transition to young adulthood are the periods during which young people are most likely to abuse drugs, alcohol, and tobacco (Tucker, Ellickson, Orlando, Martino, & Klein, 2005). Alcohol consumption peaks between age 25 and 44 for both men and women and declines steadily thereafter; and smoking is most prevalent between the ages of 18 to 24 and then declines with age (Adams & Schoenborn, 2006). Heavy alcohol and cigarette consumption have adverse effects on health and increase mortality risk (Thun et al., 1995). On the other hand, young adults are most likely to be physically active and least likely to be overweight or obese. According to national longitudinal data from Americans' Changing Lives Survey (1986–2001), about one out of two young adults aged 24–30 are *often* engaged in some kind of active sport or exercise and that frequency of participation in exercise or athletic events decreases with age during adulthood.

Many studies show that marriage in young adulthood may trigger important changes in health behavior (see Lewis et al., 2006). Overall, empirical evidence suggests that the married are less likely than the unmarried to engage in risky health behaviors (Tucker & Anders, 2001), although, as we discuss below, the evidence is not always in the expected direction depending on the particular health behavior examined (Grzywacz & Marks, 1999).

Drinking and Smoking. The married exhibit dramatically lower levels of alcohol and cigarette consumption than their unmarried counterparts, and this is particularly true for men (Merline, O'Malley, Schulenberg, Bachman, & Johnston, 2004). A longitudinal study among young adults between 21 and 30 finds that the transition into marriage is associated with a reduction in alcohol disorders, while remaining single and becoming divorced signal higher risk for the onset of alcohol disorders (Chilcoat & Breslau, 1996). Young married adults are also less likely than young adults who are unmarried or separated to use marijuana or cocaine or to misuse prescription drugs (Merline et al., 2004).

A number of studies suggest that spouses often attempt to regulate one another's health behaviors. For example, one partner may tell or remind the other partner to quit/reduce smoking or drinking to protect his/her health (Tucker & Anders, 2001). Having a spouse may also facilitate self-regulation of health behaviors by fostering a sense of responsibility to others (Tucker & Anders, 2001). At the same time, negative health behaviors, such as substance use, may affect young adults' chances of getting married. Indeed, adults with more alcohol/drug consumption are less likely to get married than others (Fu & Goldman, 1996).

Exercise and Body Weight. Unlike the apparent beneficial effects of marriage on smoking, alcohol, and substance abuse, marriage appears to increase the risk of being overweight and to reduce the amount of time spent on exercise (Grzywacz & Marks, 1999). This contradicts the general argument that marriage is a panacea for health. Research shows that the transition into marriage is associated with weight gain, while the transition out of marriage is associated with weight loss (Sobal, Rauschenbach, & Frongillo, 2003). Evidence about gender differences in the association between marriage and body mass/exercise is inconsistent (Sobal et al., 2003). Some studies find that entering/leaving a marriage is associated with weight gain/loss for women but not for men (Jeffery & Rick, 2002), while others find that this effect is more salient for men than for women (Sobal et al., 2003).

According to the causation perspective, marriage increases body mass through a number of psychosocial mechanisms. For example, newly married couples devote considerable effort to eating together and people tend to eat more in the presence of others (Sobal & Nelson, 2003). Getting or being married may also facilitate more food consumption through the planning and scheduling of meals with a partner (Jeffery & Rick, 2002). Having a partner to cook for you may facilitate greater food consumption for both partners. This is especially true for men. Research also suggests that marriage reduces time spent on exercise due to greater time commitment to family roles (Nomaguchi & Bianchi, 2004) and diminishing concerns about staying slim (Sobal et al., 2003). On the other hand, according to the selection perspective, being obese or overweight is less attractive to the opposite sex and influences the chances of young adults entering into marriage. Several studies support this selection argument by finding that those with higher body weight, especially women, are less likely to get married (Fu & Goldman, 1996).

Prevention and Treatment of Marital Problems

While marriage may positively shape young adults' well-being, this protective effect largely depends on the quality of marriage (Horwitz, Mclaughlin, & White, 1997). The prevention and treatment of marital problems, hence, may be particularly germane to the health and well-being of young married adults. It is generally agreed that clinical-based marital therapy is effective in improving marital quality and reducing marital distress, at least in the short term (Bray & Jouriles, 1995). Different types of marital therapy have proved efficacious. One of the most often utilized is behavioral marital therapy (BMT). This approach is largely skill oriented. It involves training couples in communication and problem-solving skills in order to improve relationship quality. Other types of marital therapy, such as emotionally focused therapy (EFT) (e.g., helping couple to strengthen emotional bonds), have also been found to be effective in relieving marital discord (see a review on different types of marital therapy in Mead, 2002). Positive outcomes from marital therapy—usually assessed by self-reported questionnaires—include a variety of components, such as improving marital satisfaction, reducing marital conflict, promoting couples' friendship, and enhancing positive affect and caring, depending on the specific intervention (Gottman & Ryan, 2005).

As opposed to marital therapy that is more clinically oriented and helps couples already experiencing marital problems, prevention programs are aimed at maintaining marital satisfaction and preventing marital dysfunction and divorce for couples with little or no marital distress. Although some studies suggest that some prevention programs (e.g., Prevention and Relationship Enhancement Program) may have a beneficial effect on relationship quality in the short term (Sayers, Kohn, & Heavey, 1998), their long-term effects on prevention of marital separation and divorce are not yet fully understood (Bray & Jouriles, 1995). These interventions may prove to be particularly helpful for young couples who are establishing lifelong relationship skills.

Conclusions

Marriage is the most studied relationship in the social science literature—this has been the case since the earliest sociological studies and continues today with studies of marriage that rely on up-to-date, sophisticated statistical techniques and longitudinal data (House, Landis, & Umberson, 1988). This intimate relationship has received so much theoretical and empirical attention because it is a fundamental institutional unit in society and because substantial research evidence shows that involvement in marriage is associated with improved mental health, physical health, and health behaviors, and with lower rates of mortality (Waite & Gallagher, 2000). In this chapter, we have reviewed predictors and consequences of marriage and identified important trends among young adults.

KEY POINTS

- Young Americans are experiencing remarkable changes in marriage that distinguish them from their parents' and grandparents' generations. In particular, compared to their older counterparts, young adults are more likely to delay their first marriage and experience premarital cohabitation and divorce.

- Although the meanings and significance of marriage have changed for young adults in the context of rapid social movement, the positive association between marriage and mental health, especially when comparing the married with the previously married, is still robust but depends on a host of social factors. As alternatives to marriage become more common and socially acceptable, mental health of the never-married young adults may become more similar to their married counterparts than ever before.
- Marriage may encourage individuals to engage in a healthier lifestyle, especially in terms of smoking and drinking behaviors. This benefit appears to be greater for men than women. However, marriage may also encourage some negative health behaviors. The married spend less time exercising and are more likely to be overweight compared to the unmarried.

PRACTICE GUIDELINES

- Young adults in today's America are different from those several decades ago. With the meanings and experiences of marriage and gender changing for younger cohorts, the relative distribution of the benefits of marriage for men and women are quite likely to undergo transformation (see Williams, 2003). Although some research points to potential changes in the relationship between marriage and mental health across birth cohorts (Simon, 2002), few empirical studies have directly tested this possibility. An historical change perspective on the relationship between marriage and mental health should shed light on the nature of marital change among young adults and has important implications for population health.
- Depending on gender, race, socioeconomic status, and other characteristics, the meanings and consequences of marriage may differ among young adults. Future research should focus more on these group differences. Young adults are also different from one another in terms of how they express distress, making it difficult to generalize the effects of marriage on mental well-being. Before we can draw any conclusions about group differences in the psychological reaction to marriage among young adults, future research must identify the ways that different groups express distress and develop measures for those expressions.
- Although most studies emphasize the positive consequences of marriage on mental health, a few researchers direct attention to the potential negative effects of social ties and social control associated with marriage (Tucker & Anders, 2001). Marriage may increase psychological distress through eliciting feelings of "guilt and indebtedness" and "resentment and irritation" (Tucker & Anders, 2001, p. 469). Moreover, poor marital quality has significant adverse effects for mental and physical health (Umberson, Williams, Powers, Liu, & Needham, 2006). Policies and therapeutic approaches that advocate

(Practice Guidelines continued)

for marriage while ignoring these costs may actually contribute to greater mental and physical morbidity. Young adults have more options than ever before in terms of establishing long-term intimate relationships with others. Although these options, in the form of cohabitation and gay and lesbian committed partnerships, may be not as protective as marriage for young adults' well-being (Kim & McKenry, 2002), these differences may diminish as cohabitation and same-sex partnerships become more common and accepted (Hull, 2006). Within this new and changing context, the potential benefits and costs of marriage and its alternatives represent new opportunities for social scientists to forge greater understanding of the links between intimate relationships and individual health and well-being. The transformation of the institution of marriage may pose new opportunities for individuals wishing to create meaningful, sustaining intimate relationships outside of marriage.

References

Adams, P. F., & Schoenborn, C. A. (2006). *Health behaviors of adults: United States, 2002-2004.* National Center for Health Statistics. *Vital Health Statistics, 10*(230); 1–140.

Bernard, J. (1972). *The future of marriage.* New Haven, CT: Yale University Press.

Bird, C. E. (1997). Gender differences in the social and economic burdens of parenting and psychological distress. *Journal of Marriage and the Family, 59*(4), 809–823.

Bramlett, M. D., & Mosher, W. D. (2002). *Cohabitation, marriage, divorce, and remarriage in the United States.* National Center for Health Statistics. *Vital Health Statistics, 23*(22). 1–93.

Bray, J. H., & Jouriles, E. N. (1995). Treatment of marital conflict and prevention of divorce. *Journal of Marital and Family Therapy, 21,* 461–473.

Brines, J., & Joyner, K. (1999). The ties that bind: Principles of cohesion in cohabitation and marriage. *American Sociological Review, 64,* 333–355.

Brown, S. L. (2000). The effect of union type on psychological well-being: Depression among cohabitors versus marrieds. *Journal of Health and Social Behavior, 41,* 241–255.

Casper, L., & Bianchi, S. (2001). *Continuity and change in the American family.* San Francisco: Sage.

Chilcoat, H. D., & Breslau, S. (1996). Alcohol disorders in young adulthood: Effects of transition into adult roles. *Journal of Health and Social Behavior, 37,* 339–349.

Dohrenwend, B. P., & Dohrenwend, B. S. (1976). Sex differences and psychiatric disorders. *The American Journal of Sociology, 81*(6), 1447–1454.

Elliott, S., & Umberson, D. (2004). Recent demographic trends in the US and implications for well-being. In J. L. Scott, J. Treas, & M. Richards (Eds.), *The Blackwell companion to the sociology of families.* Malden, MA: Blackwell.

Erickson, R. J. (2005). Why emotion work matters: Sex, gender, and the division of household labor. *Journal of Marriage and Family, 67,* 337–351.

Feng, D., Giarrusso, R., Bengtson, V. L., & Frye, N. (1999). Intergenerational transmission of marital quality and marital instability. *Journal of Marriage and the Family, 61,* 451–463.

Forthofer, M. S., Kessler, R. C., Story, A. L., & Gotlib, I. H. (1996). The effects of psychiatric disorders on the probability and timing of first marriage. *Journal of Health and Social Behavior, 37,* 121–132.

Fu, H., & Goldman, N. (1996). Incorporating health into models of marriage choice: Demographic and sociological perspectives. *Journal of Marriage and the Family, 58*(3), 740–758.

Goldstein, J. R. (1999). The leveling of divorce in the United States. *Demography, 36,* 409–414.

Gottman, J. M., & Ryan, K. D. (2005). The mismeasure of therapy: Treatment outcomes in marital therapy research. In W. M. Pinsof & J. Lebow (Eds.), *Family psychology: The art of the science* (pp. 65–90). Oxford, England: Oxford University Press

Gove, W. R., & Tudor, J. F. (1973). Adult sex roles and mental illness. *The American Journal of Sociology, 78*(4), 812–835.

Grzywacz, J. G., & Marks, N. F. (1999). Family solidarity and health behaviors. *Journal of Family Issues, 20,* 243–268.

Heaton, T. B. (2002). Factors contributing to increasing marital stability in the United States. *Journal of Family Issues, 23*, 392–409.

Horwitz, A. V., Mclaughlin, J., & White, H. R. (1997). How the negative and positive aspects of partner relationships affect the mental health of young married people. *Journal of Health and Social Behavior, 39*, 124–136.

Horwitz, A. V., & White, H. R. (1998). The relationship of cohabitation and mental health: A study of young adult cohort. *Journal of Marriage and the Family, 60*, 505–514.

Horwitz, A. V., White, H. R., & Howell-White, S. (1996a). The use of multiple outcomes in stress research: A case study of gender differences in responses to marital dissolution. *Journal of Health and Social Behavior, 37*, 278–291.

Horwitz, A. V., White, H. R., & Howell-White, S. (1996b). Becoming married and mental health: A longitudinal study of a cohort of young adults. *Journal of Marriage and the Family, 58*, 895–907.

House, J. S., Landis, K. R., & Umberson, D. J. (1988). Social relationships and health. *Science, 241*, 540–545.

Hull, K. E. (2006). *Same-sex marriage: The cultural politics of love and law*. Cambridge, England: Cambridge University Press.

Jeffery, R. W., & Rick, A. M. (2002). Cross-sectional and longitudinal associations between body mass index and marriage-related factors. *Obesity Research, 10*, 809–815.

Joung, I. M., Van de Mheen, H. D., Stronks, K., Van Poppel, F. W., & Mackenbach, J. P. (1998). A longitudinal study of health selection in marital transitions. *Social Science & Medicine, 46*(3), 425–435.

Joyner, K., & Udry, J. R. (2000). You don't bring me anything but down: Adolescent romance and depression. *Journal of Health and Social Behavior, 41*, 369–391.

Kim, H. N., & McKenry, P. C. (2002). The relationship between marriage and psychological well-being. *Journal of Family Issues, 23*, 885–911.

Lewis, M. A., McBride, C. M., Pollak, K. I., Puleo, E., Butterfield R. M., & Emmons, K. M. (2006). Understanding health behavior change among couples: An interdependence and communal coping approach. *Social Science & Medicine, 62*, 1369–1380.

Marks, N. F. (1996). Flying solo at midlife: Gender, marital status, and psychological well-being. *Journal of Marriage and the Family, 58*(4), 917–933.

Marks, N. F., & Lambert, J. D. (1998). Marital status continuity and change among young and midlife adults - Longitudinal effects on psychological well-being. *Journal of Family Issues, 19*(6), 652–686.

McHale, S. M., & Huston, T. L. (1985). The effect of the transition to parenthood on the marriage relationship: A longitudinal study. *Journal of Family Issues, 6*, 409–434.

Mead, D. E. (2002). Marital distress, co-occurring depression, and marital therapy: A review. *Journal of Marital and Family Therapy, 28*, 299–314.

Merline, A. C., O'Malley, P. M., Schulenberg, J. E., Bachman, J. G., & Johnston, L. D. (2004). Substance use among adults 35 years of age: Prevalence, adulthood predictors, and impact of adolescent substance use. *American Journal of public Health, 94*, 96–102.

Mirowsky, J., & Ross, C. E. (2003). *Education, social status, and health*. New York: Aldine De Gruyter.

Mosher, W. D., Chandra, A., & Jones, J. (2005). *Sexual behavior and selected health measures: Men and women 15-44 years of age, United States, 2002*. Hyattsville, MD: National Center for Health Statistics.

Musick, K., & Bumpass, L. (2006). *Cohabitation, marriage and trajectories in well-being and relationships*. California Center for Population Research On-Line Working Paper Series. http://www.ccpr.ucla.edu/asp/papers.asp; accessed March 19, 2009

Myers, S. M., & Booth, A. (1999). Marital strains and marital quality: The role of high and low locus of control. *Journal of Marriage and the Family, 61*, 423–436.

Nomaguchi, K. M., & Bianchi, S. M. (2004). Exercise time: Gender differences in the effects of marriage, parenthood and employment. *Journal of Marriage and Family, 66*, 413–430.

Oppenheimer, V. K. (1997). Women's employment and the gain to marriage: The specialization and trading model. *Annual Review of Sociology, 23*, 431–453.

Ostermann, J., Sloan, F. A., & Taylor, D. H. (2005). Heavy alcohol use and marital dissolution in the USA. *Social Science & Medicine, 61*, 2304–2316.

Price, I. R., & Lavercombe, L. J. (2000). Depression in early adolescence: Relation to externalising and internalising behavior. *Perceptual and Motor Skills, 90*, 723–730.

Raley, K., & Bumpass, L. (2003). The topography of the plateau in divorce: Levels and trends in union stability after 1980. *Demographic Research, 8*, 246–258.

Rosenfield, S. (1999). Splitting the difference: Gender, the self, and mental health. In C. Anaschensel & J. Phelan (Eds.), *Handbook of the sociology of mental health*. New York: Plenum.

Ross, C. E., Mirowsky, J., & Goldsteen, K. (1990). The impact of family on health: The decade in review. *Journal of Marriage and the Family, 52*, 1059–1078.

Sayers, S. L., Kohn, C. S., & Heavey, C. (1998). Prevention of marital dysfunction: Behavioral approaches and beyond. *Clinical Psychology Review, 18*, 713–744.

Simmons, T., & Dye, J. (2004). *What has happened to median age at first marriage data?* Paper presented at the Annual Meeting of the American Sociological Association, San Francisco, CA.

Simon, R. W. (2002). Revisiting the relationships among gender, marital status, and mental health. *American Journal of Sociology, 107*, 1065–1096.

Skinner, K. B., Bahr, S. J., Crane D. R., & Call, V. R. A. (2002). Cohabitation, marriage, and remarriage. *Journal of Family Issues, 23*, 74–90.

Smock, P. (2000). Cohabitation in the United States: An appraisal of research themes, findings, and implications. *Annual Review of Sociology, 26*, 1–20.

Sobal, J., & Nelson, M.K. (2003). Commensal eating patterns: A community study. *Appetite, 41*, 181–190.

Sobal, J., Rauschenbach, B., & Frongillo, E. A. (2003). Marital status changes and body weight changes: a US longitudinal analysis. *Social Science & Medicine, 56*, 1543–1555.

Strohschein, L., McDonough, P., Monette, G., & Shao, Q. (2005). Marital transitions and mental health: Are there gender differences in the short-term effects of marital status change? *Social Science & Medicine, 61*, 2293–2303.

Sweeney, M. (2002). Two decades of family change: The shifting economic foundations of marriage. *American Sociological Review, 67*(1), 132–147.

Teachman, J. D., Tedrow, L. M., & Kyle, D. (2000). The changing demography of America's families. *Journal of Marriage and Family, 62*, 1234–1246.

Thun, M. J., Peto, R., Lopez, A. D., Monaco, J. H., Henley, S. J., Heath, C. W., & Doll, R. (1995). Alcohol consumption and mortality among middle-aged and elderly U.S. adults. *New England Journal of Medicine, 333*, 677–685.

Tucker, J., & Anders, S. (2001). Social control of health behaviors in marriage. *Journal of Applied Social Psychology, 31*, 467–485.

Tucker, J. S., Ellickson, P. L., Orlando, M., Martino, S. C., & Klein, D. J. (2005). Adolescence to emerging adulthood: A comparison of smoking, binge drinking, and marijuana use. *Journal of Drug Issues, 35*(2), 307–332.

Umberson, D., Chen, M. D., House, J. S., Hopkins, K., & Slaten, E. (1996). Social relationships and their effects on psychological well-being: Are men and women really so different? *American Sociological Review, 61*, 836–856.

Umberson, D., & Williams, K. (1999). Family status and mental health. In Carol S. Aneshensel & Jo C. Phelan (Eds.), *Handbook of the sociology of mental health* (pp.225–253). New York: Plenum.

Umberson, D., Williams, K., Powers, D. P., & Chen, M. D. (2005). As good as it gets? A life course perspective on marital quality. *Social Forces, 84*, 493–511.

Umberson, D., Williams, K., Powers, D. P., Liu, H., & Needham, B. (2006). You make me sick: Marital quality and health over the life course. *Journal of Health and Social Behavior, 47*, 1–16.

U.S. Bureau of the Census. (2001). America's families and living arrangements: Population characteristics 2000. *Current Population Reports*, Series P20–537. Author: Washington, DC.

VanLaningham, J., Johnson, D. R., & Amato, P. (2001). Marital happiness, marital duration, and the U-shaped curve: Evidence from a five-wave panel study. *Social Forces, 79*, 1313–1341.

Wade, T. J., & Pevalin, D. J. (2004). Marital transitions and mental health. *Journal of Health and Social Behavior, 45*, 155–170.

Waite, L. J., & Gallagher, M. (2000). *The case for marriage: Why married people are happier, healthier, and better off financially.* New York: Doubleday.

Walzer, S. (1998). *Thinking about the baby: Gender and transitions into parenthood.* Philadelphia: Temple University Press.

Wickrama, K. A. S., Lorenz, F. O., & Conger, R. D. (1997). Marital quality and physical illness: A latent growth curve analysis. *Journal of Marriage and the Family, 59*, 143–155.

Williams, K. (2003). Has the future of marriage arrived? A contemporary examination of gender, marriage, and psychological well-being. *Journal of Health and Social Behavior, 44*, 470–487.

Williams, K., & Umberson, D. (2004). Marital status, marital transitions, and health: A gendered life course perspective. *Journal of Health and Social Behavior, 45*, 81–98.

Chapter 12

Developmental Pathways to Parenting

Thomas J. McMahon

Maureen was an intellectually bright, socially reserved girl who grew up in an urban, blue-collar neighborhood in southern New England with her father, mother, and an older brother. Her parents worked hard to support their children emotionally and financially while setting clear, reasonable behavioral expectations. Although close with her mother, Maureen had a special relationship with her father, who, as she got older, spent a lot of time teaching her to play basketball. Maureen sometimes quarreled with her older brother, but he always looked after her and took pride in being her older brother.

During elementary school, Maureen had a close friendship with Amy, a more gregarious girl who lived down the street and, like Maureen, did well in school academically. Amy lived with her mother, two older half-sisters, and a younger half-brother. Her father had only lived with her mother briefly when Amy was an infant, and she rarely saw him. When Amy did see her father, he and her mother usually quarreled about money, and he would not return for an extended period of time. Despite his absence, Amy only spoke positively about him. During elementary school, two men with whom Amy's mother had brief romantic relationships had also lived with the family. While growing up, Maureen noticed that Amy and her mother frequently quarreled in a frightening manner, and she noticed that Amy's mother did not seem to worry about Amy the way her mother worried about her.

During 5th grade, Amy began gaining weight and developing breasts. Just before the end of the school year, Amy proudly announced that she had begun menstruating, and she began teasing Maureen about her tall, lanky body and the delay in her pubertal development. As they entered middle school, the two girls began drifting apart as Amy began spending time with boys in 8th grade and began bragging that she was learning how to kiss with her mouth open. As they moved through middle school, Maureen began feeling increasingly uncomfortable as Amy talked constantly about her sexual experiences with one boyfriend after the other. Although she had begun to menstruate a year later, Maureen still felt uncomfortable when alone with a boy. The idea of kissing one seemed exciting but also frightening. She was spending more time with a small group of friends that now included boys who were also good students and enjoyed playing basketball, but she still preferred to spend time her free time with her family and a few close girlfriends.

During high school, Maureen and Amy migrated to completely different circles of friends. Maureen continued to study hard and play basketball. She continued to spend most of her free time with a few close girlfriends, but she became increasingly comfortable talking to boys. During her junior year, she developed a romantic interest in a tall, quiet boy who also played basketball for the high school. After clumsily flirting with him for several months, she eventually asked him to spend time some time alone with her. About the same time, her older brother withdrew from community college and left home for the military. Maureen missed him terribly but found that she felt better when with her new boyfriend, who

181

seemed to understand how she felt. Over the next year, Maureen and her boyfriend spent a lot of time together, and they developed a close relationship that included a lot of hand-holding, kissing, and petting. Although they frequently talked about someday having sexual intercourse, they agreed that they were not ready to have more intimate sexual relations.

Throughout high school, Maureen repeatedly heard gossip about Amy. She heard that Amy had lost her virginity soon after they began high school during a single encounter with a senior boy while at a party where everyone was drinking. Friends frequently told her that Amy always seemed to have a new boyfriend who she was madly in love with, and everyone seemed to know that she was having sexual relations. Her boyfriend told Maureen that a friend on the basketball team told him that Amy had been bragging that her current boyfriend would never leave her because she regularly and expertly provided him with oral sex. One night during her senior year, Maureen's mother told her that there were rumors Amy had gotten pregnant during her second year of high school and had an elective abortion. Her mother also made an alarming remark about a man Amy's mother had lived with who had to leave because he had been caught kissing Amy.

During the summer after graduation, Maureen and her boyfriend spent a lot of time talking about being separated to attend college. Maureen planned to attend a small, private college, where she hoped to continue playing basketball. She thought that she might like to be a teacher. Her boyfriend planned to attend a large, state university. He hoped to go to law school. They intended to talk over the telephone every day and visit each other on the weekends. As a couple, they talked for the first time about getting married and someday having children.

Before going off to college Maureen and her boyfriend began having sexual intercourse. Together, they had decided that a camping trip with some friends to celebrate their graduation would be the best time to begin having sexual relations. Suspicious she was considering becoming sexually active, Maureen's mother had helped her secure contraception. Although the discussion was tense, Maureen told her mother that she thought she loved her boyfriend and wanted to share herself with him. Her mother encouraged her to wait but also acknowledged that the decision was hers. They agreed it was probably best that her father not know the details of her decision.

Just before leaving for college, Maureen met Amy in the local shopping mall and learned that she had a newborn daughter. Amy told her that she had been engaged to marry the baby's father, but he had ended the relationship soon after she became pregnant. She now had a new boyfriend who was promising to help support her and her child financially because her previous boyfriend had promised that he would not. Amy said that she was planning to live with her new boyfriend and have another child with him as soon as possible. She and her 20-year-old half-sister who now had two children planned to share responsibility for child care so they could both work part time at a local grocery store. Maureen felt somewhat awkward talking with Amy, and she said good-bye feeling as though there was something left unsaid. Later that evening, she found herself crying while telling her boyfriend how sad she felt about the way things had turned out for her childhood friend.

Over the course of the past 10 years, there has been growing attention to the concept of emerging adulthood as a unique developmental period falling between adolescence and early adulthood. Conceptually, Arnett (2004) defined *emerging adulthood* as a transitional period when young people approximately 18 to 24 years of age cannot accurately be thought of as either adolescents or young adults. Emphasizing the integration of psychological and sociological considerations, Arnett argued that emerging adulthood is a distinct phase of development in postindustrial cultures best characterized as a period of exploration and instability that precedes the transition to adulthood. Although the nature of this transition varies somewhat across technologically advanced cultures, socioeconomic context seems to shape the manner in which young people negotiate this transition in the United States (Tanner, 2006), and when compared with young people living in other modern cultures, young people in the United States seem to negotiate elements of this transition sooner and in a more homogeneous manner (Fussell, Gauthier, & Evans, 2007).

As social, economic, and technological changes occurring in modern cultures have reshaped the transition to adulthood, young people have been delaying marriage and parenthood while exploring the nature of love, sexual relations, and commitment (Arnett, 2004). Demographic trends reflecting ongoing change in developmental pathways to adulthood suggest that becoming a parent before 25 years of age must now be considered early when examined from a normative perspective. Increasingly, young people are delaying parenthood while preparing for the social, psychological, and economic independence that typically comes with being an adult (Arnett, 2004).

As emerging adulthood has been redefined as a developmental phase incompatible with parenthood, questions once asked about teenage parents have been extended to young people who become parents before 25 years of age (e.g., see Gest, Mahoney, & Cairns, 1999; Woodward, Fergusson, & Horwood, 2006). Within this literature, the fundamental question is: Why do some young people like Maureen delay having sexual intercourse and avoid early parenthood while they acquire the social, psychological, and economic resources needed to successfully negotiate being a parent later in life, while young people like Amy begin having sexual relations early only to become a parent long before they are adequately prepared to be a parent? This chapter will address that question by examining the utility of a life history perspective on reproductive behavior that emphasizes the potential impact of early developmental experiences on risk for early birth of a first child. The primary goal is to illustrate how life history theory and attachment theory can be used to inform understanding of a broad developmental pathway to early parenthood that, in the context of changing norms, may complicate the transition to adulthood.

Emerging Adulthood: New Developmental Norms

Longitudinal investigations of psychosocial development during the transition from adolescence to adulthood suggest that emerging adulthood has become a time to continue exploring questions about the nature of sexual partnerships that typically begins during adolescence. As young people move through adolescence toward adulthood, romantic relationships become much more common, they become more enduring, and they involve more psychological intimacy (Arnett, 2004). They also involve more sexual intercourse, and they are more likely to result in periods of cohabitation (Arnett, 2004). Although a majority of young people now marry before they reach 30 years of age, they usually do so after being involved in several serious romantic relationships (Arnett, 2004).

Ironically, although young people agree that emerging adulthood represents a period of exploration in the context of more intimate, more enduring sexual partnerships, most young people do not list parenthood as a developmental task to be met during this time of their lives (Arnett, 2004). Surveys of the general population indicate that parenthood becomes more common as young people move toward early adulthood (Lefkowitz & Gillen, 2006). However, there has, over the past 30 years, been a dramatic decline in parenthood during this time of life, and birth rates for individuals less than 25 years of age continue to decline (Chandra, Martinez, Mosher, Abma, & Jones, 2005; Martinez, Chandra, Abma, Jones, & Mosher, 2006). Recent surveys of the general population indicate that less than 2% of men and 8% of women 16 to 19 years of age have had a first child. Less than 18% of men and 33% of women have had a first child by 25 years of age (Chandra et al., 2005; Martinez et al., 2006).

Moreover, research on the psychosocial consequences of early parenthood suggests that becoming a parent before 25 years of age represents risk for poor developmental outcomes as young people make the transition to adulthood. Building upon the work of Hogan and Astone (1986), researchers (e.g., Pears, Pierce, Kim, Capaldi, & Owen, 2005; Sigle-Rushton, 2005) have argued that the early birth of a first child affects performance as a parent because young people lack the psychosocial resources needed to successfully negotiate this important developmental transition. Early parenthood may also affect the successful negotiation of developmental tasks more clearly associated with emerging adulthood, and the early birth of a first child may affect development far into adulthood (Pears et al., 2005; Sigle-Rushton, 2005).

Although some researchers have argued that the consequences of early parenthood may not be as dramatic as originally thought (for a discussion, see Moore & Brooks-Gunn, 2002), the impact of early parenthood may actually become more marked as social and economic changes demand that young people have this period to prepare for the transition to adulthood.

At this time, there is a relatively extensive literature on the consequences of early parenthood for young women. Understanding of the consequences for young men is much more limited. There is also more information about the consequences of parenthood beginning during adolescence than there is information about the consequences of parenthood beginning during emerging adulthood, and there is relatively little information about the ways risks may vary with social context (Moore & Brooks-Gunn, 2002). Given the focus of this chapter, it is also important to note that there is much more information about the social consequences of early parenthood than there is information about the psychological consequences (Moore & Brooks-Gunn, 2002). It is clear that there are social costs associated with early parenthood, but it is less clear how the early birth of a first child affects psychological development as young people make the transition to adulthood. This gap in the literature is important because research suggests that young people believe that the psychological changes that typically occur during emerging adulthood are just as important as the social role transitions (Arnett, 2004).

Despite the limitations, there is substantial evidence that, even after allowance for differences that represent risk for early pregnancy, the psychosocial adjustment of young mothers tends to be poorer than that of their peers as they move through adulthood (for reviews, see Luster & Haddow, 2005; Moore & Brooks-Gunn, 2002). Although there is tremendous variability in developmental outcomes, young mothers tend to have poorer educational achievement, poorer employment, and less stable sexual partnerships following the early birth of a first child. They are also more likely to have additional children, they are more likely to be psychologically dependent on their mothers, and their psychological development is likely to be dominated by concern about their role as a mother. They are also more likely to have problems parenting their children, and their children are more likely to experience psychosocial difficulty.

Similarly, there is accumulating evidence that, even after allowance for differences that represent risk for early birth of a first child, the psychosocial adjustment of young fathers tends to be poorer than that of their peers as they move through adulthood (e.g., see Sigle-Rushton, 2005). Although some researchers (e.g., Sigle-Rushton, 2005) have suggested that there may actually be more variability in developmental outcomes among young men, young fathers tend, like young mothers, to have poorer educational achievement, poorer employment, and less stable sexual partnerships following the early birth of a first child (e.g., see Berrington, Cobos Hernandez, Ingham, & Stevenson, 2005; Nock, 1998; Sigle-Rushton, 2005). When compared with their peers who delay fatherhood, young fathers are also less likely to live with their children (e.g., see Berrington et al., 2005; Jaffee, Caspi, Moffitt, Belsky, & Silva, 2001), they are less likely to provide financial support (Berrington et al., 2005), and they are less likely to see their children regularly (Berrington et al., 2005). They are also more likely to remain involved in illegal activity (Stouthamer-Loeber & Wei, 1998), they are more likely to be receiving public entitlements (Berrington et al., 2005), and they are more likely to be living in a second family with children they did not conceive (Berrington et al., 2005).

Life History Theory

Given the social, psychological, and economic problems commonly associated with the early birth of a first child, researchers interested in family process occurring across generations (e.g., Belsky, Steinberg, & Draper, 1991) have begun to consider how life history theory may inform understanding of risk for early parenthood. Life history theory is a broad conceptual framework that examines individual variation in reproductive milestones as trade-offs associated with the distribution of resources to support competing life functions (Charnov, 1993; Roff, 1992; Stearns, 1992). Life history theory broadly distinguishes between *somatic effort* representing resources devoted to the survival of the individual and *reproductive effort* representing resources devoted to the production and parenting of children. Reproductive effort involves a balance between *mating effort* involving resources devoted to the recruitment and retention of sexual partners and *parenting effort* involving resources devoted to childrearing.

Although the immediate goal of mating effort may be sexual satisfaction, reproduction is the more distal, often unconscious, goal of all mating effort when it is examined from an evolutionary perspective. Individual differences in the allocation of mating versus parenting effort define the *reproductive strategy* being pursued by a specific individual. Reproductive strategy is defined by a cluster of individual characteristics representing (1) pubertal timing, (2) a strategy for the selection of sexual partners, (3) the stability of sexual relationships, (4) patterns of reproduction, and (5) investment in parenting (Belsky et al., 1991).

According to life history theory, individuals shape their reproductive strategy in response to prevailing circumstances in their immediate environment. That is, individuals consciously or unconsciously tailor their reproductive strategy to accommodate the demands of the local ecology. From an evolutionary perspective, the reproductive strategy pursued by an individual should insure, as much as possible, that children have access to the resources that they need to survive in their ecological niche.

Attachment Theory and Reproductive Behavior

Since publication of the provocative paper on adult attachment written by Hazan and Shaver (1987), researchers have been interested in the idea that the attachment system so critical to early child development continues to shape the nature of close relationships across the life span. Writing from an attachment perspective, this group of scholars (e.g., Fraley & Shaver, 2000; Hazan & Shaver, 1994; Hazan & Zeifman, 1999) has highlighted ways basic needs for affection, protection, and stimulation activate behavioral systems that cause children to seek contact with their primary caretakers. Simultaneously, the basic needs of children activate a reciprocal behavioral system in parents organized around caregiving. Over time, children develop internal working models of themselves in caregiving systems that guide the quality of their interactions with their primary caretakers.

Although discussion continues about the organization and influence of different psychological representations, this group of researchers (e.g., Fraley & Shaver, 2000; Hazan & Shaver, 1994; Hazan & Zeifman, 1999) believes that internal working models of early relationships with caretakers become more elaborate during childhood and adolescence. During childhood, psychological representations of self in caretaking relationships become templates that guide interaction with peers and other adults. During adolescence, they become the foundation for more elaborate representations of self as a sexual partner and a potential parent. As individuals move through adolescence, attachment, caregiving, and sexual behavior systems become consolidated in the development of romantic attachments that involve the expression of openness to caretaking, capacity for caretaking, and sexual expression. Although the process begins during infancy, continues during childhood, and accelerates dramatically with the onset of puberty, the consolidation of romantic attachments typically occurs during emerging adulthood.

Psychosexual Acceleration Hypothesis

Over time, scholars interested in evolutionary perspectives on contemporary human behavior have begun to outline developmental formulations of reproductive behavior that represent an integration of concepts drawn from life history theory and attachment theory (for reviews, see Simpson, 1999; Simpson & Belsky, in press). Writing from this perspective, Belsky et al. (1991) outlined a very influential life history theory that emphasized ways quality of early relationships with primary caretakers interact with contextual factors to influence pair bonding, production of children, and quality of parenting across generations. This work has since been elaborated upon (e.g., see Belsky, 1997, 1999; Chisholm, 1993, 1996), revised (e.g., see Ellis, 2004, 2005), and contrasted with competing positions (e.g., see Buss & Greiling, 1999; Kirkpatrick, 1998; Simpson, 1999). The original theory proposed by Belsky et al. (1991)

has also informed a new generation of research on the development of reproductive behavior as young people move through adolescence toward adulthood (e.g., see Belsky et al., 2007; Ellis & Essex, 2007).

Drawing upon principles outlined in both life history theory and attachment theory, Belsky et al. (1991) argued that reproductive strategy evolves over time largely outside conscious awareness. Like other scholars interested in life history theory, they distinguished between a *short-term reproductive strategy* and a *long-term reproductive strategy*. A short-term reproductive strategy is characterized by the rapid production of multiple children with different partners with minimal effort devoted to parenting. Because this reproductive strategy is characterized by an emphasis on mating effort over parenting effort, it is defined as a quantity over quality approach to insuring the survival of children. Conversely, a long-term reproductive strategy is characterized by the production of fewer children with a single partner over a more extended period of time with maximal effort devoted to parenting. Because this reproductive strategy is characterized by an emphasis on parenting effort over mating effort, it is defined as a quality over quantity approach to insuring the survival of children.

When examining reproductive behavior from an evolutionary perspective, Belsky et al. (1991) argued that early experiences with primary caretakers influence psychosocial development during childhood in ways that set the stage for later pursuit of a reproductive strategy that is always adaptive from the perspective of the individual. That is, early experience with primary caretakers produces psychological orientations that guide mating and parenting later in the life cycle. Although described in a linear fashion, Belsky et al. argued that the impact of developmental ecology on child development is cumulative and probabilistic as individuals move through childhood into adolescence.

A Broad Developmental Pathway to Later Parenthood

Within this conceptual model, Belsky et al. (1991) proposed a broad developmental pathway that evolves out of sensitive, responsive parenting occurring in the context of a stable family environment that, over time, promotes pursuit of a long-term reproductive strategy. When parents believe that the social environment is stable, they consciously or unconsciously parent children in a manner designed to communicate that sense of stability. From an early age, sensitive, responsive parenting fosters the development of stable psychological representations concerning the importance of self, the dependability of others, and the predictability of the environment.

When early experiences confirm the responsiveness of others, a positive sense of self, and a sense of predictability in the environment, individuals typically pursue a long-term reproductive strategy. In this developmental ecology, *(1)* the onset of puberty typically comes later, *(2)* pair bonding begins later, *(3)* sexual intercourse is delayed, *(4)* relationships with sexual partners are reciprocal and enduring, *(5)* fewer children come later in the life cycle when socioeconomic and psychological resources are more stable, and *(6)* parents, particularly fathers, invest more in the care of children. Clearly, her early developmental experiences had put Maureen on this broad developmental pathway.

A Broad Developmental Pathway to Early Parenthood

Within this conceptual model, Belsky et al. (1991) also proposed a broad, alternate developmental pathway that evolves out of harsh, critical, insensitive parenting occurring in the context of an unstable family environment that, over time, promotes pursuit of a short-term reproductive strategy. When parents believe that the social environment is not stable, they consciously or unconsciously parent children in a manner designed to communicate a sense of unpredictability. Moreover, situational stress that taxes the psychological resources of parents contributes to harsh, rejecting, inconsistent parenting behavior. From an early age, unresponsive, insensitive parenting fosters the development of stable psychological representations involving negative images of self, mistrust of others, and the unpredictable, unsupportive nature of the environment.

When early experiences promote a negative sense of self, the insensitive nature of others, and a sense of unpredictability in the environment, individuals typically pursue a short-term reproductive strategy. In this developmental ecology, disruption of parent–child relationships, exposure to negative parenting, and chronic adversity contribute to the development of an opportunistic psychological orientation and an acceleration of pubertal development. When puberty begins early in the context of largely negative psychological representations of self and others, *(1)* pair bonding begins early, *(2)* sexual intercourse begins sooner, *(3)* relationships with sexual partners are not enduring, *(4)* multiple children come earlier in the life cycle when social, psychological, and economic resources are not stable, and *(5)* parents, particularly fathers, do not invest in the care of children. Clearly, her early developmental experiences had put Amy on this broad developmental pathway.

Extending the original work, Chisholm (1996) outlined more specific developmental pathways to early parenthood based on the nature of early, insecure attachment representations. From his perspective, the reproductive strategy pursued by parents directly influences the reproductive strategy that their children will pursue, at least in part, by producing distinct variations in attachment style. Consistent with this, Chisholm argued that the reproductive strategy pursued by an individual with an ambivalent attachment style should be different from that pursued by an individual with an avoidant attachment style because differences in attachment style represent longer-term psychological adaptations to qualitatively different early family environments.

Defining ambivalent attachment as adaptation to a parenting style characterized by inconsistency, Chisholm (1996) argued that children living in environments where adults are willing, but not always able, to invest resources in the future develop demanding, self-centered behavioral predispositions at an early age. Consequently, the reproductive strategy of children with an ambivalent attachment style should be characterized by early sexual maturation, early pair bonding with concern about abandonment, early sexual intercourse to promote closeness and avoid rejection, and unstable sexual partnerships that result in the conception of multiple children with multiple partners with some investment in parenting but difficulty consistently providing sensitive caregiving. Again, her early developmental experiences seemed to have put Amy on this more clearly defined developmental pathway.

Defining avoidant attachment as adaptation to a parenting style characterized largely by rejection, Chisholm (1996) argued that children living in environments where adults are able, but not willing, to invest resources in the future develop self-reliant, opportunistic behavioral predispositions at an early age. Consequently, the reproductive strategy of children with an avoidant attachment style should be characterized by discomfort with intimacy, difficulty developing stable, reciprocal sexual partnerships, and a selfish, opportunistic approach to sexual relations that, over time, should result in the conception of multiple children with multiple partners with little investment in parenting.

Empirical Support for the Psychosocial Acceleration Hypothesis

Reviews of existing research (e.g., Belsky et al., 1991; Chisholm, 1993, 1996) were originally used to support the initial development of the psychosocial acceleration hypothesis. Moreover, empirical investigations of reproductive behavior based on the early work of Belsky et al. (1991) have confirmed elements of the original theory. At this time, there is accumulating evidence that quality of early relationships with parents and exposure to psychosocial stress affect the onset of puberty, but the evidence confirming a link between early caretaking, psychosocial stress, and acceleration of pubertal development is clearer for girls (for reviews, see Ellis, 2004, 2005).

In one of the more comprehensive, longitudinal investigations of life history theory in girls, Ellis and Essex (2007) found that positive early relationships with parents were associated with a delay in the onset of puberty. They also found that, when combined with higher socioeconomic status, positive mother–daughter relationships were associated with the most dramatic delay in pubertal development. In one of the few longitudinal investigations of life history theory to include both boys and girls, Belsky et al. (2007) found that, in contrast to Ellis and Essex who found that positive parent–child relationships seemed to be associated with delay in pubertal development, negative parenting during early to middle childhood, particularly harsh mothering, was more clearly associated with early menarche in girls. Although Kim and his colleagues (Kim & Smith, 1998, 1999; Kim, Smith, & Palermiti, 1997) found evidence that a retrospective description of early family environment by boys was associated with timing of sexual maturation in cross-sectional research designs, Belsky et al. found that quality of early family environments did not seem to influence the pubertal development of boys.

Within the attachment literature, there is also support for the idea that psychological representations of early caregiving may influence psychosexual development. Although there is empirical evidence of some degree of continuity in attachment representations from early childhood to early adulthood, the evidence across longitudinal studies is equivocal (Grossman, Grossman, & Waters, 2005). Sroufe, Egeland, Carlson, and Collins (2005) recently suggested that attachment representations evolve more dynamically over time through successive transactions between the individual and the social environment such that there may be both continuity in attachment representations when social environments remain stable and lawful discontinuity when social environments change. That said, it is interesting that Sroufe and his colleagues (Roisman, Collins, Sroufe, & Egeland, 2005; Roisman, Madsen, Henninghausen, Sroufe, & Collins, 2001) have shown that attachment behavior present during early childhood and psychological representation of early caregiving present during early adolescence are clearly associated with psychological representations of romantic relationships during emerging adulthood.

Empirical support for elements of the theory proposed by Belsky et al. (1991) can also be found in the literature on romantic attachment styles. Although the data are somewhat limited, researchers have shown that psychological representations of romantic relationships derived, at least in part, from how psychological representations of early caregiving correlate with individual differences in psychosexual development during adolescence and emerging adulthood. Over time, researchers have shown that the three most common attachment styles are consistently associated with differences in psychosexual development that represent differential risk for early parenthood.

For example, Tracy, Shaver, Albino, and Cooper (2003) found that, when compared with teens who demonstrate an insecure attachment style, teens like Maureen who demonstrate a secure attachment style confirm romantic and sexual experiences that reflect a positive view of self, a positive view of a sexual partner, and interest in psychological and sexual intimacy. A secure attachment style is also usually associated with more frequent dating and more participation in romantic relationships. When compared with their peers, these teens are (1) more interested in love, (2) more likely to be involved in a romantic relationship, (3) more likely to view sex as a way to express their love for their partner, (4) more likely to experience positive emotions during sexual relations, and (5) less likely to experience negative emotions during sexual relations. They are also less likely to be sexually aggressive, less likely to be the target of sexual aggression, and less likely to use alcohol or drugs during sexual encounters.

When the psychosexual adjustment of teens reporting insecure attachment styles was examined, Tracy et al. (2003) found that teens like Amy who demonstrate an anxious attachment style are more likely to describe romantic relationships colored by fears of abandonment. When compared with their peers, they report that they have been in love more often, they usually have more idealized views of their romantic relationships, they begin having sexual relations at a younger age, and once sexually active, they have sex more frequently. Although they report having sex to express love for their partner, they are more likely to have sexual relations to please their partner because they fear being abandoned. They also do not enjoy sexual relations as much, and they are more likely to use alcohol or drugs during sexual encounters.

Likewise, Tracy et al. (2003) found that, when compared with teens reporting a secure or anxious attachment style, teens who demonstrate an avoidant attachment style are less likely to have ever have had a romantic relationship, they report having been in love the fewest number of times, they have had fewer serious romantic relationships, and they are less likely to be involved in a romantic relationship. Teens with an avoidant attachment style are also less likely to have ever had sexual relations, and they are more likely to be interested in having sexual relations to lose their virginity without much desire for psychological intimacy. When they have been sexually active, these teens are less likely to experience positive emotions during sexual relations, they are likely to consider the event less important, they report being less confident in their sexual competence, and they are more likely to use alcohol or drugs during sexual encounters.

Consistent with the conceptual model outlined by Belsky et al. (1991), researchers have also shown that differences in psychosexual adjustment associated with attachment style evident during adolescence persist into emerging adulthood. Mikulincer and Shaver (2007) recently prepared a comprehensive review of this literature. When examining the relationship between attachment style and attitudes concerning sexual partnerships during emerging adulthood, researchers have shown that, when compared with young people confirming an insecure attachment orientation, young people like Maureen who demonstrate a secure attachment style are more likely to believe in romantic love, and they are more positive about the prospect of maintaining love for a sexual partner over an extended period of time. Consistent with their attitudes, these young people tend to be more invested in romantic relationships, and they tend to more easily make the transition from secure relationships with primary caretakers to a secure relationship with a sexual partner. They also tend to seek some balance in the degree of closeness versus autonomy within their romantic relationships, they tend to view their romantic partners as more predictable, more dependable, and more faithful, and during emerging adulthood, their sexual partnerships tend to be more enduring.

Moreover, researchers have also shown that young people like Amy who demonstrate an anxious attachment style believe that people easily fall in love, they are also more likely to prefer a sexual partner with a secure or anxious attachment style, and they typically seek security and reassurance within a romantic relationships in a manner that insures the relationship does not endure. When sexual behavior has been examined, women with anxious attachment representations are more likely to have sexual relations for the first time at an early age, while men with anxious attachment representations are more likely to have sexual relations for the first time at a later age. Young people with anxious attachment representations also tend to be obsessed with their romantic partners, and they more frequently suffer from intense feelings of jealousy. They also more frequently have sexual relations to assuage feelings of insecurity, secure reassurance, promote emotional closeness, and reduce tension.

Like Amy, these young people tend to idealize sexual partnerships early in the relationship, readily commit themselves to a long-term relationship, and then quickly devalue and end the relationship when conflict occurs. They may also be prone to displays of intense anger that hasten the deterioration of romantic relations. Young people with an anxious attachment style are also less likely to consistently use contraception, they are more likely to continue using alcohol or drugs during sexual encounters, and they are more likely to have an unplanned pregnancy. When compared with young people with a secure attachment orientation, the sexual partnerships of these young people are, as might be expected, less likely to continue over time.

Similarly, researchers have shown that young people with an avoidant attachment style report attitudes reflecting less acceptance of romantic love, less confidence in the enduring nature of sexual partnerships, and greater acceptance of casual sex. They are also more likely to report being interested in having sexual relations for enhancement or affirmation of self, they are more likely to prefer a sexual partner with an avoidant or anxious attachment style, and they are less likely to confirm interest in having children. Consistent with reports of their attitudes, these young people initiate sexual partnerships motivated to limit closeness and maximize independence. When compared with young people with a secure or anxious attachment orientation, the sexual partnerships of these young people are, as might be expected, more likely to be tumultuous over time.

Longitudinal investigations of risk for early parenthood have also produced broad support for elements of the developmental pathways outlined by Belsky et al. (1991). For example, Cooper and her colleagues (2006) recently examined relationships involving attachment style, motives to engage in sexual relations, and sexual behavior during the transition from adolescence to adulthood. Consistent with positions outlined by Chisholm (1996), Cooper et al. found that an anxious attachment style in women during adolescence was associated with interest in engaging in sexual relations to affirm self-esteem and please a partner with more infidelity in romantic relationships during emerging adulthood. An anxious attachment style in men during adolescence was associated with interest in engaging in sexual relations to affirm self-esteem and diminish emotional distress with less infidelity in romantic relationships during emerging adulthood. Similarly, an avoidant attachment style during adolescence in both men and women was associated with self-serving motives to engage in sexual relations that seemed to encourage casual, promiscuous sexual behavior during emerging adulthood.

Finally, Woodward et al. (2006) found that *(1)* socioeconomic status of family, *(2)* maternal age at birth of first child, *(3)* single-parent family structure, *(4)* exposure to parental conflict, *(5)* exposure to punitive parenting, *(6)* exposure to sexual abuse, *(7)* quality of parent–child relations during adolescence, and *(8)* early sexual intercourse were associated with elevated risk for parenthood before 25 years of age for both boys and girls living in New Zealand. In a multivariate statistical analysis, *(1)* socioeconomic status of family, *(2)* exposure to punitive parenting, and *(3)* early sexual intercourse emerged as the most salient developmental correlates of risk for boys, and *(1)* socioeconomic status of family, *(2)* maternal age at birth of first child, *(3)* inconsistency in the presence of primary caretakers, *(4)* exposure to punitive parenting, and *(5)* early sexual intercourse emerged as the most salient developmental correlates for girls. Developmental correlates of risk for parenthood during adolescence compared with the developmental correlates of risk for parenthood during emerging adulthood.

Limitations of the Psychosocial Acceleration Hypothesis

Although there is growing empirical support for elements of the life history theory originally proposed by Belsky et al. (1991), it is important to note that some researchers have argued for other conceptualizations of reproductive development. For example, Ellis (2004) reviewed conceptual and empirical support for the life history theory outlined by Belsky et al. and proposed a revision that emphasized the role quality of father–daughter relationships during early childhood seems to play in pubertal timing for girls. Ellis and Essex (2007) found some support for that position; Belsky et al. (2007) did not. Ellis (2004) also argued that quality of early relationships with parents and exposure to psychosocial stress may accelerate the onset of puberty, but an early onset of puberty may not necessarily be associated with pursuit of a short-term reproductive strategy.

Disagreeing with elements of the psychosocial acceleration hypothesis, MacDonald (1997, 1999) argued that physical and psychosocial stress during childhood should delay, rather than accelerate, the onset of puberty and reproductive behavior. Consistent with this, Malo and Tremblay (1997) found that boys exposed to punitive parenting in the context of paternal alcoholism demonstrated a delay in pubertal development. More recently, other researchers (e.g., Ellis, 2004) have argued that different forms of biopsychosocial stress may have differential, and possibly opposite, effects on pubertal development. For example, serious physical illness or severe nutritional deprivation may delay pubertal development, but in the context of good physical health, psychosocial stress may accelerate pubertal development (for further discussion, see Ellis, 2004).

Similarly, Rowe (2000a, 2000b) has argued that the psychosocial acceleration hypothesis overstates the importance of early social experience and fails to acknowledge the role genetic influences play in determining life history traits. Considering this, Ellis and Essex (2007) included age of menarche for mother as a crude marker of genetic variability in pubertal timing for girls and found that, after allowance for maternal age of menarche, quality of parental investment still added to the prediction of menarche. Belsky et al. (2007) reported a similar finding. Focusing more on expectations of resource development, MacDonald (1997, 1999) has proposed that perception of upward socioeconomic mobility may be an important determinant of reproductive strategy independent of any evolutionary process.

Conclusions

Social, economic, and technological changes in postindustrial nations have begun to redefine normative developmental pathways to parenthood during the transition from adolescence to adulthood. Increasingly, the developmental period from 18 to 24 years of age is being defined as a time for young people to defer parenthood while accumulating the social, psychological, and economic resources needed to successfully negotiate the transition to adulthood. From a life history perspective, the critical developmental issue for young people as they move through adolescence toward adulthood still involves questions about when to shift from acquiring resources to support personal growth to using resources to produce and parent children. Increasingly, the answer to that question in postindustrial nations is later in the second decade of life.

As early parenthood becomes more problematic for both parents and their children, researchers need to expand understanding of the genetic, psychological, familial, and social influences that put children like Amy on developmental pathways to early parenthood that adversely affect their ability to successfully negotiate the transition from adolescence to adulthood. When doing so, they need to consider ways that genetic and environmental influences may interact to influence risk for early parenthood (for a discussion, see Belsky, 2000), they need to expand understanding of psychosocial influences that allow children at risk to avoid early parenthood (for a discussion, see Masten, Obradovic, & Burt, 2006), and they need to expand understanding of psychosocial influences that allow some young people to successfully negotiate early parenthood (for a discussion, see Moore & Brooks-Gunn, 2002). Moreover, as researchers better delineate the biological, psychological, and social factors that create risk for early birth of a first child, professionals working with young people throughout the human service system need to define more effective ways of preventing early parenthood and more effective ways to support young people like Amy who become parents during this critical developmental period.

KEY POINTS

- Social, economic, and technological changes in postindustrial nations have extended the transition from adolescence to adulthood such that most young people are delaying the birth of a first child until sometime after 25 years of age.
- Evolutionary, demographic, and developmental approaches to examining reproductive behavior can be used to support dynamic conceptualizations of risk for early parenthood that acknowledge the complex, multidetermined nature of reproductive development.
- Through reciprocal exchange with the social environment, children may, over time, develop psychological orientations that, with the onset of puberty, put them on developmental pathways to early parenthood that represents risk for poorer psychosocial adjustment as an adult.

> **PRACTICE GUIDELINES**
>
> - Professionals working with young people in human service systems should be sensitive to the biopsychosocial influences that represent risk for young people to pursue a socially undesirable, short-term reproductive strategy that results in the rapid birth of multiple children with different sexual partners without the social, psychological, and economic resources needed to successfully parent children.
> - Professionals working with young people in human service systems should do everything they can to help young people delay the birth of a first child until they have developed the social, psychological, and economic resources necessary to adequately parent a child.
> - Professionals working with young people in human service systems should do everything they can to minimize the extent to which the early birth of a first child disrupts psychosocial development as young people move through the transition from adolescence to adulthood.

References

Arnett, J. J. (2004). *Emerging adulthood: The winding road from the late teens through the twenties.* New York: Oxford University Press.

Belsky, J. (1997). Attachment, mating, and parenting: An evolutionary interpretation. *Human Nature, 8,* 361–381.

Belsky, J. (1999). Modern evolutionary theory and patterns of attachment. In J. Cassidy & P. R. Shaver (Eds.), *Handbook of attachment: Theory, research, and clinical applications* (pp. 141–161). New York: Guildford Press.

Belsky, J. (2000). Conditional and alternative reproductive strategies: Individual differences in susceptibility to rearing experiences. In J. L. Rodgers, D. C. Rowe, & W. B. Miller (Eds.), *Genetic influences on human fertility and sexuality: Theoretical and empirical contributions from the biological and behavioral sciences* (pp. 127–146). Boston: Clair Academic Publishing.

Belsky, J., Steinberg, L., & Draper, P. (1991). Childhood experience, interpersonal development, and reproductive strategy: An evolutionary theory of socialization. *Child Development, 62,* 647–670.

Belsky, J., Steinberg, L., Houts, R., Friedman, S. L., DeHart, G., Cauffman, E., Roisman, G. I., Halpern-Felsher, B., Susman, E. & NICHD Early Child Care Research Network. (2007). Family rearing antecedents of pubertal timing. *Child Development, 78,* 1302–1321.

Berrington, A., Cobos Hernandez, M. I., Ingham, R., & Stevenson, J. (2005). *Antecedents and outcomes of young fatherhood: Longitudinal evidence from the 1970 British Birth Cohort Study.* University of Southampton Statistical Sciences Institute Applications and Policy Working Paper no 05/09. Retrieved June 17, 2008, from http://eprints.soton.ac.uk/18182

Buss, D. M., & Greiling, H. (1999). Adaptive individual differences. *Journal of Personality, 67,* 209–243.

Chandra A., Martinez, G. M., Mosher, W. D., Abma, J. C., & Jones, J. (2005). *Fertility, family planning, and reproductive health of U.S. women: Data from the 2002 National Survey of Family Growth* (DHHS Publication No. PHS 2006-1977). Hyattsville, MD: U.S. Department of Health and Human Services, Centers for Disease Control and Prevention, National Center for Health Statistics.

Charnov, E. L. (1993). *Life history invariants: Some explanations of symmetry in evolutionary ecology.* Oxford, England: Oxford University Press.

Chisholm, J. S. (1993). Death, hope, and sex: Life-history theory and the development of reproductive strategies. *Current Anthropology, 34,* 1–24.

Chisholm, J. S. (1996). The evolutionary ecology of attachment organization. *Human Nature, 7,* 1–38.

Cooper, M. L., Pioli, M., Levitt, A., Talley, A., Micheas, L., & Collins, N. (2006). Attachment style, sex motives, and sexual behavior: Evidence for gender specific expressions of attachment dynamics (pp. 243–274). In M. Mikulincer & G. S. Goodman (Eds.), *Dynamics of romantic love: Attachment, caregiving, and sex.* New York: Guilford Press.

Ellis, B. J. (2004). Timing of pubertal maturation in girls: An integrated life history approach. *Psychological Bulletin, 130,* 920–958.

Ellis, B. J. (2005). Determinants of pubertal timing: An evolutionary developmental approach. In B. J. Ellis

& D. F. Bjorklund (Eds.), *Origins of the social mind: Evolutionary psychology and child development* (pp. 164–188). New York: Guilford Press.

Ellis, B. J., & Essex, M. J. (2007). Family environments, adrenarche, and sexual maturation: A longitudinal test of a life history model. *Child Development, 78*, 1799–1817.

Fraley, R. C., & Shaver, P. R. (2000). Adult romantic attachment: Theoretical developments, emerging controversies, and unanswered questions. *Review of General Psychology, 4*, 132–154.

Fussell, E., Gauthier, A. H., & Evans, A. (2007). The transition to adulthood in Australia, Canada, and the United States: A comparative perspective. *European Journal of Population, 23*, 389–414.

Gest, S. D., Mahoney, J. L., & Cairns, R. B. (1999). A developmental approach to prevention research: Configural antecedents of early parenthood. *American Journal of Community Psychology, 27*, 543–565.

Grossman, K., Grossman, K., & Waters, E. (Eds.). (2005). *Attachment from infancy to adulthood: The major longitudinal studies.* New York: Guilford Press.

Hazan, C., & Shaver, P. R. (1987). Romantic love conceptualized as an attachment process. *Journal of Personality and Social Psychology, 52*, 511–524.

Hazan, C., & Shaver, P. R. (1994). Attachment as an organizational framework for research on close relationships. *Psychological Inquiry, 5*, 1–22.

Hazan, C., & Zeifman, D. (1999). Pair bonds as attachments: Evaluating the evidence. In J. Cassidy & P. Shaver (Eds.), *Handbook of attachment theory and research* (pp. 336–354). New York: Guilford Press.

Hogan, D. P., & Astone, N. (1986). The transition to adulthood. *Annual Review of Sociology, 12*, 109–130.

Jaffee, S. R., Caspi, A., Moffitt, T. E., Belsky, J., & Silva, P. (2001). Why are children born to teen mothers at risk for adverse outcomes in young adulthood? Results from a 20-year longitudinal study. *Development and Psychopathology, 13*, 377–397.

Kim, K., & Smith, P. K. (1998). Retrospective survey of parental marital relations and child reproductive development. *International Journal of Behavioral Development, 22*, 729–751.

Kim, K., & Smith, P. K. (1999). Family relations in early childhood and reproductive development. *Journal of Reproductive and Infant Psychology, 17*, 133–148.

Kim, K., Smith, P. K., & Palermiti, A. (1997). Conflict in childhood and reproductive development. *Evolution and Human Behavior, 18*, 109–142.

Kirkpatrick, L. A. (1998). Evolution, pair-bonding, and reproductive strategies: A reconceptualization of adult attachment. In J. A. Simpson & W. S. Rholes (Eds.), *Attachment theory and close relationships* (pp. 353–393). New York: Guilford Press.

Lefkowitz, E. S., & Gillen, M. M. (2006). "Sex is just a normal part of life": Sexuality in emerging adulthood. In J. J. Arnett & J. L. Tanner (Eds.), *Emerging adults in America: Coming of age in the 21st century* (pp. 235–255). Washington, DC: American Psychological Association.

Luster, T., & Haddow, J. L. (2005). Adolescent mothers and their children: An ecological perspective. In T. Luster & L. Okagaki (Eds.), *Parenting: An ecological perspective* (2nd ed., pp. 73–101). Mahwah, NJ: Erlbaum.

MacDonald, K. B. (1997). Life history theory and human reproductive behavior: Environmental/contextual influences and heritable variation. *Human Nature, 8*, 327–359.

MacDonald, K. B. (1999). An evolutionary perspective on human fertility. *Population and Environment, 21*, 223–246.

Malo, J., & Tremblay, R. E. (1997). The impact of paternal alcoholism and maternal social position on boys' school adjustment, pubertal maturation and sexual behavior: A test of two competing hypotheses. *Journal of Child Psychology and Psychiatry and Allied Disciplines, 38*, 187–197.

Martinez, G. M., Chandra, A., Abma, J. C., Jones, J., & Mosher, W. D. (2006). *Fertility, contraception, and fatherhood: Data on men and women from Cycle 6 (2002) of the National Survey of Family Growth.* (DHHS Publication No. PHS 2006-1978). Hyattsville, MD: U.S. Department of Health and Human Services, Centers for Disease Control and Prevention, National Center for Health Statistics.

Masten, A. S., Obradovic, J., & Burt, K. B. (2006). Resilience in emerging adulthood: Developmental perspectives on continuity and transformation. In J. J. Arnett & J. L. Tanner (Eds.), *Emerging adults in America: Coming of age in the 21st century* (pp. 173–190). Washington, DC: American Psychological Association.

Mikulincer, M., & Shaver, P. R. (2007). *Attachment in adulthood: Structure, dynamics, and change.* New York: Guilford Press.

Moore, M. R., & Brooks-Gunn, J. (2002). Adolescent parenthood. In M. H. Bornstein (Ed.), *Handbook of parenting. Volume 3: Being and becoming a parent* (2nd ed., pp. 173–214). Mahwah, NJ: Erlbaum.

Nock, S. L. (1998). The consequences of premarital fatherhood. *American Sociological Review, 63*, 250–263.

Pears, K. C., Pierce, S. L., Kim, H. K., Capaldi, D. M., & Owen, L. D. (2005). The timing of entry into fatherhood in young, at-risk men. *Journal of Marriage and Family, 67*, 429–447.

Roff, D. A. (1992). *The evolution of life histories: Theory and analysis.* New York: Chapman & Hall.

Roisman, G. I., Collins, W. A., Sroufe, L. A., & Egeland, B. (2005). Predictors of young adults' representations of and behavior in their current romantic relationship: Prospective tests of the prototype hypothesis. *Attachment and Human Development, 7*, 105–121.

Roisman, G. I., Madsen, S. D., Hennighausen, K. H., Sroufe, L. A., & Collins, W. A. (2001). The coherence of dyadic behavior across parent-child and romantic relationships as mediated by the internalized representation of experience. *Attachment and Human Development, 3*, 156–172.

Rowe, D. C. (2000a). Environmental and genetic influences on pubertal development: evolutionary life history traits? In J. L. Rodgers, D. C. Rowe, & W. B. Miller (Eds.), *Genetic influences on human fertility and sexuality: Theoretical and empirical contributions from the biological and behavioral sciences* (pp. 147–168). Boston: Clair Academic Publishing.

Rowe, D. C. (2000b). Death, hope, and sex: Steps to an evolutionary ecology of mind and morality. *Evolution and Human Behavior, 21*, 352–364.

Sigle-Rushton, W. (2005). Young fatherhood and subsequent disadvantage in the United Kingdom. *Journal of Marriage and the Family, 67*, 735–753.

Simpson, J. A. (1999). Attachment theory in modern evolutionary practice. In J. Cassidy & P. R. Shaver (Eds.), *Handbook of attachment: Theory, research, and clinical applications* (pp. 115–140). New York: Guilford Press.

Simpson, J. A., & Belsky, J. (in press). Attachment theory within a modern evolutionary framework. In P. R. Shaver & J. Cassidy (Eds.), *Handbook of attachment: Theory, research, and clinical applications* (2nd ed.). New York: Guilford Press.

Sroufe, L. A., Egeland, B., Carlson, E., & Collins, W. A. (2005). Placing early attachment experiences in developmental context. In K. E. Grossmann, K. Grossmann, & E. Waters (Eds.), *Attachment from infancy to adulthood: The major longitudinal studies* (pp. 48–70). New York: Guilford Press.

Stearns, S. C. (1992). *The evolution of life histories.* Oxford, England: Oxford University Press.

Stouthamer-Loeber, M., & Wei, E. H. (1998). The precursors of young fatherhood and its effects on delinquency of teenage males. *Journal of Adolescent Health, 22*, 56–65.

Tanner, J. L. (2006). Recentering during emerging adulthood: A critical turning point in life span human development. In J. J. Arnett & J. L. Tanner (Eds.), *Emerging adults in America: Coming of age in the 21st century* (pp. 21–55). Washington, DC: American Psychological Association.

Tracy, J. L., Shaver, P. R., Albino, A. W., & Cooper, M. L. (2003). Attachment styles and adolescent sexuality. In P. Florsheim (Ed.), *Adolescent romance and sexual behavior: Theory, research, and practical implications* (pp. 137–159). Mahwah, NJ: Erlbaum.

Woodward, L. J., Fergusson, D. M., Horwood, L. J. (2006). Gender differences in the transition to early parenthood. *Development and Psychopathology, 18*, 275–294.

Chapter 13

Barriers to Mental Health Service Use in Young Adulthood

Deborah A. Perlick, Yariv Hofstein and Lesley A. Michael

Chris, a 21-year-old physics major at a southwestern university, sought treatment for symptoms of depression after breaking up with his girlfriend. Entitled to six free sessions at the university counseling center, he was dismayed when his therapist, a certified Substance Abuse Counselor, ignored his acute distress and concerns about his choice of partners to focus on his recreational drinking, which Chris perceived was below the norm for his campus. In addition, the counselor made persistent inquiries into his parents' and grandparents' substance use. Frustrated that his immediate grief symptoms were not being addressed, Chris dropped out of treatment after three sessions.

Tom, a 26-year-old apprentice electrician, moved in with his girlfriend of 2 years. His girlfriend, age 27, was eager to marry and start a family, but Tom was insecure about his career and finances and felt unprepared to take these steps. Arguments became more frequent, and Tom became a regular at the local bar after work, finding that alcohol made it easier to ignore the growing tensions in his relationship. When his girlfriend suggested he had a drinking problem and that one or both of them should see a therapist, he responded he was just doing a normal "guy thing" and was not going to see someone for "crazy people."

Amy, a 19-year-old student, left college in her sophomore year due to a growing sense of alienation from her friends and sorority sisters. She had begun hearing voices warning her to stay away from certain sisters, but she confided in no one.

Dismayed by their daughter's choice, her parents refused to support her. Amy lived by taking on temporary work. She felt increasingly depressed and began cutting herself but had no health insurance or sufficient income to seek treatment.

Young adulthood is a time of multiple and often competing demands relating to pursuit of education and career training, and the imperative to make decisions about career, relationships/marriage, and lifestyle that will have far-reaching consequences. These daunting tasks and choices occur at a time when young men and women are disengaging further from the protective influence of parents (Arnett & Tanner, 2006) and grappling with personal identity issues relating to religion, sexual preference, and political affiliation, all in the context of limited economic resources. These tasks represent psychosocial stressors that frequently lead to psychological distress, and national surveys have shown the incidence of serious mental disorders is high in individuals age 18–34 relative to those in younger or older age groups. Disturbingly, studies have also shown that mental health service utilization is lowest for these age groups, and that the percentage of young adults with unmet mental health needs is highest (National Survey on Drug Use and Health Report; Office of Applied Studies, 2007).

In this chapter we discuss two sets of barriers to mental health treatment that we hypothesize explain the gap between need for and actual use of services (Figure 13-1): *(1)* barriers relating to normative influences, which dissuade young

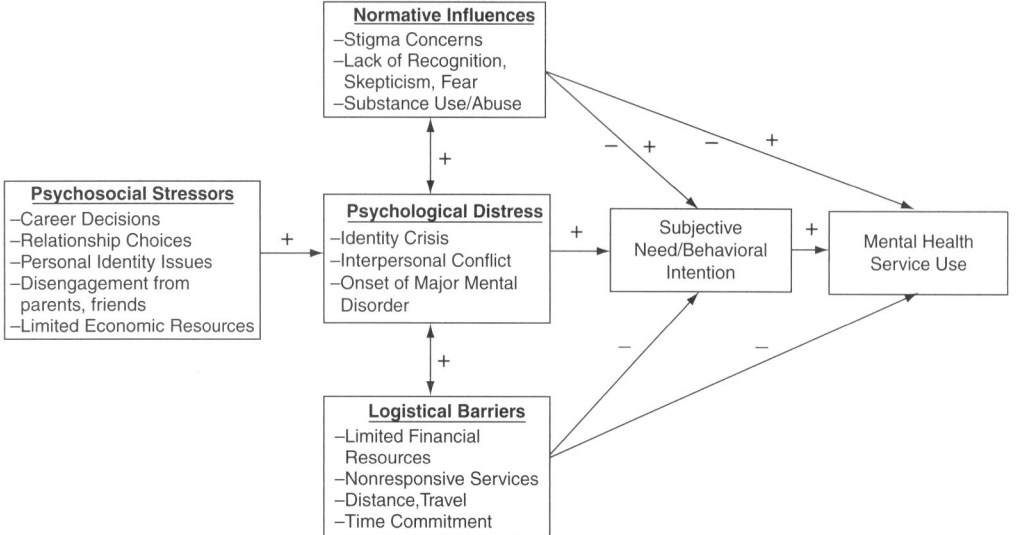

Figure 13-1. Impact of psychosocial stressors, psychological distress, normative influences, and logistical barriers on mental health service use in young adulthood.

adults from seeking treatment and/or suggest alternate ways of dealing with stress and distress; and *(2)* logistical barriers, which either preclude use of services or limit their effectiveness.

These barriers are hypothesized to mediate the relationship between psychological distress and mental health service use. They are hypothesized to exert both direct effects on service use and indirect effects, via their impact on the individual's subjective sense of need and intention to seek treatment. Because earlier chapters have addressed the psychosocial stressor and manifestations of psychological distress among young adults, we will not discuss these in detail here. We begin with a brief overview of data on the epidemiology of mental disorders and frequency of service use in this age group, and then we discuss barriers in detail.

Data on Mental Disorders and Mental Health Service Use

In 2006, more than 11% of adults 18 or older (24.9 million) were estimated to have serious mental illness in the past year (Office of Applied Studies, 2007). The rate of serious mental illness in the past year was highest among young adults between ages 18–25 (17.7%), compared to adults between ages 26–49 (13%) or 50+ (6.9%). In 2006, 6.4% of males and 11.7% of females between the ages of 18–25 reported at least one major depressive episode (MDE) in that year. Furthermore, 15% of people between 18–25 reported at least one MDE in their lifetime, the highest reported for any age group.

A recent epidemiological survey of nearly 136,000 adults found that the group least likely to receive treatment for any mental health problem was that between the ages of 18–25 (10.8%) (Office of Applied Studies, 2007). Consistent with this finding, adults between the ages of 18–25 reported the highest percentage of perceived unmet need for mental health treatment and counseling among all other adult age groups (Office of Applied Studies, 2007). The gap between the heightened prevalence of depression and other mental disorders among young adults, and their disproportionately low use of mental health services, underscores the urgency of understanding and remedying the barriers that young adults experience in seeking treatment.

Barriers to Service Use

Normative Influences

Our model incorporates three types of social norms that negatively impact, that is, interfere with the tendency of distressed young adults to perceive the need for and actively seek mental health services: *(1)* concerns about being perceived as a member of a stigmatized group, that is, "the mentally ill"; *(2)* a peer culture that endorses avoidance of emotional and/or psychological problems; and *(3)* the tendency to deal with emotional problems through use and abuse of alcohol and other substances, particularly pronounced in young adulthood. We discuss each of these influences, which are not mutually exclusive, below.

Stigma Concerns. Goffman (1963) defined a "stigma" as a nonnormative personal characteristic that "deeply discredits" the individual such that s/he is denied the basic respect granted to individuals without this undesirable characteristic. More recently, Link and Phelan (2001; Link, Yang, Phelan, & Collins, 2004) expanded upon this definition to emphasize the impact of stigmatization on the individual in society, that is, the discrimination and exclusion that he/she experiences and its results. Their model describes a process in which stigma exists when a series of interrelated components converge: *(1)* distinction and labeling of human differences; *(2)* linkage of labeled persons to undesirable traits, that is, negative stereotyping; *(3)* cognitive separation in which labeled individuals, that is, "them" are viewed as fundamentally different from "us"; *(4)* emotional reactions of the stigmatizer (e.g., anger, anxiety, pity, fear) and stigmatized (e.g., embarrassment, shame, alienation, anger); and *(5)* discrimination and status loss for labeled individuals, leading to unequal outcomes. In line with this theory, research has demonstrated that individuals diagnosed as having mental illness are socially stigmatized or discriminated against on several dimensions by key individuals in their social networks and communities. For example, studies have found that employers (Farina & Felner, 1973; Farina, Murray, & Groh, 1978; Olshansky, Grob, & Malamud, 1958), families of consumers (Struening et al., 2001), mental health workers (Cohen & Struening, 1962), and prospective landlords (Page, 1977) all endorsed devaluing statements about or discriminated against mentally ill individuals. Consistent with the above findings, large-scale surveys have found that "stigmatizing" beliefs about mental illness and mentally ill individuals are widely endorsed in the United States For example, a survey of 1,444 U.S. citizens found that 47% and 63% of participants reported a "desire for social distance" from people with major depressive disorder and schizophrenia, respectively (Link, Phelan, Bresnahan, Stueve, & Pescosolido, 1999). Similarly, among a representative sample of 1,507 adults in the United States, Struening, Moore, Link, Schwartz, & Stueve (1992) found that 60% believed fearing people with mental illnesses was "only natural," and 70% agreed that people with mental illness "may be dangerous."

Link and colleagues (1987, 1989) have demonstrated that individuals experiencing emotional problems respond to anticipated discrimination with secrecy and withdrawal. Studies of young adults show similar results. For example, in a study of 311 college students, attitudes reflecting the stigmatization of mental illness, such as, "It is a sign of personal weakness or inadequacy to see a psychologist for emotional or interpersonal problems" and "It is advisable for a person to hide from people that he/she has seen a psychologist" were associated with less favorable attitudes toward seeking psychological help (Komiya, Good, & Sherod, 2000). In another study using a questionnaire to evaluate students' thoughts about psychotherapy, the authors found a factor, the "Image Concerns" factor, which loaded high on such items as, "Whether my friends will think I'm abnormal for coming." Higher scores on this factor were associated with current nonuse of services despite higher levels of psychological distress. Interestingly, females showed higher image concerns than males. Pipes, Schwartz, and Crouch (1985) found similar results in an earlier study of college students, and anecdotal evidence from our interviews supports the view that stigma concerns are a barrier to service use. One young woman said it was a deterrent that the University Counseling Center was boldly labeled as such and located directly in the center of campus, creating a risk that one's friends or classmates would find out and think less of the service user. A young man expressed a similar concern that seeking treatment for symptoms of anxiety would be found out by his coach and buddies on the football team and would cost him his place on the team. Finally, in a qualitative study of the college experience of 35 young adults with psychiatric disabilities, 36% cited social isolation relating to either perceived avoidance by other students, or withdrawal from other students because of feared rejection (Megivern, Pellerito, & Mowbray, 2003). Statements made by participants included, "I always feel discriminated against and stigmatized." Because studies have also found that the general public devalues individuals who have sought or received mental health services (e.g., Farina, Holland, & Ring, 1966; Philips, 1963; Sibicky & Dovidio, 1986), the stigma concerns expressed in the above studies appear substantiated.

Perceived mental illness stigma has also been identified as a barrier to help-seeking and/or treatment adherence among adults (Corrigan, 2004; Perlick, Rosenheck, & Clarkin, 2004; Sirey et al., 2001). A recent report from the National Survey on Drug Use and Health (Office of Applied Studies, 2007) found that 22.7% of individuals 18 or older who perceived an unmet need for treatment for mental health problems cited stigma as a reason for the unmet need. Strikingly, stigma was more frequently reported as a treatment barrier by young adults in this sample: 29.7% of adults aged 18–25 reported stigma as a reason for not getting treatment, compared to 24.8% of those aged 26–34, 21.8% of those aged 35–49, and 12% of those aged 50 or older. Young adults may be particularly susceptible to stigma concerns as they are in the process of establishing themselves in several arenas, including work, relationships, and economic independence, and are thus more potentially susceptible to devaluation from peers or employers based on mental illness stigmatization. For example, the risk of denial of health insurance coverage due to having a mental health diagnosis based on past mental health service use, reported by 30% of respondents in a large-scale study, may present a particular barrier for young adults who are not yet secure financially. Studies have in fact shown that young adults are more susceptible to peer influence and judgment compared to their older adult counterparts (Bartolow, Sher, & Krull, 2003). Peer influence can also serve to alleviate stigma concerns when peers are supportive of seeking treatment. In a Web-based survey of 2,785 students attending a large public university, Eisenberg, Golberstein, and Gollust (2007) found that having a close friend or immediate family member who has sought professional help was associated with current use of services by students who screen positive for depression or anxiety.

Lack of Recognition, Skepticism, and Fear. Lack of recognition of symptoms associated with psychological disorders, and fear, skepticism, or avoidance of addressing perceived problems in treatment also serve as barriers to treatment for young adults. Examining the reasons for not seeking treatment among college students with positive screens for anxiety disorders and/or depression, Eisenberg et al. (2007) found that 51% of 2,785 college students reported believing that "stress is normal in college/graduate school" and 37% believed that the problem would get better by itself. Other studies have also identified a lack of recognition of psychological problems as a barrier to treatment seeking for young adults (e.g., Golan, 1969). In a revealing study, Jorm et al. (1997) found that 28% of 2,531 adult participants in a household survey in Australia given a vignette describing an individual with depression and 16% given a vignette describing a person with schizophrenia failed to recognize the presence of a mental health problem.

Even individuals who recognize they need help may avoid seeking help either because they are skeptical they can be helped or want to avoid confronting painful feelings. Thirty-seven percent of college students with positive screens for anxiety disorders and depression said they did not use services because they felt no one "can understand my problems" (Eisenberg et al., 2007). The majority of students in this same study expressed the belief that therapy and medication are only somewhat helpful or not at all helpful for students with depression. Similar skepticism about the potential helpfulness of therapy and therapist responsiveness, in particular, differentiated 92 students who used college counseling services from 526 who did not (Kushner & Sher, 1989). Therapist responsiveness concerns endorsed by nonusers included not knowing "whether the therapist will be honest with me" and "whether the therapist will take my problem seriously."

Nonusers in this study also endorsed concerns relating to what they might be pushed to think, do, or say against their will, such as, "whether I will be pressured into talking about things that I don't want to" or "whether I will lose control of my emotions while in therapy." Interestingly, those who reported higher levels of psychological distress also reported higher levels of concerns, suggesting that as the need for treatment is higher, the concerns and fears intensify, creating a conflict for the individual in need, wherein he/she is afraid to do what he/she feels he needs. Concerns about maintaining emotional control also predicted attitudes about help-seeking behavior in a study of 311 college students (Komiya et al., 2000). Other researchers have similarly identified a reluctance to self-disclose (Hinson & Swanson, 1993) and a tendency to conceal distressing personal material (Kelly & Achter, 1995) as reasons associated with reluctance to seek help. Among male college students, stronger endorsement of traditional male gender roles, which prohibit self-disclosure of weaknesses, and gender role conflict are associated with more negative attitudes toward help-seeking (Good & Wood, 1995).

Substance Use/Abuse. Alcohol use is at its peak in young adulthood. According to the National Survey on Drug Use and Health (Substance Abuse and Mental Health Services Administration [SAMSHA], 2003), in 2002 nearly 70% of 21- to 25-year-olds used alcohol in the past month, a higher percentage than any other age group. Binge drinking was also highest among 21- to 25-year-olds (44%) and second highest among 18- to 20-year-olds, relative to older age groups. Illicit drug use in the past month was highest among 18- to 20-year-olds (23%), with 21- to 25-year-olds close behind (19%).

The association between substance use and service use is complex. Data from the National Comorbidity Study show an increased use of services by individuals diagnosed with a pure or comorbid alcohol disorder compared to those with other or no psychiatric disorder in the 18–26 and 27–35 age groups. However these data pertain to individuals who met diagnostic criteria for an actual alcohol disorder and are not representative of the relationship between social use of alcohol and service use.

Clinical observations suggest that individuals casually drink to alleviate distress associated with everyday problems or symptoms of depression (e.g., Berger & Adesso, 1991; Freed, 1978), and evidence suggests that for some of young adults self-medication may be a means to cope with psychological distress that is more socially acceptable than using mental health services. Drinking has been associated with depressive symptoms among college students (Miller et al., 2002), and it has also been shown to alleviate depressive symptoms, particularly for male college students who consume more alcohol than female college students (e.g., Bachman et al., 1997). A potential gender-specific use of alcohol to self-medicate may also explain reduced use of services by young adult males relative to females (Good & Wood, 1995). Additional studies of drinking in noncollege, older young adults, stratified by presence/absence of diagnostic status is needed to help understand when and why social alcohol use may increase versus reduce the use of mental health services.

Logistical Barriers

Financial Resources. Cost is universally the most frequently cited barrier to mental health treatment among young adults. While the costs of mental health services partially come from insurance benefits, the remainder (usually 50% or more) is paid directly by the service user. Young adults, in the process of schooling and choosing and establishing an occupation, are often financially constrained. They also represent the largest age group of uninsured individuals in the United States. For example, although young adults (ages 19–29) account for 17% of adults under the age of 65, they represent 30% of all uninsured Americans younger than 65 (Collins, Schoen, Kriss, Doty, & Marato, 2007). Forty-eight percent of young adults aged 20–23 were uninsured for part of the year in 2002, compared to 12% for those under 18, and 22% for those aged 20–64 (Collins et al., 2007). Large-scale surveys of service use have identified absence of insurance coverage as a predictor of reduced probability of mental health service use, particularly among individuals with psychiatric disorders (Wang et al., 2005). Thus, relative lack of insurance coverage represents a major barrier to mental health service use for young adults.

There are several reasons for this gap in coverage for young adults. First, most employer insurance policies will not cover subscribers' children over the age of 18 or 19 as dependents if they are no longer attending school full time. While the majority of young adults attending college full time are insured, those who attend college part time and those who do not attend college are vulnerable until they are able to find employment that secures continuing health insurance coverage. However, many part-time jobs or entry-level (i.e., temporary) jobs do not offer benefits at all, or they may only offer very limited coverage (Collins et al., 2005). Health insurance enrollment for college students comes either from parental coverage (50%), employment (7%), or a college health plan (18%) (Collins et al., 2005). However, if a student attends a school in a different state than their family, some smaller plans may have more restrictions on out-of-network referrals.

Young adulthood represents a time of transition, moving from a state of dependence to independence, from school to work environments; however, this is seldom a seamless transition (Arnett, 2000, 2004). Thus, current third-party payer models that link health insurance coverage to affiliation with discrete institutions (i.e., work, school), discriminate against young adults who are often transitioning from school to work (or vice versa), affording a lapse in coverage and a high rate of uninsurance for young adults relative to that observed for younger, dependent children or adults who have established their careers and/or marriage and successfully transitioned to full adulthood. Considering the gaps in insurance coverage for young adults, it is not surprising that a National Institute of Healthcare Management Foundation study found that 250 college students between the ages of 18–24 reported inability to pay for services as one of the main reasons why they did not seek mental health treatment (Baber, 2006). Survey responses cited included inability to afford treatment, lack of health insurance coverage for mental health services, insufficient health insurance coverage for mental health services, and lacking health insurance entirely.

Discrimination in mental health care coverage is particularly problematic for socioeconomically disadvantaged young adults. Recent changes in public health insurance programs (e.g., Medicaid and the State Children's Health Insurance Program) reclassify children as adults on their 19th birthday, resulting in discontinuation of benefits they received as children. According to Collins et al. (2007), "Most low-income young adults become ineligible for public programs, since eligibility for adults generally is restricted to very low-income parents of disabled adults." As a result, young adults ages 19–29 are disproportionately represented among the uninsured: although roughly 24% live in households with incomes below the poverty level, a staggering 41% of the 13.3 million adults in this age group who are uninsured live in households with income below poverty (Collins et al., 2007). Although nearly half (46%) of uninsured young adults are white, both Hispanics and African Americans are at greater risk of being uninsured: 52% of Hispanics and 34% of African Americans ages 19–29 are uninsured compared to 23% of whites. Young adults who live in families with incomes below the poverty line often lack the resources to attend college on a full-time basis and must seek employment to cover their basic living expenses and/or help support their families. However, without a college degree the jobs for which they are eligible are less likely to offer health benefits (Collins, Davis, & Ho, 2005). Unable to compete for better jobs requiring a college education, and unable to attend college full-time due to financial needs, these economically disadvantaged young adults are caught in a catch-22 which reduces or blocks their access to mental health services and, in addition, perpetuates their economic and socially disadvantaged positions in society. Inability to get treatment for disabling mental disorders further exacerbates this disparity.

An alternative option for those who are without health insurance includes community-run clinics or organizations that provide free or low-fee services. However, Kuwabara, Van Voorhees, Gollan, & Alexander (2007) found that these sources of support are usually hard to find and wrought with administrative complexities and long waiting periods before service can be provided.

Travel Issues and Time Commitment. Newly gained financial independence, generally established in young adulthood, imposes limitations on discretionary spending, as competing financial needs often outweigh available resources from entry-level salaries. These competing demands may impact not only on the ability to pay for mental health services but also the ability to pay for transportation. For example, young adults who are not living on a college campus with an on-campus counseling center or do not reside in an area with a city-wide transportation system may be unable to travel to treatment locations at convenient times if they cannot afford their own car or other means of transportation (Kuwabara et al., 2007). Travel is also time consuming, and 32% of college students with unmet needs sampled in Eisenberg et al.'s (2007) Web-based survey cited lack of time as a treatment barrier.

Symptom Constraints: The Catch-22. Symptoms of depression, anxiety, and other mental health problems may also get in the way of seeking treatment. These barriers to care, often depressogenic symptoms, make it difficult for the person in need to navigate the red tape of insurance companies, find an appropriate place to receive services, withstand the usual waiting period, and sometimes meet with different clinicians before settling on a therapist or doctor that fits the individual's needs. These symptoms may also compromise relationships with families and other supporters, who, according to anecdotal and retrospective studies, tend to promote treatment-seeking behavior. For example, in a qualitative study, young adults (ages 18–25) reported that strong levels of support were instrumental in encouraging them to seek help for psychological symptoms (Kuwabara et al., 2007). Similarly, a retrospective study of the treatment-seeking process found that over 90% of therapy applicants talked to someone about this decision and 57.5% stated that talking to a family member or friend helped them realize that they had a problem needing clinical attention (Saunders, 1996). Thus, paradoxically and sometimes tragically, those young adults most in need of treatment may be those who experience the greatest problems in access. In addition, the symptoms of depression and other mental health disorders make it much more difficult to maintain a solid academic standing and matriculation status and/or a secured job, and lapses in academic standing or job loss serve to jeopardize health insurance accessibility. Further correlational studies of this specific group of young adults are needed to assess how much health-seeking behavior for psychological distress is dependent upon reported levels of social and familial support, as well as the logistical barriers to seeking help. In addition, the symptoms of depression and other mental health disorders make it much more difficult to maintain a solid academic standing and matriculation status and/or a secured job, and lapses in academic standing or job loss will serve to jeopardize health insurance accessibility.

Nonresponsive Services. Finding and receiving new mental health services from a friendly and approachable health care provider can be a barrier not only to engagement in treatment but also to treatment continuation. In a 2007 study of 250 undergraduates, Baber et al. (2007) reported that seeking mental health services is uncomfortable for young adults, and that finding matching characteristics in potential clinicians is often difficult and makes the process discouraging. Young adult survey respondents claimed that they valued "knowledge and competence, friendliness and approachability, credentials and reputation, being caring and compassionate." They further felt that in the services provided to them they were not adequately spoken to about depression, eating disorders, sleep problems, and other mental health issues. The universal skepticism that appears prototypical of many young adults makes finding a compatible and competent clinician more vital to ensuring a trusting environment. Many times a troubled young adult may give up treatment seeking if he or she is initially matched up with a therapist who is not able to establish an appropriate rapport and level of understanding.

Another problem occurs when appropriate services are offered but not readily available. On college campuses, where the majority of full-time students are insured, getting mental health services can still be difficult. In the 2006 survey of National Counseling Center Directors (from 367 universities), 25% of students referred for treatment were on psychotropic medications, but only 58% of centers offered psychiatric services on campus (Gallagher, 2006). On average, a full-time counselor is expected to have only 23 client contact hours per week, yet 82 of the counseling directors reported extended wait list problems and 232 directors cited "a growing demand for services without an appropriate increase in resources" (Gallagher, 2006). Given that 40% of student clients are judged to have "severe" psychological problems and 32% have "severe problems" than can be treated with available modalities, the availability of resources and limits imposed seems inadequate. In 2006, of the 142 cases of suicide reported on college campuses, only 9.8% (14) of these students were currently utilizing or had utilized counseling center services (Gallagher, 2006), suggesting that either the level or type of services offered is not reaching, or adequately containing, these very troubled individuals.

For young adults outside of a university setting, locating responsive services can be even more taxing. Not only do they similarly face the problem of finding a therapist that is appropriate for their situation, they first have to look for a place offering counseling services. With or without insurance, this task usually consists of numerous phone calls, referrals, and waiting periods. For someone suffering from distress, these tasks more than likely make services feel less responsive.

Conclusion

In this chapter, we have discussed multiple and varied barriers to young adults using mental health services, ranging from concerns of being stigmatized by ones' peers to the lack of insurance and other economic resources that characterize this age group. The total array and magnitude of these barriers is both impressive and troubling, in light of the high prevalence of major depression and other mental disorders that characterize this phase of life.

Many or most of these barriers are deeply engrained in the fabric of the psychosocial and economic realities of the United States today and will take major efforts from multiple stakeholders to overcome. We do not wish to minimize these barriers or imply that they can easily be overcome. However, we conclude this chapter with some suggestions for beginning to address them, both at the individual and societal level.

KEY POINTS

- Stigmatization of people with mental disorders, and even those who use mental health services to cope with relatively minor symptoms, is endemic to the culture and must be confronted in order to encourage greater mental health service use.
- Addressing the disparities in health and mental health insurance coverage between young adults and other age groups is necessary and likely requires a campaign to restructure financing and delivery of health care at the national level. Young adults will be less likely to seek mental health treatment if it remains unaffordable.
- Studies have repeatedly shown that choice is the most significant factor in treatment outcome (Calsyn et al., 2000, 2003; Laugharne & Priebe, 2006). Young adults need to be able to "own" their own treatments more, if they are to be effective. The process of seeking help must be more streamlined and confidential.

> **PRACTICE GUIDELINES**
>
> - Strategic groups and organizations (i.e., religious institutions, college mental health services) might sponsor development of programs featuring young adults describing the adjustment problems and psychological symptoms/disorders they experience and how use of mental health services helped them to cope better and make positive life decisions.
> - Mental health awareness days sponsored by health or educational institutions help to increase recognition of symptoms of depression and other disorders and reduce fears and other concerns regarding treatment through normalizing these symptoms and their treatment.
> - Those services that are available to young adults free of charge, such as college counseling centers, might increase their effectiveness at reaching those students in the most need by expediting their intake procedures and offering a broader array of services from which students can select to meet their needs.

References

Arnett, J. J. (2000). Emerging adulthood: A theory of development from the late teens through the twenties. *American Psychologist, 55,* 469–480.

Arnett, J. J. (2004). *Emerging adulthood: The winding road from the late teens through the twenties.* New York: Oxford University Press.

Arnett, J. J., & Tanner, J. L. (2006). *Emerging adults in America: Coming of age in the 21st century.* Washington, DC: American Psychological Association.

Baber, K. M., Bean, G., & Harrington, L. (2006). College students' perception about health care and care providers (poster). Accessed march 19, 2009. http://www.adolescence.unh.edu/HYHabstract.pdf

Baber, K. M., Bean, G., & Harrington, L. (2007). Older youths' opinions about their healthcare and their care providers. *Journal of Adolescent Health, 40*(2), S38–S38.

Bachman, J.G.; Wadsworth, K.N.; O'Malley, P.M.; Johnston, L .D.; & Schulenberg, J. E. (1997). *Smoking, Drinking, and Drug Use in Young Adulthood: The Impacts of New Freedoms and New Responsibilities.* Mahwah, NJ: Lawrence Erlbaum Associates.

Bartholow, B. D., Sher, K. J., & Krull, J. L. (2003). Changes in heavy drinking over the third decade of life as a function of collegiate fraternity and sorority involvement: A prospective multilevel analysis. *Health Psychology, 22,* 616–626.

Berger, B. D., & Adesso, V. J. (1991). Gender differences in using alcohol to cope with depression. *Addictive Behaviors, 16*(5), 315–327.

Calsyn, R. J., Morse, G. A., Yonker, R. D., Winter, J. P., Pierce, K. J., & Taylor, M. J. (2003). Client choice of treatment and client outcomes. *Journal of Community Psychology, 31*(4), 339–348.

Calsyn, R. J., Winter, J. P., & Morse, G. A. (2000). Do consumers who have a choice of treatment have better outcomes? *Community Mental Health Journal, 36*(2),149–160.

Cohen, J., & Struening, E. L. (1962). Opinions about mental illness in the personnel of two large mental hospitals. *Journal of Abnormal Psychology, 64,* 349–360.

Collins, S. R., Davis, K., & Ho, A. (2005). A shared responsibility: U.S. employers and the provision of health insurance to employees. *Inquiry, 42*(1), 6–15.

Collins, S. R., Schoen, C., Kriss, J. L., Doty, M. M., & Marato, B. (2007, August). *Rite of passage? Why young adults become uninsured and how new policies can help.* New York: The Commonwealth Fund.

Corrigan, P. (2004). How stigma interferes with mental health care. *American Psychologist, 59,* 614–625.

Druss, B. G., Hoff, R. A., & Rosenheck, R. A. (2000). Underuse of antidepressants in major depression: Prevalence and correlates in a national sample of young adults. *Journal of Clinical Psychiatry, 61*(3), 234–237.

Eisenberg, D., Golberstien, E., & Gollust, S. (2007). Help-seeking and access to mental health care in a university student population. *Medical Care, 45*(7), 594–601.

Farina, A., & Felner, R. D. (1973). Employment interviewer reactions to formal mental patients. *Journal of Abnormal Psychology, 82,* 268–272.

Farina, A., Holland, C. H., & Ring, K. (1996). Role of stigma and set in interpersonal interaction. *Journal of Abnormal Psychology, 71*, 421–428.

Farina, A., Murray, P., & Groh, T. (1978). Sex and worker acceptance of a former mental patient. *Journal of Consulting and Clinical Psychology, 46*, 887–891.

Freed, E. X. (1978). Alcohol and mood: An updated review. *International Journal of Addiction, 13*(2), 173–200.

Gallagher, R. P. (2006). *National survey of counseling center directors.* The International Association of Counseling Services, Inc, Alexandria, VA. accessed March 19, 2009; http://www.education.pitt.edu/survey/nsccd/archive/2006/monograph.pdf

Goffman, E. (1963). *Stigma: Notes on the management of a spoiled identity.* Englewood Cliffs, NJ: Prentice-Hall.

Golan, N. (1969). When is a student in crisis? *Social Casework, 50*, 389–394.

Good, G. E., & Wood, P. K. (1995). Male gender role conflict, depression, and help-seeking: Do college men face double jeopardy? *Journal of Counseling and Development, 74*(1), 70–75.

Hinson, J. A., & Swanson, J. L. (1993). Willingness to seek help as a function of self-disclosure and problem severity. *Journal of Counseling and Development, 71*(4), 465–470.

Jorm, A. F., Korten, A. E., Jacomb, P. A., Christensen, H., Rodgers, B., & Pollitt, P. (1997). Public beliefs about causes and risk factors for depression and schizophrenia. *Social Psychiatry and Psychiatric Epidemiology, 32*, 143–148.

Kelly, A. E., & Achter, J. A. (1995). Self-concealment and attitudes toward counseling in university students. *Journal of Counseling Psychology* 42, 40–46.

Komiya, N., Good, G. E., & Sherrod, N. B. (2000). Emotional openness as a predictor of college students' attitudes toward seeking psychological help. *Journal of Counseling Psychology, 47*, 138–143.

Kushner, M. G., & Sher, K. J. (1989). Fear of psychological treatment and its relation to mental health service avoidance. *Professional Psychology: Research and Practice, 20*, 251–257.

Kuwabara, S. A., Van Voorhees, B. W., Gollan, J. K., & Alexander, G. C. (2007). A qualitative exploration of depression in emerging adulthood: Disorder, development, and social context. *General Hospital Psychiatry, 29*(4), 317–324.

Laugharne, R., & Priebe, S. (2006). Trust, choice and power in mental health. *Social Psychiatry and Psychiatric Epidemiology, 41*(11), 843–852.

Link, B. G., Cullen, F. T., Frank, J., & Wozniak, J. F. (1987). The social rejection of former mental patients: Understanding why labels matter. *American Journal of Sociology, 92*, 1461–1500.

Link, B. G., Cullen, F. T., Struening, E. L., Shrout, P. E., & Dohrenwend, B. P. (1989). A modified labeling theory approach to mental disorders: An empirical assessment. *American Sociology Review, 54*, 400–423.

Link, B. G., & Phelan, J. C. (2001). Conceptualizing stigma. *Annual Review of Sociology, 27*, 363–385.

Link, B. G., Phelan, J. C., Bresnahan, M., Stueve, A., & Pescosolido, B. A. (1999). Public conceptions of mental illness: Labels, causes, dangerousness, and social distance. *American Journal of Public Health, 89*, 1328–1333.

Link, B. G., Yang, L. H., Phelan, J. C., & Collins, P. Y. (2004). Measuring mental illness stigma. *Schizophrenia Bulletin, 30*, 511–541.

Megivern, D., Pellerito, S., & Mowbray, C. T. (2003). Barriers to higher education for individuals with psychiatric disabilities. *Psychiatric Rehabilitation Journal, 26*, 217–231.

Miller, E. T., Neal, D. J., Roberts, L. J., Baer, J. S., Cressler, S. O., Metrik, J., & Marlatt, G. A. (2002). Test-retest reliability of alcohol measures: Is there a difference between internet-based assessment and traditional methods? *Psychology of Addictive Behavior, 16*(1), 56–63.

Office of Applied Studies, Substance Abuse, and Mental Health Services Administration. (2007). Results from the 2006 National Survey on Drug Use and Health. Rockville, MD:Substance Abuse and Mental Health Services Administration, Office of Applied Studies.

Olshansky, S., Grob, S., & Malamud, I. T. (1958). Employers' attitudes and practices in the hiring of ex-mental patients. *Mental Hygiene, 42*, 391–442.

Page, S. (1977). Effects of the mental illness label in attempts to obtain accommodation.*Canadian Journal of Behavioral Science, 9*, 85–90.

Perlick, D. A., Rosenheck, R. A., & Clarkin, J. F. (2004). Impact of family burden and affective response on clinical outcome among patients with bipolar disorder. *Psychiatric Services, 55*, 1029–1035.

Pipes, R. B., Schwarz, R., & Crouch, P. (1985). Measuring client fears. *Journal of Consulting and Clinical Psychology, 53*, 933–934.

Phillips, D. L. (1963). Rejection: A possible consequence of seeking help for mental disorders. *American Sociological Review, 28*(6), 963–972.

Saunders, S. (1996). Applicants' experience of social support in the process of seeking psychotherapy. *Psychotherapy: Theory, Research, & Practice, 33*(4), 617–627.

Sibicky, M., & Dovidio, J. F. (1986). Stigma of psychological therapy: Stereotypes, interpersonal reactions, and the self-fulfilling prophecy. *Journal of Counseling Psychology, 33*, 148–154.

Sirey, J. A., Bruce, M. L., Alexopoulos, G. S., Perlick, D. A., Friedman, S. J., & Meyers, B. S. (2001). Stigma as a barrier to recovery: Perceived stigma and patient-rated severity of illness as predictors of antidepressant drug adherence. *Psychiatric Services*, *52*(12), 1615–1620.

Struening, E. L, Moore, R. E, Link, B. G., Schwartz, S., & Stueve, A. (1992). Perceived dangerousness of the homeless and the homeless mentally ill. Presented at the annual meeting of the American Public Health Association, Washington, DC.

Struening, E. L., Perlick, D. A., Link, B. G., Hellman, F., Herman, D., & Sirey, J. A. (2001). The extent to which caregivers believe most people devalue consumers and their families. *Psychiatric Services*, *52*, 1633–1638.

Substance Abuse and Mental Health Services Administration [SAMSHA]. (2003). National Survey on Drug Use and Health. Accessed March 19, 2009. http://www.oas.samhsa.gov/nhsda/2k3nsduh/2k3Results.htm

Vredenberg, K., & Krames, L. (1986). Sex differences in the clinical expression of depression. *Sex Roles*, *14*(1–2), 37–49.

Wang, P. S., Lane, M., Olfson, M., Pincus, H. A., Wells, K. B., & Kessler, R. C. (2005). Twelve-month use of mental health services in the Unites States. *Archives of General Psychiatry*, *62*, 629–640.

Wu, L. T., Kouzis, A. C., & Leaf, P. J. (1999). Influence of comorbid alcohol and psychiatric disorders on utilization of mental health services in the national comorbidity survey. *American Journal of Psychiatry*, *156*, 1230–1236.

Chapter 14

Psychiatric Disorders in Young Adults: Depression Assessment and Treatment

Carlos A. Zarate, Jr.

Mr. A, a 19-year-old single white male with treatment-resistant major depression, had the onset of his illness at the age of 16. There was no history of hypomania, mania, psychosis, or other Axis I disorder. His family history was unremarkable. He had previously failed to respond to several selective serotonin reuptake inhibitors (SSRIs), bupropion, venlafaxine, mirtazapine, tricyclic antidepressants (TCAs), and tranylcypromine; many of these were augmented unsuccessfully with either stimulants, thyroid hormone, lithium, or several atypical antipsychotic drugs. He also failed to respond to the combinations of venlafaxine with mirtazapine, an SSRI with a TCA, and to 17 electroconvulsive therapy treatments (unilateral and bilateral) with liothyronine, bupropion, and venlafaxine. Admission medications included phenelzine (75 mg/day), modafanil (300 mg/day), and inositol (3 g/day). On admission, his clinical picture was that of severe psychomotor retardation and insomnia, social withdrawal, anhedonia, without psychotic features. These symptoms had been present and unremitting for over 12 months prior to admission. Medical work-up, laboratory tests, and MRI were unremarkable. Montgomery-Asberg Depression Rating Scale (MADRS) score on admission was 39 and remained unchanged after a 2-week drug-free period. Within 3 days of riluzole (an inhibitor of glutamate release and enhancer of AMPA [alpha-amino-3-hydroxy-5-methyl-4-isoxazole propionic acid] trafficking and glutamate transporter expression) treatment he has noted to be significantly more animated and conversing with other patients (30% improvement in the MADRS total score from baseline), and within 7 days of beginning riluzole (50 mg BID), he met remission criterion (MADRS ≤ 10). The patient and family observed that this was the best he had felt and functioned since the onset of his illness. Six months later he was still taking riluzole and doing well.

Introduction

Major depressive disorder (MDD) in adults is a serious, debilitating, life-shortening illness that affects the lives of millions worldwide irrespective of age and background. Individuals afflicted with this disorder generally experience high rates of relapse, chronicity, lingering residual symptoms, cognitive and functional impairment, psychosocial disability, and diminished well-being.

Depressive illnesses also carry significant risks of morbidity and mortality. The World Health Organization's (WHO) Global Burden of Disease study ranked unipolar depression as the fourth leading cause of disability in 1990, and it is projecting unipolar depression to increase in rank to become the second leading cause of disability worldwide by 2020 (Murray & Lopez, 1996). MDD often strips individuals of their ability of becoming productive members of society by having poor work productivity (Kessler et al., 2006; Lerner et al., 2004).

With respect to mortality, both major depression and residual depressive symptoms are associated with at least a doubling in risk of subsequent cardiac events later in life, even when standard cardiac risk factors, including left ventricular ejection fraction and number of blocked coronary arteries, are taken into account. In fact, several large, longitudinal community-based studies show that depression often precedes the development of clinically evident coronary artery disease by many years (Frasure-Smith et al., 1993). It is estimated that about 15% of patients with a mood disorder commit suicide (Bostwick & Pankratz, 2000), and approximately 90% of those who suicide in the United States have a mental illness diagnosis most often being major depression.

In recent years, increased attention has been giving to the study of MDD in young adults in an effort to more accurately identify the precise pathophysiology and better understand the course of disease by reducing the confounds of long-term medication exposure and the chronicity of the illness. Few efforts have been made to summarize the extant literature on young adults with major depression, defined for this review as individuals aged 18 to 24 years.

For many young adults with MDD, the onset commences in adolescence, and the disorder then usually persists, and transitions unabated, into young adulthood (Dunn & Goodyer, 2006). Early age of onset of a mood disorder has been reported to predict a more severe, chronic, and recurrent form of the illness. Evidence for the increasing recognition of mental disorders, particularly mood disorders, in young adults involves studies of treatment prevalence. An increasing and alarming trend in general hospital discharges involving serious mental illness, particularly that of young adults, has been reported. Discharges per 10,000 of adults 18 to 24 years of age increased from 19.9 in 1995 to 42.3 in 2002 (Watanabe-Galloway & Zhang, 2007). Further evidence of the importance of mood disorders in this young population comes from data indicating a secular increase of comorbid substance-use disorders among first admissions for mood disorder, especially in young males (Minnai et al., 2006).

An early start of the illness often deprives individuals of developing as adults. Young adulthood is one of the most critical periods of educational, occupational, and social development; the consequence of depression at this critical juncture often leads to lifelong disability. Not surprisingly, unipolar depression is the leading cause of disability among all noncommunicable medical illnesses in individuals ages 15 to 44 years in the Western Hemisphere (Murray & Lopez, 1996). Individuals with MDD with an onset in adolescence or young adulthood spend an average of a decade of their lives in episodes of illness. Research of MDD in young adults has increased at a rapid pace in recent years partly in an effort to more accurately identify the precise pathophysiology of the disease by minimizing confounds such as long-term medication use and unremitting illness. Additionally, a disorder that begins in early adult years may differ from one beginning later in adulthood with respect to efficacy of treatments and the subsequent pathophysiology of the disorder itself. Another key reason for the increased research of mood disorders in young adulthood is that this age group is believed to be a key period for both prevention and treatment of mental disorders to avoid chronicity of symptoms (Newman et al., 1996; Wang et al., 2005).

Classification of Mood Disorders

The mood disorders include the depressive disorders (MDD, dysthymic disorder, and depressive disorder not otherwise specified); the bipolar disorders (bipolar I disorder, bipolar II disorder, cyclothymic disorder, and bipolar disorder not otherwise specified), mood disorder due to a medical condition, substance-induced mood disorder, and mood disorder not otherwise specified. The definition and nosology of mood disorders in early adult years is the same as in middle adulthood. The criteria for the mood disorders are briefly review here.

The following classification of mood disorders is based on DSM-IV (*Diagnostic and Statistical Manual of Mental Disorders* (4th ed.), American Psychiatric Association, 1994). A *major depressive episode*, which is the identical for a patient with MDD or bipolar disorder, consists of a minimum of five symptoms of depression that have been present for at least 2 weeks coincident with a change in the previous level of functioning. The symptoms must cause significant distress or functional impairment.

According to DSM-IV, *dysthymic disorder* is defined by a depressed mood for most of the day, for most days, for a period of at least 2 years. At least two additional depressive symptoms must be present in dysthymic disorder. These include change in sleep (insomnia or hypersomnia), appetite, decreased energy, low self-esteem, poor concentration or difficulty making decisions, helplessness, or hopelessness. To meet the criteria for dysthymic disorder, the mood symptoms cannot be absent for more than 2 months at a time. *Depressive disorder not otherwise specified* includes disorders with depressive features that do not meet the criteria for other depressive disorders or adjustment disorders with disturbances of mood.

Epidemiology

Major Depressive Disorder

Major depressive disorder (MDD) is among the most common afflictions for which patients present to their physicians. Depression is twice as common in women as in men. The mean age at onset of major depressive disorder is 30 years. The hazard for age of onset of MDD increases sharply increases between ages 18–29 through 45–64 and then declines in subjects ≥65 years (Hasin et al., 2005) (Table 14-1). Lifetime rates (and odds) of MDD appear higher among older than young (18- to 29-year-old) adults, in contrast to earlier surveys showing highest rates in the youngest cohorts (Kessler et al., 1994; Kessler et al., 2003). The findings suggest that the post-World War II increase in lifetime prevalence of MDD may be tapering off and may ultimately be a specific age-period effect rather than a permanent increase (Hasin et al., 2005).

Another nationally representative prevalence estimate of mood disorders is based on the Third National Health and Nutrition Examination Survey (NHANES III) and compares these estimates to the Epidemiologic Catchment Area Study (ECA) conducted 10 years earlier. NHANES III, conducted from 1988 to 1994, surveyed a large nationally representative cross-sectional sample of the United States. In a population-based sample of 8,602 men and women 17–39 years of age, lifetime prevalence estimates were 8.6% for major depressive episode, 7.7% for severe major depressive episode, 6.2% for dysthymia 6.2%, 3.4% for major depressive episodes with dysthymia, 1.6% for any bipolar disorder, and 11.5% for any mood disorder. With the exception of the estimate for major depressive episode, all estimates were significantly higher than comparable ECA ones (Jonas et al., 2003).

The lifetime prevalence of MDD in an epidemiologically defined population of 1,197, predominately poor, African American 19- to 22-year-olds, living in the greater Baltimore, MD metropolitan was 9.4%, whereas the last year and last month prevalence estimates were 6.2% and 2.7%, respectively. Females as compared to males were approximately 1.6 times more likely to report a lifetime episode of MDD. MDD was highly comorbid with substance disorders (Ialongo et al., 2004).

Suicide

In the United States, the United Kingdom, and Europe in general, suicide is more common among males at every age, apart from the rare young childhood death by suicide. In patients participating in the Sequenced Treatment Alternatives to Relieve Depression (STAR*D) trial, for those with a past history of suicide attempt versus those who never had a suicide attempt, the onset of MDD occurred approximately 9 years earlier in life on average (Claassen et al., 2007). In Asia and some Latin American countries, suicide rates are equally distributed by gender or are higher in female adults. Racial, ethnic, and cultural factors influence suicidal behavior. In the United States, suicide rates are more common among whites than among other racial groups, with the exception of certain Native American groups. A significant gender difference in the risk factors for attempted suicide has been found among young adults. Data from 3,357 men and 4,004 women in young adults aged 17 to 39 years, as a part of the NHANES III, found that the lifetime prevalence

Table 14-1. Prevalence of 12-Month and Lifetime DSM-IV Major Depressive Disorder

Age in Years	12-Month MDD, % (SE)	Lifetime MDD % (SE)
18–29	6.39 (0.35)	12.02 (0.49)
30–44	5.52 (0.26)	14.03 (0.46)
45–64	5.62 (0.28)	15.91 (0.50)
≥65	2.69 (0.22)	8.19 (0.38)

MDD, major depressive disorder; SE, standard error.
Source: From Hasin et al. (2005).

of attempted suicides was 7.6% in women and 3.7% in men. In men, low income and smoking were associated with attempted suicide, whereas attempted suicide in women was linked with poor self-evaluated health, low educational achievement, and drug use (Zhang et al., 2005).

Factors Associated with Depression in Young Adulthood

Genetic Factors

Genetics contribute substantially to the etiology of mood disorders. By modeling data from affected individuals and their relatives, genetic epidemiological studies can provide information about the familial and genetic natures of a disorder (e.g., depression). Such studies have provided much information about the genetic transmission of mood disorders. The three types of studies that have been used to determine the role of genetic factors in mood disorders are as follows: *(1)* family studies; *(2)* twin studies; and *(3)* adoption studies. These studies have largely focused on the overall adult population and have not specifically examined the subgroup of young adults. A recent genomewide linkage scan examining age of onset of recurrent MDD was completed, the results of which are described below.

Family Studies. Family studies determine whether the rate of depression in the family members of the probands with the disorder is greater than that of the general population. The studies conducted in families of probands with unipolar depression reveal morbid risks for depressive disorders among first-degree relatives that are two to three times those of the general population. These data suggest a genetic contribution to mood disorders. However, family studies cannot establish that a disorder is hereditary, as familial aggregation of a disorder (e.g., major depression) may reflect a shared environment (Pardes et al., 1989). Other types of genetic studies address some of the limitations of family studies. Family studies of suicide and suicide attempts show a several-fold increased rate of suicidal behavior in the relatives of either suicide completers or attempters, compared to relatives of controls (Brent et al., 2002; Johnson et al., 1998).

A positive family history of mood disorder has been reported to be associated with younger age of onset of MDD in the proband (Nierenberg et al., 2007). Controversy exists regarding the occurrence of the phenomenon of anticipation in mood disorders. Anticipation posits that MDD in the parental generation will be associated with MDD in the offspring, typically occurring at a younger age. To further assess this hypothesis on the unipolar pattern of the disease, 21 two-generation pairs of first- and second-degree relatives with unipolar recurrent major depression were studied. A significant difference in the age at onset and episode frequency between parental and offspring generation was observed. The median age at onset of the parental generation was 37 years compared to 22 years in the offspring generation. The offspring generation also experienced an episode frequency two times greater than the parent generation. Anticipation was demonstrated in 95% of pairs regarding age at onset and in 84% of pairs in episode frequency (Papadimitriou et al., 2005).

Twin Studies. Although family study data indicate that mood disorders are familial, they cannot distinguish whether genetic or environmental factors are accountable for familial transmission. Families might share environmental factors that could "pass on" the illness, and young adults may be exposed to that environment before they become independent. Such factors might be frequent exposure to a particular culture, diet, behavior, virus, toxin, or other brain insult. Twin studies provide a powerful approach for dissecting genetic from environmental contributions. Twin studies compare the concordance rate for illness in pairs of monozygotic (identical) twins with that in dizygotic (nonidentical twins). The rationale is that monozygotic twins share identical genes, whereas dizygotic twins share only half their genes. Usually, twin pairs are selected who have been raised together, so that many environmental factors are shared equally. The marked difference in concordance rates between monozygotic and dizygotic twins strongly supports the hypothesis of a major genetic contribution to the development of unipolar depression (Kendler et al.,

1993; McGuffin et al., 1996). These studies find that the concordance rate for mood disorder in monozygotic twins is two to four times greater than in dizygotic twins. Since the concordance rate for monozygotic twins is not 100%, other nonheritable environmental factors probably exist and might contribute significantly to mood disorders. Although monozygotic twins have the same genetic composition, if one twin succumbs to depression, there is approximately a 50%–60% risk of the other twin for becoming ill. Twin studies show a much greater concordance for attempted and completed suicide among monozygotic than among dizygotic twins (Roy & Segal, 2001; Statham et al., 1998). Major depression and comorbid alcohol use disorders commonly co-occur. Whether they share a common or distinct pathophysiology is unclear. One way of addressing this problem is with the use of twin studies and is discussed below.

Adoption Studies. Adoption studies provide an attempt to parse the genetic and environmental factors in familial transmission (Shih et al., 2004). Mendlewicz and Rainer (1977) found a two-fold increase in the rate of MDD in biological relatives. Similarly, Wender and colleagues (Wender et al., 1986) found evidence for a genetic effect on the transmission of major depression. However, not all studies found an increase in mood disorders in the biological parents of adoptees with mood disorders. This method of research has not been pursued much with modern diagnostic criteria in the last few decades, thus limiting the amount of data with which to make any firm conclusions.

GenomeLinkage Scan. A recent genomewide linkage scan was conducted to identify chromosomal regions likely to contain genes that contribute to susceptibility to recurrent early-onset MDD. Microsatellite DNA markers were studied in 656 families with two or more such cases (onset before age 31 in probands and age 41 in other relatives). Suggestive evidence for linkage was observed in regions of chromosomes 15q, 17p, and 8p; genes from these regions might contribute to susceptibility to major depression. Evidence for linkage has been reported independently in the same regions of chromosome 15q for major depression (Holmans et al., 2007).

Environmental Factors

In contrast to genetic studies where there have been few if any studies conducted specifically in young adulthood, there have been several studies examining the effects of adverse life events in this young population.

Family Interactions. Family interactions with regard to the development of depression in an adolescent and young adult are complicated and difficult to interpret. Children who are raised in family environments characterized by high levels of parental depression, conflict, neglect, unavailable parents, or harsh parenting styles have been linked to a variety of psychiatric disorders. More specifically, depressed parents may model negative cognitive styles and low self-esteem, resulting in poor coping strategies in adolescents and young adults. Marital discord and lack of an adequate support system for the family represent additional risks for development of depression. Overall, risk for depression in children of depressed patients is highest when parental illness is of earlier onset, is recurrent, and disrupts parental functioning.

Adverse Life Events. The adult literature and a number of studies with adolescents document a correlation between stressful life events and depressive symptoms. In young adulthood, child abuse and neglect were associated with an increased risk for current MDD and children who were physically abused or experienced multiple types of abuse were at increased risk of lifetime MDD. A history of childhood sexual abuse alone without other types of neglect or abuse was not associated with an elevated risk of MDD (Widom et al., 2007). Another study found that here is a higher likelihood of developing MDD if a trauma is suffered during childhood than if the trauma occurs in adolescence (Maercker et al., 2004).

Adolescent life events (e.g., changes in romantic relationships or family composition, changes in school or occupational status, changes in physical health, as well as legal or financial troubles) predict an increased risk for MDD diagnosis in young adults (Pine et al., 2002). In one longitudinal study examining predictors of MDD in a sample of 128 young women, a history of three variables predicted firstonset MDD: having witnessed family violence before age 16, having a parent with a psychiatric disorder, and having a non-mood Axis I disorder (Daley et al., 2000).

Genotype–Environment Interactions

Biological vulnerability (including genetic composition) may predispose a person to a particular illness that may not appear until the person is exposed to a stress of sufficient magnitude. Traumatic experiences, such as violence, incest, and other highly unfavorable situations recurring for long periods in childhood, can inflict severe and detrimental stress. Such harmful stress may results in depression if left untreated and may do so via influencing specific structures in the brain (e.g., reduction of hippocampal volume) (Sheline et al., 2003). When the environment is perceived as extremely stressful and the susceptible person cannot adequately cope with the external stress, depression, anxiety, a sense of helplessness, hopelessness, and suicidal ideation may ensue. However, it appears that in most cases, stress alone will not lead to recurrent or severe MDD; a genetic susceptibility may be necessary as well. A recent investigation found that an allelic variant of the gene coding for the serotonin transporter (5-HTTLPR or *SLC6A4*) is an important predictor of onset of major depression following multiple adverse life events. Adverse life events appear to have a significantly greater impact on the onset of depression for individuals with the s/s genotype (Wilhelm et al., 2006).

Suicide affects approximately 1 million people each year worldwide. The causes of suicide are multifaceted and no simple explanation exists for its occurrence. Frequently, environmental factors such as negative life events (i.e., traumatic experiences) may contribute considerably to suicidal behavior. However, in many cases the exposure to the same environmental stress does not result in increased suicidality. Hence, as with MDD, there is evidence of a significant genetic component with suicidal behavior. This next section summarizes these data.

Multiple studies are examining genetic variants with respect to correlates (personality, psychiatric diagnosis, etc.) of suicidal behavior so as to better understand the relationship between suicidal behavior and genetic variation, stress, and life trauma. For example, serotonergic neurotransmission has been implicated in suicidal behavior. A relatively consistent finding is low cerebrospinal fluid (CSF) levels of 5-hydroxy-indole-acetic-acid (5HIAA) among suicide attempters (Asberg et al., 1976; Mann & Malone, 1997; Roy et al., 1986). Studies are not only investigating for genetic markers of "risk" for suicidal behavior but also for genetic markers of "protection" against the risk this type of behavior, particularly among those who have experienced substantial stress and life trauma. Suicidal behaviors are associated with not only serotonergic genetic variants but also with other genes such as those relating to the noradrenergic system. Some serotonergic candidate genes include those coding for tryptophan hydroxylase (TPH) (Abbar et al., 2001; Geijer et al., 2000; Kirov et al., 1999; Mann et al., 1997;), which codes for the rate-limiting enzyme of the metabolic pathway of serotonin, particularly TPH2 (Zill et al., 2004); the serotonin transporter (SERT) (Lin & Tsai, 2004); and the serotonergic receptors HTR1A, HTR1B, and HTR2A (Lemonde et al., 2003). Within the noradrenergic system, a genetic variation in the noradrenergic tyrosine hydroxylase gene was linked with the angry/hostility personality trait and susceptibility to stress (Persson et al., 2000). Other recent findings include variations in genes coding for components of the stress-related hypothalamic pituitary adrenocortical axis and corticotropin releasing hormone receptor 1, all of which showed association and linkage to high anger/hostility personality trait and suicide attempt (Wasserman et al., 2007a, 2007b).

Substance Use Disorders

Substance use disorders appear to be associated with the development of depression in early adulthood. In a cohort of about 3,000 Australian young adults followed from birth to the age of 21, it was found that individuals who began using cannabis before the age of 15 years and used it often at 21 years were more likely to endorse symptoms of anxiety and depression in early adulthood. The relationship between early-onset and frequent use of cannabis and symptoms of anxiety appears to be independent of individual and family background. Repeated cannabis use is associated with increased anxiety and depression in young adults independently of whether the person also uses other illicit drugs. The direction of the association remains to be determined; that is, whether cannabis is a risk factor for anxiety and depression or whether the latter symptoms predispose an adolescent and young adult to begin using cannabis (Hayatbakhsh et al., 2007). Substance use disorders represent a large public health problem (Swartz et al., 2000) that is increasing in younger cohorts (Somers et al., 2004). Clarifying the relationship between MDD and DSM-IV substance use disorders remains an important goal. Genetic studies are identifying factors underlying the comorbidity of alcohol dependence and MDD (Nurnberger et al., 2001; Wang et al., 2004). Given the strong association of MDD with drug dependence, exploration of the genetic and environmental factors for this link will be vital. Another central issue is whether alcohol dependence precedes or follows the onset of MDD; the study of adolescents and young adults offers the prospect to attend to this crucial question. Several of the investigations performed to date have had methodological limitations that make it difficult to interpret the results. One way of addressing these limitations is using a genetically informative study design. In this type of study, Kuo and colleagues (Kuo et al., 2006) used a genetically informative population-based twin sample to examine the age-at-onset distributions and the temporal relationship of alcohol dependence and MDD. They found that the age-at-onset distributions of alcohol dependence and MDD differed substantially. Most onsets of alcohol dependence were in young adulthood, whereas MDD had a flatter distribution across age. Prior MDD significantly affected risk for developing alcohol dependence, and this risk decreased over time. By contrast, previous alcohol dependence had insignificant effects on the risk for future MDD (Kuo et al., 2006).

Depression and anxiety in adolescence and medical illness have also been reported to be risk factors for the development of MDD in young adulthood. More information is provided on the presence of depression and anxiety in adolescence and subsequent risk for MDD in young adults in the outcome and prognosis section below.

Anxiety, Depressive, and Medical Disorders

In a prospective longitudinal study, the Early Developmental States of Psychopathology (EDSP) study, anxiety disorders (e.g., social phobia, agoraphobia, generalized anxiety disorder) at baseline predicted an increased risk for the onset of MDD in young adults at follow-up (Bittner et al., 2004). Depressive symptoms in adolescence predicted early adulthood depressive disorders (MDD and dysthymia) (Aalto-Setala et al., 2002). In a cross-sectional observation study of individuals with HIV seeking treatment at local infectious disease clinics in Philadelphia, younger adults were more likely to have a mental health/substance condition compared to older adults, and were particularly more likely to be in treatment for depression (Zanjani et al., 2007).

Factors Associated with Suicide in Young Adulthood

As previously discussed, MDD and alcohol dependence commonly co-occur. The presence of a substance use disorder also appears to confer a greater risk for aggression. Among patients ages 18–26 years, depressed suicide attempters with comorbid alcohol use disorders had higher aggression and impulsivity scale scores compared to the depressed suicide attempters without a history of any substance abuse/dependence. It appears that those with comorbid alcohol use disorders are more impaired with regard to aggressiveness and impulsivity compared to persons without comorbid alcohol abuse/dependence (Sher et al., 2007). The presence of anxiety disorders also confers a greater risk of suicidal behavior in young adults, and thus clinicians should carefully evaluate patient for such comorbidity and address it accordingly (Boden et al., 2007).

Biological Studies of Depression in Young Adulthood

Most biological research conducted among young adults with MDD consists of neuroimaging and neuropsychological studies. The next two studies summarize the biological investigations performed in young adults with depression.

Neuroimaging Studies

Prefrontal impairments have been hypothesized to be most strongly related to cognitive and emotional dysfunction in depression. A volumetric reduction in left subgenual prefrontal cortex has been described in early-onset depression (17–23 years old) (Botteron et al., 2002). The microstructural integrity of whole-brain white matter as evaluated by diffusion tensor imaging in first-episode, treatment-naive young adults with MDD revealed lower fractional anisotropy values than found in healthy comparison subjects in the white matter of the right middle frontal gyrus, the left lateral occipitotemporal gyrus, and the subgyral and angular gyri of the right parietal lobe (Ma et al., 2007). These findings suggest that abnormalities of brain white matter may be present early in the course of MDD, and they support the concept that white matter lesions may disrupt the neural circuits involved in mood regulation, thus contributing to the neuropathology of MDD (Li et al., 2007; Ma et al., 2007). Another retrospective, cross-sectional investigation found that young depressed adults with periventricular white matter intensities as determined by MRI were more likely to have a history of suicide attempts (Ehrlich et al., 2005).

Previous research examining amygdala and hippocampal volumes in MDD present seemingly contradictory findings (Drevets, 2003). In one study, depressive young women were found to have a considerably enlarged amygdala size and reduced hippocampal size compared with matched controls (Weniger et al., 2006). Furthermore, depressive subjects were significantly impaired in learning emotional facial expressions, with deficits being most pronounced for fearful, surprised, and disgusted faces. The investigators speculate that amygdala enlargement in young MDD subjects is correlated with amygdalar over-activation and resolves with anti-depressant treatment (Weniger et al., 2006). However, it is possible that amygdalar volume may be influenced by familial or genetic influences rather than simply by chronicity of illness or long-term medication use. Another study also supports the finding of an enlarged amygdala volume and reduced hippocampal volume in young women with MDD (Lange & Irle, 2004). However, a recent study did not find changes in amygdala volume. In this neuroimaging study, 29 twin pairs in which one twin per pair had a lifetime history of MDD were compared with 18 age-matched control twin pairs who had no lifetime history of MDD. No significant differences were found in amygdala volumes between depressed, high-risk, or control subjects. The investigators hypothesize that there are familial, perhaps genetic, influences on amygdala volumes which might account for the discrepancies among the studies (Munn et al., 2007). With regard to studies examining both hippocampal volume and function in major depression, MacQueen and colleagues found that both first- (average age: 28 years) and multiple-episode depressed patients had hippocampal dysfunction apparent on several tests of recollection memory. Only those patients with multiple depressive episodes had hippocampal volume reductions (MacQueen et al., 2003).

Neurocognition Studies

There is growing evidence for cognitive dysfunction in depressive disorders, and presence of impaired cognition following remission could be a potential objective marker of disease and treatment response (Gallagher et al., 2007). Most studies examining the connection between depression and cognitive dysfunction have been conducted in middle-aged and elderly patients (for a review, see Kindermann & Brown, 1997). The neuropsychological profile of young adult patients has not received much attention. In a review, Castaneda and colleagues found that cognitive impairments are fairly common in young adults with MDD, mostly in executive functioning; these findings are suggestive of mild to moderate disruption in prefrontal functions in recurrent MDD (Steele et al., 2007). Attentional deficits (Egeland et al., 2003; Smith et al., 2006), short-term and working memory impairment in verbal and visual tasks (Fossati et al., 1999), and dysfunction in psychomotor skills (Hill et al., 2004) occur in young adults with MDD. However, not all studies observe the finding of verbal memory deficits in young adults with MDD (Wang et al., 2006). Apparent discrepancies in findings might reflect methodological differences (e.g., cross-sectional vs. longitudinal design, use of medications that might obscure any differences, etc).

Another central question is whether the neuropsychological findings are state versus trait dependent. One study found that young adults with mood disorders continue to have neurocognitive impairment during the euthymic phases of the illness. Patients with bipolar spectrum disorder were significantly more affected than MDD patients and controls on tests of executive function and verbal memory. MDD patients did not differ appreciably from controls on verbal memory function but performed less well on a test of executive function (Smith et al., 2006).

Endocrine and Immunological Studies

Numerous studies propose that increased central drive to the hypothalamic-pituitary adrenal (HPA) axis occurs in patients with MDD. Abnormal cortisol secretion in adults with MDD was demonstrated with overall elevation of 24-hour basal secretion, nonsuppression on a dexamethasone challenge test (DST), blunting of normal diurnal rhythms, and increased normal cortisol secretion. However, few of these types of investigations have been conducted specifically in young adults to confirm whether the same types of endocrinological findings also occur in this population. This section proceeds to summarize the few neuroendocrine studies conducted in young adults.

A recent study found elevated concentrations of cortisol and pro-inflammatory cytokines and an increased cortisol/DHEA ratio in young adults with comorbid MDD and borderline personality disorder. However a limitation of this study was that there was no comparison group with current MDD without borderline personality disorder. This makes it difficult to make a distinction on whether the observed alterations are an effect of depression alone or an interaction between depression and borderline personality disorder or its respective risk factors (Kahl et al., 2006). Low bone density, high concentrations of TNF-alpha, low concentrations of osteoprotegerin, and high rates of bone turnover markers (osteocalcin) were found in young female patients with current MDD and lifetime anorexia nervosa, indicating high rates of bone-turnover osteopenia (Kahl et al., 2005). Another study found no difference in the pattern of growth hormone secretion during the menstrual cycle in healthy and depressed young women (Kasa-Vubu et al., 2005). In a study examining urinary free cortisol among younger adults with mild to moderate MDD, male patients had higher mean urinary free cortisol levels than female patients. Significant interactions between age and severity were found among men, but not women (Grant et al., 2007). Thus, neuroendocrine contributions to MDD in young adults seem complex, although studies to date are limited.

Electrophysiological Studies

Event-related potentials are an objective parameter reflecting cognitive functions. Among event-related potentials, the P300 component (amplitude and latency) has been reported to be abnormal in adults with MDD. In 130 female subjects ages 14 to 20 years with a lifetime history of MDD, a decrement in P300 amplitude was observed in the depressed group as compared to girls with no history of depression, and the difference between the depressed and nondepressed groups was maximal in the right prefrontal region (Houston et al., 2003).

Psychological Studies of Depression in Young Adulthood

In a study of psychosocial development, a childhood sibling relationship was a strong predictor of MDD in adulthood. Poorer relationships with siblings prior to age 20 and a family history of depression independently predicted both the occurrence of MDD and the frequency of use of mood-altering drugs by age 50, even after adjustment for the quality of childhood relationships with parents (Waldinger et al., 2007).

Another psychological issue is the consequence of abortion and whether this event may have an impact on the future diagnosis of MDD and suicidal behavior. One study suggests that those having an abortion had elevated rates of subsequent mental health problems, including depression, anxiety, suicidal behaviors, and substance use disorders in young adulthood (Fergusson et al., 2006).

Another investigation examined the correlates of depression in a general population sample of young adults (20–24 years; n = 443) as part of the Finnish Health Care Survey. Drunkenness at least twice a month or once a month, not being married, and infrequent physical exercise were found to be related to MDD (Haarasilta et al., 2004).

Comorbidity

The co-occurrence of MDD and psychiatric and medical illnesses is reviewed here. Substance use disorders were previously reviewed above. In a prospective longitudinal cohort study from birth to age 32 years, 12% of the cohort had comorbid generalized anxiety disorder plus MDD, of whom 66% had recurrent MDD, 47% had recurrent generalized anxiety disorder, 64% reported using mental health services, 47% took psychiatric medication, 8% were hospitalized, and 11% attempted suicide (Moffitt et al., 2007).

Social anxiety disorder is frequently comorbid with major depression, and in such cases, almost always precedes it. Data from a prospective, longitudinal epidemiologic study of adolescents and young adults (aged 14–24 years) in Munich, Germany, found that social anxiety disorder in nondepressed persons at baseline was associated with an increased probability of depressive disorder onset during the follow-up period. In addition, comorbid social anxiety disorder and depressive disorder at baseline was associated with a worse prognosis (compared with depressive disorder without comorbid SAD at baseline) (i.e., greater likelihood of depressive disorder persistence or recurrence and attempted suicide) (Stein et al., 2001; Beesdo et al., 2007).

The sequenced treatment alternatives to relieve depression (STAR*D) study, found that those with pre-adult-onset MDD compared to adult-onset (>18 years) MDD were more likely to be women, experience a more chronic, severe, and disabling form of depression, have higher rates of family history of depression, make more past suicide attempts, and exhibit lower rates of obsessive compulsive and panic disorder (Zisook et al., 2007).

In a prospective community-based single-age cohort study of young adults (n = 591) followed between the ages of 19 and 40, MDD was found to predict an increase in body weight variability in young adults irrespective of antidepressant medication (Hasler et al., 2005). Given increasing evidence for a link between MDD and both diabetes and cardiovascular disease, further research on depression, body weight variability, and negative health outcomes is warranted (Hasler et al., 2005).

Finally, major depressive episode has been reported to be related to migraine among young adults (Breslau & Davis, 1993; Haarasilta et al., 2005; Pine et al., 1996).

Transition from Adolescence to Young Adulthood and Factors Associated with Outcome and Prognosis

In adults, it has been proposed that an initial episode of a MDD sensitizes an individual to future episodes. Presence of dysthymic disorder at the onset of MDD, "double depression," predicts decreased length of episode, with the baseline being the dysthymic disorder. Factors that predict relapse and recurrence of major depression among adults include the severity of the index episode, psychotic features, earlier age of onset, family history, multiple past episodes, a history of double depression, and nonadherence to prescribed treatment.

Factors related to the recurrence of MDD during young adulthood (19–23 years of age) in a community sample of formerly depressed adolescents included female gender, multiple MDD episodes in adolescence, higher proportion of family members with recurrent MDD, elevated borderline personality disorder symptoms, and conflict with parents (females only) (Lewinsohn et al., 2000). In terms of the postpartum period, a recent report found that childbearing women with avoidant, dependent, and obsessive-compulsive personality disorders have increased risk of new-onset MDD during the postpartum period (Akman et al., 2007).

Among adolescents, severe depression characterized by psychomotor retardation, delusional symptoms, and pervasive anhedonia is associated with the highest risk for future manic episodes. Among young adults, the development of future hypomanic episodes (bipolar II disorder) has been associated with atypical depression, early onset of depression, seasonal affective disorder, and comorbid substance abuse. The risk of "switching" from unipolar depression to bipolar disorder is highest in young adulthood, occurring at a rate of about 3% to 5% per year; it then decreases by the late 30s, at which point it flattens out to about 1% per year.

Added complications of MDD in adolescents and young adults include the persistence of social impairment and the perception of being socially secluded. While social disturbance is not restricted to mood disorders, depression in youth is linked with increased risk of tobacco and substance use and sustained negative attributions, all of which affect social functioning.

A recent study examined the linkages between suicidal ideation and attempt in adolescence and subsequent suicidal behaviors and mental health in young adulthood. In this 25-year longitudinal study of a birth cohort of 1,265 New Zealand children, suicide attempt in adolescence was associated with greater risks of subsequent suicidal ideation, suicide attempt, and MDD in young adulthood (Fergusson et al., 2005).

Evidence suggests that MDD taking place at any time during the transition to adulthood (ages 18–26) compromises future adult functioning. The transitional period requires the achievement of vital developmental tasks, such as establishing a career and forming and maintaining romantic partnerships (Arnett, 2000). However, suffering from depression during these developmental years may hinder age-appropriate functioning in critical areas (Rao et al., 1995; Lewinsohn et al., 1999). One study found that psychosocial impairment was not restricted to those actively depressed at the time functioning was assessed. Young adults with prior depressive episodes experience deficits across numerous areas of functioning, signifying possible long-term adjustment problems and a vulnerability to future depressive episodes and other psychiatric disorders (Lewinsohn et al., 1999; Birmaher et al., 2002). Males and females afflicted with depression during the transition to adulthood manifest comparable difficulties (Paradis et al., 2006). Young adults with depression view themselves as having poorer behavioral functioning, less unified families, and needing more social support than those without depression from ages 18 to 26 (Paradis et al., 2006). There is considerable psychosocial instability in affective disturbance from adolescence to adulthood. Young women with MDD during the post-high school transition had more negative functional outcomes in school and intimate romantic relationships (Rao et al., 1999).

Parental depression appears to affect the psychiatric course from adolescence to young adulthood. In a longitudinal study of 244 subjects (average age: 24 years) who had experienced MDD by 19 years, maternal MDD was associated with MDD recurrence, chronicity and severity, anxiety disorders, and (among sons only) lower psychosocial functioning (Rohde et al., 2005). Maternal MDD was related to MDD recurrence, chronicity and severity, anxiety disorders, and (among sons only) lower psychosocial functioning in offspring between the ages of 19 and 24. Paternal MDD was associated with lower functioning. Sons of depressed fathers had elevated suicidal ideation and attempt rates in young adulthood. Recurrent paternal MDD was linked with depression recurrence in daughters but not sons.

The personality dimensions of harm avoidance and self-directedness have been widely associated with depression, and there is preliminary evidence that they may represent trait markers for liability to recurrent MDD in young adults (Smith et al., 2005). Among a sample of college freshmen with a history of remitted MDD, 42% experienced a recurrence of MDD by the end of their sophomore year. In this study, exploratory survival analyses indicated that dimensional score on Cluster B (dramatic/emotional/erratic) was positively associated with increased risk of MDD recurrence (Hart et al., 2001).

Diagnosis and Clinical Features

Currently no compelling evidence exists for specific clusters of symptoms occurring more regularly in young adults with MDD compared with older adults. As described above, some clinical presentations may be associated with a greater risk for developing bipolar disorder.

Pathology and Laboratory Examination

Since no specific laboratory tests serve as direct measures of mood disorders or suicide risk, the clinical history, medical history, and psychiatric interview continue to be the most significant sources of arriving at a diagnosis. A physical examination and a screening blood panel for blood count and electrolyte concentrations are usually indicated at the start of a course of pharmacotherapy. A pregnancy test or a reliable history of absence of sexual activity is needed before any female of child bearing potential is given a medication that may have teratogenic effects.

Thyroid function tests that measure serum thyroxine, triodothyronine resin uptake, thyroid-stimulating hormone (TSH), and triodothyronine may be useful with a young adult with a psychiatric disorder because of the high frequency of thyroid dysfunction in this population and the potential overlap of mood disorder symptoms with those of thyroid disease. Thyroid function testing is not helpful as a diagnostic tool for the diagnosis of depression. Dexamethasone suppression test (DST) and the thyrotropin-releasing hormone (TRH) stimulation test have little practical value in the clinic.

Toxicology for drugs of abuse including opioids, cannabinoids, amphetamines, barbiturates, and cocaine are prudent on admission of young adult psychiatric inpatients. This substance abuse panel may be useful in clarifying contributing causes of a new onset of psychosis, mood changes, and aggressive behavior. Toxicology screening may, however, reveal past exposure rather than current use (e.g., positive results several weeks following cannabis, within days to a week of cocaine use and 48 hours after use of amphetamines).

Brain-imaging techniques, including MRI, computed tomography (CT), positron emission tomography (PET), and single-photon emission computed tomography (SPECT), are being used investigatively in psychiatry; the clinical value of routinely obtaining imaging tests has been debated. MRI and CT scans should be obtained where there are accompanying neurological signs and symptoms present (Wahlund et al., 1992). Clinical indications for the use of MRI or CT are to rule out signs of intracranial pressure or other neurological conditions. PET scans and SPECT have no current indication for their use diagnostically for young adults. Electroencephalography is also not of use diagnostically, especially since up to 15% of the general population displays abnormal EEG findings.

Except for TCAs, which are generally not used as first line treatments in major depression, the use of laboratory testing has little value as other antidepressants levels are not monitored. If the patient is going to begin treatment with a TCA, regular monitoring of the electrocardiogram (ECG), pulse, and blood pressure is required. Psychological testing, including tests of intelligence quotient, are not useful diagnostically, although they may help to identify a person's relative strengths and weaknesses.

Differential Diagnosis

The main psychiatric disorders from which MDD should be distinguished from include anxiety disorders and substance use disorders. Both of these conditions commonly co-occur in patients with MDD. Caution should also be giving to misdiagnosing bipolar disorder as unipolar depression or vice versa. In some clinical studies, between 40% and 60% of patients with bipolar disorder appear to have been misdiagnosed with unipolar depression in both inpatient and outpatient psychiatric settings (Benazzi, 1999). Hence, careful consideration to the differential diagnosis of bipolar disorder and unipolar depression is fundamental. Lack of insight regarding hypomania or mania is often cited as a reason for misdiagnosis. Thus, the need to obtain information from family members or other collateral sources is vital in assessing the bipolar disorder diagnosis. Of relevance to diagnosing bipolar diagnosis is a self-report questionnaire, the Mood Disorder Questionnaire (MDQ), which was developed as a screening instrument for bipolar disorder (Hirschfeld et al., 2000). The questionnaire reflects DSM-IV criteria. Patients are asked to report whether they have experienced those symptoms, whether the symptoms occurred simultaneously, and whether they led to significant social and occupational dysfunction. However, the primary goal involves improving clinicians' skill at recognizing clinical and historical features of bipolar diagnosis as screening instruments do not always lead to an accurate assessment (Phelps & Ghaemi, 2006). Certain aspects of the course of illness may indicate a greater likelihood of a bipolar disorder diagnosis; for example, the occurrence of depressive episodes before manic episodes in the onset of the illness (false unipolar depression or pseudounipolar depression) (Benazzi et al., 2004). Thus, in any depressed young adult, the index of suspicion for bipolar disorder should be high, as opposed to depressed individuals in their 30s or older. Furthermore, a distinction should be made on whether the current episode is accompanied or not by psychotic symptoms. The former type of depression (i.e., bipolar depression, psychotic depression) requires different treatment approaches. Clinicians should also seek to gather information on the age of onset, episode frequency, family history, and treatment response. Factors that point to a possible diagnosis of bipolar disorder include an earlier age of onset, a greater number of major depressive episodes, a positive family history of bipolar disorder, and response to lithium.

Treatment

Mental Health Services

Among Canadians, it was estimated that in young adults aged 19 to 24 with depression or suicidality, nearly half had not used any mental health services (Cheung & Dewa, 2007). The reasons young adults do not pursue treatment are unclear. A recent study found that negative beliefs and attitudes about either a biological or counseling-based explanation or treatment approach for depression, social norms, and past treatment behavior predicted low perceived depression treatment need (Van Voorhees et al., 2006). The trouble in seeking treatment is similar in other parts of the world. In the Finnish Health Care Survey of 1996, among 15 to 24-year-olds with a major depressive episode, 52% were estimated to be in need of treatment while 21% had actually sought care for depression during the preceding year. Only 14% reported recent use of antidepressant medication (Haarasilta et al., 2003).

In the United States, epidemiologic studies have also reported disturbingly low rates of treatment for MDD. Between 1988 and 1994, 7,589 individuals aged 17–39 years as part of the NHANES III were studied to determine the use of antidepressant treatment for those who had current MDD. A total of 312 individuals, or 4.1% of the sample, met DSM-III criteria for current MDD. Only 7.4% of those with current MDD were being treated with an antidepressant. Being insured and having a primary care provider each predicted a 4-fold increase in odds of antidepressant treatment; telling the primary provider about depressive symptoms predicted a 10-fold increase in treatment (Druss et al., 2000). In another study, just under 10% of those who had experienced an episode of MDD within the last year reported receiving mental health specialty services within the same time period (Ialongo et al., 2004)

Antidepressant Therapy

Treatment with antidepressants is a favored strategy in patients who have moderate to severe major depression. A number of guidelines have been proposed for the treatment of MDD and the reader is encouraged to refer to them for more detailed information on assessing and managing MDD (Anderson et al., 2000; Crismon et al., 1999; Kennedy et al., 2001). The rate of response to an antidepressant trial is approximately 60% after the first trial and increases to 70%–80% with the second trial in the case the first antidepressant is ineffective. Response signifies some degree of improvement of depressive symptoms. In recent years, there has been an emphasis on achieving greater improvements and achieving remission, which means virtual absence of depressive symptoms and return to baseline. A recent large effectiveness study in outpatients with MDD (STAR*D) found that less than one-third of patients achieved remission with an adequate trial of a standard antidepressant after approximately 10–14 weeks of treatment. Even more worrisome is that it often takes two antidepressant trials and close to 24 weeks for half of patients with MDD to remit.

Perhaps one of the greatest challenges in treating depression in young adulthood is nonadherence to the prescribed antidepressant treatment (Bambauer et al., 2007). Patients should be educated on the use of the medications. They should be told that it often takes time to improve on antidepressants, strict adherence to the prescribed treatment is important, side effects are probable and frequently short lived, and symptoms of depression usually do not start to improve until the patient has received an adequate dosage of medication for a minimum of 2 to 4 weeks. Furthermore, they should realize that remission may take even longer, between 3 and 6 months for most patients. Patients should also be informed that recovery is typically choppy or "saw-tooth" in nature in that as they continue to improve, they may have occasional days of feeling depressed and that they will need to remain on antidepressant treatment well beyond achieving remission. Finally, it is important to alert young adults ages 18 to 24 during the first 1 to 2 months of starting an antidepressant that there is an increased risk of suicidal thinking and behavior. The risk has been reported to be three-fold greater than other age groups and for that reason weekly visits are recommended when initiating an antidepressant in this age group.

There are well over 20 antidepressants that are commercially available and are classified based on their chemical structure or mechanism of function. These include tricyclic antidepressants (TCAs), monoamine oxidase inhibitors (MAOIs), selective serotonin-reuptake inhibitors (SSRIs), serotonin-norepinephrine reuptake inhibitors (SNRIs), and others. Table 14-2 summarizes the currently commonly prescribed antidepressants and the recommended daily dose. In general, there has been no consistent evidence that any antidepressant medication is superior to another one. The choice of antidepressant is usually based on the side effect profile. A better tolerated drug and one that is safer in overdose is preferably prescribed as a first-line treatment. The TCAs are generally not among the first-choice antidepressants because of the risk of cardiac arrhythmias and considerable lethal potential in overdose. Instead, SSRIs have become the drugs of choice for mood disorders because of the better side-effect profile (i.e., minimal risk of cardiac arrhythmias and considerably lower lethal potential in overdose) than older generation ones (e.g., TCAs, MAOIs). The SSRIs are summarized in Table 14-2 and include fluoxetine (Prozac), paroxetine (Paxil), sertraline (Zoloft), fluvoxamine (Luvox), and citalopram (Celexa). These drugs all have a relatively benign adverse-effect profile, with low lethality after overdose. Dosage-related adverse effects include headache and nausea. There have been no indications thus far that plasma levels correlate with expected responses. Additional potential adverse effects of these drugs include insomnia, restlessness, and agitation that can be ameliorated by decreasing the dose.

Table 14-2. Common Antidepressant Medications

Drug	Adult (Daily Dose Range)	Comments
First Generation (TCAs)		
Phenelzine	45–90 mg	Hypertensive crisis is a risk; MAOI diet required. Risk of hypotension, insomnia; potential for significant drug interactions
Nortriptyline	25–150 mg	Therapeutic level is 50–150 ng/ml
Second Generation (SSRIs)		
Fluoxetine	10–80 mg	Generic available. May be activating
Paroxetine	10–60 mg	Generic available. Increased risk for anticholinergic side effects
Sertraline	50–200 mg	
Citalopram	20–60 mg	Generic available. Few significant drug interactions
Escitalopram	10–30 mg	Few significant drug interactions
Third Generation (SNRIs, Others)		
Bupropion	75–450 mg	Use with caution in seizure disorders
Mirtazapine	15–45 mg	Weight gain/sedation at lower doses (<30 mg)
Trazodone	50–300 mg	Risk of priapism and orthostasis
Venlafaxine	75–375 mg	Monitor for hypertension
Duloxetine	40–60 mg	

Please check with the PDR for detailed information on prescribing. Each patient requires careful assessment and individualized prescribing based on medical and psychiatric needs.

Other antidepressants include bupropion (Wellbutrin), a noradrenergic and dopaminergic drug; venlafaxine (Effexor), which blocks serotonin and norepinephrine reuptake; mirtazapine (Remeron), a serotonin, plus norepinephrine reuptake inhibitor; and the MAOIs phenelzine (Nardil) and tranylcypromine (Parnate). Bupropion is an antidepressant with stimulant-like properties that has few anticholinergic side effects, produces virtually no sedation, weight gain, or sexual dysfunction, and is a much safer in overdose than the TCAs. The most common adverse effects of venlafaxine include nausea, anorexia, nervousness, and sexual dysfunction. Despite its potential to induce nervousness, there are reports of its efficacy in the treatment of anxiety disorders such as generalized anxiety disorder. MAOIs have been shown to be effective in adults with MDD and those with atypical depression. MAOIs require strict adherence to a restricted diet (no cheese [except cottage cheese or cream cheese], processed meats, caviar, cured fish, overripe fruits, avocados, fava beans, yeast extracts, Chianti or burgundy wine, beers containing yeast, or over-the-counter cold preparations, especially decongestants and inhalers). Aside from these restrictions (which potentially result in hypertensive crises and death if ingested), other adverse effects of the drugs include orthostatic hypotension, nervousness, and sleep disturbances. Such diet restrictions may not be favored among young adults.

Predictors of Efficacy and Side Effects from SSRIs. No clear biological predictors of side effects or efficacy have emerged from the literature. Efforts are underway to determine whether pharmacogenomics might be used as a tool in determining a priori side effects and efficacy with an antidepressant. In a recent study, an association between treatment-emergent suicidal ideation with citalopram and polymorphisms near cyclic adenosine monophosphate response element binding protein in the STAR*D study was found; however, age did not seem to confer an increased risk (Perlis et al., 2007).

A lesser adverse effect burden resulting from citalopram treatment was associated with the high-expression, gain-f-function L_A allele. L_A allele predicts increased *SLC6A4* transcription and increased serotonin transporter levels in brain and other tissues (Hu et al., 2007).

To determine whether age/gender-based differences in efficacy exist between bupropion and the selective serotonin reuptake inhibitors for MDD, analyses of data from 10 double-blind studies comparing bupropion with a selective serotonin reuptake inhibitor were conducted. No difference in antidepressant efficacy was noted in younger (less than 40) versus older adults (Papakostas et al., 2007).

Some basic guidelines on the prescribing of an antidepressant are as follows:

- *Previously effective antidepressants.* It is preferable to restart an antidepressant that was previously efficacious and well tolerated rather than starting a new one.
- *Side effect profile.* The choice of an antidepressant may be influenced by the patient having a particular preference to avoid a certain side effect profile. Some possible side effects may be more or less problematic for particular individuals, especially young adults (e.g., weight gain, sexual dysfunction).
- *Safety.* For severely depressed patients at risk for suicide, generally avoid (unless the patients can be monitored in an inpatient setting) TCAs and MAOIs. Instead, first consideration should be given to prescribing SSRIs as they are safer in overdose. Weekly visits are recommended when initiating an antidepressant because of the increased risk of suicidal ideation/behavior in this age group with this type of drugs.
- *Drug interactions.* Some significant drug interactions could occur if potential interactions with other drugs are not monitored for when starting an antidepressant (e.g., MAOIs). In the case a patient is taking multiple medications for medical problems, SSRIs may be safer than other classes of antidepressants.
- *Cost.* The costs of antidepressant may vary considerably from one antidepressant to another. Some of the SSRIs are now available in generic form (Table 14-2).
- *Maintenance treatment.* For a first bout of MDD, maintenance treatment is for at least 9–12 months of achieving remission. The more bouts of major depression a patient has had, the longer the patient should continue taking an antidepressant.

Monotherapy versus Augmentation. Approximately 60% of patients with MDD or a dysthymic disorder will have a clinical response to an adequate trial (3–6 weeks) of an antidepressant. However, if there is no response after 3 weeks, the probability of obtaining a response is less than 20% (Nierenberg et al., 1995), and a switch to an antidepressant of a different chemical class should be contemplated.

If after 3–6 weeks, there is a partial response but not full resolution of depressive symptoms, the clinician should consider either raising the dose of the antidepressant (if the patient can tolerate a higher dose with minimal side effects) or augmentation. The addition of lithium (Bauer & Dopfmer, 1999) or liothyronine sodium (Altshuler et al., 2001) has been reported to possibly help convert a partial responder into a full responder in about 25% of patient. However, a recent large study found that remission rates with these augmentation strategies for patients who experienced unsatisfactory results with two prior medication treatments were modest at best (Nierenberg et al., 2006). There are an increased number of studies exploring the efficacy and safety of atypical antipsychotic drugs added to antidepressants. Similarly, there are studies underway in adults to examine the efficacy of combining two antidepressants at the initiation of treatment in order to accelerate time to, and increased rates of, response and remission.

Switching Antidepressants. If there is no or incomplete response to an adequate antidepressant trial and increasing the dose or augmentation is either ineffective or not appropriate, then choosing between cognitive therapy, augmenting treatment, or switching to a different antidepressant are suitable tactics (Thase et al., 2007). One study found that pharmacologic augmentation was more rapidly effective than cognitive therapy augmentation of an SSRI, whereas switching to cognitive therapy was better tolerated than switching to a different antidepressant (Thase et al., 2007).

Most clinicians will defer a trial of a TCA or MAOI until at least 2–3 trials of newer medications have proven ineffective (Fava et al., 2006; McGrath et al., 2006). For the most part, there is no need to discontinue one antidepressant before starting a second drug trial, and typically the dosage of the first drug is tapered as the new antidepressant is started. Classic MAOIs are the exception, requiring a 2-week washout period before therapy with another antidepressant can be initiated. If the patient has not tolerated the first drug well, then a washout period may be sensible to minimize the risk of side effects before a second trial.

Special Considerations. There are few noteworthy drug–drug interactions with the newer antidepressants (i.e., SSRIs, SNRIs). All antidepressants are metabolized by one or more of the cytochrome P450 (CYP450) hepatic isoenzymes. For patients with depression taking several other medications, antidepressants that have minimal CYP450 inhibitions (e.g., citalopram, venlafaxine, and mirtazapine) should be considered.

In pregnant and breast-feeding women, one should be vigilant of certain factors. There is growing evidence that antidepressants are fairly safe during pregnancy, that they do not significantly increase the risk of teratogenesis, and that the risk of depressive relapse may be as high as 75% in pregnancy women who stop their antidepressant medication (Cohen et al., 2006; Pearson et al., 2007). These data should be incorporated into discussions with pregnant women as they consider the benefits and risks of maintenance treatment. Information on the use of antidepressants during breast-feeding is incomplete, and long-term developmental effects on the fetus are not known with certainty. Preliminary safety data do not contraindicate the use of several TCAs and SSRIs (Pearson et al., 2007; Stowe et al., 2003).

Maintenance Therapy. Most patients will have a recurrence of depression during their lifetime. Current guidelines suggest that, after recovery occurs, antidepressant therapy should be continued at the therapeutic dosage for at least 6–9 months to appreciably lessen the risk of relapse. Longer duration of maintenance treatment with antidepressant should be considered in the presence of additional factors (e.g., two or more episodes of depression in 5 years, difficult-to-treat episodes). The clinician should evaluate in detail with the patient the benefits (prevention of recurrence) and risks (e.g., cost, side effects) of treatment. If antidepressant therapy is discontinued, the dosage should be tapered gradually to avoid discontinuation symptoms (Baldwin et al., 2007).

Electroconvulsive Therapy. Electroconvulsive therapy (ECT) is a potentially efficacious treatment for mood disorders. Between 60% and 80% of all depressed patients who receive a course of ECT respond to this treatment (Potter & Rudorfer, 1993; Eitan & Lerer, 2006). A typical course of ECT is 6 to 12 treatments, with 2 to 3 treatments given per week. Improvements are typically noted after the fourth treatment. ECT should be considered a first-line treatment in depressed patients with psychotic or melancholic features, actively suicidal patients, and patients who have not responded to, or cannot tolerate, antidepressants (Brown, 2007).

Light Therapy. Phototherapy is a well-known and useful treatment for MDD with a seasonal variation, mostly fall/winter depressions (Lam et al., 2006; Lewy et al., 2006). Phototherapy is an option to antidepressant therapy in mild to moderate seasonal depression. The usual treatment is at least 30 minutes per day of light therapy with a standard phototherapy device (delivering 10,000 lx of full spectrum white light) throughout the fall/winter period.

Psychological Treatment. There are different types of psychotherapeutic treatments, and they can be classified as those that focus on the individual and those that involve multiple individuals. It is important to note that there have been few of these techniques specifically studied in young adults. Most of the psychotherapies have been studied in the other age groups. The types of therapies include individual psychotherapies, psychoanalytic treatment, cognitive-behavioral treatment, behavior therapy, interpersonal therapy, family treatment, and group treatment. Here we briefly review individual and cognitive-behavioral therapies.

In addition to supportive and psychoeducation techniques, specific psychotherapeutic interventions are as effective as antidepressant therapy in mild to moderate major depression and dysthymic disorders (Keller et al., 2000). Cognitive behavioral therapy and interpersonal therapy are treatment interventions with proven efficacy (Thase et al., 2007). Both therapies require specialized therapists and usually necessitate 8 to 16 weekly sessions for efficacy.

Individual psychotherapy focuses on the individual with the goal of changing patterns of thinking, expression of affect, and behavior. It is beyond the scope of this chapter to review the different theoretical paradigms and intervention techniques. Overall, these therapies do not focus on changing the individual's environment as the psychotherapeutic intervention is suppose to facilitate the individual in adapting to his/her environment.

Cognitive-behavioral therapy is increasing in popularity and is being systematically studied in outcomes research in different age groups. The goal is to use this psychotherapeutic technique to effect change in emotional, cognitive, and behavioral profile in individuals. In contrast to individual psychotherapies, cognitive-behavioral therapy focuses on both the external environment and the individual's internal processing of environmental situations. This intervention focuses on strengthening the individual's behavioral control and cognitive skills with the goal of changing faulty logic processing. Controlled studies have shown that this therapeutic intervention is effective in a time-limited number of sessions to treat both adolescents and adults with mood and anxiety disorders.

The choice of treatment should be based on patient preference, clinician judgment, and cost, as well as the practical issue of availability of psychotherapy. Furthermore, patients who have not responded to their preferred treatment modality should be encouraged to try other interventions.

Cognitive-behavioral and psychopharmacological may target deficits in psychosocial functioning, symptom reduction, and the use of social support networks. A study of young impoverished minority women with MDD (Miranda et al., 2003) found that both the medication intervention (antidepressant paroxetine or bupropion) and the psychotherapy intervention (8 weeks of manual-guided cognitive behavioral therapy) reduced depressive symptoms. In addition, the psychotherapy intervention resulted in improved social functioning.

Family treatment develops intrafamilial communication, behavior, and routines to help ensure that the young adults' sense of identity, social values, and future goals are recognized and addressed. From late adolescence to young adulthood, there are important transitions; at this stage, psychosocial transition is paramount. An important aspect of this transition is to promote new choices of school, occupation, and interpersonal relationships. Family therapy aims to facilitate this transition from adolescence to early adulthood behavior in seeking individual and societal responsibility and insights about future life expectations.

Other Interventions. Although current data are limited in young adults, potential new interventions for the treatments of mood disorders may include exercise regiments (Blumenthal et al., 2007), sleep deprivation (Wirz-Justice & Van den Hoofdakker, 1999), psychosurgery (Anderson & Arciniegas, 2004), vagal nerve stimulation (Ressler & Mayberg, 2007), and transcranial magnetic stimulation (O'Reardon et al., 2007). Other experimental treatments under investigation for mood disorders in adults are reviewed elsewhere (Sanacora et al., 2008; Zarate & Manji, 2008).

KEY POINTS

- Mood disorders in young adults are common and can be quite impairing if there is not early intervention. Early age of onset of a mood disorder generally predicts a more severe, chronic, and recurrent form of the illness.
- Young adulthood is one of the most critical periods of education, occupation, and social development; the consequence of depression at this critical juncture often leads to lifelong disability. For that reason, early intervention is important.
- Identifying comorbid psychiatric conditions (e.g., substance use disorders, anxiety disorders, etc.) is crucial as they may adversely influence the course of depression.

PRACTICE GUIDELINES

- There is the possibility of a diagnostic shift (e.g., transition from MDD to bipolar disorder) and for that reason close monitoring and frequent follow-up and longitudinal assessments is paramount in young adults.
- Young adults being treated with antidepressants should be evaluated on a weekly basis for the possibility of a suicidal ideation de novo or a worsening of preexisting suicidal ideation. Adults 18–24 years of age have a three-fold greater risk of suicidal behavior than other age groups.
- For depression of moderate severity or greater, combined pharmacotherapy and psychotherapy with familial involvement offers the best chance of a successful outcome.

Acknowledgments

We would like to acknowledge the support of the Intramural Research Program of the National Institute of Mental Heath and NARSAD.

References

Aalto-Setala, T., Marttunen, M., Tuulio-Henriksson A, Poikolainen K, Lönnqvist J. (2002). Depressive symptoms in adolescence as predictors of early adulthood depressive disorders and maladjustment. *American Journal of Psychiatry*, 159(7), 1235–1237.

Abbar, M., Courtet, P., Bellivier F, Leboyer M, Boulenger JP, Castelhau D, Ferreira M, Lambercy C, Mouthon D, Paoloni-Giacobino A, Vessaz M, Malafosse A, Buresi C.. (2001). Suicide attempts and the tryptophan hydroxylase gene. *Molecular Psychiatry*, 6(3), 268–273.

Akman, C., Uguz, F., Kaya N.. (2007). Postpartum-onset major depression is associated with personality disorders. *Comprehensive Psychiatry*, 48(4), 343–347.

Altshuler, L. L., Bauer, M., Frye MA, Gitlin MJ, Mintz J, Szuba MP, Leight KL, Whybrow PC (2001). Does thyroid supplementation accelerate tricyclic antidepressant response? A review and meta-analysis of the literature. *American Journal of Psychiatry*, 158(10), 1617–1622.

Anderson, C. A., & Arciniegas, D. B. (2004). Neurosurgical interventions for neuropsychiatric syndromes. *Current Psychiatry Reports*, 6(5), 355–363.

Anderson, I. M., Nutt, D. J., Deakin JF (2000). Evidence-based guidelines for treating depressive disorders with antidepressants: A revision of the 1993 British Association for Psychopharmacology guidelines. British Association for Psychopharmacology. *Journal of Psychopharmacology*, 14(1), 3–20.

Arnett, J. J. (2000). Emerging adulthood. A theory of development from the late teens through the twenties. *American Journal of Psychology*, 55(5), 469–480.

Asberg, M., Traskman, L., Thorén P. (1976). 5-HIAA in the cerebrospinal fluid. A biochemical suicide predictor? *Archives of General Psychiatry*, 33(10), 1193–7.

Baldwin, D. S., Montgomery, S. A., Nil R, Lader M (2007). Discontinuation symptoms in depression and anxiety disorders. *International Journal of Neuropsychopharmacology*, 10(1), 73–84.

Bambauer, K. Z., Soumerai, S. B., Adams AS, Zhang F, Ross-Degnan D (2007). Provider and patient characteristics associated with antidepressant nonadherence: The impact of provider specialty. *Journal of Clinical Psychiatry*, 68(6), 867–873.

Bauer, M., & Dopfmer, S. (1999). Lithium augmentation in treatment-resistant depression: Meta-analysis of placebo-controlled studies. *Journal of Clinical Psychopharmacology*, 19(5), 427–434.

Beesdo, K., Bittner, A., Pine DS, Stein MB, Höfler M, Lieb R, Wittchen HU. (2007). Incidence of social anxiety disorder and the consistent risk for secondary depression in the first three decades of life. *Archives of General Psychiatry*, 64(8), 903–912.

Benazzi, F. (1999). Bipolar II disorder is common among depressed outpatients. *Psychiatry and Clinical Neuroscience*, 53(5), 607–609.

Benazzi, F., Koukopoulos, A., Akiskal HS. (2004). Toward a validation of a new definition of agitated depression as a bipolar mixed state (mixed depression). *European Journal of Psychiatry*, 19(2), 85–90.

Birmaher, B., Arbelaez, C., Brent D. (2002). Course and outcome of child and adolescent major depressive disorder. *Child and Adolescent Psychiatric Clinics of North America*, 11(3), 619–637, x.

Bittner, A., Goodwin, R. D., Wittchen HU, Beesdo K, Höfler M, Lieb R. (2004). What characteristics of primary anxiety disorders predict subsequent major depressive disorder? *Journal of Clinical Psychiatry*, 65(5), 618–626, quiz 730.

Blumenthal, J. A., Babyak, M. A., Doraiswamy PM, Watkins L, Hoffman BM, Barbour KA, Herman S, Craighead WE, Brosse AL, Waugh R, Hinderliter A, Sherwood A. (2007). Exercise and pharmacotherapy in the treatment of major depressive disorder. *Psychosomatic Medicine*, 69, 587–596.

Boden, J. M., Fergusson, D. M., Horwood LJ. (2007). Anxiety disorders and suicidal behaviours in adolescence and young adulthood: Findings from a longitudinal study. *Psychological Medicine*, 37(3), 431–440.

Bostwick, J. M., & Pankratz, V. S. (2000). Affective disorders and suicide risk: A reexamination. *American Journal of Psychiatry*, 157(12), 1925–1932.

Botteron, K. N., Raichle, M. E., Drevets WC, Heath AC, Todd RD (2002). Volumetric reduction in left subgenual prefrontal cortex in early onset depression. *Biological Psychiatry*, 51(4), 342–344.

Brent, D. A., Oquendo, M., Birmaher B, Greenhill L, Kolko D, Stanley B, Zelazny J, Brodsky B, Bridge J, Ellis S, Salazar JO, Mann JJ. (2002). Familial pathways to early-onset suicide attempt: Risk for suicidal behavior in offspring of mood-disordered suicide attempters. *Archives of General Psychiatry*, 59(9), 801–807.

Breslau, N., & Davis, G. C. (1993). Migraine, physical health and psychiatric disorder: A prospective epidemiologic study in young adults. *Journal of Psychiatric Research*, 27(2), 211–221.

Brown, W. A. (2007). Treatment response in melancholia. *Acta Psychiatrica Scandinavica Supplementum* 433, 125-129.

Cheung, A. H. & Dewa, C. S. (2007). Mental health service use among adolescents and young adults with major depressive disorder and suicidality. *Canadian Journal of Psychiatry*, 52(4), 228-232.

Claassen, C. A., Trivedi, M. H., Rush AJ, Husain MM, Zisook S, Young E, Leuchter A, Wisniewski SR, Balasubramani GK, Alpert J.. (2007). Clinical differences among depressed patients with and without a history of suicide attempts: Findings from the STAR*D trial. *Journal of Affective Disorders*, 97(1-3), 77-84.

Cohen, L. S., Altshuler, L. L., Harlow BL, Nonacs R, Newport DJ, Viguera AC, Suri R, Burt VK, Hendrick V, Reminick AM, Loughead A, Vitonis AF, Stowe ZN. (2006). Relapse of major depression during pregnancy in women who maintain or discontinue antidepressant treatment. *Journal of the American Medical Association*, 295(5), 499-507.

Crismon, M. L., Trivedi, M., Buchanan RW, Buckley PF, Chiles JA, Conley RR, Crismon ML, Ereshefsky L, Essock SM, Finnerty M, Marder SR, Miller DD, McEvoy JP, Rush AJ, Saeed SA, Schooler NR, Shon SP, Stroup S, Tarin-Godoy B. (1999). The Texas Medication Algorithm Project: Report of the Texas Consensus Conference Panel on Medication Treatment of Major Depressive Disorder. *Journal of Clinical Psychiatry*, 60(3), 142-156.

Daley, S. E., Hammen, C., Rao U. (2000). Predictors of first onset and recurrence of major depression in young women during the 5 years following high school graduation. *Journal of Abnormal Psychology*, 109(3), 525-533.

Drevets, W. C. (2003). Neuroimaging abnormalities in the amygdala in mood disorders. *Annals of the New York Academy of Sciences*, 985, 420-444.

Druss, B. G., Hoff, R. A., Rosenheck RA. (2000). Underuse of antidepressants in major depression: Prevalence and correlates in a national sample of young adults. *Journal of Clinical Psychiatry*, 61(3), 234-237; quiz 238-239.

Dunn, V., & Goodyer, I. M. (2006). Longitudinal investigation into childhood- and adolescence-onset depression: Psychiatric outcome in early adulthood. *British Journal of Psychiatry*, 188, 216-222.

Egeland, J., Rund, B. R., Sundet K, Landrø NI, Asbjørnsen A, Lund A, Roness A, Stordal KI, Hugdahl K. (2003). Attention profile in schizophrenia compared with depression: Differential effects of processing speed, selective attention and vigilance. *Acta Psychiatrica Scandinavica*, 108(4), 276-284.

Ehrlich, S., Breeze, J. L., Hesdorffer DC, Noam GG, Hong X, Alban RL, Davis SE, Renshaw PF (2005). White matter hyperintensities and their association with suicidality in depressed young adults. *Journal of Affective Disorders*, 86(2-3), 281-287.

Eitan, R. & Lerer, B. (2006). Nonpharmacological, somatic treatments of depression: Electroconvulsive therapy and novel brain stimulation modalities. *Dialogues in Clinical Neuroscience*, 8(2), 241-258.

Fava, M., Rush, A. J., Wisniewski SR, Nierenberg AA, Alpert JE, McGrath PJ, Thase ME, Warden D, Biggs M, Luther JF, Niederehe G, Ritz L, Trivedi MH.. (2006). A comparison of mirtazapine and nortriptyline following two consecutive failed medication treatments for depressed outpatients: A STAR*D report. *American Journal of Psychiatry*, 163(7), 1161-1172.

Fergusson, D. M., Horwood, L. J., Ridder EM, Beautrais AL (2005). Suicidal behaviour in adolescence and subsequent mental health outcomes in young adulthood. *Psychological Medicine*, 35(7), 983-993.

Fergusson, D. M., Horwood, L. J., Ridder EM. (2006). Abortion in young women and subsequent mental health. *Journal of Child Psychology and Psychiatry*, 47(1), 16-24.

Fossati, P., Amar, G., Raoux N, Ergis AM, Allilaire JF. (1999). Executive functioning and verbal memory in young patients with unipolar depression and schizophrenia. *Psychiatry Research*, 89(3), 171-187.

Frasure-Smith, N., Lesperance, F., Talajic M (1993). Depression following myocardial infarction. Impact on 6-month survival. *Journal of the American Medical Association*, 270(15), 1819-1825.

Gallagher, P., Robinson, L. J., Gray JM, Porter RJ, Young AH (2007). Neurocognitive function following remission in major depressive disorder: potential objective marker of response? *Australian and New Zealand Journal of Psychiatry*, 41(1), 54-61.

Geijer, T., Frisch, A., Persson ML, Wasserman D, Rockah R, Michaelovsky E, Apter A, Jönsson EG, Nöthen MM, Weizman A. (2000). Search for association between suicide attempt and serotonergic polymorphisms. *Psychiatry and Genetics*, 10(1), 19-26.

Grant, M. M., Friedman, E. S., Haskett RF, Riso LP, Thase ME. (2007). Urinary free cortisol levels among depressed men and women: differential relationships to age and symptom severity? *Archives in Womens Mental Health*, 10(2), 73-78.

Haarasilta, L., Marttunen, M., Kaprio J, Aro H. (2003). Major depressive episode and health care use among adolescents and young adults. *Social Psychiatry and Psychiatric Epidemiology*, 38(7), 366-372.

Haarasilta, L. M., Marttunen, M. J., Kaprio JA, Aro HM. (2004). Correlates of depression in a representative nationwide sample of adolescents (15-19 years) and young adults (20–24 years). *European Journal of Public Health*, *14*(3), 280–285.

Haarasilta, L., Marttunen, M., Kaprio JA, Aro HM. (2005). Major depressive episode and physical health in adolescents and young adults: Results from a population-based interview survey. *European Journal of Public Health*, *15*(5), 489–493.

Hart, A. B., Craighead, W. E., Craighead, L. W. (2001). Predicting recurrence of major depressive disorder in young adults: A prospective study. *Journal of Abnormal Psychology*, *110*(4), 633–643.

Hasin, D. S., Goodwin, R. D., Stinson FS, Grant BF (2005). Epidemiology of major depressive disorder: Results from the National Epidemiologic Survey on Alcoholism and Related Conditions. *Archives of General Psychiatry*, *62*(10), 1097–1106.

Hasler, G., Lissek, S., Ajdacic V, Milos G, Gamma A, Eich D, Rössler W, Angst J. (2005). Major depression predicts an increase in long-term body weight variability in young adults. *Obesity Research*, *13*(11), 1991–1998.

Hayatbakhsh, M. R., Najman, J. M., Jamrozik K, Mamun AA, Alati R, Bor W. (2007). Cannabis and anxiety and depression in young adults: A large prospective study. *Journal of the American Academy of Child and Adolescent Psychiatry*, *46*(3), 408–417.

Hill, S. K., Keshavan, M. S., Thase ME, Sweeney JA (2004). Neuropsychological dysfunction in antipsychotic-naive first-episode unipolar psychotic depression. *American Journal of Psychiatry*, *161*(6), 996–1003.

Hirschfeld, R. M., Williams, J. B., Spitzer RL, Calabrese JR, Flynn L, Keck PE Jr, Lewis L, McElroy SL, Post RM, Rapport DJ, Russell JM, Sachs GS, Zajecka J. (2000). Development and validation of a screening instrument for bipolar spectrum disorder: The Mood Disorder Questionnaire. *American Journal of Psychiatry*, *157*(11), 1873–1875.

Holmans, P., Weissman, M. M., Zubenko GS, Scheftner WA, Crowe RR, Depaulo JR Jr, Knowles JA, Zubenko WN, Murphy-Eberenz K, Marta DH, Boutelle S, McInnis MG, Adams P, Gladis M, Steele J, Miller EB, Potash JB, Mackinnon DF, Levinson DF. (2007). Genetics of recurrent early-onset major depression (GenRED): Final genome scan report. *American Journal of Psychiatry*, *164*(2), 248–258.

Houston, R. J., Bauer, L. O., Hesselbrock VM. (2003). Depression and familial risk for substance dependence: A P300 study of young women. *Psychiatry Research*, *124*(1), 49–62.

Hu, X. Z., Rush, A. J., Charney D, Wilson AF, Sorant AJ, Papanicolaou GJ, Fava M, Trivedi MH, Wisniewski SR, Laje G, Paddock S, McMahon FJ, Manji H, Lipsky RH. (2007). Association between a functional serotonin transporter promoter polymorphism and citalopram treatment in adult outpatients with major depression. *Archives of General Psychiatry*, *64*(7), 783–792.

Ialongo, N., McCreary, B. K., Pearson JL, Koenig AL, Schmidt NB, Poduska J, Kellam SG (2004). Major depressive disorder in a population of urban, African-American young adults: Prevalence, correlates, comorbidity and unmet mental health service need. *Journal of Affective Disorders*, *79*(1–3), 127–136.

Johnson, B. A., Brent, D. A., Bridge J, Connolly J. 1998). The familial aggregation of adolescent suicide attempts. *Acta Psychiatrica Scandinavica*, *97*(1), 18–24.

Jonas, B. S., Brody, D.,Roper M, Narrow WE(2003). Prevalence of mood disorders in a national sample of young American adults. *Social Psychiatry and Psychiatric Epidemiology*, *38*(11), 618–624.

Kahl, K. G., Bens, S., Ziegler K, Rudolf S, Dibbelt L, Kordon A, Schweiger U. (2006). Cortisol, the cortisol-dehydroepiandrosterone ratio, and pro-inflammatory cytokines in patients with current major depressive disorder comorbid with borderline personality disorder. *Biological Psychiatry*, *59*(7), 667–671.

Kahl, K. G., Rudolf, S., Dibbelt L, Stoeckelhuber BM, Gehl HB, Hohagen F, Schweiger U (2005). Decreased osteoprotegerin and increased bone turnover in young female patients with major depressive disorder and a lifetime history of anorexia nervosa. *Osteoporos International*, *16*(4), 424–429.

Kasa-Vubu, J. Z., Dimaraki, E. V., Young EA (2005). The pattern of growth hormone secretion during the menstrual cycle in normal and depressed women. *Clinical Endocrinology (Oxford) 62*(6), 656–660.

Keller, M. B., McCullough, J. P., Klein DN, Arnow B, Dunner DL, Gelenberg AJ, Markowitz JC, Nemeroff CB, Russell JM, Thase ME, Trivedi MH, Zajecka J. (2000). A comparison of nefazodone, the cognitive behavioral-analysis system of psychotherapy, and their combination for the treatment of chronic depression. *New England Journal of Medicine*, *342*(20), 1462–1470.

Kendler, K. S., Pedersen, N., Johnson L, Neale MC, Mathé AA (1993). A pilot Swedish twin study of affective illness, including hospital- and population-ascertained subsamples. *Archives of General Psychiatry*, *50*(9), 699–700.

Kennedy, S. H., Lam, R. W., Cohen NL, Ravindran AV; CANMAT Depression Work Group. (2001). Clinical guidelines for the treatment of depressive disorders. IV. Medications and other biological treatments. *Canadian Journal of Psychiatry*, *46*(Suppl. 1), 38S–58S.

Kessler, R. C., Akiskal, H. S., Ames M, Birnbaum H, Greenberg P, Hirschfeld RM, Jin R, Merikangas KR, Simon GE, Wang PS. (2006). Prevalence and effects of mood disorders on work performance in a nationally representative sample of U.S. workers. *American Journal of Psychiatry*, 163(9), 1561–1568.

Kessler, R. C., Berglund, P., Demler O, Jin R, Koretz D, Merikangas KR, Rush AJ, Walters EE, Wang PS; National Comorbidity Survey Replication. (2003). The epidemiology of major depressive disorder: results from the National Comorbidity Survey Replication (NCS-R). *Journal of the American Medical Association*, 289(23), 3095–3105.

Kessler, R. C., McGonagle, K. A., Zhao S, Nelson CB, Hughes M, Eshleman S, Wittchen HU, Kendler KS. (1994). Lifetime and 12-month prevalence of DSM-III-R psychiatric disorders in the United States. Results from the National Comorbidity Survey." *Archives of General Psychiatry*, 51(1), 8–19.

Kindermann, S. S., & Brown, G. C. (1997). Depression and memory in the elderly: a meta-analysis. *Journal of Clinical and Experimental Neuropsychology*, 19(5), 625–642.

Kirov, G., Owen, M. J., Jones I, McCandless F, Craddock N. (1999). Tryptophan hydroxylase gene and manic-depressive illness. *Archives of General Psychiatry*, 56(1), 98–99.

Kuo, P. H., Gardner, C. O., Kendler KS, Prescott CA. (2006). The temporal relationship of the onsets of alcohol dependence and major depression: Using a genetically informative study design. *Psychological Medicine*, 36(8), 1153–1162.

Lam, R. W., Levitt, A. J., Levitan RD, Enns MW, Morehouse R, Michalak EE, Tam EM. (2006). The Can-SAD study: A randomized controlled trial of the effectiveness of light therapy and fluoxetine in patients with winter seasonal affective disorder. *American Journal of Psychiatry*, 163(5), 805–812.

Lange, C., & Irle, E. (2004). Enlarged amygdala volume and reduced hippocampal volume in young women with major depression. *Psychological Medicine*, 34(6), 1059–1064.

Lemonde, S., Turecki, G., Bakish D, Du L, Hrdina PD, Bown CD, Sequeira A, Kushwaha N, Morris SJ, Basak A, Ou XM, Albert PR. (2003). Impaired repression at a 5-hydroxytryptamine 1A receptor gene polymorphism associated with major depression and suicide. *Journal of Neuroscience*, 23(25), 8788–8799.

Lerner, D., Adler, D. A., Chang H, Lapitsky L, Hood MY, Perissinotto C, Reed J, McLaughlin TJ, Berndt ER, Rogers WH. (2004). Unemployment, job retention, and productivity loss among employees with depression. *Psychiatric Services*, 55(12), 1371–1378.

Lewinsohn, P. M., Rohde, P., Klein DN, Seeley JR. (1999). Natural course of adolescent major depressive disorder: I. Continuity into young adulthood. *Journal of the American Academy of Child and Adolescent Psychiatry*, 38(1), 56–63.

Lewinsohn, P. M., Rohde, P., Seeley JR, Klein DN, Gotlib IH (2000). Natural course of adolescent major depressive disorder in a community sample: Predictors of recurrence in young adults. *American Journal of Psychiatry*, 157(10), 1584–1591.

Lewy, A. J., Lefler, B. J., Emens JS, Bauer VK. (2006). The circadian basis of winter depression. *Proceedings of the National Academy of Sciences USA*, 103(19), 7414–7419.

Li, L., Ma, N., Tan L, Liu J, Gong G, Shu N, He Z, Jiang T, Xu L. (2007). Prefrontal white matter abnormalities in young adult with major depressive disorder: A diffusion tensor imaging study. *Brain Research*, 1168, 124–128.

Lin, P. Y., & Tsai, G. (2004). Association between serotonin transporter gene promoter polymorphism and suicide: Results of a meta-analysis. *Biological Psychiatry*, 55(10), 1023–1030.

Ma, N., Li, L., Shu N, Liu J, Gong G, He Z, Li Z, Tan L, Stone WS, Zhang Z, Xu L, Jiang T.. (2007). White matter abnormalities in first-episode, treatment-naive young adults with major depressive disorder. *American Journal of Psychiatry*, 164(5), 823–826.

MacQueen, G. M., Campbell, S. McEwen BS, Macdonald K, Amano S, Joffe RT, Nahmias C, Young LT. (2003). Course of illness, hippocampal function, and hippocampal volume in major depression. *Proceedings of the National Academy of Sciences USA*, 100(3), 1387–1392.

Maercker, A., Michael, T., Fehm L, Becker ES, Margraf J. (2004). Age of traumatisation as a predictor of post-traumatic stress disorder or major depression in young women. *British Journal of Psychiatry*, 184, 482–487.

Mann, J. J., & Malone, K. M. (1997). Cerebrospinal fluid amines and higher-lethality suicide attempts in depressed inpatients. *Biological Psychiatry*, 41(2), 162–171.

Mann, J. J., Malone, K. M., Nielsen DA, Goldman D, Erdos J, Gelernter J. (1997). Possible association of a polymorphism of the tryptophan hydroxylase gene with suicidal behavior in depressed patients. *American Journal of Psychiatry*, 154(10), 1451–1453.

McGrath, P. J., Stewart, J. W., Fava M, Trivedi MH, Wisniewski SR, Nierenberg AA, Thase ME, Davis L, Biggs MM, Shores-Wilson K, Luther JF, Niederehe G, Warden D, Rush AJ. (2006). Tranylcypromine versus venlafaxine plus mirtazapine following three failed antidepressant medication trials for depression: a STAR*D report. *American Journal of Psychiatry*, *163*(9), 1531–1541; quiz 1666.

McGuffin, P., Katz, R., Watkins S, Rutherford J (1996). A hospital-based twin register of the heritability of DSM-IV unipolar depression. *Archives of General Psychiatry*, *53*(2), 129–136.

Mendlewicz, J., & Rainer, J. D. (1977). Adoption study supporting genetic transmission in manic-depressive illness. *Nature*, *268*(5618), 327–329.

Minnai, G. P., Tondo, L. Salis P, Ghiani C, Manfredi A, Paluello MM, Baethge C, Baldessarini RJ. (2006). Secular trends in first hospitalizations for major mood disorders with comorbid substance use. *International Journal of Neuropsychopharmacology*, *9*(3), 319–326.

Miranda, J., Chung, J. Y., Green BL, Krupnick J, Siddique J, Revicki DA, Belin T. (2003). Treating depression in predominantly low-income young minority women: A randomized controlled trial. *Journal of the American Medical Association*, *290*(1), 57–65.

Moffitt, T. E., Harrington, H., Caspi A, Kim-Cohen J, Goldberg D, Gregory AM, Poulton R. (2007). Depression and generalized anxiety disorder: cumulative and sequential comorbidity in a birth cohort followed prospectively to age 32 years. *Archives of General Psychiatry*, *64*(6), 651–660.

Munn, M. A., Alexopoulos, J., Nishino T, Babb CM, Flake LA, Singer T, Ratnanather JT, Huang H, Todd RD, Miller MI, Botteron KN. (2007). Amygdala volume analysis in female twins with major depression. *Biological Psychiatry*, *62*(5), 415–422.

Murray, C. J., & Lopez, A. D. (1996). Evidence-based health policy—Lessons from the Global Burden of Disease Study. *Science*, *274*(5288), 740–743.

Newman, D. L., Moffitt, T. E., Caspi A, Magdol L, Silva PA, Stanton WR. (1996). Psychiatric disorder in a birth cohort of young adults: Prevalence, comorbidity, clinical significance, and new case incidence from ages 11 to 21. *Journal of Consulting and Clinical Psychology*, *64*(3), 552–562.

Nierenberg, A. A., Fava, M. Trivedi MH, Wisniewski SR, Thase ME, McGrath PJ, Alpert JE, Warden D, Luther JF, Niederehe G, Lebowitz B, Shores-Wilson K, Rush AJ. (2006). A comparison of lithium and T(3) augmentation following two failed medication treatments for depression: A STAR*D report. *American Journal of Psychiatry*, *163*(9), 1519–1530; quiz 1665.

Nierenberg, A. A., McLean, N. E., Alpert JE, Worthington JJ, Rosenbaum JF, Fava M. (1995). Early nonresponse to fluoxetine as a predictor of poor 8-week outcome. *American Journal of Psychiatry*, *152*(10), 1500–1503.

Nierenberg, A. A., Trivedi, M. H., Fava M, Biggs MM, Shores-Wilson K, Wisniewski SR, Balasubramani GK, Rush AJ. (2007). Family history of mood disorder and characteristics of major depressive disorder: A STAR*D (sequenced treatment alternatives to relieve depression) study. *Journal of Psychiatric Research*, *41*(3–4), 214–221.

Nurnberger, J. I., Jr., Foroud, T., Flury L, Su J, Meyer ET, Hu K, Crowe R, Edenberg H, Goate A, Bierut L, Reich T, Schuckit M, Reich W. (2001). Evidence for a locus on chromosome 1 that influences vulnerability to alcoholism and affective disorder. *American Journal of Psychiatry*, *158*(5), 718–724.

O'Reardon J, P., Solvason, H. B., Janicak PG, Sampson S, Isenberg KE, Nahas Z, McDonald WM, Avery D, Fitzgerald PB, Loo C, Demitrack MA, George MS, Sackeim HA. (2007). Efficacy and safety of transcranial magnetic stimulation in the acute treatment of major depression: A multisite randomized controlled trial. *Biological Psychiatry*, *62*(11), 1208–1216.

Papadimitriou, G. N., Souery, D. Lipp O, Massat I, Mahieu B, Van Broeckhoven C, Mendlewicz J. (2005). In search of anticipation in unipolar affective disorder. *European Journal of Neuropsychopharmacology*, *15*(5), 511–516.

Papakostas, G. I., Kornstein, S. G., Clayton AH, Soares CN, Hallett LA, Krishen A, Tucker VL. (2007). Relative antidepressant efficacy of bupropion and the selective serotonin reuptake inhibitors in major depressive disorder: Gender-age interactions. *International Journal of Clinical Psychopharmacology*, *22*(4), 226–229.

Paradis, A. D., Reinherz, H. Z., Giaconia RM, Fitzmaurice G (2006). Major depression in the transition to adulthood: The impact of active and past depression on young adult functioning. *Journal of Nervous and Mental Disorders*, *194*(5), 318–323.

Pardes, H., Kaufmann, C. A., Pincus HA, West A. (1989). Genetics and psychiatry: Past discoveries, current dilemmas, and future directions. *American Journal of Psychiatry*, *146*(4), 435–443.

Pearson, K. H., Nonacs, R. M., Viguera AC, Heller VL, Petrillo LF, Brandes M, Hennen J, Cohen LS. (2007). Birth outcomes following prenatal exposure to antidepressants. *Journal of Clinical Psychiatry*, *68*(8), 1284–1289.

Perlis, R. H., Purcell, S., Fava M, Fagerness J, Rush AJ, Trivedi MH, Smoller JW (2007). Association between treatment-emergent suicidal ideation with citalopram and polymorphisms near cyclic adenosine monophosphate response element binding protein in the STAR*D study. *Archives of General Psychiatry*, *64*(6), 689–697.

Persson, M. L., Wasserman, D., Jönsson EG, Bergman H, Terenius L, Gyllander A, Neiman J, Geijer T.

(2000). Search for the influence of the tyrosine hydroxylase (TCAT)(n) repeat polymorphism on personality traits. *Psychiatry Research*, 95(1), 1–8.

Phelps, J. R., & Ghaemi, S. N. (2006). Improving the diagnosis of bipolar disorder: predictive value of screening tests. *Journal of Affective Disorders*, 92(2–3), 141–148.

Pine, D. S., Cohen, P., Brook J. (1996). The association between major depression and headache: results of a longitudinal epidemiologic study in youth. *Journal of Child and Adolescent Psychopharmacology*, 6(3), 153–164.

Pine, D. S., Cohen, P., Johnson JG, Brook JS. (2002). Adolescent life events as predictors of adult depression. *Journal of Affective Disorders*, 68(1), 49–57.

Potter, W. Z., & Rudorfer, M. V. (1993). Electroconvulsive therapy—A modern medical procedure. *New England Journal of Medicine*, 328(12), 882–883.

Rao, U., Hammen, C., Daley SE. (1999). Continuity of depression during the transition to adulthood: A 5-year longitudinal study of young women. *Journal of theAmerican Academy of Child and Adolescent Psychiatry*, 38(7), 908–915.

Rao, U., Ryan, N. D., Birmaher B, Dahl RE, Williamson DE, Kaufman J, Rao R, Nelson B (1995). Unipolar depression in adolescents: Clinical outcome in adulthood. *Journal of the American Academy of Child and Adolescent Psychiatry*, 34(5), 566–578.

Ressler, K. J., & Mayberg, H. S. (2007). Targeting abnormal neural circuits in mood and anxiety disorders: From the laboratory to the clinic. *Nature Neuroscience*, 10(9), 1116–1124.

Rohde, P., Lewinsohn, P. M., Klein DN, Seeley JR (2005). Association of parental depression with psychiatric course from adolescence to young adulthood among formerly depressed individuals. *Journal of Abnormal Psychology*, 114(3), 409–420.

Roy, A., Agren, H., Pickar D, Linnoila M, Doran AR, Cutler NR, Paul SM. (1986). Reduced CSF concentrations of homovanillic acid and homovanillic acid to 5-hydroxyindoleacetic acid ratios in depressed patients: Relationship to suicidal behavior and dexamethasone nonsuppression. *American Journal of Psychiatry*, 143(12), 1539–1545.

Roy, A., & Segal, N. L. (2001). Suicidal behavior in twins: A replication. *Journal of Affective Disorders*, 66(1), 71–74.

Sanacora, G., Zarate, C. A., Krystal JH, Manji HK. (2008). Targeting the glutamatergic system to develop novel, improved therapeutics for mood disorders. *Nature Reviews Drug Discovery*, 7(5), 426–437.

Sheline, Y. I., Gado, M. H., Kraemer HC. (2003). Untreated depression and hippocampal volume loss. *American Journal of Psychiatry*, 160(8), 1516–1518.

Sher, L., Sperling, D., Stanley BH, Carballo JJ, Shoval G, Zalsman G, Burke AK, Mann JJ, Oquendo MA. (2007). Triggers for suicidal behavior in depressed older adolescents and young adults: do alcohol use disorders make a difference? *International Journal of Adolescent Medicine and Health*, 19(1), 91–98.

Shih, R. A., Belmonte, P. L., Zandi, P.P. (2004). A review of the evidence from family, twin and adoption studies for a genetic contribution to adult psychiatric disorders. *International Review of Psychiatry*, 16(4), 260–283.

Smith, D. J., Duffy, L., Stewart ME, Muir WJ, Blackwood DH. (2005). High harm avoidance and low self-directedness in euthymic young adults with recurrent, early-onset depression. *Journal of Affective Disorders*, 87(1), 83–89.

Smith, D. J., Muir, W. J., Blackwood DH. (2006). Neurocognitive impairment in euthymic young adults with bipolar spectrum disorder and recurrent major depressive disorder. *Bipolar Disorder*, 8(1), 40–46.

Somers, J. M., Goldner, E. M., Waraich P, Hsu L. (2004). Prevalence studies of substance-related disorders: A systematic review of the literature. *Canadian Journal of Psychiatry*, 49(6), 373–384.

Statham, D. J., Heath, A. C., Madden PA, Bucholz KK, Bierut L, Dinwiddie SH, Slutske WS, Dunne MP, Martin NG. (1998). Suicidal behaviour: An epidemiological and genetic study. *Psychological Medicine*, 28(4), 839–855.

Steele, J. D., Currie, J., Lawrie SM, Reid I. (2007). Prefrontal cortical functional abnormality in major depressive disorder: A stereotactic meta-analysis. *Journal of Affective Disorders*, 101(1–3), 1–11.

Stein, M. B., Fuetsch, M., Müller N, Höfler M, Lieb R, Wittchen HU. (2001). Social anxiety disorder and the risk of depression: A prospective community study of adolescents and young adults. *Archives of General Psychiatry*, 58(3), 251–256.

Stowe, Z. N., Hostetter, A. L., Owens MJ, Ritchie JC, Sternberg K, Cohen LS, Nemeroff CB. (2003). The pharmacokinetics of sertraline excretion into human breast milk: Determinants of infant serum concentrations. *Journal of Clinical Psychiatry*, 64(1), 73–80.

Swartz, J. A., Lurigio, A. J., Goldstein P (2000). Severe mental illness and substance use disorders among former Supplemental Security Income beneficiaries for drug addiction and alcoholism. *Archives of General Psychiatry*, 57(7), 701–707.

Thase, M. E., Friedman, E. S., Biggs MM, Wisniewski SR, Trivedi MH, Luther JF, Fava M, Nierenberg AA,

McGrath PJ, Warden D, Niederehe G, Hollon SD, Rush AJ. (2007). Cognitive therapy versus medication in augmentation and switch strategies as second-step treatments: A STAR*D report. *American Journal of Psychiatry*, 164(5), 739–752.

Van Voorhees, B. W., Fogel, J., Houston TK, Cooper LA, Wang NY, Ford DE. (2006). Attitudes and illness factors associated with low perceived need for depression treatment among young adults. *Social Psychiatry and Psychiatric Epidemiology*, 41(9), 746–754.

Wahlund, L. O., Agartz, I., Sääf J, Wetterberg L, Marions O (1992). MRI in psychiatry: 731 cases. *Psychiatry Research*, 45(2), 139–140.

Waldinger, R. J., Vaillant, G. E., Orav EJ. (2007). Childhood sibling relationships as a predictor of major depression in adulthood: A 30-year prospective study. *American Journal of Psychiatry*, 164(6), 949–954.

Wang, C. E., Halvorsen, M., Sundet K, Steffensen AL, Holte A, Waterloo K. (2006). Verbal memory performance of mildly to moderately depressed outpatient younger adults. *Journal of Affective Disorders*, 92(2–3), 283–286.

Wang, J. C., Hinrichs, A. L., Stock H, Budde J, Allen R, Bertelsen S, Kwon JM, Wu W, Dick DM, Rice J, Jones K, Nurnberger JI Jr, Tischfield J, Porjesz B, Edenberg HJ, Hesselbrock V, Crowe R, Schuckit M, Begleiter H, Reich T, Goate AM, Bierut LJ. (2004). Evidence of common and specific genetic effects: Association of the muscarinic acetylcholine receptor M2 (CHRM2) gene with alcohol dependence and major depressive syndrome. *Human Molecular Genetics*, 13(17), 1903–1911.

Wang, P. S., Berglund, P., Olfson M, Pincus HA, Wells KB, Kessler RC (2005). Failure and delay in initial treatment contact after first onset of mental disorders in the National Comorbidity Survey Replication. *Archives of General Psychiatry*, 62(6), 603–613.

Wasserman, D., Geijer, T., Sokolowski M, Rozanov V, Wasserman J. (2007a). Genetic variation in the hypothalamic-pituitary-adrenocortical axis regulatory factor, T-box 19, and the angry/hostility personality trait. *Genes Brain Behavior*, 6(4), 321–328.

Wasserman, D., Geijer, T., Sokolowski M, Rozanov V, Wasserman J. (2007b). Nature and nurture in suicidal behavior, the role of genetics: Some novel findings concerning personality traits and neural conduction. *Physiological Behavior*, 92(1–2), 245–249.

Watanabe-Galloway, S., & Zhang, W. (2007). Analysis of U.S. trends in discharges from general hospitals for episodes of serious mental illness, 1995–2002. *Psychiatric Services*, 58(4), 496–502.

Wender, P. H., Kety, S. S., Rosenthal D, Schulsinger F, Ortmann J, Lunde I. (1986). Psychiatric disorders in the biological and adoptive families of adopted individuals with affective disorders. *Archives of General Psychiatry*, 43(10), 923–929.

Weniger, G., Lange, C., Irle E. (2006). Abnormal size of the amygdala predicts impaired emotional memory in major depressive disorder. *Journal of Affective Disorders*, 94(1–3), 219–229.

Widom, C. S., DuMont, K., Czaja SJ. (2007). A prospective investigation of major depressive disorder and comorbidity in abused and neglected children grown up. *Archives of General Psychiatry*, 64(1), 49–56.

Wilhelm, K., Mitchell, P. B., Niven H, Finch A, Wedgwood L, Scimone A, Blair IP, Parker G, Schofield PR. (2006). Life events, first depression onset and the serotonin transporter gene. *British Journal of Psychiatry*, 188, 210–215.

Wirz-Justice, A., & Van den Hoofdakker, R. H. (1999). Sleep deprivation in depression: What do we know, where do we go? *Biological Psychiatry*, 46(4), 445–453.

Zanjani, F., Saboe, K., Oslin D. (2007). Age difference in rates of mental health/substance abuse and behavioral care in HIV-positive adults. *AIDS Patient Care STDS*, 21(5), 347–355.

Zarate, C. A., Jr., & Manji, H. K. (2008). Bipolar disorder: Candidate drug targets. *Mt Sinai Journal of Medicine*, 75(3), 226–247.

Zhang, J., McKeown, R. E., Hussey JR, Thompson SJ, Woods JR. (2005). Gender differences in risk factors for attempted suicide among young adults: Findings from the Third National Health and Nutrition Examination Survey. *Annals of Epidemiology*, 15(2), 167–174.

Zill, P., Buttner, A., Eisenmenger W, Möller HJ, Bondy B, Ackenheil M. (2004). Single nucleotide polymorphism and haplotype analysis of a novel tryptophan hydroxylase isoform (TPH2) gene in suicide victims. *Biological Psychiatry*, 56(8), 581–586.

Zisook, S., Rush, A. J., Lesser I, Wisniewski SR, Trivedi M, Husain MM, Balasubramani GK, Alpert JE, Fava M. (2007). Preadult onset vs. adult onset of major depressive disorder: A replication study. *Acta Psychiatrica Scandinavica*, 115(3), 196–205.

Chapter 15

Anxiety Disorders

Brian L. Odlaug, Waqar Mahmud, Andrew Goddard and Jon E. Grant

Anxiety disorders affect approximately 40 million adults in the United States with current (past 12 months) and lifetime prevalence rates of 18.1% and 28.2%, respectively, and are among the most common psychiatric disorders (APA, 2000; Kessler et al., 2005; Kessler, Chiu, Demler, Merikangas, & Walters, 2005). According to the *Diagnostic and Statistic Manual for Mental Disorders* (4th ed.) (DSM-IV), the anxiety disorders include obsessive-compulsive disorder, generalized anxiety disorder, social anxiety disorder, panic disorder (both with and without agoraphobia), posttraumatic stress disorder, acute stress disorder, specific phobia, substance-induced anxiety disorder, and anxiety disorders not otherwise specified (APA, 2000). Per year, their estimated cost (directly and indirectly) to the United States is over $42 billion. More than 50% of these expenses are due to clinical care stemming from misdiagnosis, inadequate treatment, and emergency care (including psychiatric and nonpsychiatric hospitalization), the net effect of which is reduced productivity and absenteeism from the workplace (Lepine, 2002).

Anxiety disorders have a substantial impact on pediatric, adolescent, and adult populations. Their negative effects are seen not only in emotional and physical health but also through impairments in educational, social, and occupational functioning, as well as in overall quality of life. A review of over 1,000 subjects aged 16–25 with anxiety disorders found that those with anxiety disorders had a 5.85 times higher rate of suicide attempts (Boden, Fergusson, & Horwood, 2007) than those without an anxiety disorder. Although extremely common, anxiety disorders often go undiagnosed and untreated. Paradoxically, while young adults can be profoundly affected by clinical anxiety, they are the least likely to seek clinical care, with only one-third of patients utilizing mental health services through either psychiatric or primary care facilities (Suvisaari et al., 2008).

The goal of this chapter is to discuss the aspects of certain anxiety disorders not elsewhere discussed in this publication. Specifically, we will be discussing the impact of social anxiety disorder, panic disorder, generalized anxiety, and posttraumatic stress disorder on young adult mental health, with particular emphasis on their epidemiology, etiology, clinical presentation, current treatment guidelines, and future directions for research.

Social Anxiety Disorder

Case Vignette

Cindy is a 21-year-old, single, female college student presenting to her university's counseling service with difficulties managing and completing her coursework. A review of her history uncovered that she received high marks in school and was first chair flute in her high school's top band, but that she also endorsed feelings of ineptitude as a teenager and was labeled as "shy" as a child. Due to her musical prowess, Cindy is on a full scholarship at the university; however, she reports that performing in front of an audience is becoming increasingly difficult due to thoughts that people are judging her negatively or that she might do something embarrassing. She reports feeling extremely anxious immediately preceding a performance in front of an audience, but she experiences no anxiety when practicing alone in her dorm room. Her anxiety symptoms have begun to affect her overall grades, as live performance is an essential element of her coursework. Although she feels as though music is her major of choice, she believes that she should switch majors because of her inability to perform. Cindy also reports feeling anxious in social situations, fearing that she might say or do something that will make her appear foolish. In order to decrease potential anxiety symptoms at social gatherings, Cindy reports drinking alcohol at home before going out so that she can relax and interact with others.

Clinical Characteristics

Social anxiety disorder (SAD), also referred to as social phobia, is the fourth most commonly diagnosed psychiatric disorder, with lifetime and current prevalence rates of 12.1% and 6.8%, respectively, in the general population (Magee, Eaton, Wittchen, McGonagle, & Kessler, 1996; Kessler et al., 2005a; Kessler, Chiu, Demler, Merikangas, & Walters, 2005). The most severe form of SAD is generalized SAD (GSAD), in which individuals fear and avoid numerous social situations as opposed to only a few situations in SAD. GSAD is believed to affect about two-thirds of individuals with SAD and appears to be more common in women (15.5%) than men (11.1%) (Kessler et al., 1994; Kessler, Stein, & Berglund, 1998). Generally, SAD begins in the early teen years and typically maintains a chronic course (Bruce et al., 2005; Wittchen & Beloch, 1996). Because individuals with SAD experience anxiety and fear in social situations, many also report reduced quality of life in personal and professional areas (Wittchen, Fuetsch, Sonntag, Müller, & Liebowitz, 1999). As a result, the clinical presence of SAD, or its variant GSAD, can become a significant burden to young adults and can be detrimental to both career development and the establishment of long-term relationships.

Comorbidity

Co-occurring psychiatric conditions are the rule, not the exception, in patients with SAD (Grant et al., 2005) and may result in marked morbidity if left untreated (Wittchen & Beloch, 1996). High rates of depression, alcohol dependence, and other anxiety disorders have been documented in people with SAD and have been found to be detrimental to recovery (Bruce et al., 2005; Grant et al., 2005; Lecrubier & Weiller, 1997). In the case of co-occurring alcohol dependence, the onset of SAD often predates the onset of alcohol dependence. In addition, alcohol dependence in those with SAD is generally more severe than those without SAD and causes greater functional impairment and overall health problems (Buckner et al., 2008).

Etiology

Overall, there is accumulating evidence that either abnormal conditioning (e.g., stimulus overgeneralization) and/or extinction failure may contribute to the genesis of social phobias in humans. Abnormalities in conditioning and extinction processes suggest dysfunction within cortico-limbic circuits (Davidson, Marshall, Tomarken, & Henriques, 2000). For example, there is pathophysiological evidence of delayed extinction of the conditioned response in GSAD patients relative to controls, supporting the concept that extinction failure could contribute to the maintenance of social fears in GSAD patients (Hermann, Ziegler, Birbaumer, & Flor, 2002). Research on these circuits has identified that the excessive anxiety experienced prior to, for example, a speaking task by people with social phobia, is associated with excessive EEG activation in the right anterior cortex (Davidson, Marshall, Tomarken, & Henriques, 2000). In addition, controlled exposure to a social stimulus (i.e., slides of faces) is accompanied by excessive amygdala activation (an increased fMRI signal) (Birbaumer et al., 1998; Stein, Goldin, Sareen, Zorrilla, & Brown, 2002). Another fMRI study illustrated that SAD patients demonstrate excessive orbitofrontal and amygdala activation upon face presentation, while reverse patterns are observed in antisocial personality disorder patients (Veit et al., 2002). Classical conditioning (pairing a neutral face with an aversive odor) has been associated with increased activation of both the amygdalar and hippocampal regions of the brain as measured by fMRI in SAD patients, while controls demonstrate the reverse of this activation pattern (Schneider et al., 1999).

On a neurochemical level, two extensive reviews (Hollander et al., 1998; Nutt, Bell, & Malizia, 1998) speculate that serotonin, GABA, and dopamine may all play key roles in the pathophysiology of SAD. There is also some evidence that oxytocin (anxiolytic effect) and vasopressin (anxiogeneic) are involved in the etiology of social behavior, aggression, and interaction (Heinrich & Domes, 2008).

Treatment

Psychological Treatments. Cognitive behavioral therapy (CBT) is an evidence-based psychotherapy for individuals with anxiety disorders (Acarturk, Cuijpers, van Straten, & de Graaf, 2008; Hoffman & Smits, 2008) and, in particular, SAD (Rodebaugh, Holaway, & Heimberg, 2004). CBT involves strategically and repeatedly practicing changing maladaptive behaviors and thoughts by using graded exposure to feared situations, applied relaxation, cognitive restructuring, and learning social skills. Research has demonstrated that CBT is effective in reducing SAD symptomology and may be associated with lower relapse rates (17%) than pharmacotherapy alone, which has demonstrated relapse rates of 30%–60% in a number of studies (Liebowitz, 1999; Rodebaugh, Holaway, & Heimberg, 2004).

Results from meta-analyses have suggested that group CBT (GCBT) and individual CBT (ICBT) yield similar treatment results (Liber et al., 2008; Manassis et al., 2002; Rodebaugh, Holaway, & Heimberg, 2004) in adolescents with GSAD. In one study, researchers randomized 73 adolescents (ages 12–17) to either ICBT, GCBT, or psychoeducational-supportive therapy (PST). Results indicated that all three conditions had comparable and significant reductions in anxiety symptomology and functional impairment at posttreatment with improvements in social skills and similar overall recovery rates. Despite these similarities, however, those in the GCBT condition maintained treatment gains at 6-month follow-up in 54% of subjects compared to only 15% in the ICBT group and 19% in the PST group, suggesting that the group environment afforded to subjects in the GCBT group may result in more long-term treatment gains (Herbert et al., 2008). A similar study of 78 children (ages 8–12) diagnosed with SAD and treated with either 12 weeks of GCBT or ICBT found that children with higher rates of anxiety responded preferentially to the ICBT treatment but that both groups showed significant improvements overall (Manassis et al., 2002).

Other studies have also found that individual therapy is superior in treating SAD compared to group therapy (Mortberg, Clark, Sundin, & Aberg Wistedt, 2007; Stanger, Heidenreich, Peitz, Lauterbach, & Clark, 2003). However, GCBT has been shown to be helpful versus a control condition for adolescents. A study of 35 adolescent females (mean age: 15.8 years old) examined 16 weeks of 1.5 hour sessions with no parental involvement during the therapy sessions. At posttreatment, 45% of the GCBT group no longer met criteria for SAD versus only 4% in the control group, mimicking results obtained in a previous study of five adolescents (Albano, Marten, Holt, Heimberg, & Barlow, 1995). At 1-year follow-up, however, 44% of the control group no longer met criteria for SAD versus 60% in the GCBT group, a no longer statistically significant difference (Hayward et al., 2000).

Although CBT involves exposing the subject to feared situations and has been shown to be effective in treating SAD, exposure might not be the most efficacious element of CBT. When comparing cognitive therapy (CT) to exposure therapy plus applied relaxation (EX+AR), researchers found that CT was superior at reducing social phobic symptoms compared to the EX+AR group. However, at the 1-year follow-up, more participants in the EX+AR group had received additional treatments compared to the CT group (Clark et al., 2006), suggesting that improvements in the EX+AR group may have been due to extra treatments and not the therapy conducted in the study exclusively.

A more recently developed treatment for SAD is mindfulness-based stress reduction (MBSR). In MBSR, individuals are taught how to be aware of the present moment and simultaneously reduce negative self-evaluations. One study examining the efficacy of MBSR in 53 GSAD subjects (mean age: 37.6 years old) found that subjects randomized either to MSBR or group CBT had similar clinical improvements in the areas of social anxiety, mood, and quality of life, but the group CBT had significantly higher remission and response rates relative to MBSR (Koszycki, Benger, Shlik, & Bradwejn, 2007). Since MBSR was helpful to approximately half of the individuals randomized to that condition (45% response rate), future studies should examine the efficacy of integrating mindfulness techniques into CBT.

As previously mentioned, some individuals with SAD fear being embarrassed in public and thus feel too anxious to attend therapy sessions at a counseling center. A more private version of therapy might be a better option for these individuals, such as Internet-based therapy (IBT). To investigate the effectiveness of IBT, researchers randomized 64 participants (ages 18–67) who met DSM-IV criteria for SAD into either a waitlist control or an IBT group. The IBT participants participated in a 9-week, Internet-based program with minimal therapist involvement (communication via e-mail) and had two group exposure activities in person. Compared to the waitlist control group, the IBT subjects made significant improvements in reported quality of life and significant decreases in both anxiety and depression levels (Andersson et al., 2006). However encouraging, limited research has been done in the area of Internet-based treatments, and consequently, more research needs to be conducted in order to better assess the efficacy of IBT in the treatment of SAD.

Pharmacological Treatment. Convincing young adults with SAD to consider psychotropic medications is often quite challenging. It requires significant discussions regarding medication-related side effects such as sexual dysfunction, weight gain, and suicidal thinking (McLeod, Pescosolido, Takeuchi, & White, 2004). These patients may feel awkward and burdened taking regular medications because they may believe their peers will be critical of them and have a heightened fear of being labeled as "weird" or "insane" (Pescosolido, Perry, & Martin, 2007; Schnittker, 2003).

Pharmacotherapy for SAD includes a variety of medication classes such as selective serotonin reuptake inhibitors (SSRIs), serotonin norepinephrine reuptake inhibitors (SNRIs), monoamine oxidase inhibitors (MAOIs), reversible inhibitors of monoamine oxidase type A (RIMAs), anticonvulsants, benzodiazepines, and beta-blockers.

SSRI medications such as sertraline and paroxetine are FDA-approved treatments for SAD, as is the SNRI, venlafaxine, and are considered to be the first-line medication treatment for SAD (Schneier, 2006). Several randomized, controlled studies have been conducted that report the efficacy of these medications for adolescents and young adults with SAD. In a study of 225 adolescents (ages 12–17) randomized to either paroxetine or placebo for a period of 16 weeks, 47.5% of the paroxetine group improved significantly compared to 20.7% of the placebo group (Wagner et al., 2004). A controlled study of escitalopram versus paroxetine versus placebo in 839 patients (ages 18–65) treated over a period of either 12 or 24 weeks showed a significant beneficial effect of escitalopram (20 mg) over paroxetine (20 mg) and placebo. However, both escitalopram and paroxetine proved to be significantly more efficacious treatments than placebo (Lader, Stender, Bürger, & Nil, 2004). In general, an adequate clinical trial of 8 to 12 weeks should be given before considering switching to other medications in the same class. Following stabilization, medications should generally be maintained for 12–18 months prior to discontinuation or dose tapering (Schneier, 2006).

Partial symptom improvement is the rule in SAD, and it may necessitate the addition of second-line pharmacotherapy such as benzodiazepines or off-label use of anticonvulsants (e.g., gabapentin). However, controlled studies have shown that the combination of benzodiazepines given with paroxetine or placebo results in no significant differences between the two treatment groups (Seedat & Stein, 2004). In addition, due to their potential for abuse, benzodiazepines should be prescribed with caution to younger adults and avoided in teenagers due to the likelihood of causing disinhibition. MAOI drugs should be considered as third-line agents for SAD, but they may be limited in their acceptability to the young adult population because of the restrictions of the low-tyramine diet. More novel off-label augmenting approaches may include coadministration of atypical neuroleptic agents.

Combination Psychotherapy and Psychopharmacology. Research investigating the combination of psychotherapy and psychopharmacology for SAD is limited and studies have produced mixed results. In one study of 295 subjects (mean age: 37.1 years) who met DSM-IV criteria for social phobia, researchers randomized the participants to either receive fluoxetine, CBT, CBT+fluoxetine, or CBT+placebo. At week 4, both fluoxetine-only and CBT-only were more effective at reducing social anxiety symptoms relative to the combined and placebo conditions. Yet at posttreatment (week 14), all active conditions (fluoxetine, CBT, and CBT+fluoxetine) were superior to the placebo conditions and were similar in their effectiveness in reducing social anxiety symptoms (Davidson et al., 2004).

Some studies have uncovered significant differences in treatment efficacy when comparing the combination of psychotherapy with psychopharmacology versus a placebo condition (Hoffman et al., 2006; Guastella et al., 2008). In two studies, participants received exposure therapy in addition to taking either D-Cycloserine, a glutamatergic partial N-methyl-d-aspartate (NMDA) agonist, or a placebo. When treatment was completed, researchers found that exposure plus D-Cycloserine resulted in significant reductions in social anxiety fears (Hoffman et al., 2006; Guastella et al., 2008), dysfunctional cognitions, and life impairment (Guastella et al., 2008) compared with placebo. A recent study evaluated the use of clonazepam alone versus clonazepam plus psychodynamic group therapy for 58 subjects with GSAD. After 12 weeks, the combination therapy group had significantly more improvement than the clonazepam-only group on the CGI-Improvement scale ($p = .03$) (Knijnik et al., 2008).

KEY POINTS

- As in the case of Cindy, it is not uncommon for patients with social anxiety disorder to be considered shy (Heiser, Turner, & Beidel, 2003). Most individuals with shy temperament tend to "grow out" of their shyness as they become young adults, but those with social anxiety disorder may become more shy or reclusive over time.
- Fear of social situations and being negatively evaluated are core features of SAD. These characteristic thoughts of SAD help to distinguish it from other anxiety disorders such as panic disorder (fear of panic itself is predominant) and GAD (everyday worries have become exaggerated).
- Difficulties adjusting to collegiate life are common in persons with SAD, which may result in social isolation. As demonstrated in the case vignette, self-medicating behaviors (such as using alcohol and/or drugs) are common ways to cope with the social anxiety and the desire to isolate in the young adult population. Consequently, it may be alcohol and/or drug abuse that motivates the individual to initially seek mental health care rather than the anxiety (Barry, 2005; Hsu & Alden, 2008).
- Cindy's case illustrates how a combination medication treatment may prove to be more beneficial than monotherapy. Due to the physiological response to fears about performing, a combination of CBT with controlled exposure plus an agent to control the pounding heart and sweating preperformance may prove to be beneficial for Cindy. As is seen in Cindy's case, it is important to screen for substance abuse and other psychiatric conditions, especially in the case of young adults if benzodiazepines are being considered in the treatment plan.

Panic Disorder

Case Vignette

Karrie is a 20-year-old female college student who presents with "intolerable" anxiety. She reports that she feels anxious and "panicky" when she is in closed spaces such as classrooms, theaters, and the grocery store. She describes physical manifestations of anxiety when in these places, such as increased heart rate, chest pain, sweating, headache, nausea, and a feeling of numbness in her fingers and toes. Physical examination revealed no underlying medical cause for these symptoms. In addition to somatic complaints, she reports experiencing intense urges to flee from many situations and, consequently, has had difficulty attending classes and participating in social activities. She reports that these symptoms worsened when she moved from her small hometown to a large city campus and that over the past few months, she has missed classes and her grades have fallen, something that was atypical for her in high school. Her social life also suffers, as she describes that attending places like restaurants, movies, and social gatherings is extremely difficult for her.

Clinical Characteristics

Epidemiological data suggest that panic disorder (PD) has lifetime rates of 3.5%–4.7% and current rates of 2.3%–2.7% in the general population (Kessler et al., 2005a; Kessler, Chiu, Demler, Merikangas, & Walters, 2005). Subsyndromal forms of PD occur in 7.5% of the population (Batelaan, de Graaf, van Balkom, Vollebergh, & Beekman, 2006). Women are twice as likely to be diagnosed with PD compared to men (Eaton, Kessler, Wittchen, & Magee, 1994). In addition, people who are unemployed, separated or divorced, and have lower levels of education have higher rates of PD (Faravelli & Paionni, 2001). Individuals with a history of PD often are seen in medical settings prior to seeking psychiatric care and have more frequent visits to emergency medicine, family medicine, and cardiology compared to patients with other anxiety disorders (Deacon, Lickel, & Abramowitz, 2008). Complaints of general fatigue, low productivity, and pain are often associated with PD, subsequently masking the disorder, and often result in underdiagnosis by treating physicians (Kaiya, Sugaya, Iwasa, & Tochigi, 2008; Zastrow et al., 2008). In many cases, PD often goes unrecognized, is misdiagnosed, and often times, goes untreated, causing deterioration in both the physical and mental health of an individual (Eguchi et al., 2005).

Comorbidity

Co-occurring psychiatric conditions are extremely common in individuals with PD. Studies have found high rates of comborbid anxiety (66%–93.6%), mood (50%–73.3%), impulse control (47%–59.5%), and substance use (27%–37.3%) disorders in subjects diagnosed with PD (Kessler et al., 2006). The poor quality of life secondary to PD is comparable to that reported by patients with major depressive disorder (Candilis et al., 1999).

Etiology

The onset of PD has been examined from two relevant aspects of neurobiology that integrate neuroanatomy and neurochemistry to explain the onset of PD (Goddard & Charney, 1997). The concept of a fear network in the brain has been proposed for fear induction in patients with PD. This "network" includes a variety of overly fear-sensitive mechanisms in the brain, including the prefrontal cortex, hypothalamus, amygdala, and insula (Gorman, Kent, Sullivan, & Coplan, 2000), suggesting a complex neurobiological pathway that may be implicated in patients with PD. Brain imaging studies have shown that anterior cingulate cortex (ACC) structural abnormalities may play an important role in patients with panic disorder. The insula and the ACC detect and evaluate any negative stimuli experienced from our surroundings. In response to these stimuli, the insula and ACC generate an aversive emotional response, which, in turn, generates panic-like symptoms (Graeff & Del-Ben, 2008). Researchers have found that there is reduction in the volume of the ACC with gray matter deficiency (Asami et al., 2008; Uchida et al., 2008). Other structural abnormalities include increases in gray matter volume in the insula and upper brain stem (Uchida et al., 2008) in PD subjects.

Neurochemistry also appears to play an important part in the generation of panic symptoms. Activation with NE pathways has long been associated with flight and fright response in animals and is strongly associated with increased panic-like symptoms (Shekhar, Katner, Sajdyk, & Kohl, 2002). As in other anxiety disorders and depression, reduced 5-HT1A receptor availability has been documented in PD patients though brain imaging (Nash et al., 2008) and illustrated through the effectiveness of treatment with selective-serotonin reuptake inhibitors (SSRIs). Freezing behavior in rats caused by the introduction of an unavoidable fear-inducing stimuli has shown that conditioned freezing and activation of the periaqueductal gray (PAG) may mimic the symptoms of both panic attacks and panic disorder (Brandão, Zanoveli, Ruiz-Martinez, Oliveira, & Landeira-Fernandez, 2008). Vasopressin is another neurotransmitter that plays a role in perpetuating panic symptoms and research has shown that blockage of their receptors reduces panic symptoms (Surget & Belzung, 2008). A general theory of anti-anxiety medications effect is in their ability to modulate the release of cortisol releasing factor (CRF) in the amygdala and hippocampus (Coplan, 2001). Animal models have shown a strong correlation of CRF role in panic symptoms (Sajdyk, Schober, Gehlert, & Shekhar, 1999).

Treatment

Psychological Treatment. Cognitive-behavioral therapy (CBT), which involves psychoeducation, skills for coping with and monitoring panic attacks, cognitive restructuring, and in vivo exposure, has been shown to be an effective treatment for PD. Using meta-analytic techniques on 124 articles, Mitte (2005) examined the efficacy of CBT treatment for subjects with PD with and without agoraphobia, finding an effect size of 0.87 for CBT compared to waitlist on measures of anxiety. When comparing CBT with behavioral therapy (BT), results showed that both CBT and BT were effective at reducing the anxiety associated with PD, but only CBT was associated with decreased rates of co-occurring depression (ES = 0.18) (Mitte, 2005). Another meta-analysis of 43 controlled studies of treatment interventions for PD found that studies which combined a cognitive-restructuring component along with an interoceptive exposure had the strongest effect sizes (0.88). The researchers also examined follow-up data and found that the CBT treatment effects were maintained overall by subjects in the studies examined (ES = 0.06) (Gould, Otto, & Pollack, 1995).

Other studies have further supported the efficacy of CBT while also investigating the effectiveness of more brief versions of CBT and CBT with minimal therapist involvement. In one study, 100 subjects (ages 19–65) meeting criteria for PD with agoraphobia were randomized to receive fourteen 1-hour sessions of weekly ICBT or GCBT, or seven 1-hour sessions of brief-intervention CBT every 2 weeks. All three groups showed significant improvement at therapy completion and maintained this improvement at 3-month follow-up (Roberge, Marchand, Reinharz, & Savard, 2008). In a similar randomized study that included 40 participants, results showed that four sessions of experimental cognitive therapy (an integration of traditional CBT with virtual reality exposure) was as effective as 12 sessions of traditional CBT (Choi et al., 2005).

Researchers have also examined the efficacy of Internet-based CBT with minimal therapist involvement. Studies have indicated that people with PD who participate in Internet-based CBT (Carlbring, Ekselius, & Andersson, 2003) with minimal therapist contact via e-mail or telephone (Klein, Richards, & Austin, 2006) have decreased PD symptomatology and that Internet-based CBT is equally effective as in-person therapy. One study included 49 subjects (mean age: 35.0 years) with PD (both with and without agoraphobia) who were randomized to receive either 10 weekly sessions (45–60 minutes each week) of in-person (IP), manualized therapy or an Internet-based treatment (IT), which included homework and participation in an online discussion group. At posttreatment, both groups had improved significantly on PD symptom severity measures, and 68.8% of the IP group and 61.5% of the IT group were classified as responders (Carlbring et al., 2005).

Psychodynamic psychotherapy has also demonstrated efficacy for PD in controlled studies. Panic-focused psychodynamic psychotherapy is brief and focuses on understanding the unconscious meaning of panic symptoms and resolving unconscious conflicts. In recent a clinical trial of 49 participants who met criteria for DSM-IV panic disorder, researchers found that subjects in the panic-focused psychodynamic psychotherapy group had significant reductions in symptom severity and function impairment when compared to the applied relaxation-training group (Milrod et al., 2007). To our knowledge, there are no current studies comparing the efficacy of CBT to psychodynamic psychotherapy; therefore, future research should explore this topic.

Breathing training may also be useful in controlling panic symptoms. Based on the assumption that respiratory dysregulation is a main component of PD, one study explored the efficacy of capnometry-assisted breathing therapy (BRT). The main goals of BRT include teaching subjects how to voluntarily and simultaneously reduce respiration rate and increase levels of carbon dioxide via breathing exercises. Education about the role breathing plays in the maintenance of PD symptoms is also provided to subjects. Thirty-seven participants with PD, both with and without agoraphobia, were randomized to receive 10 individual weekly sessions of BRT or a delayed-treatment control group. Researchers found that subjects in the BRT treatment significantly improved in terms of PD symptom severity, anxiety, respiratory measures, agoraphobic avoidance, and functional impairment compared to the control group (Meuret, Wilhelm, Ritz, & Roth, 2008).

Pharmacotherapy. Two SSRIs, paroxetine and sertraline, have been approved by the FDA to treat PD: however, case studies have shown that other SSRIs may also be beneficial (Goddard & Charney, 1998; Sheehan, 1999). Because of the delayed onset of action of SSRIs, a combination of both SSRIs and a benzodiazepine medication (especially longer-acting, high-potency benzodiazepines) has been shown to be beneficial in treating the symptoms of PD (Goddard et al., 2001). Other medications to consider are SNRIs (venlafaxine or venlafaxine extended release) (Sheehan, 2002) or tricyclic antidepressants (TCAs) (Andersch et al., 1991; Schweizer, Rickels, Weiss, & Zavodnick, 1993; Zitrin, Klein, Woerner, & Ross, 1983). Within the youth population, monitoring of suicidal ideation, sexual dysfunction, and potential abuse of benzodiazepines are crucial aspects of therapy. In general, TCAs and benzodiazepines should be avoided in teenagers with PD due to their potential toxicity through abuse.

In general, the acute phase of pharmacological treatment lasts up to 12 weeks. Patients who show no signs of improvement by 6–8 weeks of treatment initiation should be re-evaluated. Combination medication strategies may useful in refractory patients with PD, even though evidence for different combinations beyond SSRI and benzodiazepines is limited.

Combination Pharmacotherapy and Psychotherapy. Several studies have shown that the combination of pharmacotherapy with CBT is advantageous in reducing the symptom severity of PD. A recent study of 150 PD patients both with and without agoraphobia, examined the use of either SSRI, SSRI plus CBT, or CBT over a period of 9 months. Results indicated that all three treatments were significantly effective in treating PD, although the combination treatment was more effective than CBT alone (van Apeldoorn et al., 2008). However, differences between the combination of CBT plus SSRI group and mono-SSRI or mono-CBT were insignificant.

The combination of an SSRI or imipramine with CBT (Barlow, Gorman, Shear, & Woods, 2000; Coupland, 2008; Furukawa, Watanabe, & Churchill, 2006; Marchand et al., 2008), TCAs with CBT (Furukawa, Watanabe, & Churchill, 2006), SSRI or SNRI medications with CBT (Craske et al., 2005; Roy-Byrne et al., 2005) and benzodiazepines with exposure therapy (Cottraux et al., 1995; Marks et al., 1993) have all been shown to be beneficial for PD subjects in reducing anxiety and fear associated with the disorder. However, discontinuation of medication, even following CBT treatment, may result in limited symptom reduction and symptoms may reappear if medication is discontinued prematurely (Barlow, Gorman, Shear, & Woods, 2000; Marks et al., 1993). Consequently, further investigation regarding the efficacy of combination pharmacotherapy and psychotherapy is necessary in order to substantiate these findings.

> **KEY POINTS**
>
> - As illustrated in the case of Karrie, PD patients typically have distressing physical symptoms accompanying their anxiety, which can lead to increased fear about future physical sensations. These subjective responses to anxiety-provoking cues (i.e., physical symptoms) can cause individuals like Karrie to be wary of future panic attacks, resulting in increased anxiety of future fear.
> - People suffering from PD may often present to their primary care physician numerous times before receiving psychiatric treatment. These visits result in unnecessary medical expenses and frustration to the patient.
> - A variety of psychosocial and pharmacotherapeutic interventions have been shown to be helpful for patients with PD. Young adult patients like Karrie are common and may be unaware that treatment for their problem is available. Consequently, it is important for not only clinicians to be aware of the signs of PD but also for teachers and school administrations to be aware so that students presenting with signs of PD can find help.

Generalized Anxiety Disorder

Case Vignette

Brenda is a 22-year-old female who, over the past year, has reported feeling tremendous "stress and anxiety." She describes worrying about her job, finances, and maintaining an increasingly more difficult relationship with her fiancé. Brenda states that these worries are constantly present and associated with insomnia, fatigue, poor concentration, and memory. She describes herself as tense and irritable most of the time. She claims that she used to be outgoing and cheerful but has not felt like "herself" for approximately 1 year. After presenting to her primary care physician numerous times about her symptoms and reporting that it was not beneficial, she decided to consult with a psychiatrist due to her deteriorating mood.

Clinical Characteristics

Generalized anxiety disorder (GAD) is a syndrome characterized by excessive and constant worry over different life areas. The 1-year prevalence rate among the general population is approximately 1.6% to 3% with a lifetime prevalence of 5.1% to 6% (Kessler et al., 2005a).

Even though the mean age onset of GAD is in the mid-30s, it is a condition that affects all age groups including young adults (Kessler, Keller, & Wittchen, 2001). GAD is about twice as common in females and is more common in nonmarried people reporting a lower socioeconomic status and in racial minorities or ethnic groups (Wittchen, Zhao, Kessler, & Eaton, 1994). A majority of these individuals do not seek treatment from a psychiatrist but instead are seen by primary care physicians, cardiologists, and pulmonologists due to the physical symptoms often associated with the disorder. GAD is associated with considerable health care costs, lower work productivity, and high utilization of medical resources (Hoffman, Dukes, & Wittchen, 2008; Roy-Byrne et al., 2008).

Comorbidity

Research has shown that 90.4% of people with GAD also meet criteria for another lifetime psychiatric condition (Wittchen, Zhao, Kessler, & Eaton, 1994). Alcohol abuse, major depression, social anxiety, panic disorder, and specific phobias are among the most commonly reported comorbid conditions (Wittchen, Zhao, Kessler, & Eaton, 1994). These comorbid conditions further complicate proper diagnosis and treatment and may manifest following proper GAD treatment. Untreated, GAD has demonstrated long-term physical health effects, such as chronic fatigue, pain, and insomnia and a negative impact on overall functioning and quality of life (Roy-Byrne et al., 2008).

Etiology

There are several different biological models that have been implicated in the pathogenesis of GAD, but no singular theory can explain the complex neurobiology involved in the disorder. One proposed theory is the behavioral inhibition model (Gray, 1988), which involves the septohippocampal area, locus ceruleus, and median raphe nuclei in the brain. This model asserts that during acute stress and fear states, the hippocampus is placed on "high alert" by neurochemicals like norepinephrine and serotonin. Researchers have found that repeated activation of this area leads to hypervigilance and a chronic state of fear in the animals (Vianna, Coitinho, & Izquierdo, 2004). Two fMRI studies of children and adolescents with GAD found significant right amygdala activation in the prefrontal cortex when subjects were presented with images of threatening faces. The researchers noted a negative connectivity between the amygdala and the right ventrolateral prefrontal cortex, suggesting that increased activation in this part of the brain may be associated with less severe forms of anxiety (Monk et al., 2006; Monk et al., 2008).

Other proposed models such as the developmental vulnerability model hypothesize that the neurobiological impact of early life stressors may lead to the upregulation of CRF and the HPA axis (Nemeroff, 2004). Abnormal noradrenergic, serotonergic, and GABAergic functioning occurs in the patients with GAD (Jetty, Charney, & Goddard, 2001). Another model suggests that vasopressin also plays a role in anxiety and affective disorders and that antagonism of vasopressin reduces anxiety symptoms (Surget & Belzung, 2008).

Treatment

Psychotherapy. Psychotherapy, such as CBT and applied relaxation therapy (AR), has been clearly demonstrated to be an efficacious treatment for GAD (Canadian Psychiatric Association, 2006; Gorman, 2003; Hunot, Churchill, Teixeira, & de Lima, 2007). A recent meta-analysis (Hunot, Churchill, Teixeira, & de Lima, 2007) examined 13 studies comparing CBT to treatment as usual/wait list (TAU/WT). A significantly higher percentage (47% vs. 13%) of subjects in the CBT group clinically responded to treatment and had significantly reduced anxiety symptoms compared to TAU/WT. The same meta-analysis assessed six studies that compared CBT with supportive therapies, such as Rogerian and Gestalt therapies, transactional analysis, and discussion groups. At posttreatment and at 6-month follow-up (only three of the six studies completed a 6-month follow-up), CBT and supportive therapies did not significantly differ in clinical response rates. However, in terms of anxiety reduction, CBT was more effective than supportive therapy at post-treatment and 6-month follow-up (Hunot, Churchill, Teixeira, & de Lima, 2007). Another study provides further evidence to these results finding that CBT was superior to supportive therapies after 12 sessions of therapy. The CBT group maintained treatment gains, while subjects assigned to supportive therapy did not sustain improvements at posttreatment, 6-month, and 12-month follow-up assessments (Borkovec & Costello, 1993).

Applied relaxation (AR) is another form of therapy that has been used to treat GAD. In AR, patients learn progressive relaxation techniques, how to identify feared situations, and how to utilize relaxation skills in stressful situations (Arntz, 2003). In a study of 49 subjects with GAD, subjects were randomized to receive either AR or a waitlist control (WLC) for 12 weekly sessions. In an intention-to-treat analysis, 36% of AR patients were classified as significantly improved versus 5% of the WLC group. However, the researchers noted high dropout rates in the AR group, which affects the generalizability of the results (Conrad, Isaac, & Roth, 2008). Studies that have evaluated AR against CBT have found that both treatments are comparable in decreasing anxiety and depression (Borkovec & Costello, 1993; Ost & Breitholtz, 2000). One study suggested that AR may be more helpful than CBT in treating GAD, as evidenced by the fact that AR had higher rates of recovery than CBT at posttreatment (44.4%

compared to 35.0%). However, at the 6-month follow-up, both groups had similar recovery rates (53.3% compared to 50.0%) (Arntz, 2003), illustrating the effectiveness of both treatments.

Eye movement desensitization and reprocessing (EMDR) has also been studied in the treatment of GAD. Designed to treat trauma-related disorders, patients in EMDR focus on an emotionally upsetting event while simultaneously attending to an external stimuli, such as a laterally moving object with their eyes. In a small, noncontrolled study involving four GAD subjects treated with 15 sessions of EMDR, results showed that all subjects no longer met criteria for GAD at posttreatment and 2-month follow-up and their levels of anxiety and worry had significantly decreased (Gauvreau & Bouchard, 2008).

Pharmacotherapy. To date, there have been eight different medications that have been approved by the FDA for the treatment of GAD, including SSRIs (paroxetine, escitalopram), SNRIs (duloxetine, venlafaxine), benzodiazepines (diazepam, lorazepam, alprazolam), and an azapirone (buspirone). A meta-analysis of 39 pharmacotherapy interventions revealed an overall effect size of 0.60 for medication treatment of GAD (Gould, Otto, Pollack, & Yap, 1997). SSRIs are widely considered to be the first-line treatments for GAD (Davidson, Bose, Korotzer, & Zheng, 2004; Pollack et al., 2001); however, serotonergic antagonists such as agomelatine (an agonist of melatonergic [MT1, MT2] receptors) have recently been shown to be beneficial in treating GAD. A double-blind, placebo-controlled study randomized 121 subjects (mean age: 41.7 years old) to receive agomelatine or placebo for 12 weeks. Results indicated that agomelatine was associated with significant reductions in anxiety symptoms as measured by the CGI Improvement Scale (41.3% versus 22.4%) (Stein, Ahokas, & de Bodinat, 2008).

Benzodiazepines, such as lorazepam, alprazolam, and diazepam, which have all been FDA approved for the treatment of GAD, have been studied extensively. A meta-analysis of 23 studies using benzodiazepines revealed that diazepam had been evaluated the most (n = 11 studies) and had the largest treatment effect size (0.76) (Gould, Otto, Pollack, & Yap, 1997). These medications are generally helpful for patients taking an SSRI or SNRI where benefits may be delayed by up to 6 weeks. In addition, SNRIs may also help those with physical problems that often accompany GAD. For example, some research suggests that using an SNRI may address the neuropathic pain issues commonly associated with GAD (Allgulander et al., 2008; Hartford et al., 2008).

Similar to both SSRIs and SNRIs, buspirone, a 5-HT1A agonist or azapirone (AZA), has shown significant benefit to patients with GAD without a high side-effect profile. A review of 36 treatment studies (5,908 participants) of GAD revealed that azapirones were significantly beneficial in treating GAD, especially for patients that had not taken a benzodiazepine (Chessick et al., 2006).

Tricyclic medications such as imipramine have also been used in GAD. However, due to the lack of extensive evidence, poor tolerability, and with other options available, TCAs are rarely used to treat GAD.

In general, clinical improvement is noted at the 6- to 12-week mark after medication implementation; however, many clinicians suggest that the duration of the treatment should be at least 1 year after a good clinical response is achieved. Some studies have shown that off-label augmentation with other medications such as aripiprazole (Hoge et al., 2008; Menza, Dobkin, & Marin, 2007), olanzapine (Pollack et al., 2006), and risperidone (Simon et al., 2006) may be useful for refractory patients who do not receive desired benefit from first- or second-line pharmacotherapy. However, other studies have shown less augmentation benefit with medications such as quetiapine (Simon et al., 2008). Due to conflicting and limited data surrounding off-label augmentation, further research is necessary in order to identify viable treatments for treatment refractory patients.

Combined Psychological and Pharmacological Treatment. Few studies have examined whether combining psychosocial and pharmacological treatments improves outcome. One of the few studies to address this question demonstrated no significant difference between subjects receiving medication plus therapy versus those receiving only medication or only therapy (Lader & Bond, 1998). Another study randomized 101 GAD subjects into one of five treatment categories, one of which included diazepam plus CBT treatment, over a period of 9 weeks. Overall, 90% of subjects in the diazepam plus CBT group were classified as "very much improved" or "much improved" at the end of the 9 weeks, a significant difference from the diazepam only and CBT-only groups also included in the study (Power, Simpson, Swanson, & Wallace, 1990). However, the CBT group showed the lowest rate of follow-up treatments needed at a 6-month follow-up, regardless of whether the CBT group was with or without diazepam, suggesting that CBT alone might be as useful.

> **KEY POINTS**
>
> - As highlighted in the case above, the core features of GAD are constant worrying for more than 6 months along with the presence of three or more additional symptoms such as irritability, muscle tension, insomnia, fatigue, and poor concentration.
> - Issues that complicate the assessment of GAD are symptoms that overlap with affective disorder symptoms, such as fatigue, poor concentration, and irritability and the patient's tendency to under-report symptoms because of their chronic nature.
> - With many of the added pressures to adolescents and young adults to succeed in school and be involved in numerous activities, it is not uncommon for people to attribute their GAD symptoms to environmentally induced stress. Patients such as Brenda are examples of this attribution and, as a result, in many cases, do not seek treatment.

Posttraumatic Stress Disorder

Case Vignette

Meghan is a 30-year-old female graduate student who presented to her university mental health clinic for depressive symptoms. At her initial visit, Meghan reported feeling sad, tired, and anxious and reported that these symptoms had been affecting her schoolwork and social life. When asked about precipitating factors that she could attribute these feelings to, she reported that she had been sexually assaulted 2 months ago in a parking garage close to her current residence. She also stated that on occasion, she would have "flashbacks" of the attack, especially when getting her vehicle out of her home garage or while walking to her classes. In addition, Meghan described having vivid dreams of the incident and said that she was afraid to leave her home after dark. Because of this fear of leaving her residence and another reported fear of being around groups of people, she stated that she had stopped participating in most of the activities that she enjoyed prior to the attack. Over the past month, Meghan recounted feeling hopeless and hyper-vigilant. She endorsed frequent sleeping problems and a substantial problem concentrating. As a result, health and academic problems have become pervasive. During the interview, she cried repeatedly when describing the attack and said that she had not told anyone of the incident due to feelings of shame. She reported that she felt as though she should have been "more careful" in the garage and that the attack was essentially her fault.

Clinical Characteristics

Epidemiological data suggest that the lifetime prevalence rate for posttraumatic stress disorder (PTSD) is 6.8%, with a current prevalence of 3.6% in the general population (Kessler et al., 2005). With ongoing conflicts in Iraq and Afghanistan, a substantial amount of research on the rates of PTSD in young adult soldiers returning from combat has been conducted. A study of 2,530 Iraq/Afghanistan army veterans interviewed before deployment (86% between the ages of 18–29) and 3,671 Iraq/Afghanistan veterans interviewed 3–4 months following their return (83% between the ages of 18–29) demonstrated PTSD rates of 12.9% and 6.2% in these two groups, respectively (Hoge et al., 2004). Larger studies of 103,788 Iraq and Afghanistan war veterans found a prevalence rate of 13% and noted that younger veterans (ages 18–24) had a higher risk of PTSD and other psychiatric diagnoses (Seal, Bertenthal, Miner, Sen, & Marmar, 2007). These numbers are consistent with other war veteran groups. A study of 3.1 million Vietnam veterans conducted in 1990 found that 30% of Vietnam veterans had developed PTSD after returning home from combat and that up to 15% of those soldiers still had PTSD symptoms up to 19 years later (Kulka et al., 1990; Kulka et al., 1991). Significant morbidity and mortality is associated with PTSD, and overall, almost over half of male Vietnam veterans currently suffering from PTSD have been arrested and or jailed at least once, 34.2% more than once, and 11.5% have a felony conviction.

Within the general population, PTSD is usually caused by violent road traffic accidents, physical assaults, rape, or witnessing a murder. Among the victims of sexual assault, including rape in females, a much higher prevalence of around 50% is noted compared to nonsexual assault victims where the occurrence of PTSD is 30.8% (Foa, Rothbaum, Riggs, & Murdock, 1991). In fact, reports of PTSD symptoms in rape victims 1 week after the traumatic event have been reported in as high as 94% of victims (Foa, Rothbaum, Riggs, & Murdock, 1991).

Comorbidity

Co-occurring psychiatric conditions are extremely common in those with PTSD. Studies have shown that substance use problems and PTSD may be related to one another (Back, Brady, & Waldrop, 2008), with one study illustrating that comorbid substance use and PTSD comprised 52% of the sample (Kessler, Sonnega, Bromet, Hughes, & Nelson, 1995). In fact, a recent study of 988 young adult patients (ages 19–24) who had been exposed to trauma only or had PTSD found that PTSD, not trauma only, was predictive of substance abuse or dependence (Reed, Anthony, & Breslau, 2007). Major depressive disorder (48%), conduct disorder (43%), and phobias (31%) are common in men affected by PTSD (Vojvoda & Southwich, 2007).

Both men and women with PTSD have high rates of co-occurring disorders. One study found that 88% of men and 79% of women with PTSD also had a co-occurring psychiatric disorder, most commonly major depressive and alcohol use disorders (Kessler, Sonnega, Bromet, Hughes, & Nelson, 1995). Co-occurring anxiety disorders are also common in patients with PTSD with studies showing lifetime rates of panic disorder in 7%–21% of women and 7%–28% in men with PTSD (Orsillo, Raja, & Hammond, 2002).

Etiology

Several studies have established a relationship between PTSD and limbic system dysfunctions. Neuroimaging studies using proton magnetic resonance spectroscopy have supported this dysfunction and showed either neuronal loss or dysfunction in the hippocampus and anterior cingulated gyrus (Mahmutyazicioğlu et al., 2005). fMRI studies have also implicated neuronal abnormalities in the hippocampus and the anterior cingulated gyrus in dysfunctions of working memory (Moores et al., 2008). Animal models have established the role of the amygdala in PTSD, where experiments on rats exposed to prolonged stress caused morphological and neurochemical changes in its neuronal architecture (Cui, Samamoto, Higashi, & Kawata, 2008). Apart from structural changes, alterations in the neuroendocrine system may manifest as the core symptoms associated with PTSD. One such system is hypothalamic-pituitary-adrenal axis system and suggests increased sensitivity to stimuli, increased responsiveness of the glucocorticoid receptors, and decreased levels of cortisol (Young & Breslau, 2004) as possible underlying mechanisms (Brimes, Escande, Gourdy, & Schmitt, 2000).

Response to stress is an important part of functioning, but prolonged, repeated, and excessive stresses may cause profound changes/alterations in brain structures such as the amygdala,

ACG, hippocampus, and the HPA axis (Siegmund, Kaltwasser, Holsboer, Czisch, & Wotjak, 2008). Impact may also occur at the level of neurotransmitters like NE, serotonin, dopamine, and benzodiazepine. The net effect of alterations to memory, learning, and stress response may be poor outcomes in perceived quality of life (Vermetten & Bremner, 2002).

Treatment

Psychotherapy. Early intervention with supportive therapy, psychoeducation, and case management have been shown to be effective in the treatment of PTSD. Studies have suggested that certain aspects of CBT can be effective in treating trauma victims (Mueser et al., 2008). Studies have shown that exposure therapy, first used for phobia treatment, can also be used to treat those with PTSD. Techniques such as prolonged exposure and stress inoculation training (Foa, Rothbaum, Riggs, & Murdock, 1991) that involve focusing on specific details of the traumatic event have been helpful in treating PTSD in female victims of rape (Foa, Rothbaum, Riggs, & Murdock, 1991). Over time, the anxiety caused by remembering the traumatic event decreases. These techniques have also been shown to be helpful for combat veterans (Cooper & Clum, 1989).

Another form of therapy, called cognitive processing therapy (CPT), has been used to treat both PTSD and trauma-induced depression. It has been shown to be beneficial in treating rape victims (Resnick & Schnicke, 1992) and victims of childhood sexual abuse (Chard, 2005). Throughout therapy sessions, the patient first works on distorted beliefs about themselves and then works on an exposure component where subjects write descriptive accounts of their specific traumatic event. After these events are written down, they are then read aloud to the therapist. During this exposure component, distorted logic is addressed and patients are encouraged to openly express emotions (Resnick & Schnicke, 1992). This method differs from another therapeutic intervention known as "flooding" because subjects read the script aloud to the therapist. In the case of flooding, the traumatic event(s) is read aloud by the therapist, not the patient, in an effort to confront the most disturbing events and thoughts, until toleration and eventual extinction of the negative emotions occurs (Cooper & Clum, 1989).

More recently, virtual reality methods have been used to treat combat veterans and victims of the September 11, 2001 attack on the World Trade Center (Difede et al., 2007; Reger & Gahm, 2008). A study using 14 weeks of weekly virtual reality (VR) exposure therapy for 9 patients with PTSD who had limited symptom improvement through previous treatment with imaginal exposure compared to 11 subjects in a waitlist control (WL), found that 5 of 8 subjects who completed the VR therapy no longer met criteria for PTSD posttreatment. Furthermore, the effect size between VR and WL groups was 1.53 (Difede et al., 2007). Another study found that a period of six, 90-minute sessions where a simulation of combat missions in Iraq was presented to an Iraq veteran in his early 30s experiencing combat-related PTSD resulted in significant reductions in both psychological distress and PTSD (Reger & Gahm, 2008). These studies show the potential for the use of VR in the treatment of PTSD, and this needs to be explored further in future studies.

Group therapy has also been demonstrated to be beneficial for PTSD. A recent study of 127 adolescents (ages 13–19) exposed to war in Bosnia who met PTSD criteria were assigned to receive either manual-based group therapy or a control condition that consisted of psychoeducation and skill training. Researchers found that both groups improved significantly at both posttreatment and a 4-month follow-up on measures of both PTSD symptoms and depression scores. However, significantly more students in the manual-based group showed higher rate reduction of PTSD (81% versus 48%) and depressive (61% versus 47%) symptoms compared to the control group (Layne et al., 2008).

Group therapy was also shown to be an effective form of treatment for 102 war veterans treated over a period of up to 18 weeks. Each patient attended the two 3-hour groups per week. The study found that 81% of patients had clinically significant reductions in PTSD symptoms at the end of treatment (Ready et al., 2008).

Pharmacotherapy. SSRIs have shown some efficacy in double-blind, controlled studies where the core symptoms (avoidance, numbing, hypervigilance, and reexperiencing) associated with PTSD are treated (Brady et al., 2000; Davidson et al., 2001; Martenyi, Brown, Zhang, Prakash, & Koke, 2002; Tucker et al., 2001; Zohar et al., 2002). Currently, sertraline and paroxetine are the only FDA-approved medications for the treatment of PTSD. As such, SSRIs are consisted to be first-line medication treatments for PTSD. Research has shown that the SSRIs reduce the depressive symptoms associated with PTSD but are less advantageous in reducing parasypathetic responses commonly reported by subjects who report the re-experiencing of the traumatic event (Asnis, Kohn, Henderson, & Brown, 2004).

Consequently, it appears that noradrenergic blockage may help in managing the many physiological responses associated with PTSD (Blanchard, Kolb, Pallmeyer, & Gerardi, 1982; Debiec & LeDoux, 2006). Adrenergic-1 antagonists such as prazosin, have been shown to be beneficial in treating disturbing dreams associated with PTSD for combat veterans (Raskind et al., 2003). Alpha-2 receptor agonists such as clonidine and beta-adrenergic receptor blockers such as propranolol have been shown to be beneficial in reducing both the physiologic responses associated with traumatic events reported by both combat trauma-induced and civilian trauma-induced PTSD but also helpful in reducing PTSD-associated nightmares and depression (Boehnlein & Kinzie, 2007; Brunet et al., 2008; Taylor et al., 2008).

A recent study of 329 subjects with PTSD randomized to the SNRI venlafaxine or placebo for 6 months showed significant reductions in reexperiencing and avoidance for the venlafaxine group compared to placebo (Davidson et al., 2006).

Other medications such as MAOIs and tricyclic antidepressants have also been shown to be beneficial (Asnis, Kohn, Henderson, & Brown, 2004; Ursano et al,, 2004). Double-blind studies of imipramine, desipramine, and amitriptyline have all illustrated positive results in treating the symptoms of PTSD (Davidson et al., 1990; Kosten, Frank, Dan, McDougle, & Giller, 1991; Reist et al., 1989). In addition, medications such as anticonvulsants (carbamazepine, valproate, lamotrigine, gabapentin, topiramate) and antipsychotics (olanzapine, quetiapine, risperidone) have been shown to be helpful especially targeting the reexperiencing symptoms associated with PTSD (Berlin, 2007). Other medication trials have been conducted with a variety of results. A double-blind, placebo-controlled trial of the NMDA agonist, D-cycloserine, showed no significant improvements in PTSD symptoms compared to placebo (Heresco-Levy et al., 2002).

KEY POINTS

- Young females are in a higher risk group of trauma. The patient above is experiencing the typical symptoms of PTSD; she is very fearful and helpless at the occurrence of the traumatic incident. These feelings are followed by recurrent thoughts and dreams of the trauma, causing her immense psychological and physiological distress.
- Avoidance, sense of detachment, poor concentration, hypervigilance, and insomnia are the core symptoms of the disorder as depicted in the above clinical case.
- Meghan is currently in the acute occurrence stage of the PTSD as the duration of symptoms is less than 3 months. The condition is considered chronic if the duration is 6 months or more and delayed onset if the symptoms is expressed after 6 months of the stressor.
- Acute stress disorder (ASD), though a separate clinical diagnosis based on the DSM-IV-TR version, is clinically similar to PTSD. The main caveat is that the duration of the symptoms last for a minimum of 2 days to 4 weeks and occurs within the 4 weeks of the traumatic event. It

(Key Points continued)

emerges sooner at the exposure of the trauma and abates quickly. In addition, the patient experiences a subjective sense of detachment, dazed, derealization, depersonalization, and dissociative amnesia. If left untreated, it is likely to progress to PTSD.
- Due to the high morbidity and mortality rate associated with PTSD, it is extremely important for clinicians, teachers, military officers, and others within the community to recognize and provide treatment resources to those who have either witnessed or suffered a trauma. Research has shown that both psychosocial and pharmacotherapeutic interventions are helpful in treating the symptoms of PTSD and must be introduced to patients as soon as possible following the traumatic event in order to begin the recovery process.

PRACTICE GUIDELINES

- A combination of psychotherapy plus medication may be most beneficial for anxiety disorders.
- Clinicians need to screen for substance use disorders when benzodiazepines are being considered for treatment.
- Not all anxiety disorders are the same and careful diagnosis is needed as both pharmacological and psychosocial treatments differ depending upon which anxiety disorder is being treated.

Conclusions/Future Directions

Due to the high prevalence of anxiety disorders in the general population and their overlap with other areas of medicine, both clinician-based and public education is necessary (Goldner & Bilsker, 1995). Education may be helpful to not only fight against the negative stigma of anxiety disorders (Bekker & Mens-Verhulst, 2007), especially in young adults, but it may also potentially benefit insurance coverage for mental health. Continued research is necessary to evaluate the impact of psychiatric disorders upon gender differences (Bekker & Mens-Verhulst, 2007; Grant & Potenza, 2007). Areas such as neuroimaging (SPECT or fMRI) (Roth, 2008), molecular psychiatry, animal models (including translational research) (Glasgow, Magid, Beck, Ritzwoller, & Estabrooks, 2005; Roth, 2008), innovative clinical trials (Tunis, Stryer, & Clancy, 2003), pharmacogenetics (Broich & Möller, 2008), and refining different modes of psychotherapy and combining them with pharmacological interventions (Foa, Franklin, & Moser, 2002; Hyland, 1991) are all beneficial in learning more about these disorders. These types of expansions in the field of psychiatry can be achieved by bringing members of academia, public policy, and the community organizations together in order to increase awareness of these disorders and to work in harmony and as a team identifies further effective treatments (Vos et al., 2005). Furthermore, increased awareness of these disorders within the community may translate into more applied care in collegiate, military, and other settings where young adults populate.

References

Acarturk, C., Cuijpers, P., van Straten, A., & de Graaf, R. (2008). Psychological treatment of social anxiety disorder: A meta-analysis. *Psychological Medicine, 28*, 1–14.

Albano, A. M., Marten, P. A., Holt, C. S., Heimberg, R. G., & Barlow, D. H. (1995). Cognitive-behavioral group treatment for social phobia in adolescents.

A preliminary study. *Journal of Nervous and Mental Disease, 183*(10), 649–656.

Allgulander, C., Nutt, D., Detke, M., Erickson, J., Spann, M., Walker, D., Ball, S. G., & Russell, J. M. (2008). A non-inferiority comparison of duloxetine and venlafaxine in the treatment of adult patients with generalized anxiety disorder. *Journal of Psychopharmacology, 22*(4), 417–425.

American Psychiatric Association (APA). (2000). *Diagnostic and statistical manual of mental disorders* (4th ed.), Text Revision. Washington, DC: Author.

Andersch, S., Rosenberg, N. K., Kullingsjö, H., Ottosson, J. O., Bech, P., Bruun-Hansen, J., Hanson, L., Lorentzen, K., Mellergård, M., & Rasmussen, S. (1991). Efficacy and safety of alprazolam, imipramine and placebo in treating panic disorder. A Scandinavian multicenter study. *Acta Psychiatrica Scandinavica Supplementum, 365*, 18–27.

Andersson, G., Carlbring, P., Homström, A., Sparthan, E., Furmark, T., Nilsson-Ihrfelt, E., Buhrman, M., & Ekselius, L. (2006). Internet-based self-help with therapist feedback and in vivo group exposure for social phobia: A randomized controlled trial. *Journal of Consulting and Clinical Psychology, 74*, 677–686.

Arntz, A. (2003). Cognitive therapy versus applied relaxation as treatment of generalized anxiety disorder. *Behavior Research and Therapy, 4*, 633–646.

Asami, T., Hayano, F., Nakamura, M., Yamasue, H., Uehara, K., Otsuka, T., Roppongi, T., Nihashi, N., Inoue, T., & Hirayasu, Y. (2008). Anterior cingulate cortex volume reductions in patients with panic disorder. *Psychiatry and Clinical Neuroscience, 62*(3), 322–330.

Asnis, G. M., Kohn, S. R., Henderson, M., & Brown, N. L. (2004). SSRIs versus non-SSRIs in PTSD: An update with recommendations. *Drugs, 64*(94), 338–404.

Back, S. E., Brady, K. T., Waldrop, A. E., Yeatts, S. D., McRae, A. L., & Spratt, E. (2008). Early trauma and sensitivity to current life stressors in the individuals with and without cocaine addiction. *American Journal of Drug and Alcohol Abuse, 34*(4), 389–396.

Barlow, D. H., Gorman, J. M., Shear, K., & Woods, S. W. (2000). Cognitive behavior therapy, imipramine or their combination for panic disorder. *Journal of the American Medical Association, 283*, 2529–2536.

Barry, D. T. (2005). Measuring acculturation among male Arab immigrants in the United States: An exploratory study. *Journal of Immigration Health, 7*(3), 179–184.

Batelaan, N. M., De Graaf, R., Van Balkom, A. J., Vollebergh, W. A., & Beekman, A. T. (2006). Epidemiology of panic. *Tijdschr Psychiatry (Netherlands), 48*(3), 195–205.

Bekker, M. H., & van Mens-Verhulst, J. (2007). Anxiety disorders: Sex differences in prevalence, degree and background but gender neutral treatment. *Gender Medicine, 4*(Suppl. B), S178–S193.

Berlin, H. A. (2007). Antiepileptic drugs for the treatment of post-traumatic stress disorder. *Current Psychiatry Reports, 9*(4), 291–300.

Birbaumer, N., Grodd, W., Diedrich, O., Klose, U., Erb, M., Lotze, M., Schneider, F., Weiss, U., & Flor, H. (1998). fMRI reveals amygdala activation to human faces in social phobics. *Neuroreport, 9*(6), 1223–1226.

Blanchard, E. B., Kolb, L. C., Pallmeyer, T. P., & Gerardi, R. J. (1982). A psychophysiological study of post traumatic stress disorder in Vietnam veterans. *Psychiatry Quarterly, 54*(4), 220–229.

Boden, J. M., Fergusson, D. M., & Horwood, L. J. (2007). Anxiety disorders and suicidal behaviours in adolescence and young adulthood: Findings from a longitudinal study. *Psychological Medicine, 37*(3), 431–440.

Boehnlein, J. K., & Kinzie, J. D. (2007). Pharmacologic reduction of CNS noradrenergic activity in PTSD: The case for clonidine and prazosin. *Journal of Psychiatric Practice, 13*(2), 72–78.

Borkovec, T. D., & Costello, E. (1993). Efficacy of applied relaxation and cognitive-behavioral therapy in the treatment of generalized anxiety disorder. *Journal of Consulting and Clinical Psychology, 61*, 611–619.

Brady, K., Pearlstein, T., Asnis, G. M., Baker, D., Rothbaum, B., Sikes, C. R., & Farfel, G. M. (2000). Efficacy and safety of sertraline treatment of PTSD: A randomized controlled trial. *Journal of the American Medical Association, 283*(14), 1837–1844.

Brandão, M. L., Zanoveli, J. M., Ruiz-Martinez, R. C., Oliveira, L. C., & Landeira-Fernandez, J. (2008). Different patterns of freezing behavior organized in the periaqueductal gray of rats: Association with different types of anxiety. *Behavioral Brain Research, 188*(1), 1–13.

Brimes, P., Escande, M., Gourdy, P., & Schmitt, L. (2000). Biological factors in PTSD: Neuroendocrine aspects. *L'Encephale, 26*(6), 55–61.

Broich, K., & Möller, H. J. (2008). Pharmacogenetics, pharmacogenomics and personalized psychiatry: Are we there yet? *European Archives of Psychiatry and Clinical Neuroscience, 258*(Suppl. 1), 1–2.

Bruce, S. E., Yonkers, K. A., Otto, M. W., Eisen, J. L., Weisberg, R. B., Pagano, M., Shea, M. T., & Keller, M. B. (2005). Influence of psychiatric comorbidity on recovery and recurrence in generalized anxiety disorder, social phobia, and panic disorder: A 12-year prospective study. *American Journal of Psychiatry, 162*(6), 1179–1187.

Brunet, A., Orr, S. P., Tremblay, J., Robertson, K., Nader, K., & Pitman, R. K. (2008). Effect of post-retrieval propranolol on psychophysiologic responding during subsequent script-driven traumatic imagery in post-traumatic stress disorder. *Journal of Psychiatric Resesrach, 42*(6), 503–506.

Buckner, J. D., Timpano, K. R., Zvolensky, M. J., Robertson, K., Nader, K., & Pitman, R. K. (2008). Implications of comorbid alcohol dependence among individuals with social anxiety disorder. *Depression and Anxiety* [Epub ahead of print].

Canadian Psychiatric Association (2006). Clinical practice guidelines: Management of anxiety disorders. *Canadian Journal of Psychiatry, 51*(8, Suppl. 2), 9S–91S.

Candilis, P. J., Mclean, R. Y., Otto, M. W., Manfro, G. G., Worthington, J. J. 3rd, Penava, S. J., Marzol, P. C., & Pollack, M. H. (1999). Quality of life in patients with panic disorder. *Journal of Nervous and Mental Disorders, 187*(7), 429–434.

Carlbring, P., Ekselius, L., & Andersson, G. (2003). Treatment of panic disorder via the internet: A randomized trial of CBT vs. applied relaxation. *Journal of Behavior Therapy and Experimental Psychiatry, 34*, 129–140.

Carlbring, P., Nilsson-Ihrfelt, E., Waara, J., Kollenstam, C., Buhrman, M., Kaldo, V., Söderberg, M., Ekselius, L., & Andersson, G. (2005). Treatment of panic disorder: Life therapy vs. self-help via the internet. *Behavior Research and Therapy, 43*, 1321–1333.

Chard, K. M. (2005). An evaluation of cognitive processing therapy for the treatment of posttraumatic stress disorder related to childhood sexual abuse. *Journal of Consulting and Clinical Psychology, 73*(5), 965–971.

Chessick, C. A., Allen, M. H., Thase, M., Batista Miralha da Cunha, A. B., Kapczinski, F. F., de Lima, M. S., & dos Santos Souza, J. J. (2006). Azapirones for generalized anxiety disorder. *Cochrane Database System Reviews, 3*, CD006115.

Choi, Y. H., Vincelli, F., Riva, G., Wiederhold, B. K., Lee, J. H., & Park, K. H. (2005).Effects of group experiential cognitive therapy for the treatment of panic disorder with agoraphobia. *Cyberpsychology & Behavior, 8*, 387–393.

Clark, D. M., Ehlers, A., Hackmann, A., McManus, F., Fennell, M., Grey, N., Waddington, L., & Wild, J. (2006). Cognitive therapy versus exposure and applied relaxation in social phobia: A randomized controlled trial. *Journal of Counseling and Clinical Psychology, 74*, 568–578.

Conrad, A., Isaac, L., & Roth, W. T. (2008). The psychophysiology of generalized anxiety disorder: 2. Effects of applied relaxation. *Psychophysiology, 45*(3), 377–388.

Cooper, N. A., & Clum, G. A. (1989). Imaginal flooding as a supplementary treatment for PTSD in combat veterans: A controlled study. *Behavior Therapy, 20*, 381–391.

Coplan, J. D. (2001). Novel perspectives of central CRF/HPA axis dysfunction across a spectrum of clinical conditions and experimental primate model. *CNS Spectrum, 6*(7), 554.

Cottraux, J., Note, I. D., Cungi, C., Legeron, P., Heim, F., Chneiweiss, L., Bernard, G., & Bouvard, M. (1995). A controlled study of cognitive behavior therapy with buspirone or placebo in panic disorder with agoraphobia. *British Journal of Psychiatry, 167*, 635–641.

Coupland, N. (2008). Combined antidepressants and CBT for panic disorder with agoraphobia. *Journal of Psychiatry and Neuroscience, 33*, E1.

Craske, M. G., Golinelli, D., Stein, M. B., Roy-Byrne, P., Bystritsky, A., & Sherbourne, C. (2005). Does the addition of cognitive behavioral therapy improve panic disorder treatment outcome relative to medication alone in the primary-care setting. *Psychological Medicine, 35*, 1645–1654.

Cui, H., Sakamoto, S. H., Higashi, S., & Kawata, M. (2008). Effects of single prolonged stress on neurons and their afferent inputs in the amygdala. *Neuroscience, 152*(3), 703–712.

Davidson, J., Baldwin, D., Stein, D. J., Kuper, E., Benattia, I., Ahmed, S., Pedersen, R., & Musgnung, J. (2006). Treatment of posttraumatic stress disorder with venlafaxine extended release: A 6-month randomized controlled trial. *Archives of General Psychiatry, 63*(10),1158–1165.

Davidson, J. R., Bose, A., Korotzer, A., & Zheng, H. (2004). Escitalopram in the treatment of generalized anxiety disorder: Double-blind, placebo controlled, flexible-dose study. *Depression and Anxiety, 19*(4), 234–240.

Davidson, J. R. T., Foa, E. B., Huppert, J. D., Keefe, F. J., Franklin, M. E., Compton, J. S., Zhao, N., Connor, K. M., Lynch, T. R., & Gadde, K. M. (2004). Fluoxetine, comprehensive cognitive behavioral therapy, and placebo in generalized social phobia. *Archives of General Psychiatry, 61*, 1005–1013.

Davidson, J., Kudler, R., Smith, S. L., Mahorney, S. L., Lipper, S., Hammett, E., Saunders, W. B., & Cavenar, J. O. Jr. (1990). Treatment of posttraumatic stress disorder with amitriptyline and placebo. *Archives of General Psychiatry, 47*(3), 259–266.

Davidson, R. J., Marshall, J. R., Tomarken, A. J., & Henriques, J. B. (2000). While a phobic waits: Regional brain electrical and autonomic activity in social phobics during anticipation of public speaking. *Biological Psychiatry, 47*(2), 85–95.

Davidson, J., Pearlstein, T., Londborg, P., Brady, K. T., Rothbaum, B., Bell, J., Maddock, R., Hegel M. T., & Farfel, G. (2001). Efficacy of sertraline in preventing relapse of posttraumatic stress disorder: Results of a 28-week double-blind, placebo-controlled study. *American Journal of Psychiatry, 158*(12), 1974–1981.

Deacon, B., Lickel, J., & Abramowitz, J. S. (2008). Medical utilization across the anxiety disorders. *Journal of Anxiety Disorders, 22*(2), 344–350.

Debiec, J., & LeDoux, J. E. (2006). Noradrenergic signaling in the amygdala contributes to the reconsolidation of fear memory: Treatment implications for PTSD. *Annals of the New York Academy of Sciences, 1071*, 521–524.

Difede, J., Cukor, J., Jayasinghe, N., Patt, I., Jedel, S., Spielman, L., Giosan, C., & Hoffman, H. G. (2007). Virtual reality exposure therapy for the treatment of posttraumatic stress disorder following September 11, 2001. *Journal of Clinical Psychiatry, 68*(11), 1639–1647.

Eaton, W. W., Kessler, R. C., Wittchen, H. U., & Magee, W. J. (1994). Panic and panic disorder in the United States. *American Journal of Psychiatry, 151*, 413–420.

Eguchi, M., Noda, Y., Nakano, Y., Kanai, T., Yamamoto, I., Watanabe, N., Lee, K., Ogawa, S., Ietsugu, T., Sasaki, M., Chen, J., & Furukawa, T. A. (2005). Quality of life and social role functioning in Japanese patients with panic disorder. *Journal of Nervous and Mental Disorders, 193*(10), 686–689.

Faravelli, C., & Paionni, A. (2001). Panic disorder: Clinical course, morbidity and comorbidity. In E. J. L. Griez, C. Faravelli, D. Nutt, and J. Zohar (Eds.), *Anxiety disorders: An introduction to clinical management and research*. Chichester, England: John Wiley & Sons.

Foa, E. B., Franklin, M. E., & Moser, J. (2002). Context in the clinic: How well do cognitive behavioral therapies and medications work in combination? *Biological Psychiatry, 52*(10), 987–997.

Foa, E. B., Rothbaum, B. O., Riggs, D. S., & Murdock, T. B. (1991). Treatment of posttraumatic stress disorder in rape victims: A comparison between cognitive-behavioral procedures and counseling. *Journal of Consulting and Clinical Psychology, 59*(5), 715–723.

Furukawa, T. A., Watanabe, N., & Churchill, R. (2006). Psychotherapy plus antidepressant for panic disorder with or without agoraphobia. *British Journal of Psychiatry, 188*, 305–312.

Gauvreau, P., & Bouchard, S. (2008). Preliminary evidence for the efficacy of EMDR in treating generalized anxiety disorder. *Journal of EMDR Practice and Research, 2*, 26–40.

Glasgow, R. E., Magid, D. J., Beck, A., Ritzwoller, D., & Estabrooks, P. A. (2005). Practical clinical trials for translating research to practice: Design and measurement recommendations. *Medical Care, 43*(96), 551–517.

Goddard, A. W., Brouette, T., Ahmad, A., Jetty, P., Woods, S. W., & Charney, D. (2001). Early coadminstration of clonazepam with sertraline for panic disorder. *Archives of General Psychiatry, 58*(7), 681–686.

Goddard, A. W., & Charney, D. S. (1997). Toward an integrated neurobiology of panic disorder. *Journal of Clinical Psychiatry, 58*(Suppl. 2), 4–11.

Goddard, A. W., & Charney, D. S. (1998). SSRIs in the treatment of panic disorder. *Depression and Anxiety, 8*(Suppl. 1), 114–120.

Goldner, E. M., & Bilsker, D. (1995). Evidence-based psychiatry. *Canadian Journal of Psychiatry, 40*(2), 97–101.

Gorman, J. M. (2003). Treating generalized anxiety disorder. *Journal of Clinical Psychiatry, 64*(Suppl. 2), 24–29.

Gorman, J. M., Kent, J. M., Sullivan, G. M., & Coplan, J. D. (2000). Neuroanatomical hypothesis of panic disorder, revised. *American Journal of Psychiatry, 157*(4), 493–505.

Gould, R. A., Otto, M. W., & Pollack, M. H. (1995). A meta-analysis of treatment outcome for panic disorder. *Clinical Psychology Review, 15*(8), 819–844.

Gould, R. A., Otto, M. W., Pollack, M. H., & Yap, L. (1997). Cognitive behavioral and pharmacological treatment of generalized anxiety disorder: A preliminary meta-analysis. *Behavior Therapy, 28*, 285–305.

Graeff, F. G., & Del-Ben, C. M. (2008). Neurobiology of panic disorder: From animal models to brain neuroimaging. *Neuroscience and Biobehavioral Reviews, 32*(7), 1326–1335.

Grant, B. F., Hasin, D. S., Blanco, C., Stinson, F. S., Chou, S. P., Goldstein, R. B., Dawson, D. A., Smith, S., Saha, T. D., & Huang, B. (2005). The epidemiology of social anxiety disorder in the United States: Results from the National Epidemiologic Survey on Alcohol and Related Conditions. *Journal of Clinical Psychiatry, 66*(11), 1351–1361.

Grant, J. E., & Potenza, M. N. (2007). *Textbook of men's mental health*. Washington, DC: American Psychiatric Association.

Gray, J. A. (1988). The neuropsychological basis of anxiety. In G. C. Last (Ed.), *Handbook of anxiety disorders*. New York: Pergamon.

Guastella, A. J., Richardson, R., Lovibond, P. F., Rapee, R. M., Gaston, J. E., Mitchell, P., & Dadds, M. R. (2008). A randomized controlled trial of D-Cycloserine enhancement of exposure therapy for social anxiety disorder. *Biological Psychiatry, 63*(6), 544–549.

Hartford, J. T., Endicott, J., Kornstein, S. G., Allgulander, C., Wohlreich, M. M., Russell, J. M., Perahia, D. G. S., & Erickson, J. S. (2008). Implication of pain in generalized anxiety disorder: Efficacy of duloxetine. *Journal of Clinical Psychiatry, 10*(3), 197–204.

Hayward, C., Varady S., Albano, A. M., Thienemann, M., Henderson, L., & Schatzberg, A. F. (2000). Cognitive-behavioral group therapy for social phobia in female adolescents: Results of a pilot study. *Journal of the American Academy of Child and Adolescent Psychiatry, 39*(6), 721–726.

Heinrich, M., & Domes, G. (2008). Neuropeptides and social behaviour: Effects of oxytocin and vasopressin in humans. *Progress in Brain Research, 170,* 337–350.

Heiser, N. A., Turner, S. M., & Beidel, D. C. (2003). Shyness: Relationship to social phobia and other psychiatric disorders. *Behavior and Research Therapy, 41*(2), 209–221.

Herbert, J. D., Gaudiano, B. A., Rheingold, A. A., Moitra, E., Myers, V. H., Dalrymple, K. L., & Brandsma, L. L. (2008). Cognitive behavior therapy for generalized social anxiety disorder in adolescents: A randomized controlled trial. *Journal of Anxiety Disorders* [Epub ahead of print].

Heresco-Levy, U., Kremer, I., Javitt, D. C., Goichman, R., Reshef, A., Blanaru, M., & Cohen, T. (2002). Pilot-controlled trial of D-cycloserine for the treatment of PTSD. *International Journal of Neuropsychopharmacology, 5*(4), m301–307.

Hermann, C., Ziegler, S., Birbaumer, N., & Flor, H. (2002). Psychophysiological and subjective indicators of aversive pavlovian conditioning in generalized social phobia. *Biological Psychiatry, 52*(4), 328–337.

Hoffman, D. L., Dukes, E. M., & Wittchen, H. U. (2008). Human and economic burden of generalized anxiety disorder. *Depression and Anxiety, 25*(1), 72–80.

Hoffman, S. G., Meuret, A. E., Smits, J. A, Simon, N. M., Pollack, M. H., Eisenmenger, K, Shiekh, M., & Otto, M. W. (2006). Augmentation of exposure therapy with D-Cycloserine for social anxiety disorder. *Archives of General Psychiatry, 63*(3), 298–304.

Hoffman, S. G., & Smits, J. A. (2008). Cognitive-behavioral therapy for adult anxiety disorders: A meta-analysis of randomized placebo-controlled trials. *Journal of Clinical Psychiatry, 69*(4), 621–632.

Hoge, C. W., Castro, C. A., Messer, S. C., McGurk, D., Cotting, D. I., & Koffman, R. L. (2004). Combat duty in Iraq and Afghanistan, mental health problems, and barriers to care. *New England Journal of Medicine, 351*(1),13–22.

Hoge, E. A., Worthington, J. J. III, Kaufman, R. E., Delong, H. R., Pollack, M. H., & Simon, N. M. (2008). Aripiprazole as augmentation treatment of refractory generalized anxiety disorder and panic disorder. *CNS Spectrum, 13*(6), 522–527.

Hollander, E., Kwon, J., Weiller, F., Cohen, L., Stein, D. J., DeCaria, C., Liebowitz, M., & Simeon, D. (1998). Serotonergic function in social phobia: Comparison to normal control and obsessive-compulsive disorder. *Psychiatry Research, 79*(3), 213–217.

Hsu, L., & Alden, L. E. (2008). Cultural influence on willingness to seek treatment for social anxiety in Chinese- and European-heritage students. *Cultural Diversity and Ethnic Minority Psychology, 14*(3), 215–223.

Hunot, V., Churchill, R., Teixeira, V., & de Lima, M. S. (2007). Psychological therapies for generalised anxiety disorder. Cochrane Database of Systematic Reviews. Issue 1(CD001848).

Hyland, J. M. (1991). Integrating psychotherapy and pharmacotherapy. *Bulletin of the Menninger Clinic, 55*(2), 205–215.

Jetty, P. V., Charney, D. S., & Goddard, A. W. (2001). Neurobiology of generalized anxiety disorder. *Psychiatric Clinics of North America, 24*(1), 75–97.

Kaiya, H., Sugaya, N., Iwasa, R., & Tochigi, M. (2008). Characteristics of fatigue in panic disorder patients. *Psychiatry and Clinical Neuroscience, 62*(2), 234–237.

Kessler, R. C., Berglund, P., Demler, O., Jin, R., Merikangas, K. R., & Walters, E. E. (2005). Lifetime prevalence and age-of-onset distributions of DSM-IV disorders in the National Comorbidity Survey Replication. *Archives of General Psychiatry, 62*(6), 593–602.

Kessler, R. C., Chiu, W. T., Demler, O., Merikangas, K. R., & Walters, E. E. (2005). Prevalence, severity, and comorbidity of 12 month DSM-IV disorders in the national comorbidity survey replication. *Archives of General Psychiatry, 62*(6), 617–627.

Kessler, R. C., Chiu, W. T., Jin, R., Ruscio, A. M., Shear, K., & Walters, E. E. (2006). The epidemiology of panic attacks, panic disorder, and agoraphobia in the national comorbidity survey replication. *Archives of General Psychiatry, 63,* 415–424.

Kessler, R. C., Keller, M. B., & Wittchen, H. U. (2001). The epidemiology of generalized anxiety disorder. *Psychiatric Clinics of North America, 24*(1), 19–39.

Kessler, R. C., McGonagle, K. A., Zhao, S., Nelson, C. B., Hughes, M., Eshleman, S., Wittchen, H. U., & Kendler, K. S. (1994). Lifetime and 12-month prevalence of DSM-III-R psychiatric disorders in the United States. Results from the National Comorbidity Survey. *Archives of General Psychiatry, 51*(1), 8–19.

Kessler, R. C., Sonnega, A., Bromet, E., Hughes, M., & Nelson, C. B. (1995). Posttraumatic stress disorder in the national comorbidity survey. *Archives of General Psychiatry, 52*(12), 1048–1060.

Kessler, R. C., Stein, M. B., & Berglund, P. (1998). Social phobia subtypes in the national comorbidity survey. *American Journal of Psychiatry, 155*(5), 613–619.

Klein, B., Richards, J. C., & Austin, D. W. (2006). Efficacy of internet therapy for panic disorder. *Journal of Behavior Therapy and Experimental Psychiatry, 37*, 213–238.

Knijnik, D. Z., Blanco, C., Salum, G. A., Moraes, C. U., Mombach, C., Almeida, E., Pereira, M., Strapasson, A., Manfro, G. G., & Eizirik, C. L. (2008). A pilot study of clonazepam versus psychodynamic group therapy plus clonazepam in the treatment of generalized social anxiety disorder. *European Psychiatry* [Epub ahead of print].

Kosten, T. R., Frank, J., Dan, E., McDougle, C. J., & Giller, E. L. Jr. (1991). Pharmacotherapy for posttraumatic stress disorder using phenelzine or imipramine. *Journal of Nervous Mental Disorders, 179*(6), 366–370.

Koszycki, D., Benger, M., Shlik, J., & Bradwejn, J. (2007). Randomized trial of a meditation-based stress reduction program and cognitive behavior therapy in generalized social anxiety disorder. *Behavior Research and Therapy, 45*, 2518–2526.

Kulka, R. A., Schlenger, W. E., Fairbank, J. A., Hough, R. L., Jordan, B. K., Marmar, C. R., & Weiss, D. S. (1990). *Trauma and the Vietnam War generation*. New York: Brunner/Mazel.

Kulka, R. A., Schlenger, W. E., Fairbank, J. A., Jordan, B. K., Hough, R. L., Marmar, C. R., & Weiss, D. S. (1991). Assessment of posttraumatic stress disorder in the community: Prospects and pitfalls from recent studies of Vietnam Veterans. *Psychological Assessment: A Journal of Consulting and Clinical Psychology, 3*, 547–560.

Lader, M. H., & Bond, A. J. (1998). Interaction of pharmacological and psychological treatments of anxiety. *British Journal of Psychiatry, 173*(Suppl. 34), 165.

Lader, M., Stender, K., Bürger, V., & Nil, R. (2004). Efficacy and tolerability of escitalopram in 12- and 24-week treatment of social anxiety disorder: Randomised, double-blind, placebo-controlled, fixed-dose study. *Depression and Anxiety, 19*(4), 241–248.

Layne, C. M., Saltzman, W. R., Poppleton, L., Burlingame, G. M., Pasalić, A., Duraković, E., Musić, M., Campara, N., Dapo, N., Arslanagić, B., Steinberg, A. M., & Pynoos, R. S. (2008). Effectiveness of a school-based group psychotherapy program for war-exposed adolescents: A randomized controlled trial. *Journal of the American Academy of Child and Adolescent Psychiatry, 47*(9), 1048–1062.

Lecrubier, Y., & Weiller, E. (1997). Comorbidities in social phobia. *International Clinical Psychopharmacology, 12*(Suppl. 6), S17–S21.

Lepine, J. P. (2002). The epidemiology of anxiety disorders: Prevalence and societal cost. *Journal of Clinical Psychiatry, 63*(Suppl. 14), 4–8.

Liber, J. M., van Widenfelt, B. M., Uten, E. M., Ferdinand, R. F., Van der Leeden, A. J., Van Gastel, W., & Treffers, P. D. (2008). No differences between group versus individual treatment of childhood anxiety disorders in a randomized clinical trial. *Journal of Child Psychology and Psychiatry, 49*, 886–893.

Liebowitz, M. R. (1999). Update on the diagnosis and treatment of social anxiety disorder. *Journal of Clinical Psychiatry, 60*(Suppl. 18), 22–26.

Magee, W. J., Eaton, W. W., Wittchen, H. U., McGonagle, K. A., & Kessler, R. C. (1996). Agoraphobia, simple phobia and social phobia in the national comorbidity survey. *Archives of General Psychiatry, 53*(2), 159–168.

Mahmutyazicioğlu, K., Konuk, N., Ozdemir, H., Atasoy, N., Atik, L., & Gündoğdu, S. (2005). Evaluation of the hippocampus and the anterior cingulate gyrus by proton MR spectroscopy in patients with post-traumatic stress disorder. *Diagnostic Intervention Radiology, 11*(3), 125–129.

Manassis, K., Mendlowitz, S. L., Scapillato, D., Avery, D., Fiksenbaum, L., Freire, M., Monga, S., & Owens, M. (2002). Group and individual cognitive-behavioral therapy for childhood anxiety disorders: A randomized trial. *Journal of the American Academy of Child and Adolescent Psychiatry, 41*(12), 1423–1430.

Marchand, A., Coutu, M. F., Dupuis, G., Fleet, R., Borgeat, F., Todorov, C., & Mainguy, N. (2008). Treatment of panic disorder with agoraphobia: Randomized placebo-controlled trial of four psychosocial treatments combined with imipramine or placebo. *Cognitive Behavior Therapy, 37*(3), 146–159.

Marks, I. M., Swinson, R. P., Basoglu, M., Kuch, K., Noshirvani, H., O'sullivan, G., Lelliott, P. T., Kirby, M., McNamee, G., & Sengun, S. (1993). Alprazolam and exposure alone and combined in panic disorder with agoraphobia: A controlled study in London and Toronto. *British Journal of Psychiatry, 162*, 776–787.

Martenyi, F., Brown, E. B., Zhang, H., Prakash, A., & Koke, S. C. (2002). Fluoxetine versus placebo in posttraumatic stress disorder. *Journal of Clinical Psychiatry, 63*(3), 199–206.

McLeod, J. D., Pescosolido, B. A., Takeuchi, D. T., & White, T. F. (2004). Public attitudes towards the use of psychiatric medications for children. *Journal of Health and Social Behavior, 45*(1), 53–67.

Menza, M. A., Dobkin, R. D., & Marin, H. (2007). An open-label trial of aripiprazole augmentation for treatment-resistant generalized anxiety disorder. *Journal of Clinical Psychopharmacology, 27*(2), 207–210.

Meuret, A. E., Wilhelm, F. H., Ritz, T, & Roth, W. T. (2008). Feedback of end-tidal pCO_2 as a therapeutic approach for panic disorder. *Journal of Psychiatric Research, 42*, 560–568.

Milrod, B., Leon, A. C., Busch, F., Rudden, M., Schwalberg, M., Clarkin, J., Aronson, A., Singer, M., Turchin, W., Klass, E. T., Graf, E., Teres, J. J., & Shear, M. K. (2007). A randomized controlled clinical trial of psychoanalytic psychotherapy for panic disorder. *American Journal of Psychiatry, 164*, 265–272.

Mitte, K. (2005). A meta-analysis of the efficacy of psycho-and pharmacotherapy in panic disorder with and without agoraphobia. *Journal of Affective Disorders, 88*, 27–45.

Monk, C. S., Nelson, E. E., McClure, E. B., Mogg, K., Bradley, B. P., Leibenluft, E., Blair, R. J., Chen, G., Charney, D. S., Ernst, M., Pine, D. S. (2006). Ventrolateral prefrontal cortex activation and attentional bias in response to angry faces in adolescents with generalized anxiety disorder. *American Journal of Psychiatry, 163*(6),1091–1097.

Monk, C. S., Telzer, E. H., Mogg, K., Bradley, B. P., Mai, X., Louro, H. M., Chen, G., McClure-Tone, E. B., Ernst, M., & Pine, D. S. (2008). Amygdala and ventrolateral prefrontal cortex activation to masked angry faces in children and adolescents with generalized anxiety disorder. *Archives of General Psychiatry, 65*(5), 568–576.

Moores, K. A., Clark, C. R., McFarlane, A. C., Brown, G. C., Puce, A., & Taylor, D. J. (2008). Abnormal recruitment of working memory updating networks during maintenance of trauma-neutral information in PTSD. *Psychiatry Research, 163*(2), 156–170.

Mortberg, E., Clark, D. M., Sundin, O., & Aberg Wistedt, A. (2007). Intensive group cognitive therapy treatment and individual cognitive therapy vs. treatment as usual in social phobia: A randomized controlled trial. *Acta Psychiatrica Scandinavica, 115*, 142–154.

Mueser, K. T., Rosenberg, S. D., Xie, H., Jankowski, M. K., Bolton, E. E., Lu, W., Hamblen, J. L., Rosenberg, H. J., McHugo, G. J., & Wolfe, R. (2008). A randomized controlled trial of cognitive-behavior treatment for PTSD in severe mental illness. *Journal of Consulting and Clinical Psychology, 76*(2), 259–271.

Nash, J. R., Sargent, P. A., Rabiner, E. A., Hood, S. D., Argyropoulos, S. V., Potokar, J. P., Grasby, P. M., & Nutt, D. J. (2008). Serotonin 5-HT1A receptor binding in people with panic disorder: Positron emission tomography study. *British Journal of Psychiatry, 193*(3), 229–234.

Nemeroff, C. B. (2004). Early life adversity, CRF dysregulation and vulnerability to mood and vulnerability to mood and anxiety disorders. *Psychopharmacology Bulletin, 38*(Suppl. 1), 14–20.

Nutt, D. J., Bell, C. J., & Malizia, A. L. (1998). Brain mechanisms of social anxiety disorders. *Journal of Clinical Psychiatry, 59*(Suppl. 17), 4–11.

Orsillo, S. M., Raja, S., & Hammond, C. (2002). Gender Issues in PTSD with comorbid mental health disorders. In R. Kimerling, P. Ouimette, J. Wolfe (Eds.), *Gender and PTSD*. New York: Guilford Press.

Ost, L. G., & Breitholtz, E. (2000). Applied relaxation vs. cognitive therapy in the treatment of generalized anxiety disorder. *Behavior and Research Therapy, 38*, 777–790.

Pescosolido, B. A., Perry, B. L., & Martin, J. K. (2007). Stigmatizing attitudes and beliefs about treatment and psychiatric medications for children with mental illness. *Psychiatric Services, 58*(5), 613–618.

Pollack, M. H., Simon, N. M., Zalta, A. K., Worthington, J. J., Hoge, E. A., Mick, E., Kinrys, G., & Oppenheimer, J. (2006). Olanzapine augmentation of fluoxetine for refractory generalized anxiety disorder: A placebo controlled study. *Biological Psychiatry, 59*(3), 211–215.

Pollack, M. H., Zaninelli, R., Goddard, A. W., McCafferty, J. P., Bellew, K. M., Burnham, D. B., & Iyengar, M. K. (2001). Paroxetine in the treatment of generalized anxiety disorder: Results of a placebo-controlled, flexible-dosage trial. *Journal of Clinical Psychiatry, 62*(5), 350–357.

Power, K. G., Simpson, R. J., Swanson, V., & Wallace, L. A. (1990). Controlled comparison of pharmacological and psychological treatment of generalized anxiety disorder in primary care. *British Journal of General Practice, 40*(336), 289–294.

Raskind, M. A., Peskind, E. R., Kanter, E. D., Petrie, E. C., Radant, A., Thompson, C. E., Dobie, D. J., Hoff, D., Rein, R. J., Straits-Tröster, K., Thomas, R. G., & McFall, M. M. (2003). Reduction of nightmares and other PTSD symptoms in combat veterans by prazosin: A placebo-controlled study. *American Journal of Psychiatry, 160*(2), 371–373.

Ready, D. J., Thomas, K. R., Worley, V., Backscheider, A. G., Harvey. L. A., Baltzell. D., Rothbaum, B. O. (2008). A field test of group based exposure therapy with 102 veterans with war-related posttraumatic stress disorder. *Journal of Trauma and Stress, 21*(2), 150–157.

Reed, P. L., Anthony, J. C., & Breslau, N. (2007). Incidence of drug problems in young adults exposed to trauma and posttraumatic stress disorder: Do early life experiences and predispositions matter? *Archives of General Psychiatry, 64*(12), 1435–1442.

Reger, G. M., & Gahm, G. A. (2008). Virtual reality exposure therapy for active duty soldiers. *Journal of Clinical Psychology, 64*(8), 940–946.

Reist, C., Kauffmann, C. D., Haier, R. J., Sangdahl, C., DeMet, E. M., Chicz-DeMet, A., & Nelson, J. N.

(1989). A controlled trial of desipramine in 18 men with posttraumatic stress disorder. *American Journal of Psychiatry, 146,* 513–516.

Resnick, P. A., & Schnicke, M. K. (1992). Cognitive processing therapy for sexual assault victims. *Journal of Consulting and Clinical Psychology, 60*(5), 748–756.

Roberge, P., Marchand, A., Reinharz, D., & Savard, P. (2008). Cognitive-behavioral treatment for panic disorder. *Behavior Modification, 32,* 333–351.

Rodebaugh, T. L., Holaway, R. M., & Heimberg, R. G. (2004). The treatment of social anxiety disorder. *Clinical Psychology Review, 24,* 883–908.

Roth, W. T. (2008). Translational research for panic disorder. *American Journal of Psychiatry, 165*(7), 796–798.

Roy-Byrne, P. P., Craske, M. G., Stein, M. B., Sullivan, G., Bystritsky, A, Katon, W., Golinelli, D., & Sherbourne, C. D. (2005). A randomized effectiveness trial of CBT and medication for primary care panic disorder. *Archives of General Psychiatry, 62*(3), 290–298.

Roy-Byrne, P. P., Davidson, K. W., Kessler, R. C., Asmundson, G. J., Goodwin, R. D., Kubzansky, L., Lydiard, R. B., Massie, M. J., Katon, W., Laden, S. K., & Stein, M. B. (2008). Anxiety disorders and comorbid illness. *General Hospital Psychiatry, 30*(3), 208–225.

Sajdyk, T. J., Schober, D. A., Gehlert, D. R., & Shekhar, A. (1999). Role of corticotropin-releasing factor and urocortin within the basolateral amygdala of rats in anxiety and panic responses. *Behavioral Brain Research, 100,* 207–215.

Schneider, F., Weiss, U., Kessler, C., Müller-Gärtner, H. W., Posse, S., Salloum, J. B., Grodd, W., Himmelmann, F., Gaebel, W., & Birbaumer, N. (1999). Subcortical correlates of differential classical conditioning of aversive emotional reactions in social phobics. *Biological Psychiatry, 45*(7), 863–871.

Schneier, F. R. (2006). Clinical practice: Social anxiety disorder. *New England Journal of Medicine, 355*(10), 1029–1036.

Schnittker, J. (2003). Misgiving of medicine? African Americans' skepticism of psychiatric medication. *Journal of Healthy Social Behavior, 44*(4), 506–524.

Schweizer, E., Rickels, K., Weiss, S., & Zavodnick, S. (1993). Maintenance drug treatment of panic disorder. I. Results of a prospective, placebo-controlled comparison of alprazolam and imipramine. *Archives of General Psychiatry, 50*(1), 51–60.

Seal, K. H., Bertenthal, D., Miner, C. R., Sen, S., & Marmar, C. (2007). Bringing the war back home: Mental health disorders among 103,788 US veterans returning from Iraq and Afghanistan seen at Department of Veterans Affairs facilities. *Archives of Internal Medicine, 167*(5), 476–482.

Seedat, S., & Stein, M. B. (2004). Double-blind, placebo-controlled assessment of combined clonazepam with paroxetine compared with paroxetine monotherapy for generalized social anxiety disorder. *Journal of Clinical Psychiatry, 65*(2), 244–248.

Sheehan, D. V. (1999). Current concepts in the treatment of panic disorder. *Journal of Clinical Psychiatry, 60*(Suppl. 18), 16–21.

Sheehan, D. V. (2002). The management of panic disorder. *Journal of Clinical Psychiatry, 63*(Suppl. 14), 17–21.

Shekhar, A., Katner, J. S., Sajdyk, T. J., & Kohl, R. R. (2002). Role of norepinephrine in the dorsomedial hypothalamic panic response: An in vivo microdialysis study. *Pharmacology Biochemical Behavior, 71*(3), 493–500.

Siegmund, A., Kaltwasser, S. F., Holsboer, F., Czisch, M., & Wotjak, C. T. (2008). Hippocampal n-acetylaspartate levels before trauma predict the development of long-lasting posttraumatic stress disorder-like symptoms in mice. *Biological Psychiatry* [Epub ahead of print].

Simon, N. M., Connor, K. M., LeBeau, R. T., Hoge, E. A., Worthington, J. J. 3rd, Zhang, W., Davidson, J. R., & Pollack, M. H. (2008). Quetiapine augmentation of paroxetine CR for the treatment of refractory generalized anxiety disorder: Preliminary findings. *Psychopharmacology (Berlin), 197*(4), 675–681.

Simon, N. M., Hoge, E. A., Fischmann, D., Worthington, J. J., Christian, K. M., Kinrys, G., & Pollack, M. H. (2006). An open-label trial of risperidone augmentation for refractory anxiety disorders. *Journal of Clinical Psychiatry, 67*(3), 381–385.

Stanger, U., Heidenreich, T., Peitz, M., Lauterbach, W., & Clark, D. M. (2003). Cognitive therapy for social phobia: Individual versus group treatment. *Behavior Research and Therapy, 41,* 991–1007.

Stein, D. J., Ahokas, A. A., & de Bodinat, C. (2008). Efficacy of agomelatine in generalized anxiety disorder: A randomized, double-blind, placebo-controlled study. *Journal of Clinical Psychopharmacology, 28*(5), 561–566.

Stein, M. B., Goldin, P. R., Sareen, J., Zorrilla, L. T., & Brown, G. G. (2002). Increased amygdala activation to angry and contemptuous faces in generalized social phobia. *Archives of General Psychiatry, 59*(11), 1027–1034.

Surget, A., & Belzung, C. (2008). Involvement of vasopressin in affective disorders. *European Journal of Pharmacology, 583*(2–3), 340–349.

Suvisaari, J., Aalto-Setälä, T., Tuulio-Henriksson, A., Härkänen, T., Saarni, S. I., Perälä, J., Schreck, M., Castaneda, A., Hintikka, J., Kestilä, L., Lähteenmäki, S., Latvala, A., Koskinen, S., Marttunen, M., Aro, H., & Lönnqvist, J. (2008).

Mental disorders in young adulthood. *Psychological Medicine, 28*, 1–13.

Taylor, F. B., Martin, P., Thompson, C., Williams, J., Mellman, T. A., Gross, C., Peskind, E. R., & Raskind, M. A. (2008). Prazosin effects on objective sleep measures and clinical symptoms in civilian trauma posttraumatic stress disorder: A placebo-controlled study. *Biological Psychiatry, 63*(6), 629–632.

Tucker, P., Zaninelli, R., Yehuda, R., Ruggiero, L., Dillingham, K., & Pitts, C. D. (2001). Paroxetine in the treatment of chronic posttraumatic stress disorder: Results of a placebo-controlled, flexible-dosage trial. *Journal of Clinical Psychiatry, 62*(11), 860–868.

Tunis, S. R., Stryer, D. B., & Clancy, C. M. (2003). Practical clinical trials: Increasing the value of clinical research for decision making in clinical and health policy. *Journal of the American Medical Association, 290*(12), 1624–1632.

Uchida, R. R., Del-Ben, C. M., Busatto, G. F., Duran, F. L., Guimarães, F. S., Crippa, J. A., Araújo, D., Santos, A. C., & Graeff, F. G. (2008). Regional gray matter abnormalities in panic disorder: A voxel-based morphometry study. *Psychiatry Research, 163*(1), 21–29.

Ursano, R. J., Bell, C., Pfefferbaum, B., Eth, S., Pynoos, R. S., Friedman, M., Zatzick, D. F., Norwood, A., & Benedek, D. M. (2004). *APA practice guideline for the treatment of patients of acute stress disorder and post-traumatic stress disorder.* Washington, DC: American Psychiatric Association.

van Apeldoorn, F. J., van Hout, W. J., Mersch, P. P., Huisman, M., Slaap, B. R., Hale, W. W., Visser, S., van Dyck, R., den Boar, J. A. (2008). Is a combined therapy more effective than either CBT or SSRI alone? Results of a multicenter trial on panic disorder with or without agoraphobia. *Acta Psychiatrica Scandinavica, 117*(4), 260–270.

Veit, R., Flor, H., Erb, M., Hermann, C., Lotze, M., Grodd, W., & Birbaumer, N. (2002). Brain circuits involved in emotional learning in antisocial behavior and social phobia in humans. *Neuroscience Letters, 328*(3), 233–236.

Vermetten, E., & Bremner, J. D. (2002). Circuits and systems in stress: I. Preclinical studies. *Depression and Anxiety, 15*(3), 126–147.

Vianna, M. R., Coitinho, A. S., & Izquierdo, I. (2004). Role of the hippocampus and amygdala in the extinction of fear-motivated learning. *Current Neurovascular Research, 1*(1), 55–60.

Vojvoda, D., & Southwich, S. (2007). Postraumatic stress disorder. In J. E. Grant, M. N. Potenza (Eds.), *Textbook of men's mental health.* Washington, DC: American Psychiatric Association.

Vos, T., Habby, M. M., Magnus, A., Mihalopoulos, C., Andrews, G., & Carter, R. (2005). Assessing cost effectiveness in mental health: Helping policymakers prioritize and plan health services. *Australia and New Zealand Journal of Psychiatry, 39*(8), 701–712.

Wagner, K. D., Berard, R., Stein, M. B., Wetherhold, E., Carpenter, D. J., Perera, P., Gee, M,, Davy, K., & Machin, A. (2004). A multicenter, randomized, double-blind, placebo-controlled trial of paroxetine in children and adolescents with social anxiety disorder. *Archives of General Psychiatry, 61*(11), 1153–1162.

Wittchen, H. U., & Beloch, E. (1996). The impact of social phobia and the quality of life. *International Clinical Psychopharmacology, 11*(Suppl. 3), 15–23.

Wittchen, H. U., Fuetsch, M., Sonntag, H., Müller, N., & Liebowitz, M. (1999). Disability and quality of life in pure and comorbid social phobia—findings from a controlled study. *European Psychiatry, 14*(3), 118–131.

Wittchen, H. U., Zhao, S., Kessler, R. C., & Eaton, W. W. (1994). DSM-III-R generalized anxiety disorder in the National Comorbidity Survey. *Archives of General Psychiatry, 51*(5), 355–364.

Young, E. A., & Breslau, N. (2004). Cortisol and catecholamines in PTSD: An epidemiological community survey. *Archives of General Psychiatry, 61*(4), 394–401.

Zastrow, A., Faude, V., Seyboth, F., Niehoff, D., Herzog, W., & Löwe, B. (2008). Risk factors of symptom underestimation by physicians. *Journal of Psychosomatic Research, 64*(5), 543–551.

Zitrin, C. M., Klein, D. F., Woerner, M. G., & Ross, D. C. (1983). Treatment of phobias. I. Comparison of imipramine hydrochloride and placebo. *Archives of General Psychiatry, 40*(2), 125–138.

Zohar, J., Amital, D., Miodownik, C., Kotler, M., Bleich, A., Lane, R. M., & Austin, C. (2002). Double-blind placebo-controlled pilot study of sertraline in military veterans with posttraumatic stress disorder. *Journal of Clinical Psychopharmacology, 22*(2), 190–195.

Chapter 16

Obsessive-Compulsive Disorder in Young Adults

Maria C. Mancebo, Jane Eisen and Steven A. Rasmussen

Obsessive-compulsive disorder (OCD) is an anxiety disorder characterized by recurrent, intrusive thoughts that are experienced as senseless but distressing. For most individuals, these thoughts are accompanied by urges to perform overt or mental behaviors (compulsions) or avoid situations that have become associated with the thoughts. OCD affects all age groups and is remarkably similar across the life span. Symptoms typically start in childhood or adolescence but are thought to reach their peak in young adulthood (age 18–29). This chapter will focus on how OCD presents in young adults as well as risk factor and treatment aspects unique to this population.

Clinical Case Vignette

Jeff, a 25-year-old, single, Caucasian male presented for treatment of OCD and depressive symptoms. Jeff was a high-school teacher and had been working full time since graduating college. His decision to seek psychiatric treatment followed an onset of depressive symptoms (depressed mood, fatigue, insomnia), which resulted in missing several days from work over the past 2 months.

Jeff first noticed OCD symptoms at age 9. He recalled fears that something terrible would happen to his parents as well as occasional counting, tapping rituals, and repeating rituals. For example, he recalled tapping five times on the headboard of his bed before going to bed so that "nothing bad" would happen to his parents. However, he stated that these symptoms were intermittent, took up very little time, did not cause significant distress, and never interfered with his routine activities. Jeff recalled persistent OCD symptoms at age 16 when he gradually became preoccupied with thoughts of being responsible for a car accident. He recalled his father teaching him how to drive and emphasizing the increased responsibility that he would be taking on. Shortly after he began driving, he began to repeat routine activities such as adjusting the car seat or the rear view mirror to "just the right spot." He recalled the rituals and associated anxiety becoming more intense over time until he avoided driving his car to any place other than school. Upon starting college, he gradually began to drive his car more often but avoided adjusting anything in his car (e.g., mirror, seat, radio frequency, items in the glove compartment) for fear that any change might cause him to be distracted and get into a car accident. Jeff could also recall making up excuses not to carry passengers in his car and gradually began to avoid some social events or running out for routine errands out of fear that someone would ask him for a ride.

Jeff's symptoms waxed and waned in intensity throughout college. He was able to complete his course work with excellent grades. However, he reported that social interactions became more difficult. He described frequently being consumed with obsessive thoughts when he was around his peers and that it became increasingly more difficult to participate in conversations because he did not feel like "his normal self." He also avoided intimate relationships or dating because he was frightened that others would "catch on that I was mentally ill." In an attempt to control his anxiety, Jeff began to smoke marijuana, which he felt made the obsessions less frequent and less disturbing. He stopped smoking marijuana 6 months prior to his initial appointment after an incident when he became "paranoid" and accused his roommate of going through his closet, which resulted in a physical altercation. Jeff reported that he was too frightened to continue smoking but believed that his depression and OCD had increased during this period of abstinence.

Jeff was treated with a combination of sertraline 150 mg/day and a total of 32 sessions of cognitive-behavioral therapy (CBT) over a period of 9 months. After the first three sessions, it became evident that Jeff was drinking excessively to cope with OCD symptoms in the evening. He was initially reluctant to engage in exposure and response prevention therapy and the first 2 months of treatment focused on cognitive therapy and motivational enhancement techniques. Jeff was then agreeable to limiting his drinking to 1–2 drinks at a social event and to using exposure and response prevention techniques. Six months following his initial appointment, Jeff had minimal OCD symptoms (less than 1 hour per day), was no longer engaging in avoidance behaviors, and reported no interference due to OCD symptoms. Objective severity ratings at baseline had decreased from severe OCD and moderate depression at baseline (total Y-BOCS of 28 and BDI-II of 23) to mild OCD symptoms and minimal depression (Y-BOCS = 14 and BDI-II = 6). However, he continued to describe feelings of loneliness and hopelessness regarding dating. He described beliefs that he had "missed out" on dating in college and lacked the skills to initiate friendships or dates. He also continued to feel "different" from his peers because he believed it was "abnormal" not to have had at least one intimate relationship at his age. He continued to attend CBT sessions (as well as maintenance medication management) to develop behavioral and cognitive coping skills to address these concerns.

Prevalence of Obsessive-Compulsive Disorder

Lifetime prevalence rates of OCD (DSM-III-R or DSM-IV) range from 1% to 3% of the general population and are consistent across cultures worldwide (Rasmussen & Eisen, 2002). As shown in Table 16.1, prevalence rates across studies of adolescent populations and young adult participants of epidemiologic surveys also suggest that 1%–3% of young adults are affected by OCD. Unlike other anxiety disorders that are more common in women, OCD affects both genders relatively equally in community samples of adolescents and adults (Flament et al., 1988; Rasmussen & Eisen, 1992; Regier et al., 1993). However, males are generally overrepresented in pediatric clinical samples (Geller et al., 2001; Hanna, 1995; Masi et al., 2005; Swedo, Rapoport, Leonard, Lenane, & Cheslow, 1989).

More than 50% of adults recall an onset of OCD symptoms before the age of 20 and less than 10% report an onset after the age of 30, which suggests that risk for OCD is highest in adolescence and young adulthood (Bland, Newman, & Orn, 1988; Karno, Golding, Sorenson, & Burnam, 1988; Kessler et al., 2005). Some studies have found that males report an earlier age at onset than females (Albert et al., 2002; Fontenelle, Mendlowicz, Marques, & Versiani, 2003; Rasmussen & Tsuang, 1986), but other studies have failed to replicate this finding (Chabane et al., 2005; Pinto, Mancebo, Eisen, Pagano, & Rasmussen, 2006; Rosario-Campos et al., 2001).

Diagnosis and Assessment

OCD is classified as an anxiety disorder in the *Diagnostic and Statistical Manual of Mental Disorders* (DSM-IV-TR) (APA, 2000). Diagnostic criteria require the presence of obsessions or compulsions, recognition of symptoms as senseless or excessive, and symptoms that reach clinical significance (are time consuming, distressing, and/or significantly interfere with psychosocial functioning). Insight into OCD symptoms often varies across individuals and over the course of the disorder. To account for these fluctuations, the DSM-IV also includes a "poor insight" specifier for those individuals who do not recognize their symptoms as senseless or excessive.

It is important to screen for comorbid conditions as OCD is associated with high comorbidity rates (Pinto, Mancebo, Eisen, Pagano, & Rasmussen, 2006). Individuals often present

Table 16-1. Prevalence of DSM-III-R or DSM-IV Obsessive-Compulsive Disorder in Community Samples of Adolescents and Young Adults

Author, Year	Type of Sample	Age Range (N)	Diagnostic Instrument	Diagnostic Criteria	OCD Prevalence Past Month	OCD Prevalence Lifetime
Reinherz et al., 1993	Community/Age cohort Northeastern USA	17–18 (N = 386)	DIS	DSM-III-R	1.3%	2.1%
Zohar et al., 1992	Community/Age cohort Israel	16–17 (N = 562)	STSOB	DSM-III-R	3.6%	NR
Lewinsohn et al., 1993	High school students USA	14–18 (N = 1,710)	K-SADS	DSM-III-R	0.6%	0.6%
Douglass et al., 1995	Community/Birth cohort New Zealand	18 (N = 930)	DIS	DSM-III-R	4.0% (1 yr)	NR
Costello et al., 1996	Community/Age cohorts USA	9, 11, 13 (N = 4,500)	CAPA	DSM-III-R	0.2% (3 mo)	NR
Canals et al., 1997	Community/Age cohort Spain	18 (N = 290)	SCAN	DSM-III-R	0.7	NR
Verhulst et al., 1997	Community Holland	13–18 (N = 2,916)	DISC	DSM-III-R	1.0% (6 mo)	NR
Andrade et al., 2006	High school students Hawaii, USA	13–21 N = 7,317	DISC	DSM-III-R	8.4%	NR
Wittchen et al., 1998	Community Germany	14–24 (N = 3,021)	CIDI	DSM-IV	0.6%	0.7%
Garland et al., 2001	Youths in public systems of care USA	6–18 (N = 1,618)	DISC	DSM-IV	2.4%	NR
Costello et al., 2003	Community North Carolina, USA	9–13 (N = 1,420)	CAPA	DSM-IV	0.1%	NR
Heyman et al., 2003	Community Great Britain	5–15 (N = 10,438)	DAWBA	DSM-IV	0.3%	NR
Bland et al., 1988; Kolada et al., 1994	Community Canada	18–34 (N = 1,721)	DIS	DSM-III-R	1.6–1.8%	2.8–3.6%
Crino et al., 2005	Community Australia	18–34 (NR)	CIDI	DSM-IV	0.5% (1 yr)	NR
Kessler et al., 2005	Community (NCS-R) USA	18–29 (493)	CIDI	DSM-IV	NR	2.0

CIDI, Comprehensive International Diagnostic Interview; DAWBA, Development and Well-being Assessment; DICA, Diagnostic Interview for Children and Adolescents; DIS, Diagnostic Interview Schedule; DISC, Diagnostic Interview Schedule for Children; ECA, Epidemiologic Catchment Area; ISC, Interview Schedule for Children; NCS-R, National Comorbidity Survey; NR, not reported; SCAN, Schedules for Clinical Assessment in Neuropsychiatry; SPE, Standardized Psychiatric Examination; STSOB, Schedule for TS and Other Behavioral Disorders.

with repetitive, intrusive thoughts that must be distinguished from obsessions. For example, intrusive thoughts are also common during depressive episodes (depressive ruminations), manic or hypomanic episodes (racing thoughts), and generalized anxiety disorder (excessive worries about the future). Unlike these intrusive thoughts, obsessions are usually experienced as senseless/inappropriate thoughts that are resisted by the patient. A diagnosis of body dysmorphic disorder or an eating disorder should be considered for individuals who describe appearance or weight concerns without any other OCD symptoms.

Compulsions can be differentiated from other repetitive behaviors by assessing antecedents and consequences of the behaviors. Compulsions are purposeful and usually performed to reduce distress (usually anxiety) triggered by obsessions. Repetitive behaviors without obsessional antecedents are often seen in tic disorders or impulse control disorders (skin picking, hair pulling). Adults may have a history of motor tics (e.g., eye blinking, neck movements) or vocal tics (e.g., sniffing, throat clearing) as OCD and childhood tics are closely associated. Complex tics (spitting, complex tapping and touching patterns) can usually be ruled out if there is no history of simple tics (AACAP, 1998). Both tics and compulsions may be preceded by physical sensations, urges, or mental perceptions that persist until the behavior is completed (Leckman et al., 1994).

Similarities in phenomenology often make it difficult to differentiate between OCD and obsessive-compulsive personality disorder (OCPD) (Mancebo, Eisen, Grant, & Rasmussen, 2005). One-quarter to one-third of individuals with OCD meet criteria for both disorders (Pinto, Mancebo, Eisen, Pagano, & Rasmussen, 2006; Samuels et al., 2000). Both individuals with OCD and those with OCPD may display preoccupations with detail and engage in time-consuming tasks, such as extensive list-making, rewriting, or ordering/arranging possessions. However, individuals with OCPD features consider symptoms to be ego-syntonic (acceptable and consistent with their personality) rather than ego-dystonic (intrusive and unacceptable). For example, patients with OCD may spend time ordering/arranging possessions to neutralize fears they will be responsible for something terrible happening, address a need for symmetry, or achieve a feeling that things are "just right" (incompleteness). In contrast, a person with OCPD will justify ordering/arranging possessions with the rationale that it is a reasonable use of their time and satisfaction with the outcome (e.g., looks perfect).

Structured interviews such as the Structured Clinical Interview for DSM-IV (SCID) and the Anxiety Disorder Interview Schedule for DSM-IV (ADIS) are empirically validated methods of making an OCD diagnosis (Di Nardo, Moras, Barlow, Rapee, & Brown, 1993; First et al., 1996). More detailed information regarding OCD symptoms and severity can be gathered using clinician-administered rating scales and patient self-reports.

The Yale-Brown Obsessive Compulsive Scale (Y-BOCS) is a widely used instrument comprised of a symptom checklist and 10-item severity scale (Goodman et al., 1989a, 1989b). The scale was originally developed as a clinician-administered, semistructured interview, but a self-report version is also available (Steketee, Frost, & Bogart, 1996). The symptom checklist consists of more than 60 items grouped in thematic categories of obsessions (aggressive, contamination, sexual, hoarding, religious, symmetry, somatic) and compulsions (washing, checking, repeating, counting, ordering) and includes miscellaneous symptoms. Once the target symptoms are identified, the clinician uses the 10-item scale to assess five aspects of obsessions and compulsions: time consumed, distress, interference, degree of resistance, and control. Subscores for obsessions and compulsions are computed (range 0–20) and yield a total scores ranging from 0 (no symptoms) to 40 (extreme symptoms). More detailed descriptions of other assessment instruments and their use in clinical practice can be found elsewhere (Bjorgvinsson, Hart, & Heffelfinger, 2007; Steketee & Frost, 2007; Wilhelm & Steketee, 2006).

Clinical Characteristics of Young Adults with OCD

There have been various descriptive reports of OCD in samples of children and adolescents (Geller et al., 2001; Hanna, 1995; Swedo, Rapoport, Leonard, Lenane, & Cheslow, 1989; Thomsen & Mikkelsen, 1991), adults (Nestadt et al., 2000; Rasmussen & Eisen, 1998; Rosario-Campos et al., 2001), and the elderly (Kohn, Westlake, Rasmussen, Marsland, & Norman, 1997; Philpot & Banerjee, 1998). However, to our knowledge, there are no published descriptive papers of characteristics of young adults with OCD. In this section, we refer to data from the Brown Longitudinal OCD study (BLOCS), an ongoing observational study of the course of OCD in 400 treatment-seeking individuals (ages 6–75) who identified OCD as their most problematic psychiatric problem in their lifetime. Individuals were recruited from various mental health treatment sites, including an OCD specialty clinic, a private psychiatric hospital, a community mental health center, and several private practices (psychiatrists and cognitive-behavioral therapists) known as main referral sources for individuals seeking treatment for mood and anxiety disorders. Detailed descriptions of study methods and sample characteristics are available elsewhere (Pinto, Mancebo, Eisen, Pagano, & Rasmussen, 2006; Zohar et al., 1992). Seventy-three participants were young adults (ages 19–29) at entry into the study. Table 16.2 lists intake characteristics of the entire sample across five age groups: children (ages 6–12), adolescents (ages 13–18), young adults (ages 19–29), middle-aged adults (ages 30–59), and older adults (ages 60–75).

Demographic Characteristcs

Gender was equally distributed over the entire sample (49% male). As shown in Table 16.2, half of young adults were male, but males were *overrepresented* among children and adolescents (65% and 68%, respectively) and *underrepresented* among the elderly (30%). These results are consistent with the literature as clinical samples tend to show an equal gender distribution in adults and elevated proportions of males in juvenile samples (Geller et al., 2001, Hanna, 1995; Masi et al., 2005; Swedo, Rapoport, Leonard, Lenane, & Cheslow, 1989) and equal gender distribution in adult samples (Geller et al., 2001; Kohn, Westlake, Rasmussen, Marsland, & Norman, 1997).

The majority (80%) of young adults had not yet married and all but four had completed high school. At the time of assessment, 59% of young adults were employed and most were well-educated (44% were enrolled in college courses and 36% had earned a college degree), suggesting high premorbid functioning. However, the majority of young adults reported substantial impairment in academic, social, and occupational functioning as a result of their OCD symptoms in the month prior to study entry. Disability rates were three times as high in middle-aged adults as young adults. The discrepancies noted among young and middle-aged adults highlight important milestones in young adulthood: marriage, occupational development, and financial independence.

Age at Onset

Mean age at onset of DSM-IV OCD symptoms in the BLOCS cohort was 17.0 ± 9.7 years and increased with chronological age (see Table 16.2). Most participants recalled first noticing OCD symptoms (minor OCD symptoms) in childhood and an onset of DSM-IV OCD in late adolescence. In a recent report of adult intake characteristics, onset of OCD before the age of 18 (juvenile onset) was associated with significantly higher rates of personality disorders (45%) compared to individuals with young or late-adult onsets (27.7% and 27.3%, respectively) (Grant et al., 2007). Individuals with juvenile onset of OCD were also less likely to be married (38.1%) than those with a young adult onset (45.8%) or late onset of OCD (69.7%).

Although we found no gender differences in mean age at OCD onset among adult or juvenile participants (Mancebo et al., in press; Pinto, Mancebo, Eisen, Pagano, & Rasmussen, 2006), it is worth examining the distributions of the full sample (see Figure 16-1). The overall shape of the distribution was bimodal and strikingly similar to the original Brown cohort of adults treated at an OCD clinic described by Rasmussen and Eisen (Rasmussen & Eisen, 1998; Rasmussen & Tsuang, 1986) in which peaks in early adolescence and early adulthood were found. However, in the current sample, age at OCD onset for males appeared to be *normally distributed* with a mean of 17.1 ± 10.0 years and reports of onset *decreased* after age 22. For females, the distribution of age at OCD onset appeared to be *bimodal* with a peak between the ages of 10 (mode) and 15 and *increased* reports after age 22. Differences in age-of-onset distribution support the idea of etiological heterogeneity and different pathways which result in some individuals developing OCD around puberty and in early adulthood, particularly among women.

Obsessive-Compulsive Disorder Symptom Expression

Most individuals report multiple types of obsessions and compulsions. The most common obsessions are fears of contamination, fears of being responsible for a terrible consequence, and concerns with symmetry. The most common compulsions are cleaning, checking, and ordering/arranging rituals. Neither chronological age nor age at OCD onset appears to

Table 16-2. Characteristics of Consecutive Participants of the Brown Longitudinal Obsessive-Compulsive Disorder Study (N = 387)

	Children (n = 20)	Adolescents (n = 44)	Young Adults (n = 73)	Middle-Aged Adults (n = 230)	Older Adults (n = 20)	**Entire Sample (n = 387)**
Age at assessment, years, Range	6–12	13–18	19–29	30–59	60–75	**6–75**
Mean (SD)	10.20 (1.8)	15.43 (1.6)	23.58 (3.4)	43.1 (8.4)	65.6 (5.2)	**35.75 (15.3)**
Characteristic	N (%)	N (%)	N (%)	N (%)	N (%)	
Sex, male	13 (65.0)	30 (68.2)	37 (50.7)	104 (45.2)	6 (30.0)	**190 (49.1)**
Race/ethnicity, white/non-Hispanic	17 (85.0)	40 (90.9)	68 (93.2)	220 (95.7)	20 (100.0)	**365 (94.3)**
Marital status, never married	20 (100.0)	44 (100.0)	59 (80.8)	56 (24.3)	1 (5.0)	**180 (46.5)**
Education, college degree	0 (0.0)	0 (0.0)	26 (35.6)	148 (64.1)	9 (45.0)	**183 (47.2)**
Employed	0 (0.0)	0 (0.0)	43 (58.9)	134 (58.3)	10 (50.0)	**187 (48.3)**
Receiving occupational disability benefits for OCD	0 (0.0)	0 (0.0)	4 (5.5)	43 (18.7)	1 (5.0)	**48 (12.4)**
Sudden onset of OCD	5 (25.0)	2 (4.5)	12 (16.4)	41 (17.8)	3 (15.0)	**63 (16.3)**
	Mean (SD)	Mean (SD)	Mean (SD)	Mean (SD)	Mean (SD)	
Age first experienced minor symptoms, years	5.05 (2.3)	7.34 (3.6)	9.54 (4.5)	12.21 (6.8)	21.11 (18.1)	**11.20 (7.7)**
Age of onset of DSM-IV OCD, years	7.3 (2.5)	10.27 (3.6)	15.05 (5.2)	18.67 (9.5)	27.83 (17.9)	**16.97 (9.7)**
Duration of illness, years	2.57 (1.6)	5.16 (3.2)	8.5 (5.2)	24.56 (11.0)	38.22 (19.3)	**18.76 (13.8)**
Treatment History						
Age first received treatment, years, Mn (SD)	8.68 (2.0)	11.72 (3.4)	19.6 (4.8)	31.88 (10.0)	47.45 (17.4)	26.94 (13.1)
Years between onset and initial treatment, Mn (SD)	1.50 (2.1)	1.47 (2.1)	4.53 (4.5)	12.84 (11.1)	20.45 (17.7)	9.79 (11.0)
Received at least one SRI trial, n (%)	9 (45.0)	35 (79.5)	61 (83.6)	199 (90.5)	17 (89.5)	327 (85.6)
Number of SRI trials, Mn (SD)	0.65 (0.9)	1.77 (1.5)	1.67 (1.3)	2.09 (1.3)	1.36 (0.9)	1.95 (1.3)
Received CBT, n (%)	11 (55.0)	31 (70.5)	37 (52.1)	132 (58.4)	16 (80.0)	227 (58.7)
Received 12 CBT sessions or more, n (%)	8 (40.0)	19 (43.2)	22 (31.4)	101 (44.7)	11 (55.0)	161 (41.6)
Intake Symptom Severity (Possible Range)	Mean (SD)	Mean (SD)	Mean (SD)	Mean (SD)	Mean (SD)	
Y-BOCS (0–40)	17.55 (6.8)	21.88 (8.8)	22.42 (7.8)	20.07 (8.5)	19.2 (8.0)	20.55 (8.4)
GAF (0–100)	59.70 (12.8)	53.18 (15.3)	49.12 (11.9)	52.39 (12.0)	55.85 (12.1)	52.42 (12.6)

CBT, cognitive-behavioral therapy; OCD, obsessive-compulsive disorder; SD, standard deviation; SE, standard error; SRI, serotonin-reuptake inhibitor.

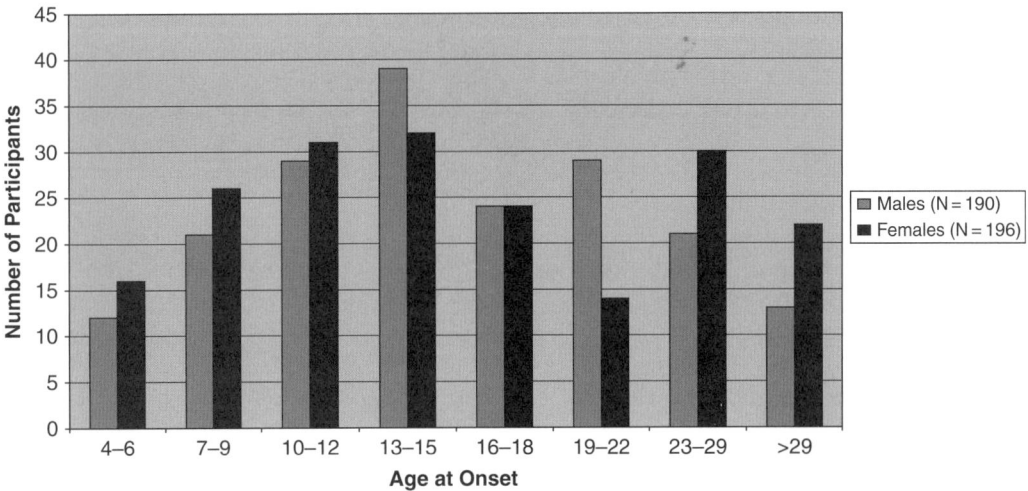

Figure 16-1. Onset of DSM-IV obsessive-compulsive disorder among BLOCS participants (n = 386).

significantly affect content of OCD symptoms (Geller et al., 2001; Mancebo et al., in press; Zohar et al., 1992). However, individuals who reported OCD onset after the age of 30 were less likely to report contamination, religious, and somatic obsessions than those who reported an earlier age at OCD onset (Grant et al., 2007). Studies comparing children, adolescents, and adults have found more similarities than differences in symptom expression. Sexual, aggressive, and religious obsessions appear to be more prevalent in adolescents and adults than in children, while adults have higher rates of mental rituals (Geller et al., 2001; Mancebo et al., in press). These differences suggest cognitive and social development influences on OCD symptom expression, especially in adolescence and adulthood. However, the lack of prospective studies precludes conclusions regarding the stability of phenomenologic subtypes over time.

Comorbidity

The majority of young adults presenting for treatment of OCD have at least one other psychiatric disorder. Ninety percent of the BLOCS adult cohort met lifetime criteria for another axis I disorder (Pinto, Mancebo, Eisen, Pagano, & Rasmussen, 2006). Adult onset of OCD was associated with lower lifetime rates of tic disorders, panic disorder, and eating disorders (Chabane et al., 2005; Pinto, Mancebo, Eisen, Pagano, & Rasmussen, 2006; Rosario et al., 2001; Zohar et al., 1992). Adults reporting a juvenile onset of OCD were more likely to be diagnosed with a personality disorder, particularly OCPD (Grant et al., 2007; Pinto, Mancebo, Eisen, Pagano, & Rasmussen, 2006). In addition, the juvenile sample also shows higher rates of tics and attention-deficit hyperactivity disorder (Geller, Biederman, Griffin, Jones, & Lefkowitz, 1996), suggesting that these comorbidities may be specific to a juvenile-onset subtype of OCD.

Course

Early retrospective reports of OCD course suggested the illness is usually chronic and lifelong (Goodwin, Guze, & Robins, 1969). In contrast, a prospective study by Skoog and Skoog (1999) of the course of OCD in 144 individuals identified as inpatients in the late 1940s and early 1950s is somewhat more optimistic. Follow-up data indicated that remission rates within the first decade were low (11% had no OCD symptoms; 17% continued to have subclinical OCD symptoms) and were slightly higher at the 40-year follow-up (20% had no OCD symptoms; 28% had subclinical symptoms), indicating that more than half of patients maintained OCD symptoms at a clinical level. Despite these low remission rates, two-thirds were improved within a decade after onset of OCD and 83% were improved at the 40-year follow-up. In the first decade after OCD onset, an episodic course (i.e., at least two symptom-free periods) was most common, while a chronic course was more typical in the later follow-up period, with 20% experiencing either no improvement or a deteriorative course over the 40 years of follow-up.

Studies of adults with OCD conducted since the 1990s, when effective treatments of OCD (namely selective serotonin reuptake inhibitors [SSRIs] and cognitive-behavioral therapy [CBT]) became widely available, have also shown favorable course patterns (Alonso et al., 2001; Catapano et al., 2006; Eisen et al., 1999; Orloff et al., 1994; Reddy et al., 2005; Steketee, Eisen, Dyck, Warshaw, & Rasmussen, 1999; Tukel et al., 2007). Among the only four prospective studies, rates of achieving at least partial remission (subclinical OCD symptoms) have ranged from 52% to 76%, while rates of full remission (no OCD symptoms) range from 17% to 43% (Eisen et al., 1999; Orloff et al., 1994; Reddy et al., 2005; Steketee, Eisen, Dyck, Warshaw, & Rasmussen, 1999). Differences in methodology may account for some of the variability in remission rates across studies. For example, highest rates of remission were reported in a study where the majority of subjects were drug-naïve at study intake (Reddy et al., 2005). Less is known about the long-term patterns of course of juveniles with OCD. In a recent review of published studies of juvenile samples, Stewart and colleagues (Stewart et al., 2004) found a high percentage of juveniles with an episodic course. The overall pooled proportion of patients (across 14 clinical samples and two community samples) who achieved at least a partial remission was 60%, indicating a significant reduction in OCD symptoms over time.

An earlier age at OCD onset and longer duration of illness have both been associated with persistence of OCD symptoms (Stewart et al., 2004). Preliminary data from our BLOCS dataset also indicate that adults with a younger age at OCD onset and a longer duration of illness were less likely to remit from OCD (i.e., no longer meet DSM-IV criteria) over the first 2 years of follow-up (Pinto, Eisen, Mancebo, & Rasmussen, 2007). However, the reverse was true for chronological age: *younger adults* were *more* likely to remit over the first 2 years of follow-up. Male gender, hoarding compulsions, and greater baseline severity of OCD were also associated with a chronic course, consistent with previous studies (Catapano et al., 2006; Kempe et al., 2007; Pinto, Eisen, Mancebo, & Rasmussen, 2007; Ravizza, Maina, & Bogetto, 1997).

Risk Factors

Studies examining the risk of developing OCD can be divided into two groups: those examining characteristics that *precede* the onset of OCD (risk factors), and those that identify characteristics that are associated with OCD but do not necessarily precede OCD onset (*correlates*) (Fontenelle & Hasler, 2007; Kraemer et al., 1997) Fontenelle and Hasler (2007) conducted a qualitative review of correlates and risk factors of OCD in epidemiological samples. Results from 90 original studies and 16 reviews that met their inclusion criteria indicated several demographic, personal, and environmental variables found to be linked with increased risk of OCD in the general population. However, only eight of these studies were designed to identify *risk factors* (Bruckl et al., 2007; Crum & Antony, 1993; Douglass, Moffitt, Dar, McGee, & Silva, 1995; Geller, Klier, & Neugebauer, 2001; Janssen, Cuisinier, Hoogduin, & de Graauw, 1996; Peterson, Pine, Cohen, & Brook, 2001; Roussos et al., 2003; Valleni-Basile et al., 1995). Older adolescents, minority racial status, and having a first-degree relative with OCD were identified as demographic and innate risk factors for the development of OCD. Childhood psychiatric antecedents to OCD included separation anxiety disorder, attention-deficit hyperactivity disorder, tics, substance abuse, and depression (Bruckl et al., 2007; Douglass, Moffitt, Dar, McGee, & Silva, 1995; Peterson, Pine, Cohen, & Brook, 2001).

Genetic Vulnerability

Several studies of clinical samples have found higher rates of OCD in individuals who have a first-degree relative with OCD (Black, Noyes, Goldstein, & Blum, 1992; Nestadt et al., 2000; Pauls, Alsobrook, Goodman, & Rasmussen, 1995). Twin and family genetic studies provide some support for the hypothesis that genetic factors play a role in the manifestation of OCD.

More recently, some studies have found that having a positive family history of OCD may predispose individuals to experience onset of OCD at a younger age, particularly in childhood (do Rosario-Campos et al., 2005; Hanna, Himle, Curtis, & Gillespie, 2005; Nestadt et al., 2000; Reddy et al., 2001). In one family study of OCD, the risk of OCD was 12% in first-degree relatives of OCD probands vs. 3% in relatives of psychiatrically healthy controls, and risk was highest (18%) in people whose siblings developed OCD before they were 18 years old (Nestadt et al., 2000). However, the evidence is more suggestive of inheritance of a general vulnerability to developing anxiety disorders than to a specific inheritance of OCD (Steketee & Barlow, 2002).

Neurobiological Factors

Neurobiological models of etiology focus on cortico-striato-pallido-thalamic (CSPT) circuitry (Raush, Whalen, Dougherty, & Jenike, 1998; Saxena, Brody, Schwartz, & Baxter, 1998). Although a primary pathological process underlying core OCD symptoms has not yet been definitively identified, functional imaging studies have established elevated metabolism in CSPT circuits in patients with OCD (especially during OC symptom provocation) and decreased activation following successful pharmacological or behavioral treatment (Hoehn-Saric et al., 2001).

Temperament

Behavioral inhibition appears to be a stable developmental personality trait shared by patients with OCD as well as others with other anxiety disorders (Kagan, Reznick, & Snidman, 1988). Toddlers with behavioral inhibition show a general fearfulness to unfamiliar stimuli/people and avoidance of novel situations that generally persists into childhood. Further, behaviorally inhibited children are at increased risk for other anxiety disorders and depression (Hirshfeld-Becker et al., 2003; Rosenbaum et al., 2000). Other OCD-specific childhood traits such as perfectionism, ambivalence, excessive devotion to work, and excessive morality have been reported by adult OCD patients but have not been systematically studied in children with OCD (Rasmussen & Eisen, 1998).

Evidence of similar personality traits across anxiety disorders supports theories of a genetic vulnerability that is shared among the anxiety disorders (Rasmussen & Eisen, 2002).

Life Events

Life events usually experienced in young adulthood have been linked to OCD onset or exacerbation of symptoms. Having a child or suffering a miscarriage is associated with greater risk for initial or recurrent onset of OCD in women and a few case reports of men (Abramowitz, Moore, Carmin, Wiegartz, & Purdon, 2001; Buttolph, Peets, & Holland, 1998; Geller, Klier, & Neugebauer, 2001). For women, elevated rates of OCD onset during the 6-week postpartum period (4%) were found in one study of 302 women who gave birth at a Turkish hospital (Uguz, Akman, Kaya, & Cilli, 2007). Women with postpartum OCD (versus OCD without a postpartum onset) had more frequent aggressive obsessions and less severe OCD symptoms. In this same study, women with avoidant and obsessive-compulsive personality disorders were at higher risk for postpartum OCD.

Traumatic and nontraumatic stressful life events are associated with increased rates of psychopathology including OCD (Boudreaux, Kilpatrick, Resnick, Best, & Saunders, 1998; Gothelf, Aharonovsky, Horesh, Carty, & Apter, 2004; Jordan et al., 1991; Maes, Mylle, Delmeire, & Altamura, 2000). At least two studies have documented that patients with OCD reported higher rates of stressful life events in the year preceding OCD onset than do unaffected control subjects (Gothelf, Aharonovsky, Horesh, Carty, & Apter, 2004; McKeon, Roa, & Mann, 1984). Experiencing a traumatic event is associated with more severe OCD symptoms (Cromer, Schmidt, & Murphy, 2007). Future work is needed examining stressful life events experienced in young adulthood (such as transitions into college, the workforce, dating and marital relationships, financial independence, and independent living) and their impact on the course of OCD symptoms.

Cognitive Vulnerabilities

Cognitive models of psychopathology speculate that dysfunctional beliefs predispose individuals to develop different types of psychopathology (Beck, 1976). Cognitive models applied to OCD (Rachman, 1997; Salkovskis, 1985) propose specific domains of empirically derived beliefs that may be implicated in the etiology and maintenance of OCD (Rachman, 1997; Salkovskis, 1985). Correlational research supports an association between OCD symptoms and the following beliefs: *(1)* inflated personal responsibility for controlling or preventing harm; *(2)* overestimation of threat; *(3)* assigning exaggerated importance to thoughts; *(4)* a need to control thoughts; *(5)* perfectionism or intolerance for mistakes; and *(6)* intolerance for uncertainty (Frost & Steketee, 2002; Obsessive Compulsive Cognitions Working Group, 1997). Studies using prospective designs are needed to test the cognitive vulnerability model in a risk sample of OCD.

Treatment Interventions

Significant evidence supports the efficacy of selective serotonin reuptake inhibitors (SSRIs) and cognitive-behavioral therapy (CBT) in reducing OCD symptoms. Clinical practice guidelines (APA, 2007; Baldwin et al., 2005; Clinical Practice Guidelines, 2006) recommend that initial treatment be selected based on five factors: *(1)* nature and severity of patient symptoms; *(2)* comorbid psychiatric and medical conditions; *(3)* past treatment history; *(4)* current medications; and *(5)* patient preferences. In addition, level of impairment, concomitant medications, and availability of treatments also need to be considered when selecting treatment strategies (Baldwin et al., 2005).

A specific form of CBT, exposure and response (ritual) prevention (E/RP), has consistently shown to be effective in reducing OCD symptoms (Abramowitz, 1997; Eddy, Dutra, Bradley, & Westen, 2004; Gava et al., 2007). During E/RP, the patient is encouraged to actively confront feared situations, thoughts, images (exposure) without engaging in anxiety-reduction behaviors (compulsions, avoidance). In theory, repeated exposures without the occurrence of feared consequences result in the habitual desensitization of anxiety over time. Individuals who complete E/RP show significantly greater reductions in symptoms than individuals who receive no treatment, usual care, or relaxation training (Gava et al., 2007; Greist et al., 2002; Lindsay, Crino, & Andrews, 1997).

Cognitive therapy is another form of CBT that has been rapidly gaining empirical support as a treatment for OCD. The primary aim of cognitive therapy is to help patients identify, challenge, and modify dysfunctional beliefs that play a central role in the maintenance of OCD symptoms (Rachman, 1997). Data support the use of cognitive techniques especially when combined with behavioral experiments (Cottraux et al., 2001; Freeston, Rheaume, & Ladouceur, 1996; Whittal, Thordarson, & McLean, 2005).

Clomipramine and SSRIs are effective in reducing OCD symptoms (Denys, 2006; Ellingrod, 1998); however, the SSRIs are recommended as the first-line pharmacological treatment for OCD due to a better adverse event profile. Pharmacological and CBT treatments have documented evidence as monotherapies as well as a combined treatment strategy. Although the optimal sequence of treatments has not yet been identified, the APA guidelines recommend E/RP monotherapy for individuals who are motivated to cooperate with E/RP demands, do not have severe depressive symptoms, or prefer not to take medications. SSRI monotherapy is recommended for individuals who are not able to engage in E/RP, report a previous response to an SSRI, or prefer medication treatments over CBT. A combination of SSRI treatment and CBT is recommended for individuals who have other comorbid conditions that could benefit from SSRI treatment (e.g., major depression, generalized anxiety disorder) or those who show an unsatisfactory response to monotherapy. Combined treatment is also recommended for individuals who prefer to take medications for the shortest possible time, as there are data from uncontrolled follow-up studies that suggest that CBT may help to prevent or delay relapse when the SSRI is discontinued (Biondi & Picardi, 2005; Hembree, Riggs, Kozak, Franklin, & Foa, 2003; Simpson et al., 2004).

In adult OCD treatment, *age at time of treatment* has generally not been found to moderate treatment outcome (Denys, 2006; Keeley, Storch, Merlo, & Geffken, 2008). In the only study to report an age effect, Foa and colleagues (1983) found that younger adults showed a greater reduction in OCD symptoms. In contrast, an *earlier age at OCD onset* and *longer duration of*

OCD were associated with a poorer response to clomipramine and SSRIs (Fineberg & Gale, 2005). Greater baseline severity of OCD and comorbid tics also associated with poorer response to clomipramine and SSRIs in adults (Fineberg & Gale, 2005; Mataix-Cols, Rauch, Manzo, Jenike, & Baer, 1999). Other possible treatment moderators have been examined such as depression, personality traits, insight, and expressed emotion. However, there is not consistent evidence that these variables affect treatment outcome.

While SSRIs and CBT treatments are highly effective in reducing OCD, studies examining broader measures of outcome (e.g., quality of life and psychosocial functioning) and long-term treatment outcome are needed (Eddy, Dutra, Bradley, & Westen, 2004; Gava et al., 2007). In light of the fact that residual symptoms are common following CBT and SSRI treatments (Abramowitz, 1998) and changes in psychosocial functioning often lag behind symptom reductions, examining quality of life and long-term functioning of young adults with OCD is critical in assessing whether these individuals are able to "catch up" to their peers or return to premorbid functioning.

Conclusion

Although OCD symptoms usually begin to develop in childhood, onset of OCD is most likely influenced by a complex system of genetic, neurobiological, and psychosocial influences that manifest in full-blown OCD symptoms in adolescence and young adulthood. The period of young adulthood is a critical point of intervention because OCD can significantly disrupt attainment of important developmental milestones necessary for success in later stages of life. OCD often interferes with forming intimate relationships, finding and keeping a job, and academic functioning. Successful OCD treatment in young adulthood could result in successful adaptation and lead to lower rates of disability in middle adulthood. More research is needed to identify developmental pathways to disability as well as protective factors. That is, why do some individuals with severe OCD return to premorbid functioning while others continue to be impaired?

OCD symptom expression is strikingly similar across the life span, but most studies are cross-sectional and the stability of OCD symptoms from adolescence through adulthood is unclear. Prospective studies are needed to understand the potential impact of cognitive and social development on OCD symptom expression and course.

SSRI and cognitive-behavioral treatments for OCD are highly effective in reducing OCD symptoms. Preliminary prospective data suggest that younger adults are more likely to remit from OCD, but it remains unclear whether early detection and treatment can improve prognosis of OCD in adolescents and young adults. Changes in functioning often lag behind symptom reductions. More work is needed to evaluate the effect of treatment interventions on long-term functioning to determine whether alternative strategies are needed to improve psychosocial outcome.

KEY POINTS

- Risk for development of OCD is highest in late adolescence and early adulthood, as the majority of individuals with OCD first experience some OC symptoms in childhood and clinically significant OC symptoms before age 25.
- Differences in age-of-onset distributions support the idea of etiological heterogeneity and different pathways, which result in some individuals developing OCD around puberty and others in early adulthood.
- Life events that typically occur in early adulthood, particularly pregnancy and miscarriage, are associated with OCD onset, exacerbation of symptoms, or recurrence.

> **PRACTICE GUIDELINES**
>
> - SSRI and CBT treatments are highly effective in reducing OCD symptoms. More work is needed to understand whether young adults accept and adhere to SSRI and CBT treatments.
> - In addition to symptom reduction, treatment interventions should focus on development of skills necessary for successful transition into adulthood and adaptive social and occupational functioning.
> - Appropriate treatment strategies may be needed during stressful life events, such as entering the workforce and having children, to prevent recurrence or exacerbation of OCD symptoms.

References

Abramowitz, J. S. (1997). Effectiveness of psychological and pharmacological treatments for obsessive-compulsive disorder: A quantitative review. *Journal of Consulting and Clinical Psychology, 65,* 44–52.

Abramowitz, J. S. (1998). Does cognitive-behavioral therapy cure obsessive compulsive disorder? A meta-analytic evaluation of clinical significance. *Behavior Therapy, 29,* 339–355.

Abramowitz, J., Moore, K., Carmin, C., Wiegartz, P. S., & Purdon, C. (2001). Acute onset of obsessive-compulsive disorder in males following childbirth. *Psychosomatics, 42,* 429–431.

Albert, U., Picco, C., Maina, G., Forner, F., Aguglia, E., & Bogetto, F. (2002). Phenomenology of patients with early and adult onset obsessive-compulsive disorder. *Epiemiologia e Psychiatria Sociale, 11,* 116–126.

Alonso, P., Menchon, J. M., Pifarre, J., Mataix-Cols, D., Torres, L., Salgado, P., Vallejo, J. (2001). Long-term follow-up and predictors of clinical outcome in obsessive-compulsive patients treated with serotonin reuptake inhibitors and behavioral therapy. *Journal of Clinical Psychiatry, 62,* 535–540.

American Academy of Child and Adolescent Psychiatry. (1998). Practice parameters for the assessment and treatment of children and adolescents with obsessive-compulsive disorder. *Journal of American Academy of Child and Adolescent Psychiatry, 37,* 27S–45S.

American Psychiatric Association. (2000). *Diagnostic and statistical manual of mental disorders* (4th ed.), text revision (DSM-IV-TR). Washington, DC: Author.

American Psychiatric Association. (2007). Practice guidelines for the treatment of patients with obsessive compulsive disorder. *American Journal of Psychiatry, 164*(Suppl. 7), 5–53.

Andrade, N. N., Hishinuma, E. S., McDermott, J. F., Jr., Johnson, R. C., Goebert, D. A., Makini, G. K., Jr., Nahulu, L. B., Yuen, N. Y., McArdle, J. J., Bell, C. K., Carlton, B. S., Miyamoto, R. H., Nishimura, S. T., Else, R. N., Guerrero, A. P., Darmal, A. & Waldron, J. A. (2006). The National Center on Indigenous Hawaiian Behavioral Health study of prevalence of psychiatric disorders in native Hawaiian adolescents. *Journal of the American Academy of Child and Adolescent Psychiatry, 45,* 26–36.

Baldwin, D. S., Anderson, I. M., Nutt, D. J, Bandelow, B., Bond, A., Davidson, J. R., den Boer, J. A., Fineberg, N. A., Knapp, M., Scott, J., & Wittchen, H. U. (2005). Evidence-based guidelines for the pharmacological treatment of anxiety disorders: Recommendations from the British Association for Psychopharmacology. *Journal of Psychopharmacology, 19,* 567–596.

Beck, A. T. (1976). *Cognitive therapy of emotional disorders.* New York: International University Press.

Biondi, M., & Picardi, A. (2005). Increased maintenance of obsessive-compulsive disorder remission after integrated serotonergic treatment and cognitive psychotherapy compared with medication alone. *Psychotherapy and Psychosomatics, 74,* 123–128.

Bjorgvinsson, T., Hart, J., & Heffelfinger, S. (2007). Obsessive-compulsive disorder: Update on assessment and treatment. *Journal of Psychiatric Practice, 13,* 362–372.

Black, D. W., Noyes, R., Jr., Goldstein, R. B., & Blum, N. (1992). A family study of obsessive-compulsive disorder. *Archives of General Psychiatry, 49,* 362–368.

Bland, R. C., Newman, S. C., & Orn, H. (1988). Age of onset of psychiatric disorders. *Acta Psychiatrica Scandinavica, 77*(Suppl. 338), 43–49.

Boudreaux, E., Kilpatrick, D. G., Resnick, H. S., Best, C. L., & Saunders, B. E. (1998). Criminal victimization, posttraumatic stress disorder, and comorbid psychopathology among a community sample of women. *Journal of Trauma and Stress, 11,* 665–678.

Bruckl, T. M., Wittchen, H. U., Hofler, M., Pfister, H., Schneider, S., & Lieb, R. (2007). Childhood separation anxiety and the risk of subsequent psychopathology: Results from a community study. *Psychotherapy and Psychosomatics, 76,* 47–56.

Buttolph, M. L., Peets, K. E., & Holland, A. D. (1998). Obsessive-compulsive disorder symptoms and medication treatment in pregnancy. In M. A. Jenike, L. Baer, & W. E. Minichiello (Eds.), *Obsessive-compulsive disorders: Practical management* (3rd ed.) (pp. 84–95). St. Louis, MO: Mosby.

Canals, J., Domenech, E., Carbajo, G., & Blade, J. (1997). Prevalence of DSM-III-R and ICD-10 psychiatric disorders in a Spanish population of 18-year olds. *Acta Psychiatrica Scandinavica, 96,* 287–294.

Catapano, F., Perris, F., Masella, M., Rossano, F., Cigliano, M., Magliano, L., & Maj, M. (2006). Obsessive-compulsive disorder: A 3-year prospective follow-up study of patients treated with serotonin reuptake inhibitors OCD follow-up study. *Journal of Psychiatric Research, 40,* 502–510.

Chabane, N., Delorme, R., Millet, B., Mouren, M. C., Leboyer, M., & Pauls, D. (2005). Early-onset obsessive-compulsive disorder: A subgroup with a specific clinical and familial pattern? *Journal of Child Psychology and Psychiatry, 46,* 881–887.

Clinical Practice Guidelines: Management of Anxiety Disorders. (2006). Obsessive-compulsive disorder. *Canadian Journal of Psychiatry, 51*(Suppl. 20), 43S–50S.

Costello, E. J., Angold, A., Burns, B. J., Stangl, D.K., Tweed, D. L., Erkanli, A., & Worthman, C. M. (1996). The Great Smoky Mountains Study of Youth: Goals, design, methods, and the prevalence of DSM-III-R disorders. *Archives of General Psychiatry, 53,* 1129–1136.

Costello, E. J., Mustillo, S., Erkanli, A., Keeler, G., & Angold, A. (2003). Prevalence and development of psychiatric disorders in childhood and adolescence. *Archives of General Psychiatry, 60,* 837–844.

Cottraux, J., Note, I., Yao, S. N., Lafont, S., Note, B., Mollard, E., Bouvard, M., Sauteraud, A., Bourgeois, M. & Dartigues, J. F. (2001). A randomized controlled trial of cognitive therapy versus intensive behavior therapy in obsessive compulsive disorder. *Psychotherapy and Psychosomatics, 70,* 288–297.

Crino, R., Slade, T., & Andrews, G. (2005). The changing prevalence and severity of obsessive-compulsive disorder criteria from DSM-III to DSM-IV. *American Journal of Psychiatry, 162,* 876–882.

Cromer, K. R., Schmidt, N. B., & Murphy, D. L. (2007). An investigation of traumatic life events and obsessive-compulsive disorder. *Behavior Research and Therapy, 45,* 1683–1691.

Crum, R. M., & Anthony, J. C. (1993). Cocaine use and other suspected risk factors for obsessive-compulsive disorder: A prospective study with data from the Epidemiologic Catchment Area surveys. *Drug and Alcohol Dependence, 31,* 281–295.

Denys, D. (2006). Pharmacotherapy of obsessive-compulsive disorder and obsessive-compulsive spectrum disorders. *Psychiatric Clinics of North America, 29,* 553–584, xi.

Di Nardo, P., Moras, K., Barlow, D. H., Rapee, R. M., & Brown, T. A. (1993). Reliability of DSM-III-R anxiety disorder categories. Using the Anxiety Disorders Interview Schedule-Revised (ADIS-R). *Archives of General Psychiatry, 50,* 251–256.

Douglass, H. M., Moffitt, T. E., Dar, R., McGee, R., & Silva, P. (1995). Obsessive compulsive disorder in a birth cohort of 18 year olds: Prevalence and predictors. *Journal of the American Academy of Child and Adolescent Psychiatry, 34,* 1424–1431.

Eddy, K. T, Dutra, L., Bradley, R., & Westen, D. (2004). A multidimensional meta-analysis of psychotherapy and pharmacotherapy for obsessive-compulsive disorder. *Clinical Psychology Review, 24,* 1011–1030.

Eisen, J. L., Goodman, W. K., Keller, M. B., Warshaw, M. G., DeMarco, L. M., Luce, D. D., & Rasmussen, S. A. (1999). Patterns of remission and relapse in obsessive-compulsive disorder: A 2-year prospective study. *Journal of Clinical Psychiatry, 60,* 346–351.

Ellingrod, V. L. (1998). Pharmacotherapy of primary obsessive-compulsive disorder: Review of the literature. *Pharmacotherapy, 18,* 936–960.

Fineberg, N. A., & Gale, T. M. (2005). Evidence-based pharmacotherapy of obsessive-compulsive disorder. *International Journal of Neuropsychopharmacology, 8,* 107–129.

First, M. B., Spitzer, R. L., & Williams, J. B. W. (1996). *Structured clinical interview for DSM-IV OCD.* Washington, DC: American Psychiatric Association.

Flament, M. F., Whitaker, A., Rapoport, J. L., Davies, M., Berg, C. J., Kalkikow, K., Sceery, W. & Shaffer, D. (1988). Obsessive compulsive disorder in adolescence: An epidemiologic study. *Journal of the American Academy of Child and Adolescent Psychiatry, 27,* 764–771.

Foa, E. B., Grayson, J. B., Steketee, G. S., Doppelt, H. G., Turner, R. M., & Latimer, P. R. (1983). Success and failure in the behavioral treatment of obsessive-compulsives. *Journal of Consulting and Clinical Psychology, 51,* 287–297.

Fontenelle, L. F., & Hasler, G. (2007).The analytical epidemiology of obsessive-compulsive disorder: Risk factors and correlates. *Progress in*

Neuropsychopharmacology and Biological Psychiatry, 32(1), 1–15.

Fontenelle, L. F., Mendlowicz, M. V., Marques, C., & Versiani, M. (2003). Early- and late-onset obsessive-compulsive disorder in adult patients: An exploratory clinical and therapeutic study. *Journal of Psychiatric Research, 37,* 127–133.

Freeston, M. H., Rheaume, J., & Ladouceur, R. (1996). Correcting faulty appraisals of obsessional thoughts. *Behavior Research and Therapy, 34,* 433–446.

Frost, R. O., & Steketee, G. (2002). *Cognitive approaches to obsessions and compulsions: Theory, assessment and treatment.* Oxford, England: Elsevier.

Garland, A. F., Hough, R. L., McCabe, K., Yeh, M., Wood, P. A., & Aarons, G. A. (2001). Prevalence of psychiatric disorders in youths across five sectors of care. *Journal of the American Academy of Child and Adolescent Psychiatry, 30,* 409–418.

Gava, I., Barbui, C., Aguglia, E., Carlino, D., Churchill, R., DeVanna, M., & McGuire, H. F. (2007). Psychological treatments versus treatment as usual for obsessive compulsive disorder (OCD). *Cochrane Database System Reviews,* CD005333.

Geller, D. A., Biederman, J., Faraone, S., Agranat, A., Cradock, K., Hagermoser, L., Kim, G., Frazier, J., & Coffey, B. J. (2001). Developmental aspects of obsessive compulsive disorder: Findings in children, adolescents, and adults. *Journal of Nervous and Mental Disease, 189,* 471–477.

Geller, D. A., Biederman, J., Griffin, S., Jones, J., & Lefkowitz, T. R. (1996). Comorbidity of juvenile obsessive-compulsive disorder with disruptive behavior disorders. *Journal of the American Academy of Child and Adolescent Psychiatry, 35,* 1637–1646.

Geller, P. A., Klier, C. M., & Neugebauer, R. (2001). Anxiety disorders following miscarriage. *Journal of Clinical Psychiatry, 62,* 432–438.

Goodman, W. K., Price, L. H., Rasmussen, S. A., Mazure, C., Delgado, P., Heninger, G. R., & Charney, D. S. (1989a). The Yale-Brown Obsessive Compulsive Scale. II. Validity. *Archives of General Psychiatry, 46,* 1012–1016.

Goodman, W. K., Price, L. H., Rasmussen, S. A., Mazure, C., Fleischman, R. L., Hill, C. L., Henninger, G. R. & Charney, D. S. (1989b). The Yale-Brown Obsessive Compulsive Scale. I. Development, use, and reliability. *Archives of General Psychiatry, 46,* 1006–1011.

Goodwin, D. W., Guze, S. B., & Robins, E. (1969). Follow-up studies in obsessional neurosis. *Archives of General Psychiatry, 20,* 182–187.

Gothelf, D., Aharonovsky, O., Horesh, N., Carty, T., & Apter, A. (2004). Life events and personality factors in children and adolescents with obsessive-compulsive disorder and other anxiety disorders. *Comprehensive Psychiatry, 45,* 192–198.

Grant, J. E., Mancebo, M. C., Pinto, A., Williams, K. A., Eisen, J. L., & Rasmussen, S. A. (2007). Late-onset obsessive compulsive disorder: Clinical characteristics and psychiatric comorbidity. *Psychiatry Research, 152,* 21–27.

Greist, J. H., Marks, I. M., Baer, L., Kobak, K. A., Wenzel, K. W., Hirsch, M. J., Mantle, J. M., & Clary, C. M. (2002). Behavior therapy for obsessive-compulsive disorder guided by a computer or by a clinician compared with relaxation as a control. *Journal of Clinical Psychiatry, 63,* 138–145.

Hanna, G. L. (1995). Demographic and clinical features of obsessive-compulsive disorder in children and adolescents. *Journal of the American Academy of Child and Adolescent Psychiatry, 34,* 19–27.

Hanna, G. L., Himle, J. A., Curtis, G. C., & Gillespie, B. W. (2005). A family study of obsessive-compulsive disorder with pediatric probands. *American Journal of Medical Genetics Part B: Neuropsychiatric Genetics, 134,* 13–19.

Hembree, E. A., Riggs, D. S., Kozak, M. J., Franklin, M. E., & Foa, E. B. (2003). Long-term efficacy of exposure and ritual prevention therapy and serotonergic medications for obsessive-compulsive disorder. *CNS Spectrums, 8,* 363–371.

Heyman, I., Fombonne, E., Simmons, H., Ford, T., Meltzer, H., & Goodman, R. (2003). Prevalence of obsessive-compulsive disorder in the British nationwide survey of child mental health. *International Review of Psychiatry, 15,* 178–184.

Hirshfeld-Becker, D. R., Biederman, J., Calltharp, S., Rosenbaum, E. D., Faraone, S. V., & Rosenbaum, J. F. (2003). Behavioral inhibition and disinhibition as hypothesized precursors to psychopathology: Implications for pediatric bipolar disorder. *Biological Psychiatry, 53,* 985–999.

Hoehn-Saric, R., Schlaepfer, T. E., Greenberg, B. D., McLeod, D. R., Pearlson, G. D., & Wong, S. H. (2001). Cerebral blood flow in obsessive-compulsive patients with major depression: Effect of treatment with sertraline or desipramine on treatment responders and non-responders. *Psychiatry Research, 108,* 89–100.

Janssen, H. J., Cuisinier, M. C., Hoogduin, K. A., & de Graauw, K. P. (1996). Controlled prospective study on the mental health of women following pregnancy loss. *American Journal of Psychiatry, 153,* 226–230.

Jordan, B. K., Schlenger, W. E., Hough, R., Kulka, R. A., Weiss, D., Fairbank, J. A., & Marmar, C. R. (1991). Lifetime and current prevalence of specific psychiatric disorders among Vietnam veterans and controls. *Archives of General Psychiatry, 48,* 207–215.

Kagan, J., Reznick, J. S., & Snidman, N. (1988). Biological bases of childhood shyness. *Science, 240,* 167–171.

Karno, M., Golding, J. M., Sorenson, S. B., & Burnam, M. A. (1988). The epidemiology of obsessive-compulsive disorder in five US communities. *Archives of General Psychiatry, 45,* 1094–1099.

Keeley, M. L., Storch, E. A, Merlo, L. J., & Geffken, G. R. (2008). Clinical predictors of response to cognitive-behavioral therapy for obsessive-compulsive disorder. *Clinical Psychology Review, 28,* 118–130.

Kempe, P. T., van Oppen, P., de Haan, E., Twisk, J. W., Sluis, A., Smit, J. H., van Dyck, R., & van Balkom, A. J. (2007). Predictors of course in obsessive-compulsive disorder: Logistic regression versus Cox regression for recurrent events. *Acta Psychiatrica Scandinavica, 116,* 201–210.

Kessler, R. C., Berglund, P., Demler, O., Jin, R., Merikangas, K., & Walters, E. E. (2005). Lifetime prevalence and age-of-onset distributions of DSM-IV disorders in the national comorbidity. *Archives of General Psychiatry, 62,* 595–602.

Kohn, R., Westlake, R. J., Rasmussen, S. A., Marsland, R. T., & Norman, W. H. (1997). Clinical features of obsessive-compulsive disorder in elderly patients. *American Journal of Geriatric Psychiatry, 5,* 211–215.

Kolada, J. L., Bland, R. C., & Newman, S. C. (1994). Epidemiology of psychiatric disorders in Edmonton. Obsessive-compulsive disorder. *Acta Psychiatrica Scandinavica, 376,* 24–35.

Kraemer, H. C., Kazdin, A. E., Offord, D. R., Kessler, R. C., Jensen, P. S., & Kupfer, D. J. (1997). Coming to terms with the terms of risk. *Archives of General Psychiatry, 54,* 337–343.

Leckman, J. F., Grice, D. E., Barr, L. C., de Vries, A.L., Martin, C., Cohen, D. J., McDougle, C. J., Goodman, W. K., & Rasmussen, S. A. (1994). Tic-related vs. non-tic-related obsessive compulsive disorder. *Anxiety, 1,* 208–215.

Lewinsohn, P. M., Hops, H., Roberts, R. E., Seeley, J. R., & Andrews, J. A. (1993). Adolescent psychopathology: I. Prevalence and incidence of depression and other DSM-III-R disorders in high school students. *Journal of Abnormal Psychology, 102,* 133–144.

Lindsay, M., Crino, R., & Andrews, G. (1997). Controlled trial of exposure and response prevention in obsessive-compulsive disorder. *British Journal of Psychiatry, 171,* 135–139.

Maes, M., Mylle, J., Delmeire, L., & Altamura, C. (2000). Psychiatric morbidity and comorbidity following accidental man-made traumatic events: Incidence and risk factors. *European Archives of Psychiatry and Clinical Neuroscience, 250,* 156–162.

Mancebo, M. C., Eisen, J. L., Grant, J. E., & Rasmussen, S. A. (2005). Obsessive compulsive personality disorder and obsessive compulsive disorder: Clinical characteristics, diagnostic difficulties, and treatment. *Annals of Clinical Psychiatry, 17,* 197–204.

Mancebo, M. C., Garcia, A. M., Pinto, A., Freeman, J. B., Przeworski, A., Stout, R., Kane, J. S., Eisen, J. L., & Rasmussen, S. A. Juvenile-onset OCD: Clinical features in children, adolescents and adults. *Acta Psychiatrica Scandinavica, 118,* 149–59.

Masi, G., Millepiedi, S., Mucci, M., Bertini, N., Milantoni, L., & Arcangeli, F. (2005). A naturalistic study of referred children and adolescents with obsessive-compulsive disorder. *Journal of the American Academy of Child and Adolescent Psychiatry, 44,* 673–681.

Mataix-Cols, D., Rauch, S. L., Manzo, P. A., Jenike, M. A., & Baer, L. (1999). Use of factor-analyzed symptom dimensions to predict outcome with serotonin reuptake inhibitors and placebo in the treatment of obsessive-compulsive disorder. *American Journal of Psychiatry, 156,* 1409–1416.

McKeon, J., Roa, B., & Mann, A. (1984). Life events and personality traits in obsessive-compulsive neurosis. *British Journal of Psychiatry, 144,* 185–189.

Nestadt, G., Samuels, J., Riddle, M., Bienvenu, O. J., Liang, K. Y., Labuda, M., Walkup, J., Grados, M., & Hoehn-Saric, R. (2000). A family study of obsessive-compulsive disorder. *Archives of General Psychiatry, 57,* 358–363.

Obsessive Compulsive Cognitions Working Group. (1997). Cognitive assessment of obsessive-compulsive disorder. *Behavior Research and Therapy, 35,* 667–681.

Orloff, L. M., Battle, M. A., Baer, L., Ivanjack, L., Pettit, A. R., Buttolph, L., & Jenike, M. A. (1994). Long-term follow-up of 85 patients with obsessive-compulsive disorder. *American Journal of Psychiatry, 151,* 441–442.

Pauls, D. L., Alsobrook, J. P., Goodman, W. K., Rasmussen, S. A., & Leckman, J. F. (1995). A family study of obsessive-compulsive disorder. *American Journal of Psychiatry, 152,* 76–84.

Peterson, B. S., Pine, D. S., Cohen, P., & Brook, J. S. (2001). Prospective, longitudinal study of tic, obsessive-compulsive, and attention-deficit/hyperactivity disorders in an epidemiological sample. *Journal of the American Academy of Child and Adolescent Psychiatry, 40,* 685–695.

Philpot, M. P., & Banerjee, S. (1998). Obsessive-compulsive disorder in the elderly. *Behavioral Neurology, 11,* 117–121.

Pinto, A., Eisen, J. L., Mancebo, M. C., & Rasmussen, S. A. (2007). A 2-year follow-up study of the course of obsessive compulsive disorder. Poster presentation at the annual meeting of the Association for Behavioral and Cognitive Therapies, Philadelphia, PA: ABCT, New York, NY.

Pinto, A., Mancebo, M. C., Eisen, J. L., Pagano, M. E., & Rasmussen, S. A. (2006). The Brown Longitudinal Obsessive Compulsive Study: Clinical features and symptoms of the sample at intake. *Journal of Clinical Psychiatry*, *67*, 703–711.

Rachman S. (1997). A cognitive theory of obsessions. *Behavior Research and Therapy*, *35*, 793–802.

Rasmussen, S. A., & Eisen, J. L. (1992). The epidemiology and clinical features of OCD. In M. A. Jenike (Ed.), *Psychiatric clinics of North America* (pp. 743–758). Philadelphia: W. B. Saunders.

Rasmussen, S. A., & Eisen, J. L. (1998). The epidemiology and clinical features of obsessive-compulsive disorder. In M. A. Jenike, L. Baer, & W. E. Minichiello (Eds.), *Obsessive-compulsive disorders: Practical management* (3rd ed.) (pp. 12–43). Boston: Mosby.

Rasmussen, S. A., & Eisen, J. L. (2002). The course and clinical features of obsessive compulsive disorder. In K. L. Davis, D. Charney, J. T. Coyle, & C. Nemeroff (Eds.), *Neuropsychopharmacology: The fifth generation of progress* (pp. 1593–1608). New York: Lippincott Williams & Wilkins.

Rasmussen, S. A., & Eisen, J. L. (2002). The course and clinical features of obsessive-compulsive disorder. In K. L. Davis, D. Charney, J. T., Coyle, & C. Nemeroff (Eds.), *Neuropsychopharmacology: The fifth generation of progress* (pp. 1593–1608). New York: Lippincott Williams & Wilkins.

Rasmussen, S. A., & Tsuang, M. T. (1986). Clinical characteristics and family history in DSM-III obsessive-compulsive disorder. *American Journal of Psychiatry*, *143*, 317–322.

Rauch, S. L., Whalen, P. J., Dougherty, D., & Jenike, M. A. (1998). Neurobiological models of obsessive-compulsive disorder. In M. A. Jenike, L. Baer, W. E. Minichiello (Eds.), *Obsessive-compulsive disorders: Practical management* (3rd ed.) (pp. 222–253). Boston: Mosby.

Ravizza, L., Maina, G., & Bogetto, F. (1997). Episodic and chronic obsessive-compulsive disorder. *Depression and Anxiety*, *6*, 154–158.

Reddy, P. S., Reddy, Y. C., Srinath, S., Khanna, S., Sheshadri, S. P., & Girimaji, S. R. (2001). A family study of juvenile obsessive-compulsive disorder. *Canadian Journal of Psychiatry*, *46*, 346–351.

Reddy, Y. C., D'Souza, S. M., Shetti, C., Kandavel, T., Deshpande, S., Badamath, S., Singisetti, S. (2005). An 11- to 13-year follow-up of 75 subjects with obsessive-compulsive disorder. *Journal of Clinical Psychiatry*, *66*, 744–749.

Regier, D. A., Farmer, M. E., Rae, D. S., Myers, J. K., Kramer, M., Robins, L. N., George, L. K., Karno, M., & Locke, B. Z. (1993). One-month prevalence of mental disorders in the United States and sociodemographic characteristics: The Epidemiologic Catchment Area study. *Acta Psychiatrica Scandinavica*, *88*, 35–47.

Reinherz, H. Z., Giaconia, R. M., Lefkowitz, E. S., Pakiz, B., & Frost, A. K. (1993). Prevalence of psychiatric disorders in a community population of older adolescents. *Journal of the American Academy of Child and Adolescent Psychiatry*, *32*, 369–377.

Rosario-Campos, M. C., Leckman, J. F., Curi, M., Quatrano, S., Katsovitch, L., Miguel, E. C., & Pauls, D. L. (2005). A family study of early-onset obsessive-compulsive disorder. *American Journal of Medical Genetics Part B: Neuropsychiatric Genetics*, *136*, 92–97.

Rosenbaum, J. F., Biederman, J., Hirshfeld-Becker, D. R., Kagan, J., Snidman, N., Friedman, D., Nineberg, A., Gallery, D. J., & Faraone, S. V. (2000). A controlled study of behavioral inhibition in children of parents with panic disorder and depression. *American Journal of Psychiatry*, *157*, 2002–2010.

Roussos, A., Francis, K., Koumoula, A., Richardson, C., Kabakos, C., Kiriakidou, T., Karagianni, S., & Karamolegou, K. (2003). The Leyton Obsessional Inventory—child version in Greek adolescents: Standardization in a national school-based survey and two-year follow-up. *European Child and Adolescent Psychiatry*, *12*, 58–66.

Salkovskis, P. M. (1985). Obsessional-compulsive problems: A cognitive-behavioural analysis. *Behavior Research and Therapy*, *23*, 571–583.

Samuels, J., Nestadt, G., Bienvenu, O. J., Costa, P. T., Riddle, M. A., Liang, K. Y., Hoehn-Saric, R., Grados, M. A. & Cullen, B. A. (2000). Personality disorders and normal personality dimensions in obsessive-compulsive disorder. *British Journal of Psychiatry*, *177*, 457–462.

Saxena, S., Brody, A. L., Schwartz, J. M., & Baxter, L. R. (1998). Neuroimaging and frontal-subcortical circuitry in obsessive-compulsive disorder. *British Journal of Psychiatry*, *Supplement*, 26–37.

Simpson, H. B., Liebowitz, M. R., Foa, E. B., Kozak, M. J., Schmidt, A. B., Rowan, V., Petkova, E., Kjernisted, K., Huppert, J. D., Fransklin, M. E., Davies, S. O., & Campeas, R. (2004). Post-treatment effects of exposure therapy and clomipramine in obsessive-compulsive disorder. *Depression and Anxiety*, *19*, 225–233.

Skoog, G., & Skoog, I. (1999). A 40-year follow-up of patients with obsessive compulsive disorder. *Archives of General Psychiatry*, *56*, 121–127.

Steketee, G., & Barlow, D. H. (2002). Obsessive-compulsive disorder. In D. H. Barlow (Ed.), *Anxiety and its disorders: The nature and treatment of anxiety and panic* (2nd ed.) (pp. 516–550). New York: Guilford.

Steketee, G., Eisen, J., Dyck, I., Warshaw, M., & Rasmussen, S. (1999). Predictors of course in obsessive-compulsive disorder. *Psychiatry Research, 89,* 229–238.

Steketee, G., & Frost, R. O. (2007). *Compulsive hoarding and acquiring.* New York: Oxford University Press.

Steketee, G., Frost, R., & Bogart, K. (1996).The Yale-Brown Obsessive Compulsive Scale: Interview versus self-report. *Behavior Research and Therapy, 34,* 675–684.

Stewart, S. E., Geller, D. A., Jenike, M., Pauls, D., Shaw, D., Mullin, B., & Faraone, S. V. (2004). Long-term outcome of pediatric obsessive-compulsive disorder: A meta-analysis and qualitative review of the literature. *Acta Psychiatrica Scandinavica, 110,* 4–13.

Swedo, S. E., Rapoport, J. L., Leonard, H., Lenane, M., & Cheslow, D. (1989). Obsessive-compulsive disorder in children and adolescents. Clinical phenomenology of 70 consecutive cases. *Archives of General Psychiatry, 46,* 335–341.

Thomsen, P. H., & Mikkelsen, H. U. (1991).Children and adolescents with obsessive-compulsive disorder: The demographic and diagnostic characteristics of 61 Danish patients. *Acta Psychiatrica Scandinavica, 83,* 262–266.

Tukel, R., Oflaz, S. B., Ozyildirim, I., Aslantas, B., Ertekin, E., Sozen, A., Alyanak, F. & Atli, H. (2007). Comparison of clinical characteristics in episodic and chronic obsessive-compulsive disorder. *Depression and Anxiety, 24,* 251–255.

Uguz, F., Akman, C., Kaya, N., & Cilli, A. S. (2007). Postpartum-onset obsessive-compulsive disorder: Incidence, clinical features, and related factors. *Journal of Clinical Psychiatry, 68,* 132–138.

Valleni-Basile, L. A., Garrison, C. Z., Jackson, K. L., Waller, J. L., McKeown, R. E., Addy, C. L., & Cuffe, S. P. (1995). Frequency of Obsessive Compulsive Disorder in a community sample of young adolescents. *Journal of the American Academy of Child and Adolescent Psychiatry, 34,* 782–791.

Verhulst, F. C., Van der Ende, J., Ferdinand, R. F., & Kasius, M. C. (1997). The prevalence of DSM-III-R diagnoses in a national sample of Dutch adolescents. *Archives of General Psychiatry, 54,* 329–336.

Whittal, M. L., Thordarson, D. S., & McLean P. D. (2005). Treatment of obsessive-compulsive disorder: Cognitive behavior therapy vs. exposure and response prevention. *Behavior Research and Therapy, 43,* 1559–1576.

Wilhelm, S., & Steketee, G. (2006). *Cognitive therapy for obsessive-compulsive disorder.* Oakland, CA: New Harbinger Publications.

Wittchen, H. U., Nelson, C. B., & Lachner, G. (1998). Prevalence of mental disorders and psychosocial impairments in adolescents and young adults. *Psychological Medicine, 28,* 109–126.

Zohar, A. H., Ratzoni, G., Pauls, D. L., Apter, A., Bleich, A., Kron, S., Rappaport, M., Weizman, A. & Cohen, D. J. (1992).An epidemiological study of obsessive-compulsive disorder and related disorders in Israeli adolescents. *Journal of the American Academy of Child and Adolescent Psychiatry, 31,* 1057–1061.

Chapter 17

Tobacco Use and Nicotine Dependence

Anne E. Smith and Suchitra Krishnan-Sarin

Betty is a 21-year-old Caucasian woman who began smoking at age 13. In adolescence she lived with her mother (a smoker) and younger brother (also a smoker) and had intermittent contact with her biological father (a nonsmoker). She initially smoked only at parties with friends but soon progressed to regular daily smoking. All of her friends smoked cigarettes. In high school, this meant smoking a cigarette at the bus stop, sneaking a cigarette in the school bathroom or behind the athletic building during the school day, and then smoking 4–8 cigarettes after school. Although Betty had been athletic and interested in team sports in elementary and middle school, she found it more and more difficult to keep up in high school and quit all sports at the beginning of her sophomore year. She reports a mild depression during that year which resolved itself without treatment, but she describes herself as generally "moody." Since graduating and moving into her own apartment, she has smoked nearly a pack a day. Betty has frequently tried to quit out of concern for her health and the expense, but she has never been successful at establishing abstinence for longer than 24 hours. She has never sought help with quitting from a doctor or other health care provider. During previous attempts to quit she felt overwhelmed by cravings to smoke, feelings of restlessness and irritability, and a diminished ability to manage her daily life. She believes that smoking cigarettes helps her calm down when stressed and helps to manage her appetite and keep her on her diet. She worries that if she quits smoking she will gain at least 15 pounds and will be unable to cope with the withdrawal symptoms, particularly the restlessness and irritability. She also admits that she is reluctant to quit because she enjoys smoking—particularly when drinking alcohol—and that many in her social circle smoke and she would feel not only tempted to smoke when they light up but also excluded and isolated from the group. She is presently motivated to quit smoking because of a new relationship with a man who does not smoke and has encouraged her to quit.

Tobacco use is one of the most serious health-related behaviors of North American young adults. Cigarette smoking is the leading preventable cause of death in the United States, accounting for approximately 1 of every 5 deaths (438,000 people) each year and estimated to be responsible for $167 billion in annual health-related economic losses in the United States (CDC, 2002a, 2004, 2005a). Tobacco use is most prevalent in young adulthood with 24.4% of 18–24 year olds reporting current cigarette use (CDC, 2006a), and despite declines in use over recent decades, data suggest that the rate of decline has slowed and positive perception of smoking is increasing once again among young people (Johnston et al., 2007).

Common features of young adult nicotine dependence are illustrated in this case study. In many ways, nicotine dependence and tobacco use follow a developmental progression from initiation in young adolescence that is strongly driven by friends' use, reduced or infrequent involvement in activities, and the presence of mood symptoms. Once established, tobacco use typically continues despite efforts to quit that are frequently motivated by health concerns and financial expense. Furthermore, tobacco use is often described as a response to stress or negative affect and for weight management. Finally, any withdrawal symptoms are anticipated to be experienced as fairly distressing and intolerable, and a cycle of dosing withdrawal symptoms with nicotine/tobacco use quickly develops.

A complex interaction of biological, behavioral, social, and psychological factors influences initiation and maintenance of tobacco use in the development of nicotine dependence. Influences on the progression and continuation of smoking include not only the aversive and rewarding influences of nicotine but also individual, social, and cultural factors such as heritability, expectancies, peer groups, and economics. This chapter discusses the epidemiology of tobacco use and dependence, briefly describes the neurobiology of nicotine dependence, identifies related issues that are particularly salient to adolescent development and the transition to adulthood, and reviews emerging evidence regarding the interaction between gene and environmental factors in the establishment of tobacco dependence. It concludes with a discussion about behavioral and pharmacological interventions and treatment guidelines.

Epidemiology

Recently young adulthood has been recognized as a critical period for tobacco use initiation (Wechsler et al., 1998). For example, 25% of 12th grade "never-smokers" initiated smoking in the year following graduation, and 39% of 12th graders increased their cigarette use in that year (Tercyak, Rodriguez, & Audrain-McGovern, 2007). Similarly, 20% of smokers tried their first cigarette after the age of 18 (Hammond, 2005). As a result, although each day an estimated 4,000 young people between the ages of 12 and 17 years initiate cigarette smoking in the United States, and an estimated 1,140 young people become daily cigarette smokers (CDC, 2006b), a considerable number of smokers initiate the behavior in young adulthood. In fact, current smoking is most prevalent among young adults than any other population subgroup, with 26%–39% reporting current tobacco use (Lawrence et al., 2007; SAMHSA, 2006). Furthermore, although cigarettes account for most reported tobacco use in young adults, the use of cigars and smokeless tobacco is also fairly common, with 8%–17% of young adults reporting either current cigar use or use of other tobacco products (Rigotti et al., 2000; SAMHSA, 2006). Rates of cigarette use differ considerably by gender, race, education, and socioeconomic status. For example, cigarette smoking is more common among men (23.9%) than women (18.1%) (CDC, 2006a), and the use of cigars and other tobacco products is significantly more common among young men than young women, with nearly 16% of young men reporting current cigar use and nearly 9% reporting current use of other products, compared with 4% and 0.4% of young women, respectively (Rigotti et al., 2000). In addition, while some reports suggest that smoking rates are highest among American Indians/Alaska Natives (33%) and whites (31%) than other racial/ethnic groups (Lawrence et al., 2007), others have found smoking prevalence estimates as high as 60% among inner-city African American young adults (Stillman et al., 2007). Less education and concurrent enrollment in school are also related to smoking prevalence among U. S. young adults. Those not enrolled in college or without a college degree have been found to be more than twice as likely to report current and daily smoking (Lawrence et al., 2007). One report found that 48% of young adults with a high school degree or less reported current smoking (Solberg et al., 2007). Data suggest that a higher educational level may increase the likelihood of a quit attempt (Green et al., 2007). However, the number of quit attempts in the past year, level of interest in quitting, and relapse rates have also been found to be similar across education level (Solberg et al., 2007). Finally, blue collar workers, the unemployed, and those reporting an annual household income of less than US$20,000 are more likely to report current, daily, and heavy smoking (Lawrence et al., 2007).

Initial tobacco use is thought to be greatly directed by social and psychological forces, but these influences are quickly reinforced by the development of nicotine dependence, which is strongly driven by the neurobiological effects of nicotine.

Nicotine Dependence

The essential characteristics of nicotine dependence include the emergence of withdrawal symptoms in response to abstinence and unsuccessful attempts to reduce use or quit tobacco use. In order to meet clinical diagnosis of nicotine dependence, a tobacco user must exhibit any three (or more) of the primary symptoms at the same time during a 12-month period. In addition to the primary characteristics described, other criteria include tolerance to the aversive effects of nicotine (i.e., nausea and lightheadedness), limiting social or occupational activities because smoking is not permitted in those settings, continued use despite significant health concerns, and greater use than intended. Withdrawal symptoms can occur within 4 to 6 hours following last nicotine use (CDC, 1988). These symptoms, including depressed mood, insomnia, irritability, anxiety, difficulty concentrating, restlessness, and increased appetite and cravings for tobacco/nicotine, can be almost immediately alleviated by tobacco use.

Neurobiology of Nicotine Dependence

Cigarette smoking—the most common form of tobacco use—quickly distributes nicotine to the brain and levels of nicotine peak within 10 seconds of inhalation (Benowitz, 1996). The effects of nicotine are thought to be mediated by the dopamine-containing neurons in the ventral tegmental area (VTA) that project to the nucleus accumbens and prefrontal cortex and form part of the brain's "reward" pathway (Laviolette & van der Kooy, 2003). This circuitry is implicated in the rewarding motivational effects of multiple addictive drugs, including cocaine (Phillips et al., 2003), alcohol (Diana et al., 2003), opiates (Nader & van der Kooy, 1997), and nicotine (Pontieri, Tanda, Orzi, & Di Chiara, 1996). Nicotinic acetylcholine (nACh) receptors located throughout the CNS stimulate neurotransmitter release (directly and indirectly) and the resultant increase in dopamine is thought to at least partially underlie the pleasure associated with smoking. Interestingly, the nature of these nACh receptors inherently contributes to a pattern of continued use. Repeated and chronic administration of nicotine—for example, smoking over the course of the day—leads to desensitization and inactivation of nACh receptors (Pidoplichko, DeBiasis, Williams, & Dani, 1997), reducing the neurochemical reward of a cigarette. However, with abstinence—for example, overnight—the receptors may resensitize and once again be responsive to nicotine (George & O'Malley, 2004), resulting in frequent positive neurochemical reinforcement of nicotine use (Benowitz, 1996).

Recent data suggest that continued use of nicotine may be a result of the multifaceted influence of nicotine on the dopamine system. For example, dopamine release may not only produce pleasurable effects but also have a role in mediating the aversive effects of nicotine (Laviolette & van der Kooy, 2003). Additionally, the increase in dopamine response to nicotine appears to generalize to behaviors and contexts associated with tobacco use: over time, associated smoking behaviors are sufficient to stimulate dopamine release and act as reinforcement of the behavior even in the absence of nicotine (Balfour, 2004). In addition, repeated exposure to nicotine may result in an increase in functional nicotinic receptors in the brain and a heightened sensitivity of the dopamine response to nicotine (Gentry & Lukas, 2002). Preclinical evidence suggests that even limited exposure to nicotine is sufficient to induce lasting changes in the reward system (Mansvelder & McGehee, 2002), and nicotine may have differential effects in adolescent and adult brains. For example, the rewarding and reinforcing effects of nicotine appear to be enhanced (Belluzzi et al., 2004; Vastola, Douglas, Varlinskaya, & Spear, 2002) and the aversive effects possibly minimized (O'Dell et al., 2006; Shram, Funk, Li, & Le, 2006) in adolescent versus adult rodents. This difference may explain the reporting of symptoms of nicotine dependence in even occasional adolescent smokers (DiFranza et al., 2000).

Once thought to require some period of regular and considerable smoking, emerging preclinical and clinical evidence suggests that symptoms of nicotine dependence, such as withdrawal and tolerance, can be established following relatively minimal administration of nicotine. For example, two-thirds of occasional adolescent smokers report at least one symptom of nicotine dependence (DiFranza et al., 2000) and nearly half of all daily young adult smokers are nicotine dependent (Breslau, Kilbey, & Andreski, 1994). In addition, considerable neurodevelopment occurs during adolescence and young adulthood (Giedd, 2004; Sowell, Thompson, Tessner, & Toga, 2001; Spear, 2000) that may create a particularly accommodating environment for the establishment of a lasting neurological impact of nicotine. For example, reduced prefrontal attentional network activity has been observed in young adult smokers compared with nonsmokers (Musso et al., 2007).

Differences in rewarding properties and withdrawal from nicotine may cause an increased vulnerability to nicotine addiction in adolescent and young adult animals and possibly in the adolescent human. Although the specifics of these neurobiological processes remain to be fully revealed, environmental influences almost certainly interact with biological vulnerabilities to result in smoking behavior in adolescence and adulthood. The following sections of the chapter discuss the influences of peers, mood, expectancies, and genetics on smoking initiation, maintenance, and cessation.

Peers and Tobacco Use

More than two decades of research have established that peer influence is a significant predictor of adolescent and young adult smoking initiation, progression, and maintenance/relapse (Conrad, Flay, & Hill, 1992; Flay, Hu, & Richardson, 1998; Leventhal & Cleary, 1980; McAlister, Krosnick, & Milburn, 1984; Sussman et al., 1998; Tyas & Pederson, 1998). Initiation of smoking generally takes place in a social context, and more than half of teens report that they smoked their first cigarette because they accepted an offer from a peer (Presti, Ary & Lichtenstein, 1992). In young adulthood, the number of high school and college friends who smoke increases the likelihood of smoking (Ridner, 2005). Recently, social smoking, that is, smoking primarily when with others or equally when alone and with others, has been found to describe the smoking behavior of more than 50% of current college student smokers (Moran, Wechsler, & Rigotti, 2004). This type of smoking behavior is associated with less use, less dependence, less intention to quit, and fewer recent attempts to quit (Moran, Wechsler, & Rigotti, 2004).

Mood and Tobacco Use

The links between mood states and smoking have been well documented. For example, in general, smokers retrospectively attribute smoking to negative affective states (Piper et al., 2004), smokers report greater overall negative affect than nonsmokers (Hall et al., 1998), and both increases in, and relative intensity of, negative affect have been identified as specific antecedents to lapse to smoking (Shiffman, 2005). In addition, negative affect has been consistently associated with relapse to smoking during a cessation attempt (e.g., Piasecki, 2006). Perhaps most clinically relevant is the fact that smokers themselves believe that their smoking ameliorates negative affect and increases positive affect (Shadel & Mermelstein, 1993). However, attempts to identify affective cues as immediate antecedents for smoking behaviors in naturalistic settings have been somewhat equivocal. There is some evidence that smoking behavior is preceded by an increased urge to smoke, feeling happy, feeling stressed, and a decrease in hunger (Shapiro, Jamner, Davydov, & James, 2002). In the presence of other smoking cues, both positive and negative affect imagery scripts can produce equivalent reports of urges to smoke (Maude-Griffin & Tiffany, 1996). In contrast, other studies have found no associations between either negative or positive affect and smoking (Shiffman et al., 2002; Shiffman, Paty, Gwaltney, & Dang, 2004).

Much of the research on affect in connection with smoking urges and behaviors has reasonably focused on negative affect, given the negative affective characteristics of withdrawal (such as dysphoria, anxiety, irritability, and restlessness). There is considerable evidence that negative affective states contribute to the smoking behaviors of adults (see Piasecki, 2006, for brief review). However, aspects of the relationship between positive affective states and smoking behaviors may be more relevant to young adult smokers. Although positive affect is less frequently associated with relapse than negative affect (Baer & Lichtenstein, 1988; Shiffman, 1986), when positive affect is predictive of relapse it is generally accompanied by other smoking-related cues (for example, the presence of other smokers smoking). In fact, this appears to be a key distinction between the influences of positive and negative affect on smoking urges: that negative affect alone produces strong urges to smoke, while positive affect appears to require additional cueing in the form of other smoking stimuli (Maude-Griffin & Tiffany, 1996). Evidence of the potentially high salience of positive affect in smoking is found in research on college age smokers. For example, heavier smokers report smoking more in response to feeling low-energy positive affect (i.e., calm, peaceful, content, or relaxed), compared to lighter smoking peers. Interestingly, the lighter smokers smoked a greater proportion of cigarettes in the presence of high-energy positive affect (i.e., happy, upbeat, cheerful, or energetic) compared to heavier smokers, and they were also significantly more likely to be influenced to smoke by having contact with another person smoking (Krukowski, Solomon, & Naud, 2005).

A primary motivation for tobacco use may be smokers' perceptions of the coping functions provided by tobacco for affect regulation—for example, to increase concentration, counter boredom, enhance positive mood, and reducing distress in anxiety-arousing conditions (Wills & Cleary, 1996). One study found that 40% of adolescent smokers reported that their primary reason for smoking was to manage negative affect (Stevens, Colwell, Smith, Robinson, & McMillan, 2005). Similarly, the majority of smoking girls in one survey reported initiating and maintaining their smoking in response to stress, and they indicated in qualitative interviews that they perceived smoking as helpful in coping with distress at home, with friends, and at school (Nichter, Nichter, Vuckovic, Quintero, & Ritenbaugh, 1997). Among adult populations, there is evidence that expectations of this coping function of tobacco use moderates the relationship of stress to smoking urges and behaviors (Shadel & Mermelstein, 1993) and that smoking helps to modulate negative affect states within "real-life" settings (Jamner, Shapiro, & Jarvik, 1999).

Genetic Influences

Tobacco smoking is a highly heritable behavior—with genetic factors accounting for up to 53% of variability in smoking and up to 67% in variability of nicotine dependence (Sullivan & Kendler, 1998). Indeed, researchers have recently identified particular chromosomes as strongly associated with nicotine dependence (Li et al., 2008). In fact, particular aspects of nicotine dependence appear more highly heritable: tolerance, withdrawal, difficulty quitting, time to first cigarette in the morning, and number of cigarettes smoked per day (Lessov et al., 2004). However, investigations into the specific genes mediating cigarette smoking are complicated by a number of different definitions of the nicotine dependence phenotype (see review by Ho and Tyndale, 2007). Investigations into the specific genes that might explain the heritability of tobacco smoking have focused on genes which influence the reward pathway. Generally, it is thought that specific genetic polymorphisms may contribute to a dopamine deficit, thereby increasing the neurochemical reward of tobacco and other substances of abuse. Indeed, smokers have been found to be more likely to have a particular polymorphism of a dopamine receptor gene (DRD2), which as been associated with lower density of dopamine receptors in the brain (Noble et al., 1994). As a result, these smokers may be more vulnerable to the rewarding aspects of nicotine, thereby increasing their likelihood for repeated use. Another genetic influence on tobacco use and dependence is related to the relative speed of metabolizing nicotine (Malaiyandi, Sellers, & Tyndale, 2005). Individuals with polymorphisms in the genes responsible for encoding the metabolic enzymes (e.g., CYP2A6) tend to smoke fewer cigarettes and are less likely to be current smokers. This may be because slower metabolism of nicotine results in longer impact of the more aversive aspects of nicotine (nausea, etc). It may also be a function of smoking greater amounts in response to faster metabolizing (Audrain-McGovern et al., 2007). Adolescents without such genetic variation (i.e., those who metabolize nicotine more rapidly) have been found to progress to nicotine dependence more quickly than those with the variation (Audrain-

McGovern et al., 2007). Additional underlying genetic predispositions or vulnerabilities may also increase risk for nicotine dependence, such as those which are associated with psychiatric or substance abuse comorbidities.

Psychiatric Comorbidity and Tobacco Use

Tobacco use is associated with a range of psychiatric diagnoses in both adults and adolescents; most commonly with depression, schizophrenia, attention-deficit hyperactivity disorder, and substance use disorders. Athough prevalence of tobacco smoking in the general population is approximately 21%, much higher rates have been observed among those with psychiatric disorders (41%) or substance abuse (67%) (Lasser et al., 2000). It is estimated that 70% of adolescent daily smokers have a comorbid psychiatric disorder (Kandel, Johnson, & Bird, 1997), and adults with mental illness consume approximately 44.3% of the cigarettes smoked in the United States (Upadhyaya, Deas, Brady, & Kruesi, 2002). Most common theoretical explanations for the strong links between psychiatric disorders and cigarette use suggest the possibility that there are shared underlying predispositions which may be genetic or environmental and influence neurobiological pathways in the brain. Relatedly, it is proposed that individuals with serious mental illness, such as schizophrenia, may be "self-medicating" and using nicotine to modulate symptoms related to their illness (again by influencing neurobiological pathways). In any case, these populations not only have higher prevalence of cigarette use but also have substantially greater difficulty quitting, with lifetime quit rates of less than half that in the general population (Lasser et al., 2000).

Depression

There is extensive evidence illustrating positive associations between depressive symptoms and diagnoses with tobacco use and nicotine dependence. Adolescents with depressive disorders are more likely to initiate experimental smoking, transition to regular use (Patton et al., 1998), and be nicotine dependent (Breslau, Felm, & Peterson, 1993) than their nondepressed counterparts. The presence of an affective disorder can increase the likelihood of nicotine dependence by 10-fold in adolescents (Dierker, Avenevoli, Merikangas, Flaherty, & Stolar, 2001). In adults, diagnoses of depression and the presence of depressive symptoms are associated with greater likelihood of use (Anda et al., 1990), more severe withdrawal symptoms (Breslau, Kilbey, & Andreski, 1992), and more difficulty with cessation (Glassman et al., 1988; Glassman et al., 1990; Glassman et al., 1993; Niaura et al., 2001). Rates of smoking among population-based samples reporting clinically significant depressive symptoms range from 40% to 60% (Anda et al., 1990). A population-based twin study of female twins suggests that the comorbidity between depression and smoking may be, in great part, due to familial factors that underlie both disorders (Kendler et al., 1999).

Schizophrenia

Cigarette smoking is highly prevalent among patients with schizophrenia—with as many as 70% to 80% of diagnosed individuals concurrently using tobacco (Degenhardt & Hall, 2001). There is evidence to suggest that nicotine improves particular deficits associated with schizophrenia, including improving attention and working memory. Nicotine and smoking also appear to remediate certain psychophysiological deficits which appear to be mediated by neurotransmission through nicotinic receptors that may function differently in schizophrenics and their first-degree relatives (Adler, Hoffer, Wiser, & Freedman,1993; Freedman et al., 1997; Leonard et al., 2002; Olincy, Ross, Young, Roath, & Freedman, 1998). In addition, nicotine may interact with the antipsychotic medications frequently prescribed to patients with schizophrenia. For example, certain aspects of motor impairment induced by neuroleptic medication may be ameliorated while other aspects are worsened—possibly by influencing dopamine systems implicated in these gross and fine motor impairments (Decina et al., 1990; Yassa, Lal, Korpassy, & Ally, 1987). Such findings would suggest that individuals with schizophrenia may be particularly prone to reinforcing effects of nicotine, by experiencing improved cognitive and motor processes, beyond the rewarding effects experienced by individuals without schizophrenia.

Attention-Deficit Hyperactivity Disorder

The links between tobacco use and attention-deficit hyperactivity disorder (ADHD) are somewhat equivocal. For example, a higher prevalence of smoking among adolescents and adults diagnosed with ADHD has been reported (Chilcoat & Breslau, 1999; Pomerleau, Downey, Stelson, & Pomerlau, 1995). However, other studies have found no increased risk for smoking related to ADHD (Dierker et al., 2001). Smokers with ADHD have been observed to have more ADHD symptoms than their nonsmoking ADHD peers (Pomerleau et al., 1995). It has been proposed that smokers with ADHD may be using nicotine as a way to improve attention by increasing the release of dopamine (Dani & Harris, 2005). This self-medicating hypothesis is supported by findings that the nicotine transdermal patch improved performance on cognitive reaction tasks in adult smokers and nonsmokers with ADHD (Conners et al., 1996; Levin et al., 1996)

Alcohol and Substance Abuse

There is significant comorbidity between tobacco use and the use of alcohol and other drugs. In young adult college students, 98% of smokers drink alcohol and up to 59% of drinkers smoke tobacco (Weitzman & Chen, 2005), and the risk for co-occurrence of use is highest among those students with the highest alcohol consumption, alcohol problems, and symptoms of alcohol abuse. Some reports have observed that more than 80% of alcohol-dependent patients are also cigarette smokers (Burling & Ziff, 1988; diFranza & Guerrera, 1990; Miller & Gold, 1998; Patten, Martin, & Owen,1996). Cigarette smoking is consistently positively, and in a bidirectional nature, associated with alcohol use. For example, smokers are more likely to drink alcohol than nonsmokers, and drinkers are more likely to smoke than nondrinkers. Data also indicate a dose-dependent relationship, with greater use of one substance related to greater use of the other (Zacny, 1990). As adolescents enter young adulthood and reach the legal age to use such substances as tobacco and alcohol, these risks are exacerbated. For example, 22% of college students report starting to engage in heavy drinking during their first semesters in college (Wechsler, Davenport, Dowdall, Moeykens, & Castillo, 1994), which increases their risk for smoking and the development of nicotine dependence.

The comorbidity of alcohol and tobacco use in young adulthood may have its roots in adolescence, as teens' vulnerability to risk for other substance use appears exacerbated by even minimal use of tobacco. For example, adolescent smokers are more likely to be heavier drinkers and have four times the risk of a comorbid alcohol use disorder than never-smokers; in fact, even those teens who experiment with cigarettes are two times more likely to have an alcohol use disorder than never-smokers (Grucza & Beirut, 2006). Interestingly, twin studies have implicated shared genetic factors as responsible for comorbid nicotine and alcohol dependence (True & Xian, 1999), suggesting an underlying biological vulnerability to dependence on both substances. Indeed, dopamine neurotransmission, particularly in the nucleus accumbens of the mesocorticolimbic system, is central to mechanisms regulating CNS effects of both nicotine and alcohol. Emerging evidence suggests both that the effects of alcohol may be regulated by the same nicotinic receptors which mediate nicotine's effect on the brain and that alcohol influences nAChR activation (Kalman, Marissette, & George, 2005).

In addition to alcohol use, evidence indicates that cigarette smoking is strongly associated with the use of other substances. Smokers are twice as likely to have ever used drugs compared with nonsmokers (Farrell & Marshall, 2006). In adults, these relationships vary as a function of nicotine dependence, with dependent smokers being at much greater risk for alcohol dependence, cocaine dependence, and cannabis dependence compared with nonsmokers and nondependent smokers. For example, nicotine-dependent smokers were found to have 11 times the risk for cocaine dependence compared with nonsmokers, but non-nicotine-dependent smokers had only 6.5 times the risk compared with nonsmokers (Breslau, 1995).

Prevention, Cessation, and Treatment

Due to the recognition that young adulthood is a period of continued risk of initiation and generally high rates of tobacco use, many college campuses have developed focused campus-wide prevention programs to support their students. These programs typically include combinations of campus policies (such as smoke-free buildings and residences), educational programming, and cessation support. Prevention-focused education programs have been linked to lower smoking rates (Borders, Xu, Bacchi, Cohen, & SoRelle-Miner, 2005), and the establishment of such campus policies as smoke-free residences has been shown to effectively prevent the initiation of tobacco use among young adults who are not already regular smokers (Wechsler, Lee, & Rigotti, 2001). However, there remains a dearth of research on the effectiveness of prevention programs targeted toward young adult smokers. The majority of research has focused on interventions for cessation of use.

Tobacco use is highly resistant to cessation: although 70% of adult smokers report a desire to quit and 42.5% have attempted to quit in the past year (CDC, 2005a), success rates in cessation are generally low, ranging from 5% without intervention to 30% with combined psychological and pharmacological treatment.

Although the overall benefits may be greater for people who stop at earlier ages, cessation is beneficial at all ages (CDC, 1990, 2001). The effects of cessation are nearly immediately beneficial with positive health impacts occurring within hours of the most recent cigarette. Smoking cessation lowers the risk for coronary heart disease, stroke, peripheral vascular disease, and lung and other types of cancer (CDC, 1990). The risk for developing cancer declines with the number of years of smoking cessation and coronary heart disease risk is considerably reduced within 2 years of quitting (CDC, 1990, 2001). Women who stop smoking before or during pregnancy reduce their risk for adverse reproductive outcomes such as infertility or having a low-birth-weight baby (CDC, 2001). However, most smokers find it highly difficult to quit, particularly because of the experience of withdrawal and cravings. In fact, the scientific consensus identifies nicotine as a powerful drug of addiction, comparable to heroin, cocaine, and alcohol (Henningfield, Miyasato, & Jasinski, 1985; Stolerman & Jarvis, 1995). It is an addiction that can require multiple repeated efforts to quit and can require a variety of interventions, including behavioral and pharmacological treatments.

Stages of Change

There is great interest among current smokers to quit smoking. Among current U. S. adult smokers, 70% report that they want to quit completely (CDC, 2006a). In 2005, an estimated 19.2 million (42.5%) adult smokers had stopped smoking for at least 1 day during the preceding 12 months because they were trying to quit (CDC, 2006a).

The extent of a smoker's motivation to make a quit attempt has been frequently assessed and described by the Stages of Change (SOC) model (Prochaska & DiClemente, 1983). The SOC model includes five progressive stages of motivation and movement toward abstinence, including precontemplation, contemplation, preparation, action, and maintenance. Precontemplation refers to a stage in which the individual has no intention or consideration regarding abstinence in the coming 6 months. Contemplation involves an intention and plan to quit in the future (i.e., in the next 2 to 6 months). Preparation includes having made recent efforts to quit and an ongoing motivation to attain abstinence in the near future (i.e., within the next 30 days). The action and maintenance stages describe individuals who have just recently attained abstinence and maintained abstinence for at least 6 months, respectively.

There is evidence that both adult (Segan et al., 2004) and adolescent smokers (Dino et al., 2004) in the preparation stage, at the initiation of a cessation intervention, are more likely to attain abstinence than those in the contemplation stages. As a result of the potential links between stage of change and cessation success, research has begun to focus on how interventions may be tailored to identify and address the issues and challenges relevant to an individual's specific stage. Indeed, such tailoring has had some success in increasing abstinence rates (e.g., Dijkstra et al., 2006). However, other research has concluded that there is little evidence that the model provides predictive power for future tobacco use or cessation (Carlson, et al., 2003). Critics of the model have argued that the stage model may minimize concepts highly relevant to addiction—such as neurological and behavioral rewards and the unpredictability of human decision making and motivation (West, 2005). Despite these critiques, the model continues to be used and promoted in the tobacco cessation field.

Certain environmental factors related to smoking that may characterize the developmental period of young adulthood, such as marrying a nonsmoker and a smoke-free workplace, have been found to increase the likelihood of long-term cessation (Macy et al., 2007). In addition, young adults appear to be sensitive to the financial cost of cigarettes. Increased smoking initiation has been observed following price reductions (Zhang, Cohen, Ferrence, & Rehm, 2006), and tobacco taxation has indicated that increased prices result in an increase in quitting (Taurus, 2004).

Interventions

Interestingly, attempts to quit can be fairly easily encouraged by brief interventions by practitioners and even minimal intervention can increase abstinence rates significantly (Fiore et al., 2000). For example, spending 3 minutes discussing smoking cessation with a practitioner can increase abstinence rates from 11% to 14.4%. A patient who spends up to 90 minutes (not necessarily at the same visit) discussing cessation with their practitioner is three times more likely to succeed in their effort to quit. Furthermore, although 90% of smokers who successfully quit do so without professional help, evidence suggests that consultation with a health care provider can nearly double the likelihood of success. Unfortunately, young adults are less likely to receive advice to quit from a health care provider than other smokers and are less likely to use pharmacotherapy (Curry, Sporer, Pugach, Campbell, & Emery, 2007). In fact, 73% of young adults who attempted to quit in the past year did not receive any assistance in their effort (Solberg et al., 2007).

Despite the apparent need for effective smoking cessation services for young adult populations and the existence of treatments specifically designed for college and university students, treatment is not frequently offered or available. In one study of college students, 77% of smokers reported that a medical professional had asked about their tobacco use, but only 56% had been advised to quit (Koontz et al., 2004). Even fewer received advice about how to quit (22%) or how to set a quit date (5%), and very few were offered follow-up care (4%). On an institutional level, although most health directors perceive smoking cessation as important, over half of surveyed sites did not offer cessation services of any kind and those who did offer some type of intervention simultaneously believed that these programs were only minimally effective (Friedman, Smith, Zhang, Perry, & Colwell, 2004). College students themselves express interest in quitting, with an average report of three attempts to quit smoking and generally moderate to high interest in intention to quit (Black, Loftus, Chatterjee, Tiffany, & Babrow, 1993). One study of factors that would entice students to participate in a smoking cessation program found that accessibility, affordability, convenience, flexibility, social support, and behavioral prompts/cues are important factors to consider (Black et al., 1993). Another found that young adults believed that programs should focus on the addictive nature of nicotine and the benefits of using nicotine replacement therapy (Staten & Ridner, 2007). However, evidence-based treatments, such as pharmacotherapy and/or behavioral counseling, are underused by the young adult population compared with the general population (Curry et al., 2007). One important barrier to treatment may be the perspective that smoking cessation messages portrayed in the media are directed at adults and/or teens, and college students or young adults may not identify with these messages (Staten & Ridner, 2007).

Innovative approaches to behavior change in young adults are in development. For example, Web-based smoking cessation programs (e.g., Escoffery, McCormick, & Bateman, 2004) and quit-to-win programs may be cost-effective and high-impact interventions that can easily target young adult populations. Other programs that incorporate individual counseling, computer-based assessments, individualized feedback, and physiological measurements (such as lung functioning) are showing promise as attractive interventions to young adults (Prokhorov et al., 2007). In addition to individual or group counseling that can be offered on campus, college and university settings have unique opportunities to establish institutional interventions that could influence smoking behaviors. A review of interventions targeted specifically toward college students found that interventions such as campus smoking restrictions, smoke-free policies, anti-tobacco messages, and cigarette pricing can reduce tobacco use (Murphy-Hoefer et al., 2005).

Behavioral Therapy

Behavioral therapies have been shown to be effective in reducing tobacco use and assisting in quit attempts, with reported success rates ranging from 7% to 20% (Lerman, Patterson, & Berrettini, 2005). These interventions have been found to be influential at increasing abstinence rates whether provided in individual or group format. Effective in both individual and group formats (Carlson, Taenzer, Koopmans, & Bultz, 2000), three primary aspects of behavioral therapy have been found to be effective in increasing abstinence rates: the provision of practical/problem-solving skills, the support provided by the practitioner during the counseling, and the assistance the smoker receives in gaining social support for a quit attempt (Fiore et al., 2000). Typically offered in addition to a pharmacological intervention, such as nicotine replacement or medication, behavioral counseling can significantly improve on the effectiveness of the pharmacological treatment (e.g., Alterman, Gariti, & Mulvaney, 2001). However, efficacy is greatly influenced by time spent in counseling, with greater length of sessions, greater number of sessions, or longer contact time resulting in higher efficacy (Niaura & Abrams, 2002).

Motivational Interviewing

Motivational interviewing is another counseling intervention that has shown to be successful in increasing abstinence rates (Butler et al., 1999; Soria, Legido, Escolano, Yeste, & Montoya, 2006). Typically administered in a brief format, the counseling emphasizes the provision of personalized feedback regarding various aspects of the individual's smoking profile (Mallin, 2002). Topics of discussion may include level and symptoms of nicotine dependence, the individual's perception of smoking norms, the relative influence of the individual's social network, the financial cost of smoking, and the impact of smoking on appearance or attractiveness to others. In addition, it might include feedback regarding lung functioning, any pulmonary symptoms, and carbon monoxide concentrations. Finally, the session focuses on how motivated the individual is to change his or her smoking behavior, addresses potential barriers to that change, and, if appropriate, assists in planning a quit attempt. However, despite success with additional risk populations, such as patients diagnosed with diabetes (Persson & Hjalmarson, 2006) or comorbid drug abuse (Richter, McCool, Catley, Hall, & Ahluwalia, 2005), other studies have found motivational interviewing not to be effective with high-risk smokers, such as those living in poverty (Okuyemi et al., 2007), pregnant women (Stotts, DeLaune, Schmitz, & Grabowski, 2004; Tappin et al., 2005), and those diagnosed with cancer (Wakefield, Olver, Whitford, & Rosenfeld, 2004). Further work to determine the efficacy of motivational interviewing on tobacco cessation is necessary (Niarua & Abrams, 2002).

Motivational Incentives

Motivational incentives, also termed contingency management (CM), involve the use of immediate, tangible, and salient rewards in response to proven abstinence from a target drug. For example, a smoker must provide a practitioner with evidence of abstinence, such as a negative level on a breath carbon monoxide assessment or a salivary cotinine measure, in order to receive a reward. Rewards may be cash payments or vouchers to be exchanged for particular goods. These procedures have been effective in increasing abstinence rates in tobacco cessation programs for adults (Stitzer, Rand, Bigelow, & Mead, 1986) and more recently in adolescents (Krishnan-Sarin et al., 2006). Although found to be less effective in reducing tobacco use than in reducing use of other substances (Prendergast, Podus, Finney, Greenwell, & Roll, 2006), this type of motivational incentive intervention may effectively supplement other treatment programs (such as cognitive-behavioral therapies, nicotine replacement interventions, or nonnicotine medications).

Quit and Win

Smoking cessation contests, in which large numbers of participants make simultaneous quit attempts during a specific time period and successful abstainers are eligible to receive prizes, have been shown to be successful in motivating quit attempts among young adult smokers. Quit and Win programs were developed in the early 1980s by the Minnesota Heart Health program and have since been implemented around the world. This type of contest may be particularly useful with young adult smokers, as research indicates that the contest tends to appeal most to younger smokers (Cummings et al., 1990; Hawk et al., 2006) and is most successful with lighter smokers (Hanewinkel, Wiborg, Isensee, Nebot, & Vartiainen, 2006). A report of use of the contest method with young adult smokers (mean age = 21 years) found an intention-to-treat success rate of almost 15% of contestants reporting abstinence at a 4-month follow-up and 7% at 12 months (Hanewinkel, Wiborg, Isensee, Nebot, & Vartiainen, 2006). Another contest held on college campuses, found that 30% of participants were abstinent at the end of 7 weeks and 12% were abstinent at a 6-month follow-up (Rooney et al., 2005). These rates compare favorably with reported typical self-initiated annual quit rates of 2%–4% (Zhu, Sun, Billings, Choi, & Malarcher, 1999).

Nicotine Replacement

Nicotine replacement therapies (NRTs) involve the administration of nicotine in order to attenuate the development of withdrawal symptoms. Considered to be "first-line" pharmacotherapy treatments, these interventions are packaged in the form of gums, lozenges, transdermal patches, inhalers, and nasal sprays and typically provide 30%–50% of the amount of nicotine provided by cigarettes. Nicotine replacement therapies are similar in efficacy to each other regardless of the method of delivery and are 1.5 to 4 times more likely than placebo treatment to result in a successful quit attempt (Fiore et al., 2000). In addition, these interventions may be combined in the event that a patient is unable to quit using a single type—for example, combining the nicotine patch (which can provide a more constant administration of nicotine) with either the nicotine gum or nicotine nasal spray when particular urges arise. Data suggest that the combining of treatment modalities can significantly increase the efficacy of treatment (Bohadana, Nilsson, Rasmussen, & Martinet, 2000).

Nonnicotine Medications

Recently nonnicotine medications such as Bupropion SR (Zyban) and Varenicline Tartrate (Chantix) have been approved for use in the treatment of nicotine dependence. Sustained-release bupropion is a prescription medication considered a first-line treatment to assist in cessation. First approved by the FDA in 1997 for the treatment of nicotine addiction, it is thought to block the reuptake of dopamine and norepinephrine and impact nicotinic receptors. This medication appears to reduce smoking by minimizing cravings and urges to smoke and can be supplemented safely by NRT. Compared with placebo, bupropion can double the odds of successfully quitting (Fiore et al., 2000). However, side effects of the medication include dry mouth, difficulty sleeping, headache, dizziness, and skin rash and the use of the medication is contraindicated for smokers with seizure conditions or eating disorders. Varenicline (Chantix) is a partial agonist of the nicotine acetylcholine receptors and was approved by the FDA in 2006. This medication acts to diminish the emergence of withdrawal symptoms and reduces the reinforcing properties of nicotine. Common side effects of varenicline are nausea, changes in dreaming, and vomiting, and it should not be used by smokers with kidney problems. Varenicline is nearly four times as effective as a placebo in determining abstinence and almost twice as effective as bupropion (Gonzales et al., 2006). Forty-four percent of patients who were administered varenicline were able to attain and maintain abstinence continuously for 4 weeks compared with only 17% of those on placebo and 29% of those administered bupropion. In addition, long-term follow-up rates are increased by varenicline (Jorenby et al., 2006), and maintenance treatment with varenicline (i.e., prolonged medication administration) can significantly reduce the likelihood of relapse (Tonstad et al., 2006).

Special Treatment Considerations

The high comorbidity of nicotine dependence and tobacco use with other psychiatric disorders requires consideration when evaluating treatment options. Typically, combined treatments that are effective at addressing both disorders are most effective. For example, intervention programs for smoking cessation (such as the use of NRTs or other medications) that included a cognitive behavioral adjunct to specifically address depression symptoms resulted in higher success rates for smokers with a lifetime history of major depression (Brown et al., 2001; Hall, Munoz, & Reus, 1994). Medications that may address both a primary psychiatric or substance abuse disorder and nicotine dependence include atypical antipsychotics for schizophrenia, antidepressants for depressive disorders, and naltrexone for alcoholism (Hall et al., 1998; Kalman et al., 2005).

As described, the prevalence of nicotine dependence among alcohol or other substance abusers is extremely high. Smoking cessation is frequently not a focus of clinical interventions for this population and at times is discouraged based on beliefs that smoking cessation may undermine attempts to quit the drug of abuse (Sussman, 2002). Smoking cessation has in fact been found to be associated with greater likelihood of abstinence from other drug use following drug treatment (Lemon, Friedman, & Stein, 2003). Similarly, continued smoking can even adversely impact treatment for marijuana dependence (Sullivan & Covey, 2002). There is evidence to suggest that timing of the cessation efforts may be important to consider: smokers who quit alcohol prior to quitting cigarettes had similar success at quitting tobacco as those who quit concurrently, but alcohol outcomes were better in those who quit cigarettes after some established period of sobriety (Joseph, Willenbring, Nugent, & Nelson, 2004). Young adults who are engaged in treatment to address alcohol or substance dependence should be assessed for tobacco use and strongly encouraged to quit—the prevalence of smoking-related morbidity makes it likely that individuals are more likely to die of smoking-related disease rather than directly from alcohol-related medical disorder or abuse of another substance (Hurt et al., 1996; Hurt & Patten, 2003).

Finally, accumulating evidence suggests that pharmacogenetics could be used to predict response to nicotine replacement and nonnicotinic therapies for smoking cessation (see Berritini & Lerman, 2005, for a review). Further advances in this exciting field may help advance therapeutic outcomes for smoking cessation for young adult smokers.

Conclusions

Young adulthood is a critical period for the initiation and establishment of tobacco use. Although great gains have been made toward greater appreciation of the needs of this population, better understanding of the potential impact of public policy to reduce initiation and increase cessation, and improved pharmacological and behavioral treatments, there remains an ongoing need for quality research on prevention and intervention for tobacco use in young adults. Indeed, future research will likely prove to be transdisciplinary and incorporate neurobiological, behavioral, psychosocial, and social aspects in the development of effective interventions.

KEY POINTS

- Tobacco use is the leading preventable cause of death in the United States—more lethal than all other major causes of death combined.
- Tobacco use is a chronic behavior that is highly resistant to cessation efforts due to the addictive nature of nicotine and the social and psychological influences on use (such as peer group, expectancies, and psychiatric comorbidities). Smokers frequently require multiple attempts to successfully quit.
- Quitting smoking improves health outcomes at any age.

PRACTICE GUIDELINES

The following are three treatment recommendations from Fiore et al. (2000):

- The single most important step in addressing tobacco use and dependence is screening for tobacco use. All clinicians should ask about tobacco use, assess the individual's willingness to quit, then provide the appropriate intervention, either by assisting the patient in quitting or by providing a motivational intervention.
- Behavioral interventions that are most helpful incorporate problem-solving skills, in-session support, and access to external social support (from family, friends, etc.).
- NRTs and nonnicotine medications are effective and useful in supporting quit attempts and can reduce discomfort associated with quitting and increase likelihood of success.

References

Adler, L. E., Hoffer, L. D., Wiser, A., & Freedman, R. (1993). Normalization of auditory physiology by cigarette smoking in schizophrenic patients. *American Journal of Psychiatry, 150*, 1856–1861.

Alterman, A. I., Gariti, P., & Mulvaney, F. (2001). Short-and long-term smoking cessation for three levels of intensity of behavioral treatment. *Psychology of Addictive Behaviors, 15*, 261–264.

Anda, R. F., Williamson, D. F., Escobedo, L. G., Mast, E. E., Giovino, G. A., & Remington, P. L.(1990). Depression and the dynamics of smoking. *Journal of the American Medical Association, 264*, 541–545.

Audrain-McGovern, J., Koudsi, N. A., Rodriguez, D., Wileyto, E. P., Shields, P. G., & R. F. Tyndale (2007). The role of CYP2A6 in the emergence of nicotine dependence in adolescents. *Pediatrics, 119*, e264–e274.

Baer, J. S., & Lichtenstein, E. (1988). Classification and prediction of smoking relapse episodes: An exploration of individual differences. *Journal of Consulting and Clinical Psychology, 56*, 104–110.

Balfour, D. J. K. (2004). The neurobiology of tobacco dependence: A preclinical perspective on the role of the dopamine projections to the nucleus accumbens. *Nicotine and Tobacco Research, 6*, 899–912.

Belluzzi J. D., Lee A. G., Oliff H. S., & Leslie F. M. (2004). Age-dependent effects of nicotine on locomotor activity and conditioned place preference in rats. *Psychopharmacology 174*(3), 389–395.

Benowitz, N. L. (1996). Pharmacology of nicotine: Addiction and therapeutics. *Annual Review of Pharmacology Toxicology, 36*, 597–613.

Berrettini, W. H., & Lerman, C. E. (2005). Pharmacotherpay and pharmacogenetics of nicotine dependence. *American Journal of Psychiatry, 162*, 1441–1451.

Black, D. R., Loftus, E. A., Chatterjee, R., Tiffany, S. T., & Babrow, A. S. (1993). Smoking cessation interventions for university students: recruitment and program design considerations based on social marketing theory. *Preventive Medicine*, 22, 388–399.

Bohadana, A. N., Nilsson, F., Rasmussen, T., & Martinet, Y. (2000). Nicotine inhaler and nicotine patch as a combination therapy for smoking cessation: A randomized double blind placebo controlled trial. *Archives of Internal Medicine*, 160, 3128–3134.

Borders, T. F., Xu, K. T., Bacchi, D., Cohen, L., & SoRelle-Miner, D. (2005). College campus smoking policies and programs and students' smoking behaviors. *BMC Public Health*, 5, 74.

Breslau, N. (1995). Psychiatric comorbidity of smoking and nicotine dependence. *Behavior Genetics*, 25, 95–101.

Breslau, N., Felm, N., & Peterson, E. L. (1993). Early smoking initiation and nicotine dependence in a cohort of young adults. *Drug and Alcohol Dependence*, 33, 129–137.

Breslau, N., Kilbey, M. M., & Andreski, P. (1992). Nicotine withdrawal symptoms and psychiatric disorders: Findings from an epidemiologic study of young adults. *American Journal of Psychiatry*, 149, 464–469.

Breslau, N., Kilbey, M., & Andreski, P. (1994). DSM-III-R nicotine dependence in young adults: Prevalence, correlates, and associated psychiatric disorders. *Addiction*, 89, 743–754.

Brown, R. A., Kahler, C. W., Niaura, R., Abrams, D. B., Sales, S. D., Ramsey, S. E., Goldstein, M. G., Burgess, E. S., Miller, I. W. (2001). Cognitive-behavioral treatment for depression in smoking cessation. *Journal of Consulting and Clinical Psychology*, 3, 471–480.

Burling, T. A., & Ziff, D. C. (1988). Tobacco smoking: a comparison between alcohol and drug abuse inpatients. *Addictive Behaviors*, 13, 185–190.

Butler, C., Rollnick, S., Cohen, D., Bachmann, M., Russell, I., & Stott, N. (1999). Motivational consulting versus brief advice for smokers in general practice: A randomized trial. *British Journal of General Practice*, 49, 611–616.

Carlson, L. E., Taenzer, P., Koopmans, J., & Bultz, B. D. (2000). Eight-year follow-up of a community-based large group behavioral smoking cessation intervention. *Addictive Behaviors*, 25, 725–741.

Carlson, L. E., Taenzer, P., Koopmans, J., & Casebeer, A. (2003) Predictive value of aspects of the Transtheoretical Model on smoking cessation in a community-based, large-group cognitive behavioral program. Addictive Behaviors, 28(4):725–740.

Centers for Disease Control and Prevention. (1988). The health consequences of smoking: nicotine addiction—A report of the Surgeon General. Rockville, MD: U. S. Department of Health and Human Services, Public Health Service.

Centers for Disease Control and Prevention. (1990). The health benefits of smoking cessation. Atlanta, GA: U.S. Department of Health and Human Services, CDC, Center for Chronic Disease Prevention and Health Promotion, Office on Smoking and Health.

Centers for Disease Control and Prevention. (2001). Women and smoking: A report of the Surgeon General. Atlanta, GA: U.S. Department of Health and Human Services, CDC, National Center for Chronic Disease Prevention and Health Promotion, Office on Smoking and Health.

Centers for Disease Control and Prevention. (2002a). Annual smoking-attributable mortality, years of potential life lost, and economic costs—United States, 1995–1999. *Morbidity and Mortality Weekly Report*, 51, 300–303.

Centers for Disease Control and Prevention. (2004). The health consequences of smoking: A report of the Surgeon General. Atlanta, GA: Department of Health and Human Services, Centers for Disease Control and Prevention, National Center for Chronic Disease Prevention and Health Promotion, Office on Smoking and Health. Washington, DC.

Centers for Disease Control and Prevention. (2005a). Annual smoking-attributable mortality, years of potential life lost, and productivity losses—United States, 1997–2001. *Morbidity and Mortality Weekly Report*, 54, 625–628.

Centers for Disease Control and Prevention. (2006a). Tobacco use among adults—United States, 2005. *Morbidity and Mortality Weekly Report*, 55, 1145–1148.

Centers for Disease Control and Prevention. (2006b). Cigarette use among high school students—United States, 1991–2005. *Morbidity and Mortality Weekly Report*, 55, 724–726.

Chilcoat H. D., & Breslau N. (1999). Pathways from ADHD to early drug use. *Journal of the American Academy of Child and Adolescent Psychiatry*. 38(11), 1347–1354.

Conners, C., Levin, E., Sparrow, E., Hinton, S., Erhardt, D., & Meck, W. (1996). Nicotine and attention in adult attention deficit hyperactivity disorder (ADHD). *Psychopharmacology Bulletin*, 32, 67–73.

Conrad, K. M., Flay, B. R., & Hill, D. (1992). Why children start smoking cigarettes: Predictors of onset. *British Journal of Addiction*, 87, 1711–1724.

Cummings, K. M., Kelly, J., Sciandra, R., DeLoughry, T., & Francois, F. (1990). Impact of a community-wide stop smoking contest. *American Journal of Health Promotion, 4*, 429–434.

Curry, S. J., Sporer, A. KPugach, O., Campbell, R. T., & Emery, S. (2007). Use of tobacco cessation treatments among young adult smokers: 2005 National Health Interview Survey. *American Journal of Public Health, 97*, 1464–1469.

Dani, J. A., & Harris, R. A. (2005). Nicotine addiction and comorbidity with alcohol abuse and mental illness. *Nature Neuroscience, 8*, 1465–1470.

Decina, P., Caracci, G., Sandik, R., Berman, W., Mukerjee, S., & Scapicchio, P. (1990). Cigarette smoking and neuroleptic-induced parkinsonism. *Biological Psychiatry, 28*, 502–508.

Degenhardt, L., & Hall, W. (2001). The relationship between tobacco use, substance use disorders and mental health: Results from the National Survey of Mental Health and Well-Being. *Nicotine and Tobacco Research, 3*, 225–234.

Diana, M., Brodie, M., Muntoni, A., Puddu, M. C., Pillolla, G., Steffensen, S., Spiga, S., & Little, H. J. (2003). Enduring effects of chronic ethanol in the CNS: Basis for alcoholism. *Alcoholism, Clinical and Experimental Research, 27*, 354–361.

Dierker, L. C., Avenevoli, S., Merikangas, K. R., Flaherty, B. P., & Stolar, M. (2001). Association between psychiatric disorders and the progression of tobacco use behaviors. *Journal of the American Academy of Child and Adolescent Psychiatry, 40*, 1159–1167.

DiFranza, J. R. & Guerrera, M. P. (1990). Alcoholism and smoking. *Journal of Studies on Alcohol, 51*, 130–135.

DiFranza, J. R., Rigotti, N. A., McNeill, A. D., Ockene, J. K., Savageau, J. A., St Cyr, D., & Coleman, M. (2000). Initial symptoms of nicotine dependence in adolescents. *Tobacco Control, 9*, 313–319.

Dijkstra, A., Conijn, B., & De Vries, H. (2006) A match-mismatch test of a stage model of behaviour change in tobacco smoking. *Addiction. 101*(7), 1035–1043.

Dino, G., Kamal, K., Horn, K., Kalsekar, I., & Fernandes, A. (2004) Stage of change and smoking cessation outcomes among adolescents. Addictive Behaviors. *29*(5), 935–940.

Escoffery, C., McCormick, L., & Bateman, K. (2004). Development and process evaluation of a web-based smoking cessation program for college smokers: Innovative tool for education. *Patient Education and Counseling, 53*, 217–225.

Farrell, M., & Marshall, E. J. (2006). Epidemiology of tobacco, alcohol and drug use. *Psychiatry, 5*, 427–430.

Fiore, M. C., Bailey, W. C., Cohen, S. J., Dorfman, S. F., Goldstein, M. G., Gritz, E. R., Heyman, R. B., Jaén C. R., Kottke, T. E., Lando, H. A., Mecklenburg, R. E., Mullen, P. D., Nett, L. M., Robinson, L., Stitzer, M. L., Tommasello, A. C., Villejo, L., & Wewers, M. E., (2000). Treating tobacco use and dependence. Rockville, MD: Department of Health and Human Services, Public Health Service.

Flay, B. R., Hu, F. B., & Richardson, J. (1998). Psychosocial predictors of different stages of cigarette smoking among high school students. *Preventive Medicine, 27*, A9–A18.

Freedman, R., Coon, H., Myles-Worsley, M., Orr-Urtreger, A., Olincy, A., Davis, A., Polymeropoulos, M., Holik, J., Hopkins, J., Hoff, M., Rosenthal, J., Waldo, M. C., Reimherr, F., Wender P, Yaw J, Young DA, Breese CR, Adams C, Patterson D, Adler LE, Kruglyak L, Leonard, S., & Byerley, W. (1997). Linkage of a neurophysiological deficit in schizophrenia to a chromosome 15 locus. *Procedures of the National Academy of Sciences USA, 94*, 587–592.

Friedman, K. E., Smith, D. W., Zhang, J. J., Perry, J., & Colwell, B. (2004). Importance of tobacco cessation services at higher education public institutions in Texas. *Journal of Drug Education, 34*, 313–325.

Gentry, C. L., & Lukas, R. J. (2002). Regulation of nicotinic acetylcholine receptor numbers and function by chronic nicotine exposure. *Current Drug Targets CNS Neurological Disorders, 1*, 359–385.

George, T. P., & O'Malley, S. S. (2004). Current pharmacological treatments for nicotine dependence. *Trends in Pharmacological Science, 25*, 42–48.

Giedd, J. N. (2004) Structural magnetic resonance imaging of the adolescent brain. *Annals of the New York Academy of Sciences, 1021*, 77–85.

Glassman, A. H., Covey, L. S., Dalack, G. W., Stetner, F., Rivelli, S. K., Fleiss, J. L., & Cooper, T. B. (1993). Smoking cessation, clonidine, and vulnerability to nicotine among dependent smokers. *Clinical Pharmacology Therapy, 54*, 670–679.

Glassman, A. H., Helzer, J. E., Covey, L. S., Cottler, L. B., Stetner, F., Tipp, J. E., & Johnson, J. (1990). Smoking, smoking cessation and major depression. *Journal of the American Medical Association, 264*, 1546–1549.

Glassman, A. H., Stetner, F., Walsh, B. T., Raizman, P. S., Fleiss, J. L., Cooper, T. B., & Covey, L. S. (1988). Heavy smokers, smoking cessation, and clonidine. Results of a double-blind, randomized trial. *Journal of the American Medical Association, 259*, 2863–2866.

Gonzales, D., Rennard, S. I., Nides, M., Oncken, C., Azoulay, S., Billing, C. B., Watsky, E. J., Gong, J., Williams, K. E., Reeves, K. R.. (2006). Varenicline, an 42 nicotinic acetylcholine receptor partial agonist, vs sustained-release bupropion and placebo for smoking cessation: A randomized controlled trial. *Journal of the American Medical Association, 296,* 47–55.

Grant, B. F., Hasin, D. S., Chou, S. P., Stinson, F. S., & Dawson, D. A. (2004). Nicotine Dependence and psychiatric disorders in the United States. Results from the National Epidemiologic Survey on Alcohol and Related Conditions. *Archives of General Psychiatry, 61,* 1107–1115.

Green, M. P., McCausland, K. L., Xiao, H., Duke, J. C., Vallone, D. M., & Healton, C. G. (2007). A closer look at smoking among young adults: Where tobacco control should focus its attention. *American Journal of Public Health, 97,* 1427–1433.

Grucza, R. A., & Bierut, L. J. (2006). Cigarette smoking and the risk for alcohol use disorders among adolescent drinkers. *Alcoholism: Clinical and Experimental Research, 30,* 2046–2054.

Hall, S. M., Munoz, R. F., & Reus, V. I. (1994). Cognitive-behavioral intervention increases abstinence rates for depressive-history smokers. *Journal of Consulting and Clinical Psychology, 62,* 141–146.

Hall, S. M., Reus, V. I., Munoz, R. F., Sees, K. L., Humfleet, G., Hartz, D. T., Frederick, S., & Triffleman, E. (1998). Nortriptyline and cognitive-behavioral therapy in the treatment of cigarette smoking. *Archives of General Psychiatry, 55,* 683–690.

Hammond, D. (2005). Smoking behaviour among young adults: Beyond youth prevention. *Tobacco Control, 14,* 181–185.

Hanewinkel, R., Wiborg, G., Isensee, B., Nebot, M., & Vartiainen, E. (2006). "Smoke-free class competition": Far-reaching conclusions based on weak data. *Preventive Medicine, 43,* 150–151.

Hawk, L. W., Higbee, C., Hyland, A., Alford, T., O'Connor, R., Cummings, K. M. (2006). Concurrent Quit & Win and nicotine replacement therapy voucher giveaway programs: Participant characteristics and predictors of smoking abstinence. *Journal of Public Health Management and Practice, 12,* 52–59.

Henningfield, J. E., Miyasato, K., & Jasinski, D. R. (1985). Abuse liability and pharmacodynamic characteristics of intravenous and inhaled nicotine. *Journal of Pharmacological Experimental Therapy, 234,* 1–12.

Ho, M. K., & Tyndale, R. F. (2007). Overview of the pharmacogenomics of cigarette smoking. *The Pharmacogenomics Journal, 7,* 81–98.

Hurt, R. D., Offord, K. P., Croghan, I. T., Gomez-Dahl, L., Kottke, T. E., Morse, R. M., & Melton, L. J. 3rd. (1996). Mortality following inpatient addictions treatment: Role of tobacco use in a community-based cohort. *Journal of the American Medical Association, 275,* 1097–1103.

Hurt, R. D., & Patten, C. A. (2003). Treatment of tobacco dependence in alcoholics. *Recent Developments in Alcoholism, 16,* 335–359.

Jamner, L. D., Shapiro, D., & Jarvik, M. E. (1999). Nicotine reduces the frequency of anger reports in smokers and nonsmokers with high but not low hostility: An ambulatory study. *Experimental and Clinical Psychopharmacology, 7,* 454–463.

Johnston, L. D., O'Malley, P. M., Bachman, J. G., & Schulenberg, J. E. (2007). *Monitoring the Future national results on adolescent drug use: Overview of key findings, 2006* (NIH Publication No. 07-6202). Bethesda, MD: National Institute on Drug Abuse.

Jorenby, D. E., Hays, J. T., Rigotti, N. A., Azoulay, S., Watsky, E. J., Williams, K. E., Billing, C. B., Gong, J., Reeves, R. (2006). Efficacy of varenicline, an $\alpha 4\beta 2$ nicotinic acetylcholine receptor partial agonist, vs placebo or sustained-release bupropion for smoking cessation: A randomized controlled trial. *Journal of the American Medical Association, 296,* 56–63.

Joseph, A. M., Willenbring, M. L., Nugent, S. M., & Nelson, D. B. (2004). A randomized trial of concurrent versus delayed smoking intervention for patients in alcohol dependence treatment. *Journal of Studies on Alcohol, 65,* 681–692.

Kalman, D., Marissette, S. B., & George, T. P. (2005). Co-morbidity of smoking in patients with psychiatric and substance use disorders. *The American Journal on Addictions, 14,* 106–123.

Kandel, D. B., Johnson, J., & Bird, H. (1997). Psychiatric disorders associated with substance use among children and adolescents: Findings from the Methods for Epidemiology of Child and Adolescent Mental Disorders (MECA) Study. *Journal of Abnormal Child Psychology, 25,* 121–132.

Kendler, K. S., Neale, M. C., Sullivan, P., Corey, L. A., Gardner, C. O., & Prescott, C. A. (1999). A population-based twin study in women of smoking initiation and nicotine dependence. *Psychological Medicine, 29,* 299–308.

Koontz, J. S., Harris, K. J., Okuyemi, K. S., Mosier, M. C., Grobe, J., Nazir, N., & Ahluwalia, J. S. (2004). Healthcare providers' treatment of college smokers. *Journal of American College Health, 53,* 117–126.

Krishnan-Sarin, S., Duhig, A., McKee, S., McMahon, T. J., Liss, T., McFetridge, A., & Cavallo, D. A. (2006). Contingency management for smoking cessation in adolescent smokers. *Experimental and Clinical Psychopharmacology, 14,* 306–310.

Krukowksi, R. A., Solomon, L. J., & Naud, S. (2005). Triggers of heavier and lighter cigarette smoking in college students. *Journal of Behavioral Medicine, 28,* 335–345.

Lasser, K., Boyd, J. W., Woolhander, S., Himmelstein, D. U., McCormick, D., & Bot, D. H. (2000). Smoking and mental illness: A population based prevalence study. *Journal of the American Medical Association, 284*, 2606–2610.

Laviolette, S. R., & van der Kooy, D. (2003). Blockade of mesolimbic dopamine transmission dramatically increases sensitivity to the rewarding effects of nicotine in the ventral tegmental area. *Molecular Psychiatry, 8*, 50–59.

Lawrence, D., Fagan, P., Backinger, C. L., Gibson, J. T., & Hartman, A. (2007). Cigarette smoking patterns among young adults ages 18-24 in the U.S. *Nicotine & Tobacco Research, 9*, 687–697.

Lemon, S. C., Friedmann, P. D., & Stein, M. D. (2003). The impact of smoking cessation on drug abuse treatment outcome. *Addictive Behaviors, 28*, 1323–1331.

Leonard, S., Gault, J., Hopkins, J., Logel, J., Vianzon, R., Short, M., Drebing, C., Berger, R., Venn, D., Sirota, P., Zerbe, G., Olincy, A., Ross, R. G., Adler, L. E., & Freedman, R. (2002). Promoter variants in the alpha-7 nicotinic acetylcholine receptor subunit gene are associated with an inhibitory deficit found in schizophrenia. *Archives of General Psychiatry, 59*, 1085–1096.

Lerman, C., Patterson, F., & Berrettini, W. (2005). Treating tobacco dependence: State of the science and new directions. *Journal of Clinical Oncology, 23*, 311–323.

Lessov C. N., Martin N. G., Statham D. J., Todorov A. A., Slutske W. S., Bucholz K. K., Heath A. C., & Madden P. A. (2004) Defining nicotine dependence for genetic research: evidence from Australian twins. *Psychological Medicine. 34*(5), 865–879.

Leventhal, H., & Cleary, P. D. (1980). The smoking problem: a review of the research and theory in behavioral risk modification. *Psychology Bulletin, 88*, 370–405.

Levin, E. D., Conners, C. K., Sparrow, E., Hinton, S. C., Erhardt, D., Meck, W. H., Rose, J. E., & March, J. (1996). Nicotine effects on adults with attention-deficit/hyperactivity disorder. *Psychopharmacology, 123*, 55–63.

Li, M. D., Ma, J. Z., Payne, T. J., Lou, X. Y., Zhang, D., Dupont, R. T., & Elston, R. C. (2008). Genome-wide linkage scan for nicotine dependence in European Americans and its converging results with African Americans in the Mid-South Tobacco Family sample. *Molecular Psychiatry, 13*, 407–416.

Macy, J. T., Seo, D. C., Chassin, L., Presson, C. C., Sherman, S. J. (2007). Prospective predictors of long-term abstinence versus relapse among smokers who quit as young adults. *American Journal of Public Health, 97*, 1470–1475.

Malaiyandi, V., Sellers, E. M., & Tyndale, R. F. (2005). Implications of CYP2A6 genetic variation for smoking behaviors and nicotine dependence. *Clinical Pharmacology and Therapeutics, 77*, 145–158.

Mallin, R. (2002). Smoking cessation: Integration of behavioral and drug therapies. *American Family Physician, 65*, 1107–1114.

Mansvelder, H. D., & McGehee, D. S. (2002). Cellular and synaptic mechanisms of nicotine addiction. *Journal of Neurobiology, 53*, 606–617.

Maude-Griffin, P. M., & Tiffany, S. T. (1996). Production of smoking urges through imagery: The impact of affect and smoking abstinence. *Experimental and Clinical Psychopharmacology, 4*, 198–202.

McAlister, A. L., Krosnick, J. A., & Milburn, M. A. (1984). Causes of adolescent cigarette smoking: Test of a structural equation model. *Social Psychology Quarterly, 47*, 24–36.

Miller, N. S., & Gold, M. S. (1998). Comorbid cigarette and alcohol addiction: Epidemiology and treatment. *Journal of Addictive Disorders, 17*, 55–66.

Moran, S., Wechsler, H., & Rigotti, N. A. (2004). Social smoking among US college students. *Journal of the American Medical Association, 114*, 1028–1034.

Murphy-Hoefer, R., Griffith, R., Pederson, L. L., Crossett, L., Iyer, S. R., & Hiller, M. D. (2005). A review of interventions to reduce tobacco use in colleges and universities. *American Journal of Preventive Medicine, 28*, 188–200.

Musso, F., Bettermann, F., Vucurevic, G., Stoeter, P., Konrad, A., & Winterer, G. (2007). Smoking impacts on prefrontal attentional network function in young adult brains. *Psychopharmacology, 191*, 159–169.

Nader, K., & van der Kooy, D. (1997). Deprivation state switches the neurobiological substrates mediating opiate reward in the ventral tegmental area. *Journal of Neuroscience, 17*, 383–390.

Niaura, R., & Abrams, D. B. (2002). Smoking cessation: Progress, priorities, and prospectus. *Journal of Consulting and Clinical Psychology, 70*, 494–509.

Niaura, R., Britt, D. M., Shadel, W. M., Goldstein, M., Abrams, D., & Brown, R. (2001). Symptoms of depression and survival experience among three samples of smokers trying to quit. *Psychology of Addictive Behaviors, 15*, 13–17.

Nichter, M., Nichter, M., Vuckovic, N., Quintero, G., & Ritenbaugh, C. (1997). Smoking experimentation and initiation among adolescent girls: Qualitative and quantitative findings. *Tobacco Control, 6*, 285–295.

Noble, E. P., St. Jeor, S. T., Ritchie, T., Fitch R. J., Brunner L., Sparkes R. S. (1994). D2 dopamine receptor gene and cigarette smoking: A reward gene? *Medical Hypotheses, 42*, 257–260.

O'Dell, L. E., Bruijnzeel, A. W., Smith, R. T., Parsons, L. H., Merves, M. L., Goldberger, B. A., Richardson, H. N., Koob, G. F., & Markou, A. (2006). Diminished nicotine withdrawal in adolescent rats: Implications for vulnerability to addiction. *Psychopharmacology, 186,* 612–619.

Okuyemi, K. S., James, A. S., Mayo, M. S., Nollen, N., Catley, D., Choi, W. S., & Ahluwalia, J. S. (2007). Pathways to health: A cluster randomized trial of nicotine gum and motivational interviewing for smoking cessation in low-income housing. *Health Education and Behavior, 34,* 43–54.

Olincy, A., Ross, R. G., Young, D. A., Roath, M., & Freedman, R. (1998). Improvement in smooth pursuit eye movements after cigarette smoking in schizophrenic patients. *Neuropsychopharmacology, 18,* 175–185.

Patten, C. A., Martin, J. E., & Owen, N. (1996). Can psychiatric and chemical dependency treatment units be smoke free? *Journal of Substance Abuse Treatment, 13,* 107–118.

Patton, G. C., Carlin, J. B., Coffey, C, Wolfe, R., Hibbert, M., & Bowes, G. (1998). Depression, anxiety, and smoking initiation: A prospective study over three years. *American Journal of Public Health, 88,* 1518–1522.

Persson, L. G., & Hjalmarson, A. (2006). Smoking cessation in patients with diabetes mellitus: results from a controlled study of an intervention programme in primary healthcare in Sweden. *Scandinavian Journal of Primary Health Care, 24,* 75–80.

Philips, P. E., Stuber, G. D., Heien, M. L., Wightman, R. M., & Carelli, R. M. (2003). Subsecond dopamine release promotes cocaine seeking. *Nature, 10,* 614–618.

Piasecki, T. M. (2006). Relapse to smoking. *Clinical Psychology Review, 26,* 196–215.

Pidoplichko, V. I., DeBiasis, M., Williams, J. T., & Dani, J. A. (1997). Nicotine activates and desensitizes midbrain dopamine neurons. *Nature, 390,* 401–404.

Piper, M. E., Piasecki, T. M., Federman, E. B., Bolt, D. M., Smith, S. S., Fiore, M. C. Baker, T. C. (2004). A multiple motives approach to tobacco dependence: The Wisconsin Inventory of Smoking Dependence (WISDM-68). *Journal of Consulting and Clinical Psychology, 72,* 139–154.

Pomerleau, O., Downey, K., Stelson, F., & Pomerleau, C. (1995). Cigarette smoking in adult patients diagnosed with attention deficit hyperactivity disorder. *Journal of Substance Abuse, 7,* 373–378.

Pontieri, F. E., Tanda, G., Orzi, F., & Di Chiara, G. (1996). Effects of nicotine on the nucleus accumbens and similarity to those of addictive drugs. *Nature, 382,* 255–257.

Prendergast, M., Podus, D., Finney, J., Greenwell, L., & Roll, J. (2006). Contingency management for treatment of substance use disorders: A meta-analysis. *Addiction, 101,* 1529–1675.

Presti, D. E., Ary, D. V., & Lichtenstein, E. (1992). The context for smoking initiation and maintenance: Findings from interviews with youths. *Journal of Substance Abuse, 4,* 35–45.

Prokhorov, A. V., Fouladi, R. T., de Moor, C., Warneke, C. L., Luca, M., Jones, M. M., Rosenblum, C., Emmons, K. M., Hudmon, K. S., Yost, T. E., & Gritz, E. R. (2007). Computer assisted, counselor delivered smoking cessation counseling for community college students: Intervention approach and sample characteristics. *Journal of Child and Adolescent Substance Abuse, 16,* 35–62.

Richter, K. P., McCool, R. M., Catley, D., Hall, M., & Ahluwalia, J. S. (2005). Dual pharmacotherapy and motivational interviewing for tobacco dependence among drug treatment patients. *Journal of Addictive Disorders, 24,* 79–90.

Ridner, S. L. (2005). Predicting smoking status in a college-age population. *Public Health Nursing, 22,* 494–505.

Rigotti, N. A., Lee, J. E., & Wechsler, H. (2000). US college students' use of tobacco products. Results of a national Survey. *Journal of the American Medical Association, 284,* 699–705.

Rooney, B. L., Silha, P., Gloyd, J., & Kreutz, R. (2005) Quit and Win smoking cessation contest for Wisconsin college students. *Wisconsin Medical Journal, 104*(4), 45–49.

Segan CJ, Borland R, Greenwood KM. What is the right thing at the right time? Interactions between stages and processes of change among smokers who make a quit attempt. Health Psychol. 2004 Jan; 23(1):86–93.

Shadel, W. G., & Mermelstein, R. J. (1993). Cigarette smoking under stress. The role of coping expectancies among smokers in a clinic-based smoking cessation program. *Health Psychology, 12,* 443–450.

Shapiro, D., Jamner, L. D., Davydov, D. M., & James, P. (2002). Situations and moods associated with smoking in everyday life. *Psychology of Addictive Behaviors, 4,* 342–345.

Shiffman, S. (1986). Cluster analytic classification of smoking relapse episodes. *Addictive Behaviors, 11,* 295–307.

Shiffman, S. (2005). Dynamic influences on smoking relapse process. *Journal of Personality, 73*(6), 1715–1748.

Shiffman, S., Paty, J. A., Gwaltney, C. J., & Dang, Q. (2004). Immediate antecedents of cigarette smoking: An analysis of unrestricted smoking patterns. *Journal of Abnormal Psychology, 113,* 166–171.

Shram, M. J., Funk, D., Li, Z., & Le, A. D. (2006). Periadolescent and adult rats respond differently in tests measuring the rewarding and aversive effects of nicotine. *Psychopharmacology, 186,* 201–208.

Solberg, L. I., Asche, S. E., Boyle, R., McCarty, M. C., & Thoele, M. J. (2007). Smoking and cessation behaviors among young adults of various educational backgrounds. *American Journal of Public Health, 97,* 1421–1426.

Soria, R., Legido, A., Escolano, C., Yeste, A. L., & Montoya J. (2006). A randomized controlled trial of motivational interviewing for smoking cessation. *British Journal of General Practice, 56,* 768–774.

Sowell, E. R., Thompson, P. M., Tessner, K. D., & Toga, A. W. (2001). Mapping continued brain growth and gray matter density reduction in dorsal frontal cortex: Inverse relationships during postadolescent brain maturation. *Journal of Neuroscience, 21,* 8819–8829.

Spear, L. P. (2000) .The adolescent brain and age-related behavioral manifestations. *Neuroscience and Biobehavioral Reviews, 24,* 417–463.

Staten, R. R., & Ridner, S. L. (2007). College students' perspectives on smoking cessation: "If the message doesn't speak to me I don't hear it." *Issues in Mental Health Nursing, 28,* 101–115.

Stevens, S. L., Colwell, B., Smith, D. W., Robinson, J., & McMillan, C. (2005). An exploration of self-reported negative affect by adolescents as a reason for smoking: Implications for tobacco prevention and intervention programs. *Preventive Medicine, 41,* 589–596.

Stillman, F. A., Bone, L., Avila-Tang, E., Smith, K., Yancey, N., Street, C., & Owings, K. (2007). Barriers to smoking cessation in inner-city African American young adults. *American Journal of Public Health, 97,* 1405–1408.

Stitzer, M. L., Rand, C. S., Bigelow, G. E., & Mead, A. M. (1986). Contingent payment procedures for smoking reduction and cessation. *Journal of Applied Behavior Analysis, 9,* 197–202.

Stolerman, I. P., & Jarvis, M. J. (1995). The scientific case that nicotine is addictive. *Psychopharmacology, 117,* 2–10.

Stotts, A. L., DeLaune, K. A., Schmitz, J. M., & Grabowski, J. (2004). Impact of a motivational intervention on mechanisms of change in low-income pregnant smokers. *Addictive Behaviors, 29,* 1649–1657.

Substance Abuse and Mental Health Services Administration. (2006). *Results from the 2005 National Survey on Drug Use and Health: National findings.* Washington, DC.

Sullivan, M. A., & Covey, L. S. (2002). Current perspectives on smoking cessation among substance abusers. *Current Psychiatry Reports, 4,* 388–396.

Sullivan, P. F., & Kendler, K. S. (1998). The genetic epidemiology of "neurotic" disorders. *Current Opinions in Psychiatry, 11,* 143–147.

Sussman, S. (2002). Smoking cessation among persons in recovery. *Substance Use & Misuse, 37,* 1275–1298.

Sussman, S., Dent, C. W., Nezami, E., Stacy, A. W., Burton, D., & Flay, B. R. (1998). Reasons for quitting and smoking temptation among adolescent smokers: Gender differences. *Substance Use and Misuse, 33,* 2705–2722.

Tappin, D. M., Lumsden, M. A., Gilmour, W. H., Crawford, F., McIntyre, D., Stone, D. H., Webber, R., MacIndoe, S., & Mohammed, E. (2005). Randomised controlled trial of home based motivational interviewing by midwives to help pregnant smokers quit or cut down. *British Medical Journal, 331,* 373–380.

Taurus, J. A. (2004). Public policy and smoking cessation among young adults in the United States. *Health Policy, 68,* 321–332.

Tercyak, K., Rodriguez, D., & Audrain-McGovern, J. (2007). High school seniors' smoking initiation and progress 1 year after graduation. *American Journal of Public Health, 97,* 1397–1398.

Tonstad, S., Tønnesen, P., Hajek, P., Williams, K. E., Billing, C. B., Reeves, K. R. (2006). Effect of maintenance therapy with varenicline on smoking cessation: A randomized controlled trial. *Journal of the American Medical Association, 296,* 64–71.

True, W. R., & Xian, H. (1999). Common genetic vulnerability for nicotine and alcohol dependence in men. *Archives of General Psychiatry, 56,* 655–661.

Tyas, S. L., & Pederson, L. L. (1998). Psychosocial factors related to adolescent smoking: A critical review of the literature. *Tobacco Control, 7,* 409–420.

Upadhyaya, H. P., Deas, D., Brady, K. T., & Kruesi, M. (2002). Cigarette smoking and psychiatric comorbidity in children and adolescents. *Journal of the American Academy of Child and Adolescent Psychiatry, 41,* 1294–1305.

Vastola, B. J., Douglas, L. A., Varlinskaya, E. I., & Spear, L. P. (2002). Nicotine-induced conditioned place preference in adolescent and adult rats. *Physiology and Behavior, 77,* 107–114.

Wakefield, M., Olver, I., Whitford, H., & Rosenfeld, E. (2004). Motivational interviewing as a smoking cessation intervention for patients with cancer: randomized controlled trial. *Nursing Research, 53,* 396–405.

Wechsler, H., Davenport, A., Dowdall, G., Moeykens, B., & Castillo, S. (1994). Health and behavioral consequences of binge drinking in college:

A national survey of students at 140 campuses. *Journal of the American Medical Association, 272,* 1672–1677.

Wechsler, H., Lee, J., & Rigotti, N. (2001). Cigarette use by college students in smoke-free housing: Results of a national study. *American Journal of Preventive Medicine, 20,* 202–207.

Wechsler, H., Rigotti, N. A., Gledhill-Hoyt, J., & Lee, H. (1998). Increased levels of cigarette use among college students: A cause for national concern. *Journal of the American Medical Association, 280,* 1673–1678.

Weitzman, E. R., & Chen, Y. Y. (2005). The co-occurrence of smoking and drinking among young adults in college: National survey results from the United States. *Drug and Alcohol Dependence, 80,* 377–386.

West, R. (2005) Time for a change: putting the Transtheoretical (Stages of Change) Model to rest. Addiction, *100*(8), 1036–1039.

Wills, T. A., & Cleary, S. D. (1996). How are social support effects mediated? A test with parental support and adolescent substance use. *Journal of Personality and Social Psychology, 71,* 937–952.

Yassa, R., Lal, S., Korpassy, A., & Ally, J. (1987). Nicotine exposure and tardive dyskinesia. *Biological Psychiatry, 30,* 109–115.

Zacny, J. P. (1990). Behavioral aspects of alcohol-tobacco interactions. *Recent Developments in Alcoholism, 8,* 205–219.

Zhang, B., Cohen, J., Ferrence, R., & Rehm, J. (2006). The impact of tobacco tax cuts on smoking initiation among Canadian young adults. *American Journal of Preventive Medicine, 30,* 474–479.

Zhu, S., Sun, J., Billings, S. C., Choi, W. S., & Malarcher, A. (1999). Predictors of smoking cessation in U.S. adolescents. *American Journal of Preventive Medicine, 16,* 202–207.

Chapter 18

Alcohol Use Disorders in Young Adulthood

Andrew K. Littlefield and Kenneth J. Sher

Zeke, aged 24 years, works intermittently as a car mechanic. He recently was charged with impaired and dangerous driving and has lost his job. He could not afford his apartment and has returned to live with his father and stepmother on the condition that he get treatment for alcohol problems. Zeke started drinking in high school at age 16. He and his friends soon became daily drinkers, often drinking at lunchtime. He had always struggled with the academic requirements of school despite average intellectual abilities, finding it difficult to maintain his interest and focus. He often forgot about or did not complete homework assignments and frequently skipped classes. Zeke was more successful with sports. During the last 2 years of high school, he and his friends typically got drunk on Friday and Saturday nights. His drinking led to considerable conflict with his parents who were concerned about him and his influence on his younger brothers.

Zeke completed high school and began a job as a car mechanic. His co-workers were frequent and heavy drinkers. Concurrently, his involvement with sports declined because he was no longer in school and living at home. He began drinking before and during work. He often arrived at work hungover and tired but felt he could "push through" and work effectively. On the night he was charged with impaired driving, Zeke crashed his car into a telephone pole and was arrested for driving while impaired.

Zeke initially did not consider himself as having a substance abuse problem. His father organized a lawyer for the driving charges who recommended a residential treatment program, to which Zeke reluctantly agreed. Although he successfully completed this program, it was years before he successfully embraced abstinence from alcohol.

Perhaps the most striking feature of the epidemiology of alcohol use disorders (AUDs; i.e., alcohol abuse and alcohol dependence) is that these disorders show a marked peak prevalence in late adolescence and early adulthood. Indeed, the remarkable rise and fall in the prevalence of disorder during this life stage suggests that it can be considered, in large part, a developmental disorder of young adulthood (Sher & Gotham, 1999). In this chapter we briefly describe the epidemiology of AUDs (and related alcohol-phenomena) and examine factors that contribute both to their manifestation early in the third decade of life and to their rapid decline soon afterward. We also discuss special considerations in the treatment of young adults with AUDs.

Conceptualizing Alcohol Involvement

Alcohol involvement can be viewed from multiple perspectives. Perhaps the most fundamental distinction concerning an individual's use of alcohol is whether he or she uses alcohol (i.e., is an abstainer). In the United States, 83% of all individuals over 18 years of age have consumed alcohol, with 70% consuming alcohol in the past year (Grant, Moore, Shepard, & Kaplan, 2003). Most initiation of alcohol use occurs prior to age 21; approximately two-thirds of 18–20 year olds report having consumed alcohol in the past year.

However, there is considerable variation across drinkers in how frequently they consume alcohol and how much they drink when they do consume. Therefore, further distinctions can be made among those who drink with respect to both their frequency and quantity of consumption. Although quantity is assessed as "typical" quantity consumed (in standard drink equivalents), individuals can and often do show high intra-individual variability, leading some researchers to measure volume/variability in order to further resolve an individual's drinking pattern. These assessments of drinking behavior include a variety of approaches, such as "graduated frequency" approaches (where individuals are queried as to how often they drink varying numbers of drinks/occasions [1–2 drinks, 3–4 drinks, 5–6 drinks, etc.]; Greenfield, 2000) various "diary" approaches (e.g., retrospective, timeline, follow-back assessments; Sobell & Sobell, 2003), and contemporaneous "diary" approaches (Carney, Tennen, Affleck, Del Boca, & Kranzler, 1998; Collins, Kashdan, & Gollnisch, 2003; Perrine, Mundt, Searles, & Lester, 1995) that provide daily (or event-specific) quantities that facilitate more detailed portrayals of drinking patterns. However, such assessments are burdensome and not practicable in many clinical and research contexts.

Consequently, measures of heavy drinking (e.g., drinking five or more drinks in one sitting) are often used to resolve drinking patterns that are likely to be associated with negative consequences. In some approaches, different thresholds are applied to men and women. The 5/4 criteria promoted by Wechsler and Austin (1998) define a "binge" episode as five drinks on an occasion for men and four drinks on an occasion for women. These different thresholds are intended to account for mean sex differences in total body water and first-pass metabolism.

Recently, the National Institute on Alcohol Abuse and Alcoholism (NIAAA; 2004) recommended defining a "binge" episode as drinking that yields a blood alcohol concentration (BAC) of .08% or more, noting the high risk of a number of alcohol-related harms that accompanies BACs at this or higher levels. This document notes that the 5/4 criteria roughly corresponds to a BAC criterion of .08% under a number of restrictive assumptions (e.g., if consumed within 2 hours, if individual is of average BMI and has an average rate of alcohol metabolism). Despite the imprecision of the 5/4 measure (or similar thresholds) for defining binge or heavy drinking, there is increasing recognition that this admittedly crude measure provides a reasonable index of excessive consumption. As we discuss below, young adults often evidence drinking patterns that are characterized by binge drinking.

Alcohol Use Disorders

The fourth edition of the *Diagnostic and Statistical Manual* (DSM-IV) of the American Psychiatric Association (1994) describes two major forms of alcohol use disorders (AUDs): *(1)* alcohol abuse, and *(2)* alcohol dependence, with alcohol dependence presumed to be the more severe disorder and its presence (or its history) excluding the diagnosis of alcohol abuse. In order for an individual to be diagnosed with dependence, three of the following seven criteria must be met: *(1)* tolerance (marked by either need for increased amounts or diminished effect with same amount of use), *(2)* withdrawal (defined by the characteristic withdrawal syndrome of the substance or substance is taken to relive/avoid withdrawal symptoms), *(3)* drinking alcohol in larger amounts or over a longer period than intended, *(4)* a persistent desire or unsuccessful efforts to cut down or control alcohol use, *(5)* a great deal of time is spent in obtaining alcohol, using it, or recovering from its effects, *(6)* giving up important social, occupational, or recreational activities because of alcohol use, and *(7)* continued use of alcohol despite knowledge that alcohol either caused or exacerbates a persistent or recurrent physical or psychological problem. Alcohol abuse is defined as a maladaptive drinking pattern characterized by one of the following: *(1)* a failure to fulfill major role obligations at work, school, or home, *(2)* recurrent alcohol use in situations in which it is physically hazardous, *(3)* recurrent alcohol-related legal problems, and *(4)* continued alcohol use despite having persistent or recurrent social or interpersonal problems caused or exacerbated by alcohol.

It should be noted at the present time that many researchers are revisiting the abuse/dependence distinction. Mixed abuse and dependence indicators can be well represented by a single factor (e.g., Hasin, Muthuen, Wisnicki, & Grant, 1994). Additionally, item-response theory-based analyses indicate that some dependence criteria (e.g., tolerance, impaired control) are prevalent (and therefore, psychometrically, less severe) and some abuse criteria relatively rare (e.g., legal difficulties) (Kahler, Strong, Hayaki, Ramsey, & Brown, 2003; Saha, Chou, & Grant, 2006). For these reasons, the validity of the category of abuse is increasingly being questioned.

Further, researchers are also reconsidering whether AUDs should be considered as *dimensional* rather than *categorical* phenotypes (Hasin, Liu, Alderson, & Grant, 2006; Muthén, 2006). Due largely to their ability to meet clinical, health-care planners', and insurance companies' needs, categorical diagnosis currently dominates DSM criteria for AUDs (Muthén, 2006). However, recent research involving nationally representative data suggests: *(1)* a continuum, rather than clear boundaries, exists among AUD criteria; *(2)* new hybrid statistical models that provide both categorical and dimensional representations of AUDs are more suitable than latent class and factor models; and *(3)* dimensional indicators of AUDs provide more information for research purposes compared to categorical classifications designed for clinical decision making (Hasin, Liu, Alderson, & Grant, 2006; Muthén, 2006). These findings are relevant to the abuse/dependence distinction that will likely be reconceputalized in the upcoming DSM-V.

The Epidemiology of Alcohol Use and Alcohol Use Disorders

Over the past 25 years, five large-scale, population-based epidemiological surveys using structured diagnostic interviews have provided estimates of alcohol use disorders in the United States. These include the Epidemiologic Catchment Area (ECA) Survey (Helzer, Burnam, & McEnvoy, 1991; Robins & Price, 1991); the National Comorbidity Survey (NCS; Kessler et al., 1994, 1997); the National Comorbidity Survey – Replication (NCS-R; Kessler, Berglund, Demler, Jin, & Walters, 2005; Kessler, Chiu, Demler, & Walters, 2005); the National Longitudinal Alcohol Epidemiologic Survey (NLAES; Grant, 1997; Grant & Pickering, 1996; Grant et al., 1994); and the National Epidemiologic Survey on Alcohol and Related Conditions (NESARC; Grant et al., 2004). Each of these major studies indicates very high past year and lifetime prevalences of AUDs in the U. S. population (13.8% lifetime and 6.8% past year DSM-III in ECA; 23.5% lifetime and 7.7% past year DSM-IIIR in NCS; 18.2 % lifetime and 7.41% past year DSM-IV in NLAES; 30.3% lifetime and 8.46% past year DSM-IV in NESARC; 18.6% lifetime and 4.4% past year DSM-IV in NCS-R).

Figure 18-1 provides representative prevalence data on DSM-IV (past 12 months) alcohol and abuse and dependence from the NESARC. As clearly indicated in this figure, there is a dramatic decline in the prevalence for both alcohol abuse and alcohol dependence in older cohorts, and this pronounced age gradient holds to a large extent across gender and as well as ethnicity (not shown). Additionally, if we subdivide the 18–29 age group into "emerging adults" (18–24) and older young adults (25–29), the age gradient is even more pronounced. This age gradient suggests either a marked developmentally limited condition that tends to remit in the third decade of life or that secular changes occur in the prevalence of AUDs that result in more recently born cohorts having higher prevalences. Comparison of estimates from NLAES (conducted in 1991–1992) and NESARC (2001–2002) reveals an overall increase in the prevalence of alcohol abuse (from 3.03% to 4.65%) and a slight decrease in the prevalence of alcohol dependence (from 4.38% to 3.81%). Of particular interest, the strong age gradient remained and was especially prominent for alcohol dependence, suggesting the age gradient is not an artifact of marked birth cohort differences. Further, large prospective studies of heavy episodic alcohol use in young adulthood (e.g., Chen & Kandel, 1995; Schulenberg, O'Malley, Bachman, Wadsworth, & Johnston, 1996) show similar patterns and suggest that the age-related decline in prevalence is primarily

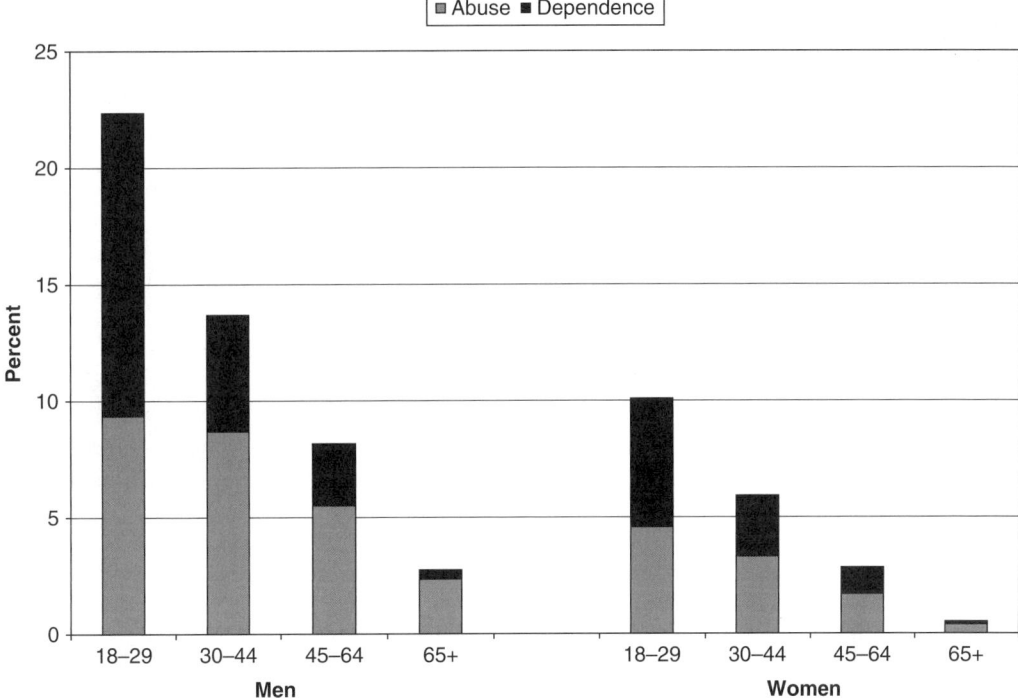

Figure 18-1. Past 12-month prevalence of alcohol abuse and dependence for men and women (as defined by the *Diagnostic and Statistical Manual of Mental Disorders* [4th ed.]. American Psychiatric Association, 1994). Data taken from the National Epidemiologic Survey on Alcohol and Related Conditions (Grant et al., 2004).

a developmental phenomenon and is not attributable to secular trends in consumption patterns (Grant, 1997; Sher & Gotham, 1999).

Are Alcohol Use Disorders in Young Adulthood Qualitatively Different Than Later in Life?

The large age gradient raises the question: Is the excess of AUDs seen in young adulthood similar to that found later in life or are they qualitatively different? More than 20 years ago, Zucker (1987; see also 1995) postulated four different subtypes of alcoholism based on developmental course: *(1)* a developmentally limited form, *(2)* an antisocial form, *(3)* a negative affect form, and *(4)* a developmentally cumulative form. Two of these would be expected to be overrepresented in young adulthood: *(1)* a developmentally limited form, and *(2)* an antisocial form. Other theorists (e.g., Babor et al., 1992; Cloninger, 1987; Knight, 1938) posited forms similar to Zucker's antisocial and negative affect forms, although these subtyping schemes did not clearly articulate the idea of a developmentally limited form of alcoholism. Indeed, the notion that some forms of alcohol dependence might be self-limiting has only recently started to gain recognition, although evidence to this effect has been accumulating for many years (Sher & Gotham, 1999).

Unfortunately, there has been a dearth of prospective studies examining factors that distinguish developmentally limited forms of AUDs from forms that have early onset but persist. The importance of behavioral dysregulation in predicting course of drinking problems has been noted in multiple studies (Zucker et al., 2006). Consistent with Zucker's taxonomy, Sher, Gotham, & Watson (2004) found that the presence of traits related to antisociality were among the few baseline (measured at age 18) traits that distinguished chronic and remitting courses of AUDs among college students who were initially diagnosed with a DSM-III AUD during the freshman year and were followed up at four additional times over the next 7 years. Although many other variables (e.g., alcohol expectancies, peer norms, and drinking motivations) are robust predictors of excessive consumption and AUDs prospectively (e.g., Baer, 2002), it is less clear how well they distinguish developmentally limited AUDs from more chronic classes when assessed as antecedent or baseline variables. Most of these variables appear to covary with course and are either likely proximal mediators of course or short-term consequences of course (Sher et al., 2004). As we discuss later in the section, *The Maturing Out Effect*, most of the research targeted at understanding processes associated with the resolution of drinking problems during the third decade of life focuses on developmental factors (especially the assumption of adult role statuses) particular to this stage of life.

One potentially important but understudied question concerns whether young adults who have AUDs show the same type of symptom patterns as older adults with AUDs. In order to address this question we conducted secondary analysis of data from the 2001 to 2002 National Epidemiologic Survey on Alcohol and Related Conditions (NESCARC), a large (n = 43,093) nationally representative sample of the U. S. population. Specifically, we compared the reported alcohol disorder symptoms experienced in the past 12 months of 18–29 year olds diagnosing with an AUD in the past year (abuse or dependence) to individuals 30 and above that also met criteria for past year AUD. Specifically, we examined the frequency of meeting each of the four abuse criteria in past-year alcohol abusers (n = 1,843) stratified by age. In a parallel way, we examined the frequency of meeting each of the seven dependence criteria in past-year alcohol dependent individuals (n = 1,484).

As can be seen in Figure 18-2a, recurrent drinking in situations in which drinking is hazardous (e.g., driving a vehicle while drinking) was the most commonly experienced symptom of alcohol abuse for those individuals meeting criteria for past year alcohol abuse, regardless of age. Younger alcohol abusers (aged 18–29) were less likely to report recurrent drinking in situations in which drinking is hazardous compared

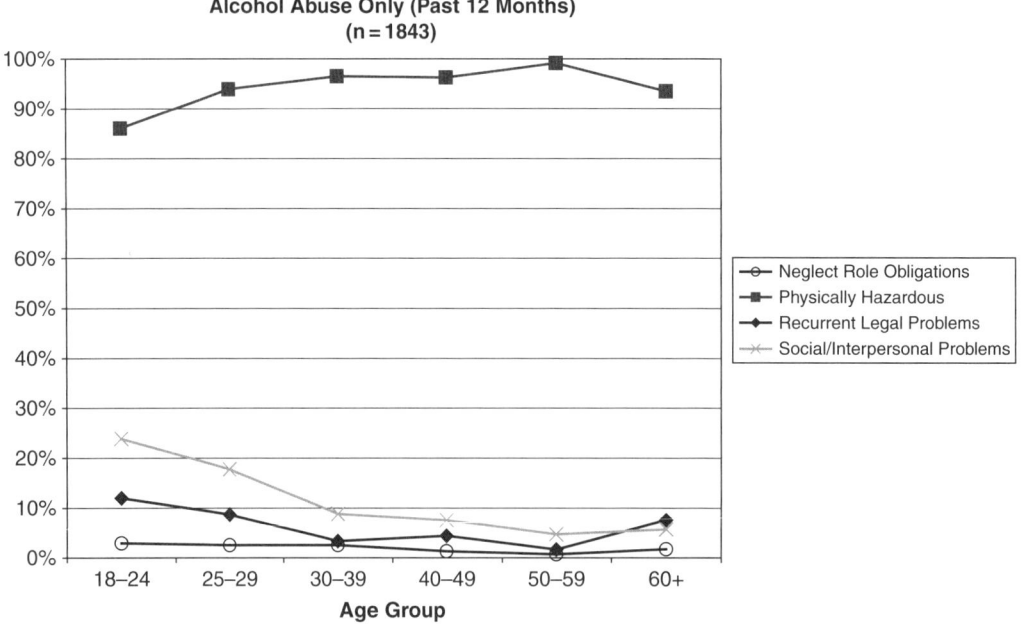

Figure 18-2a. Percent of individuals experiencing abuse symptoms in the past year who met criteria for past 12-month alcohol abuse by age.

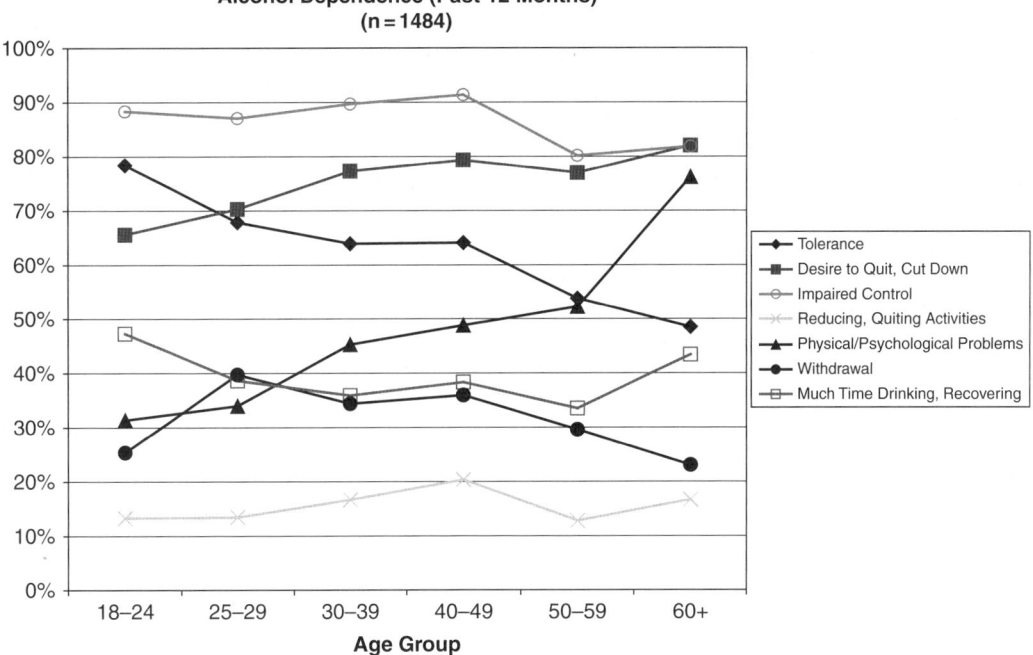

Figure 18-2b. Percent of individuals experiencing dependence symptoms in the past year who met criteria for past 12-month alcohol abuse by age.

to older alcohol abusers aged 30 and above (OR = .30; $p < .001$), but more likely to experience recurrent alcohol-related legal problems (e.g., get arrested or have other legal problems because of drinking) (OR = 2.96, $p < .001$) and to report drinking despite social or interpersonal problems caused by drinking (OR = 3.37, $p < .001$) compared to alcohol abusers over 30.

Profiles of dependence symptoms by age are displayed in Figure 18-2b. Young adults (those 18–29) with alcohol dependence were significantly more likely to experience tolerance symptoms (OR = 1.92, $p < .001$) and spend much time drinking or recovering from drinking (e.g., spent a lot of time being sick or getting over bad effects of drinking) compared to alcohol dependent individuals over 30 (OR = 1.40, $p < .02$). In contrast, these young alcohol-dependent individuals were less likely to have the desire or make unsuccessful attempts to reduce or stop drinking (e.g., more than once wanted to stop or cut down on drinking) (OR = .56, $p < .001$) and less likely to continue using alcohol despite physical or psychological problems caused by drinking (e.g., continue to drink though it was causing a health problem) (OR = .49, $p < .02$) in comparison to older individuals with alcohol dependence.

In sum, it appears that young adults with AUDs differ in their prevalence of specific alcohol disorder symptoms compared to similarly diagnosed older adults. Perhaps the most striking differences concern the relatively high rates of tolerance and spending much time engaged in drinking or getting over its effects in the younger alcohol dependents. Although one might expect younger alcohol-dependent individuals to report lower levels of tolerance (because tolerance is considered a symptom of neuroadaptation caused by excessive, chronic use), this finding has also been demonstrated in at least one prospective study (O'Neill & Sher, 2000) and so appears quite robust. The interpretation of this finding is less clear, since it is uncertain whether the strong age gradient is valid or reflects limitations of our ability to assess tolerance with standard interview and question measures (see O'Neill & Sher, 2000, for further discussion of this issue). The finding that younger adults spend more time in procuring, using, and recovering is less surprising given the relatively fewer adult responsibilities that younger adults have, potentially creating a more permissive environment for heavy drinking.

Although the younger alcohol-dependent individuals seem more severely affected than older alcohol dependents with respect to some criteria, they appear less severely affected in others. Most strikingly, younger alcohol-dependent individuals are less likely to drink despite having alcohol-related physical and psychological problems. Thus, older alcohol dependents would be more expected to come to the attention of health providers, which may partially account for the stereotype of the clinical alcoholic as a middle-aged adult with significant medical and psychiatric comorbidity.

In regard to psychiatric comorbidity, existing data regarding the associations between drinking and mood, anxiety, and personality disorders in young adults come largely from clinical samples and, to a lesser extent, general population samples (Dawson, Grant, Stinson, & Chou, 2005). Although individuals with AUDs are at a overall higher risk for a variety of Axis I and Axis II disorders, the relative strength of this association differs as a complex function of not just age but, among younger adults, whether the AUD being considered was abuse or dependence and whether they are college students (see section below). Dawson et al.'s findings are complex but, simply stated, they found that alcohol dependence was associated with extensive comorbidity in both older and younger alcohol-dependent individuals (especially for Axis I disorders and Cluster B Axis II disorders).

Are There Differences in Alcohol Involvement between College Students and Young Adult Non-College Students?

Many young adults are involved in higher education. The highly publicized reports on the rates of heavy drinking on college campuses (Wechsler, Davenport, Dowdall, Moeykens, & Castillo, 1994) and the alarming estimates of alcohol-related deaths, injuries, and sexual assaults among college students (Hingson, Heeren, Zakocs, Kopstein, & Wechsler, 2002; NIAAA, 2002) have heightened concern about the phenomenon of college student drinking (Slutske et al., 2004). However, until recently it was not clear whether these excessive levels of drinking were specific to college students or more generally characterize alcohol involvement during this stage of life regardless of student status.

Studies examining the differences between high school students who go on to attend college and their non-college-bound peers found that students who go on to attend college were less likely to be heavy drinkers in their senior year of high school than their non-college-attending peers (e.g., Bachman, Wadsworth, O'Malley, Johnston, & Schulenberg, 1997a; O'Malley & Johnston, 2002) but "catch up" to them in drinking after matriculation on some measures of alcohol involvement. Specifically, college students are typically more likely to have consumed alcohol (Crowley, 1991; Gfroerer, Greenblatt, & Wright, 1997; White, Labouvie, & Papadaratsakis, 2005) but are typically found to be as likely or less likely to binge drink compared to their non-college-attending peers (Crowley, 1991; Gfroerer et al., 1997; Muthén & Muthén, 2000; White et al., 2005). Conversely, several studies have shown that college students were more likely to report heavy drinking than their non-college-attending peers (Hingson et al., 2002; Johnston, O'Malley, & Bachman, 2002; O'Malley & Johnston, 2002). However, the studies that indicate a positive relation between college attendance and binge drinking (e.g., Hingson et al., 2002; Johnston et al., 2002; O'Malley & Johnston, 2002) did not control for background characteristics or living arrangements; when these variables are taken into account, nonsignificant or negative associations between college attendance and problematic drinking are typically found (e.g., Gfroerer et al., 1997; Muthén & Muthén, 2000; Slutske et al., 2004; White et al., 2005). Furthermore, several studies suggest that AUD prevalences for college students and their non-college-attending peers are equivalent (Dawson, Grant, Stinson, & Chou, 2004; Slutske et al., 2004; Wu, Pilowsky, Schlenger, & Hasin, 2007). In short, early, young adulthood is a time of life characterized by heavy alcohol involvement regardless of whether one is a college student.

However, some correlates of AUDs differ between college students and non-college students. For example, although both alcohol-dependent college students and nonstudent, young adults with alcohol dependence showed extensive comorbidity with a range of Axis I and Axis II conditions in NESARC, comorbidity appeared lesser in college student alcohol abusers compared to non–student age-abusers (Dawson et al., 2005). This suggests that alcohol abuse reflects less deviance in college students compared to non-students. Dawson and colleagues (2005) speculated that this could reflect norms for heavy drinking among college students, the effects of psychopathology on college matriculation and retention, greater professional and nonprofessional resources to provide various forms of behavioral and emotional support, or a tendency for college students to underutilize alcohol as an emotional regulation strategy.

Additionally, attending college appears to have a salutary effect on alcohol-related outcomes later in adulthood. White et al. (2005) found that college students were more likely to phase out of heavy drinking compared to their nonstudent peers. Though no differences were found in the extent of alcohol-related problems among those who dropped out of high school, graduated high school, or completed college at age 25, Muthén & Muthén (2000) found that individuals who dropped out of high school reported the highest rates of drinking at age 37, whereas those individuals who went to college reported the lowest rates. Similarly, Harford, Yi, and Hilton (2006), using data from a national survey, found that education beyond high school had a protective effect for alcohol dependence, whereas dropping out of high school increased the long-term risk for alcohol dependence. These findings suggest that college attendance may have a temporary effect of increasing problematic drinking during the college years but have a protective effect on problematic drinking that is manifested later in adulthood.

The finding that consumption increases can be time limited and situational (and not necessarily presage later problems) is important and highlights the fact that drinking during this stage of life appears to be highly reactive to environments that promote drinking, such as campus-based Greek letter organizations (Bartholow, Sher, & Krull, 2002). Greek drinking is associated with selection of heavier drinkers into these environments (McCabe et al., 2005; Park, Sher, & Krull, 2006), but, in turn, the environment further increases drinking. However, the environment-attributable increase in drinking does not show much persistence once an individual leaves the environment (Bartholow et al., 2002).

Related to this is the finding that one's place of residence during young adulthood (which is confounded with but separable from collegiate status) is associated with large differences in typical drinking patterns in early adulthood. Dawson et al. (2004) found differences between college students and their non-collegiate-age peers were generally smaller than differences within each group according to place of residence. The lowest levels of binge drinking were found among college students living with parents, whereas the highest rates of alcohol abuse were among college students living off campus. The high rates of alcohol abuse among off-campus college students suggest these students are more likely to engage in impaired driving, the most highly endorsed indicator of abuse (Dawson et al., 2004; see also White et al., 2005). Similarly, Bachman et al. (1997a) found among college students, living in dormitories increased the risk for heavy drinking, whereas living with a spouse decreased the risk.

Overall, both college students and non-students drink heavily. Although there seem to be some difference in drinking patterns between these groups, there is considerably more similarity. Further, the nature of one's living situation appears to be more important than whether an individual's primarily role is a student or in the labor market. Thus, as noted previously (e.g., Jackson, Sher, & Park, 2005), the high rates of heavy drinking among college students appear to reflect a "stage-of-life phenomenon." Perhaps because heavy drinking during early adulthood is relatively normative, treatment seeking in this population is low (see section on *Treatment* below). However, non-students are more likely to receive treatment for an AUD than college students (Wu et al., 2007).

"Maturing out": What Leads to De-escalation/Desistence of AUDs in Young Adulthood?

The rise in heavy drinking and AUDs during late adolescence and emerging adulthood is attributed, among other factors, to the newfound freedoms associated with leaving the parental home and identity exploration associated with this stage of life. Arnett (2006) refers to emerging adulthood as a "self-focused" time of life, where emerging adults have few social obligations and commitments to others, which grants them a great deal of autonomy in running their own lives. A large majority of these newly autonomous emerging adults who drink perceive coping and social benefits of heavy alcohol use (Schulenberg & Maggs, 2002). However, as the prevalence data indicate, this excess is relatively short lived. What factors then account for the dramatic decline in problematic alcohol use during the third decade of life?

Although there is an extensive literature on "natural recovery" (Sobell et al., 2000) describing the processes whereby many adult, alcohol-dependent individuals recognize a drinking problem and initiate various self-change strategies. However, it seems likely that much of the movement from AUDs to nondisordered drinking occurs in the absence of deliberate self-change efforts (Watson & Sher, 1998). Rather, it appears that much of the reduction in problem alcohol use arises from the natural constraints that traditional adult roles place on an individual's drinking. Role incompatibility (Yamaguchi & Kandel, 1985) is the theory that the decline of alcohol use (and other substance use) is attributable to the assumption of adult roles such as marriage and parenthood that are "incompatible" with a heavy drinking lifestyle. This theory has gained considerable empirical support in recent years. Emerging adulthood, the period intervening between adolescence and adulthood, represents in American and many other cultures a unique stage of life where the individual is relatively free of the rules and responsibilities related to his or her family of origin but where there is an extended moratorium on taking on adult responsibilities. It is at the beginning of this stage of development when the individual is at highest risk for the onset of an AUD (Grant et al., 2003; Li, Hewitt, & Grant, 2004) and the end of this stage when we begin to see a significant decline in the rate of AUDs.

Role Incompatibility

O'Malley (2004–2005) recently discussed two transitions related to the decline of heavy alcohol use among young adults: marriage and parenthood. Marriage has been shown to reduce alcohol consumption, especially problematic alcohol use (Bachman et al., 1997a; Bachman et al., 2002; Leonard & Rothbard, 1999), whereas remaining single or becoming separated/divorced is associated with increased alcohol use (Bachman, Wadsworth, O'Malley, Schulenberg, & Johnston, 1997b). Pregnant women appear to reduce their alcohol use for a number of reasons, including the belief that alcohol is harmful to the developing fetus (Coles, 1994). Furthermore, becoming a parent appears to be the key event to prompt men to reduce their drinking (Bachman et al., 1997a). Marriage and parenthood are thought to bring about reductions in social and recreational activities linked to drinking, such as attending parties and going out with friends to bars (O'Malley, 2004–2005).

The relation of social roles and substance use is thought to be underlined by two different processes: role selection and role socialization (Chassin, Presson, Sherman, & Edwards, 1992; Yamaguchi & Kandel, 1985). Role selection refers to the effects of substance use influencing later role involvement, whereas role socialization refers to the influence of adult roles on substance use behaviors. In a study designed to examine the role selection effect of AUDs on later marriage and the role socialization effect of marriage on later AUDs, Gotham, Sher, & Wood (2003) concluded that the role selection effect of AUDs on later marriage is less plausible than the socialization effect of marriage on later AUDs. Furthermore, the authors concluded that role socialization is a major contributor to the maturing-out process of problematic alcohol involvement during emerging adulthood. These findings are consistent with the maturing-out literature discussed by O'Malley (2004–2005).

Psychological Maturation

Though personality traits have traditionally been posited as inherent and static internal dispositions (McCrae et al., 2000), recent perspectives have began to view personality traits as dynamic constructs that make changes across time (e.g., Johnson, Hicks, McGue, & Iacono, 2007; Roberts, Caspi, & Moffitt, 2003). Both cross-sectional and longitudinal studies have documented systematic patterns of mean-level changes in personality traits at various ages across the life span, including during emerging and young adulthood (Caspi, Roberts, & Shiner, 2005; McCrae et al., 1999; Roberts, Walton, & Viechtbauer, 2006). A recent meta-analysis (Roberts et al., 2006) found a clear pattern of normative change across the life course, with people becoming more socially dominant, conscientious, and emotionally stable with age. Consistent with other findings (e.g., Roberts, Caspi, & Moffit, 2001), the study found that personality traits changed more often during emerging and young adulthood than during any other period of the life course, including adolescence.

Further, a normative trend toward personality structures that reflect greater self-control, risk avoidance, agreeableness, and emotional stability as people reach adulthood has been noted by several authors (e.g., Johnson et al., 2007). The tendency for individuals' personality structures to exhibit developmental adaptation to cope with the roles and tasks associated with adulthood have been labeled as the *maturity principle* (Caspi et al., 2005). Similar to the maturing-out effect discussed in the extant alcohol literature, these normative changes in personality are largely attributed to individuals undergoing role transitions associated with adulthood, such as parenthood and marriage (Helson, Kwan, John, & Jones, 2002; Roberts, Wood, & Smith, 2005; Roberts et al., 2006). Several empirical studies support this perspective, as changes in femininity and dominance have been linked to marital and family status (Roberts, Helson, & Klohnen, 2002), and emotional stability has been found to correspond with experiencing satisfying relationships (Roberts & Chapman, 2000; Robins, Caspi, & Moffitt, 2002).

Personality traits, especially those related to self-regulation/disinhibition and, to a lesser extent, those related to negative emotionality are robust risk factors for excessive drinking and AUDs. Thus, it seems very plausible that the developmentally normative changes we see in these traits in young adulthood are associated with the "maturing-out" effect. Perhaps because more researchers have assumed personality stability, there is currently a paucity of research addressing this possibility. However, researchers have shown the importance of changes in personality with changes of other important constructs in young adulthood, such as in satisfaction of social roles involving work or relationships (e.g., Roberts et al., 2002; Scollon & Diener, 2006). Thus, it would be somewhat surprising if personality change was not related to changes in drinking-related variables.

Although speculative, another possibility is that neurodevelopment of the prefrontal cortex contributes to the decline of AUDs in young adulthood. Individuals with deficits in executive functioning appear to be at risk for AUDs and other externalizing disorders in general (Giancola, 2000; Giancola & Moss, 1998). The prefrontal cortex undergoes considerable development during adolescence and emerging adulthood and this process is virtually complete by the late 20s (Casey, Galvan, & Hare, 2005; Romine & Reynolds, 2005). Coincident with these neurological changes are further development of cognitive control, self-regulation, and affect regulation (Leibenluft, Charney, & Pine, 2003). These processes are thought to be important in regulating one's behavior in general and in coping with negative emotions. Thus, although most of the extant maturing-out literature has focused on environmental changes that place individuals in life contexts that constrain drinking, these environmental contexts should be viewed in the broader framework of psychological (i.e., personality and cognitive) maturation.

Treatment of the Young Adult with an Alcohol Use Disorder

Treatment of AUDs in young adults presents special challenges. Ostensibly, the largest challenge is that self-recognition of drinking problems appears to be especially low in this group. For example, analyses conducted in the NESARC database indicate that of individuals with a past 12-month diagnosis of alcohol dependence, only 13% of individuals aged 18–29 reported that they *ever* sought help for their drinking compared to 37% of individuals aged 30 or over (OR = .25, $p < .001$). Equally important, only 8% of the younger alcohol-dependent individuals reported that during the past year that they had *thought* about getting treatment but did not, compared with 19% of similarly diagnosed individuals over 30 (OR = .37, $p < .001$).

Historically, lack of insight into the nature or extent of one's own alcohol dependence has been viewed by clinicians as "alcoholic denial." The exact meaning of the term "denial" varies as a function of theoretical orientation (Sher & Epler, 2004). Psychodynamically oriented clinicians (Freud, 1936/1966) view denial as a type of ego defense. Cognitively oriented clinicians eschew the term "denial" and might prefer to focus on those social-cognitive processes that lead to problem recognition (e.g., discrepancy between internal and external standards of behavior; Nye, Agostinelli, & Smith, 1999) and/or result in social misperceptions (e.g., Prentice & Miller, 1993; Ross, Green, & House, 1977) that facilitate the individual viewing his or her behavior as "normal." Neurobiologically oriented clinicians might focus on premorbid (Tarter, Alterman, & Edwards, 1984) and alcohol-induced (Duffy, 1995) brain dysfunction that results in limited awareness of one's deficits (a type of anosognosia). Regardless of theoretical perspective, most young adults with alcohol problems do not seek treatment and do not contemplate it.

Unfortunately, many programs utilized in alcohol treatment programs for older adults may not be compatible with the characteristics of young adults. For example, many treatment facilities commonly utilize 12-step programs, such as Alcoholics Anonymous (AA), as a primary treatment component (Mason & Luckey, 2003). Indeed, AA is the most commonly accessed source of help for an alcohol-related problem in the United States (Room & Greenfield, 1993). Although 12-step programs appear to be effective for many (e.g., Vaillant, 2005), predictors of frequent and/or long-term AA attendance, such as being older (Boscarino, 1980; Kolb, Pugh, & Gunderson, 1978) and having more severe histories of alcohol problems (Emrick, Tonigan, Montgomery, & Little, 1993; Vaillant, 1983) are the exact opposite of characteristics found in young adult treatment populations (Mason & Luckey, 2003). In a study comparing differences in characteristics and outcomes in an alcohol treatment sample between young adults aged 18–25 to similarly diagnosed older adults, Mason and Luckey (2003) found that young adults were less likely to attend AA meetings compared to the remainder of the sample. Kelly, Myers, and Brown (2002) found that adolescents who had greater substance-use problem severity were more likely to attend abstinence-focused 12-step groups, although many youths did not affiliate with AA or attended briefly before dropping out. Given that several studies suggest that 12-step approaches have a salutary association with posttreatment substance use among younger age groups (Alford, Koehler, & Leonard, 1991; Hsieh, Hoffmann, & Hollister, 1998; Kelly, Myers, & Brown, 2002), more research is needed to determine what factors may increase the motivation for young adults to attend 12-step programs (Kelly, Myers, & Brown, 2002).

Overall, young individuals who do enter treatment and remain in treatment have relatively favorable outcomes (Grella, Hser, Joshi, & Anglin, 1999). Unfortunately, relative youth has been shown to be a risk factor for dropping out of treatment (Deas, Riggs, Langenbucher, Goldman, & Brown, 2000; Joe, Simpson, & Broome, 1998). Thus, a high priority for treatment research with this population is to focus on the development of treatment programs that young adults will both seek out and remain in. Because of the documented reticence of younger alcohol-dependent individuals to seek treatment, it has been proposed that stepped-care approaches (Institute of Medicine, 1990) that titrate treatment intensity to treatment response may work particularly well with this population. Indeed, initial reports suggest that such stepped-care approaches have high retention rates and participant satisfaction among mandated college student problem drinkers (Borsari, Tevyaw, Barnett, Kahler, & Monti, 2007).

Much of what we know about the treatment of alcohol dependence in young adults comes from the college drinking literature. Although many, if not most, campuses have programs to address problems associated with alcohol, very few of these programs have been validated empirically (Sharmer, 2001; Walters, Bennett, & Noto, 2000). Larimer and Cronce (2007) recently reviewed the literature on individual-focused prevention and treatment approaches for college drinking. Interventions were organized into three broad categories: educational/awareness, cognitive/behavioral skills based, and motivational/feedback based. Education/awareness programs consisted of programs that provided information about problematic drinking (e.g., pamphlets), values clarification, and normative reeducation programs. As also concluded in an earlier review (Larimer & Cronce, 2002), no evidence emerged to support interventions based on information/knowledge alone or interventions based on values clarification. Normative reeducation programs, including personalized normative feedback, produced reductions in drinking and/or consequences, although normative reeducation interventions without personalized normative feedback had less evidence for reducing drinking.

The efficacies of cognitive and behavioral skills-based interventions were generally supported. Motivational/feedback-based interventions were also shown to be efficacious in reducing drinking and drinking-related consequences. Brief motivational interventions with personalized feedback were shown to be efficacious across a variety of treatment modalities (e.g., delivered individually, in groups, or as stand-alone feedback with no in-person contact). Importantly, the efficacy of both brief motivational interventions (e.g., Carey, Carey, Maisto, & Henson, 2006; Marlatt et al., 1998) and skills-based approaches in reducing drinking and consequences of mandated students (e.g., Fromme & Corbin, 2004) appeared promising.

Although the authors cautioned that additional research with stronger research designs and larger sample sizes is needed, they suggested campuses interested in implementing individual-focused prevention programs should consider implementing brief motivational interventions or skills-based programs. Despite the empirical support of the efficacy of skills-based programs and brief motivational interventions in reducing alcohol use and alcohol-related consequences among college students, the overwhelming majority of college students fail to receive treatment for problematic alcohol use (Wu et al., 2007).

Given that heavy consumption is strongly embedded in many critical life contexts in young adulthood, the potential value of harm reduction approaches (Marlatt & Witkiewitz, 2002) has been championed by a number of clinicians and policy makers. Such an approach promotes using behavioral strategies to avoid excessive levels of consumption (e.g., pacing drinking, setting drinking limits) and to minimize harmful consequences when intoxicated (e.g., designated driving programs; Martens et al., 2004). Harm reduction approaches have been shown to be effective and yield clinically significant outcomes in reducing drinking and drinking-related consequences in college students (Baer, Kivlahan, Blume, McKnight, & Marlatt, 2001; Roberts, Neal, Kivlaham, Baer, & Marlatt, 2000). However, critics of harm-reduction approaches warn that that it may increase alcohol use and underage drinking by making it seem acceptable or even accepted and that harm-reduction approaches discourage strict abstinence, which some view as the only acceptable treatment for problematic alcohol involvement (DuPont, 1996). Despite these criticisms, proponents maintain that harm-reduction approaches are not pro-legalization and do not discourage abstinence but rather pragmatically aim to decrease the amount of harm experienced by the individual (Marlatt, Blume, & Parks, 2001). Given that young adults are significantly more interested in reducing their drinking than abstaining, harm-reduction approaches to alcohol use are a compatible and beneficial treatment option for problematic drinkers in young adulthood.

Before concluding this section, it should be emphasized that there are now two medications (naltrexone and acamprosate) that have received FDA approval for the treatment of alcohol dependence (Garbutt, West, Carey, Lohr, & Crews, 1999) and additional promising off-label pharmacotherapies (e.g., topiramate; Johnson et al., 2007) that appear useful in alcohol treatment. Naltrexone, which has been shown to reduce craving in newly abstinent alcohol-dependent individuals (Volpicelli, Alterman, Hayashida, & O'Brien, 1992), may be an especially relevant treatment option for college students, since existing data suggest that it is most useful for early problem drinkers and people with dependence onset before age 25 (Kranzler et al., 2003; Rubio et al., 2005). However, there is a dearth of controlled outcome studies examining effectiveness in young adult treatment populations. This is unfortunate in that there appears to be a small subpopulation of young adults who do not express receptiveness to psychosocial interventions but would consider, indeed prefer, using pharmacotherapy for a drinking problem.

Summary and Future Directions

The peak prevalence and subsequent decline of AUDs that occur over the course of late adolescence and early adulthood suggests AUDs are largely a developmental disorder of young adulthood. Although there is much more similarity than differences in the symptom profiles of young and older individuals with AUDs, analyses included in this chapter reveal young adults who have AUDs differ in their prevalence of specific alcohol disorder symptoms from comparably diagnosed older adults. Most strikingly, younger alcohol-dependent individuals report higher rates of tolerance and spending more time engaged in drinking or getting over its effects and are less likely to drink despite having alcohol-related physical and psychological problems compared to older alcohol dependents. Further, although some differences in alcohol involvement have been found between college attending and nonattending young adults, there appears to be more similarity between these groups. However, attending college appears to have protective effects on alcohol-related outcomes later in adulthood, even though it appears to increase the prevalence of excessive consumption during the college years.

Declines in alcohol involvement toward the end of the third decade of life are usually attributed to individuals attaining adult role statuses incompatible with heavy drinking. Although undoubtedly true, future research should examine the role of psychological maturation (e.g., personality change, neurodevelopment) on the "maturing out" of problematic alcohol involvement given that these psychological processes are changing considerably during this period of time and almost certainly are relevant to understanding health-related behaviors.

Professionals who provide health-related services to young adults are likely to encounter relatively high levels of AUDs in this population. The overall prevalence of excessive alcohol consumption and correlated problems in this population contributes to resistance to the notion that their drinking behaviors are problematic, since many AUDs may be viewed as almost "normative." Consequently, treatment options that may increase involvement and retention rates, such as motivational interviewing and stepped-care approaches, may be especially important with this group. The appropriate role for pharmacotherapy in this population requires further investigation but may prove important to the needs of some subgroups of patients.

KEY POINTS

- A large proportion of young adults consumes alcohol, engages in binge-drinking, and meets criteria for alcohol abuse and dependence. In fact, these behaviors peak in this period of life, suggesting that alcohol use disorders (AUDs) might be conceptualized as developmental disorders involving a combination of environmental, social, and biological contributions.
- Young adults differ from older adults with respect to specific criteria of alcohol abuse, being more likely to acknowledge social and

> interpersonal problems and recurrent legal problems. Similarly, differences exist with respect to alcohol dependence, with young adults more likely to report tolerance and spending more time drinking or recovering from drinking and less likely to report a desire to cut back or quit or continuing to drink despite physical or psychological consequences.
> - Although college and non-college young adults report many similarities with respect to drinking behaviors during the early part of young adulthood, college graduates tend to experience fewer drinking-related problems later in life.

PRACTICE GUIDELINES

- Although many young adults may not view heavy drinking as problematic, it is important to obtain clinical information about alcohol use in this population.
- Young adults may benefit from specific prevention strategies (e.g., individual-focused or harm-reduction approaches).
- Young adults may benefit from specific treatments (e.g., stepped-care approaches, pharmacotherapies such as naltrexone) and may not derive as much benefit from traditional approaches (e.g., Alcoholics Anonymous attendance).

References

Alford, G., Koehler, R., & Leonard, J. (1991). Alcoholic anonymous–narcotic anonymous model of inpatient treatment of chemically dependent adolescents: A 2-year outcome study. *Journal of Studies on Alcohol, 52,* 118–126.

Arnett, J. J. (2006). Emerging adulthood: Understanding the new way of coming of age. In J. J. Arnett & J. L. Tanner (Eds.), *Emerging adults in America: Coming of age in the 21st century* (pp. 3–19). Washington, DC: American Psychological Association.

American Psychiatric Association. (1994). *Diagnostic and statistical manual of mental disorders (4th ed.).* Washington, DC: Author.

Babor, T. F., Hofmann, M., DelBoca, F. K., Hesselbrock, V., Meyer, R. E., Dolinsky, Z. S., & Rounsaville, B. (1992). Types of alcoholics: I. Evidence for an empirically derived typology based on indicators of vulnerability and severity. *Archives of General Psychiatry, 49,* 599–608.

Bachman, J. G., O'Malley, P. M., Schulenberg, J. E., Johnston, L. D., Bryant, A. L., & Merline, A. C. (2002). *The decline of substance use in young adulthood: Changes in social activities, roles, and beliefs.* Mahwah, NJ: Erlbaum.

Bachman, J. G., Wadsworth, K. N., O'Malley, P. M., Johnston, L. D., & Schulenberg, J. E. (1997a). *Smoking, drinking, and drug use in young adulthood: The impacts of new freedoms and new responsibilities.* Mahwah, NJ: Erlbaum.

Bachman, J. G., Wadsworth, K. N., O'Malley, P. M., Schulenberg, J., & Johnston, L. D. (1997b). Marriage, divorce, and parenthood during the transition to young adulthood: Impacts on drug use and abuse. In J. Schulenberg, J. Maggs, & K. Hurrelmann (Eds.), *Health risks and developmental transitions during adolescence.* (pp. 246–279). New York: Cambridge University Press.

Baer, J. S. (2002). Student factors: Understanding individual variation in college drinking. *Journal of Studies on Alcohol, 14,* 40–53.

Baer, J. S., Kivlahan, D. R., Blume, A.W., Mc Knight, P., & Marlatt, G. A. (2001). Brief intervention for heavy drinking college students: Four-year follow-up and natural history. *American Journal of Public Health, 91,* 1310–1316.

Bartholow, B. D., Sher, K. J., & Krull, J. L. (2002). Changes in heavy drinking over the third decade of life as a function of collegiate fraternity and sorority involvement: A prospective, multilevel analysis. *Health Psychology, 21,* 1–31.

Borsari, B., Tevyaw, T. O., Barnett, N. P., Kahler, C. W., & Monti, P. M. (2007). Stepped care for mandated college students: A pilot study. *The American Journal on Addictions, 16*, 131–137.

Boscarino, J. (1980). Factors related to "stable" and "unstable" affiliation with alcoholics anonymous. *International Journal of Addiction, 15*, 839–848.

Carey, K. B., Carey, M. P., Maisto, S. A., & Henson, J. M. (2006) Brief motivational interventions for heavy college drinkers: A randomized controlled trial. *Journal of Consulting and Clinical Psychology, 74*, 943–954.

Carney, M. A., Tennen, H., Affleck, G., Del Boca, F. K., & Kranzler, H. (1998). Levels and patterns of alcohol consumption using timeline follow-back, daily diaries, and real time "electronic interviews." *Journal of Studies on Alcohol, 59*, 447–454.

Casey, B. J., Galvan, A., & Hare, T. A. (2005). Changes in cerebral functional organization during cognitive development. *Current Opinion in Neurobiology, 15*, 239–244.

Caspi, A., Roberts, B. W., & Shiner, R. L. (2005). Personality development: Stability and change. *Annual Review of Psychology, 56*, 453–484.

Chassin, L., Presson, C. C., Sherman, S. J., Edwards, D. A. (1992). The natural-history of cigarette smoking and young adult social roles. *Journal of Health and Social Behaviors, 33*, 328–347.

Chen, K., Kandel, D. B. (1995). The natural history of drug use from adolescence to the mid-thirties in a general population sample. *American Journal of Public Health, 85*, 41–47.

Cloninger, C. R. (1987). Neurogenetic adaptive mechanisms in alcoholism. *Science, 236*, 410–416.

Coles, C. (1994). Critical periods for prenatal alcohol exposure. *Alcohol Health & Research World, 18*, 22–29.

Collins, R. L., Kashdan, T. B., & Gollnisch, G. (2003). The feasibility of using cellular phones to collect ecological momentary assessment data: Application to alcohol consumption. *Experimental and Clinical Psychopharmacology, 11*, 73–78.

Crowley, J. E. (1991). Educational status and drinking patterns: How representative are college students? *Journal of Studies on Alcohol, 52*(1), 10–16.

Dawson, D. A., Grant, B. F., Stinson, F. S., & Chou, S. P. (2004). Another look at heavy episodic drinking and alcohol use disorders among college and noncollege youth. *Journal of Studies on Alcohol, 65*, 477–488.

Dawson, D. A., Grant, B. F., Stinson, F. S., & Chou, P. S. (2005). Psychopathology associated with drinking and alcohol use disorders in the college and general adult populations. *Drug Alcohol Dependence, 77*, 139–150.

Deas, D., Riggs, P., Langenbucher, J., Goldman, M., & Brown, S. (2000). Adolescents are not adults: Developmental considerations in alcohol users. *Alcoholism, Clinical and Experimental Research, 24*, 232–237.

Duffy, J. D. (1995). The neurology of alcoholic denial: Implications for assessment and treatment. *Canadian Journal of Psychiatry Revue Canadienne de Psychiatrie, 40*, 257–263.

DuPont, R.L. (1996). Harm reduction and decriminalization in the United States: a personal perspective. *Substance Use & Misuse. 31*(14), 1929–1945.

Emrick, C. D., Tonigan, J. S., Montgomery, H., & Little, L. (1993). Alcoholics Anonymous: What Is Currently Known? In B. McCrady, W. R. Miller (Eds.), *Research on Alcoholics Anonymous opportunities and alternatives* (pp. 41–78). New Brunswick, NJ: Rutgers.

Freud, A. (1936/1966). *The ego and the mechanisms of defense.* London: Hogarth Press.

Fromme, K., & Corbin, W. (2004). Prevention of heavy drinking and associated negative consequences among mandated and voluntary college students. *Journal of Consulting and Clinical Psychology, 72*, 1038–1049.

Garbutt, J. C., West, S. L., Carey, T. S., Lohr, K. N., & Crews, F. T. (1999). Pharmacological treatment of alcohol dependence: a review of the evidence. *Journal of the American Medical Association, 28*, 1318–1325.

Gfroerer, J. C., Greenblatt, J. C., & Wright, D. A. (1997). Substance use in the U.S. College-Age population differences according to educational status and living arrangement. *American Journal of Public Health, 87*, 62–65.

Giancola, P. R. (2000). Neuropsychological functioning and antisocial behavior-Implications for etiology and prevention. In D. H. Fishbein (Ed)., *The science, treatment, and prevention of antisocial behaviors: Application to the criminal justice system* (pp. 11–16). Kingston, NJ: Civic Research Institute.

Giancola, P. R., & Moss, H. B. (1998). Executive cognitive functioning in alcohol use disorders. In M. Galanter (Ed), *Recent developments in alcoholism, Vol. 14: The consequences of alcoholism: Medical neuropsychiatric economic cross-cultural* (pp. 227–251). New York: Plenum Press.

Gotham, H. J., Sher, K. J., & Wood, P. K. (2003). Alcohol involvement and developmental task completion during young adulthood. *Journal of Studies on Alcohol, 64*, 32–42.

Grant, B. F. (1997). Prevalence and correlates of alcohol use and DSM-IV alcohol dependence in the United States: Results of the National

Longitudinal Alcohol Epidemiologic Survey. *Journal of Studies on Alcohol, 58*, 464–473.

Grant, B. F., & Harford, T. C. (1994). Prevalence of DSM-IV alcohol abuse and dependence: United States, 1992. *Alcohol Health & Research World, 18*, 243–248.

Grant, B. F., Moore, T. C., Shepard, J., & Kaplan, K. (2003). *Source and accuracy statement: Wave 1 National Epidemiologic Survey on Alcohol and Related Conditions (NESARC)*. Bethesda, MD: National Institute on Alcohol Abuse and Alcoholism.

Grant, B. F., & Pickering, R. P. (1996). Comorbidity between DSM-IV alcohol and drug use disorders: Results from the National Longitudinal Alcohol Epidemiologic Survey. *Alcohol Health & Research World, 20*, 67–72.

Grant, B. F., Stinson, F. S., Dawson, D. A., Chou, S., Ruan, W., & Pickering, R. P. (2004). Co-occurrence of 12-month alcohol and drug use disorders and personality disorders in the United States: Results from the National Epidemiologic Survey on Alcohol and Related Conditions. *Archives of General Psychiatry, 61*, 361–368.

Greenfield, T. K. (2000) Ways of measuring drinking patterns and the difference they make: Experience with graduated frequencies.*Journal of Substance Abuse, 12*, 33–49.

Grella, C. E., Hser, Y., Joshi, V., & Anglin, M. D. (1999). Patient histories, retention, and outcome models for younger and older adults in DATOS. *Drug and Alcohol Dependence, 57*, 151–166.

Harford, T. C., Yi, H. -Y., & Hilton, M. E. (2006). Alcohol abuse and dependence in college and non-college samples: A ten-year prospective follow-up in a national survey. *Journal of Studies on Alcohol, 67*, 803–809.

Hasin, D. S., Muthuen, B., Wisnicki, K. S., & Grant, B. (1994). Validity of the bi-axial dependence concept: a test in the US general population. *Addiction, 89*, 573–579.

Hasin, D.S., Liu, X., Alderson, D., Grant, B.F. (2006). DSM-IV alcohol dependence: a categorical or dimensional phenotype? *Psychological Medicine, 36*(12), 1695–1705.

Helson, R., Kwan, V. S. Y., John, O. P., & Jones, C. (2002). The growing evidence for personality change in adulthood: Findings from research with personality inventories. *Journal of Research in Personality, 36*, 287–306.

Helzer, J. E., Burnam, A., & McEnvoy, L. T. (1991). Alcohol abuse and dependence. In L. N. Robins & D. A. Regier (Eds.), *Psychiatric disorders in American: The Epidemiologic Catchment Area Study* (pp. 81–115). New York: Macmillan.

Hingson, R. W., Heeren, T., Zakocs, R. C., Kopstein, A., & Wechsler, H. (2002). Magnitude of alcohol-related mortality and morbidity among U.S. college students ages 18-24. *Journal of Studies on Alcohol, 63*, 136–144.

Hsieh, S., Hoffmann, N. G., & Hollister, C. D. (1998). The relationship between pre-, during-, and post-treatment factors and adolescent substance abuse behaviors. *The Journal of Addictive Behaviors, 23*, 1–12.

Institute of Medicine. (1990). *Broadening the base of treatment for alcohol problems*. Washington, DC: National Academy Press.

Jackson, K. M., Sher, K. J., & Park, A. (2005). Drinking among college students—Consumption and Consequences. In M. Galanter (Ed.), *Recent developments in alcoholism: Research on alcohol problems in adolescents and young adults* (Volume XVII) (pp. 85–117). New York: Kluwer Academic/Plenum Publishers.

Joe, G. W., Simpson, D. D., & Broome, K. M. (1998). Effects of readiness for drug abuse treatment on client retention and assessment of process. *Addiction, 93*, 1177–1190.

Johnson, W., Hicks, B., McGue, M., & Iacono, W. G. (2007). Most of the girls are alright, but some aren't: Personality trajectory groups from ages 14 to 24 and some associations with outcomes. *Journal of Personality and Social Psychology, 93*, 266–284.

Johnson, B. A., Rosenthal, N., Capece, J. A., Wiegand, F., Mao, L., Beyers, K., McKay, A., Ait-Daoud, N., Anton, R. F., Ciraulo, D. A., Kranzler, H.R., Mann, K., O'Malley, S. S., & Swift, R. M.; Topiramate for Alcoholism Advisory Board; Topiramate for Alcoholism Study Group. (2007). Topiramate for treating alcohol dependence: A randomized controlled trial. *Journal of the American Medical Association, 298*, 1641–1651.

Johnston, L. D., O'Malley, P. M., & Bachman, J. G. (2002). *National survey results on drug use from the Monitoring the Future study, 1975–2001* (Vol. Volume II: College students and young adults.). Bethesda, MD: National Institute on Drug Abuse.

Kahler C. W., Strong D. R., Hayaki J., Ramsey S. E., & Brown R. A. (2003). An item response analysis of the alcohol dependence scale in treatment-seeking alcoholics. *Journal of Studies on Alcohol, 64*, 127–136.

Kelly, J. F., Myers, M. G., & Brown, S. (2000a). A multivariate process model of adolescent 12-step attendance and substance use outcome following inpatient treatment. *Psychology of Addictive Behaviors, 14*, 376–389.

Kelly, J. F., Myers, M. G., & Brown, S. A. (2000b). A multivariate process model of adolescent 12-step attendance and substance use. *Psychology of Addictive Behaviors, 24*, 376–389.

Kelly, J. F., Myers, M. G., & Brown, S. A. (2002). Do adolescents affiliate with 12-step groups? A multivariate process model of effects. *Journal of Studies on Alcohol, 63*(3), 293–304.

Kessler, R. C., Berglund, P., Demler, O., Jin, R., & Walters, E. E. (2005a). Lifetime prevalence and age-of-onset distributions of DSM-IV disorders in the national comorbidity survey replication. *Archives of General Psychiatry, 62*, 593–602.

Kessler, R. C., Chiu, W. T., Demler, O., & Walters, E. E. (2005b). Prevalence, severity, and comorbidity of 12-month DSM-IV disorders in the National Comorbidity Survey Replication. *Archives of General Psychiatry, 62*(6), 617–627.

Kessler, R. C., Crum, R. M., Warner, L. A., & Nelson, C. B. (1997). Lifetime co-occurrence of DSM-III-R alcohol abuse and dependence with other psychiatric disorders in the National Comorbidity Survey. *Archives of General Psychiatry, 54*, 313–321.

Kessler, R. C., McGonagle, K. A., Zhao, S., Nelson, C. B., Hughes, M., Eshleman, S., Wittchen, H. U., & Kendler, K. S. (1994). Lifetime and 12-month prevalence of DSM-III-R psychiatric disorders in the United States: Results from the National Comorbidity Study. *Archives of General Psychiatry, 51*, 8–19.

Knight, R. P. (1938). The psychoanalytic treatment in a sanatorium of chronic addiction to alcohol. *Journal of the American Medical Association, 111*, 1443–1448.

Kolb, D., Pugh, W. M., & Gunderson, E. K. (1978). Prediction of posttreatmenteffectiveness in navy alcoholics. *Journal of Studies on Alcohol, 39*, 192–196.

Kranzler, H. R., Armeli, S., Tennen, H., Blomqvist, O., Oncken, C., Petry, N., & Feinn, R. (2003). Targeted naltrexone for early problem drinkers. *Journal of Clinical Psychopharmacology, 23*, 294–304.

Larimer, M. E., & Cronce, J. M. (2002). Identification, prevention, and treatment: A review of individual-focused strategies to reduce problematic alcohol consumption by college students. *Journal of Studies on Alcohol, 14*, 148–163.

Larimer, M. E., & Cronce, J. M. (2007). Identification, prevention, and treatment revisited: Individual-focused college drinking prevention strategies 1999–2006. *Addictive Behaviors, 32*, 2439–2468.

Leibenluft, E., Charney, D. S., & Pine, D. S. (2003). Researching the pathophysiology of pediatric bipolar disorder. *Biological Psychiatry, 53*, 1009–1020.

Leonard, K. E., & Rothbard, J. C. (1999). Alcohol and the marriage effect. *Journal of Studies on Alcohol, 13*, 139–146.

Li, T. K., Hewitt, B., & Grant, B. F. (2004). Alcohol use disorders and mood disorders: ANational Institute on Alcohol Abuse and Alcoholism Perspective. *Biological Psychiatry, 56*, 718–720.

Marlatt, G. A., Baer, J. S., Kivlahan, D. R., Dimeff, L. A., Larimer, M. E., Quigley, L. A., Somers, J. M., & Williams, E. (1998). Screening and brief intervention for high-risk college student drinkers: Results from a two-year follow-up assessment. *Journal of Consulting and Clinical Psychology, 66*, 604–615.

Marlatt, G.A., Blume, A.W., & Parks, G.A. (2001). Integrating harm reduction therapy and traditional substance abuse treatment. *Journal of Psychoactive Drugs, 33*(1), 13–21.

Marlatt, G. A., & Witkiewitz, K. (2002). Harm reduction approaches to alcohol use: Health promotion, prevention, and treatment. *Addictive Behaviors, 27*, 867–886.

Martens, M. P., Taylor, K. K., Damann, K. M., Page, J. C., Mowry, E. S., & Cimini, M. D. (2004). Protective factors when drinking alcohol and their relationship to negative alcohol-related consequences. *Psychology of Addictive Behaviors, 18*, 390–393.

Mason, M. J., & Luckey, B. (2003). Young adults in alcohol-other drug treatment: An understudied population. *Alcoholism Treatment Quarterly, 21*(1), 17–32.

McCabe, S. E., Schulenberg, J. E., Johnston, L. D., O'Malley, P. M., Bachman, J. G., & Kloska, D. D. (2005). Selection and socialization effects of fraternities and sororities on U.S. college student substance use: A multi-cohort national longitudinal study. *Addiction, 100*, 512–524.

McCrae, R. R., Costa, P. T., Jr., Lima, M. P., Simoes, A., Ostendorf, F., Angleitner, A., Marusić, I., Bratko, D., Caprara, G. V., Barbaranelli, C., Chae, J. H., Piedmont, R. L. (1999). Age differences in personality across the adult life span: Parallels in five countries. *Developmental Psychology, 35*, 466–477.

McCrae, R. R., Costa, P. T., Jr., Ostendorf, F., Angleitner, A., Hrebickova, M., Avia, M. D., Sanz, J., Sánchez-Bernardos, M. L., Kusdil, M. E., Woodfield, R., Saunders, P. R., & Smith, P. B. (2000). Nature over nurture: Temperament, personality, and life span development. *Journal of Personality and Social Psychology, 78*, 173–186.

Muthén, B. (2006). Should substance use disorders be considered as categorical or dimensional? *Addiction, 101* (Suppl 1), 6–16.

Muthén, B. O., & Muthén, L. K. (2000). The development of heavy drinking and alcohol-related problems from ages 18 to 37 in a U. S. national sample. *Journal of Studies on Alcohol, 61*(2), 290–300.

National Institute on Alcohol Abuse and Alcoholism (NIAAA). (2002). *A call to action: Changing the culture of drinking at U. S. colleges.* Final Report of the Task Force on College Drinking. NIH Pub. No. 02-5010. Rockville, MD.

National Institute on Alcohol Abuse and Alcoholism (2004). NIAAA Council approves definition of binge drinking. NIAAA Newsletter, No. 3. National Institute on Alcohol Abuse and Alcoholism, Bethesda, MD.

Nye, E. C., Agostinelli, G., & Smith, J. E. (1999). Enhancing alcohol problem recognition: A self-regulation model for the effects of self-focusing and normative information. *Journal of Studies on Alcohol, 60,* 685–693.

O'Malley, P. (2004/2005). Maturing out of problematic alcohol use. *Alcohol Research and Health, 28,* 202–204.

O'Malley, P. M., & Johnston, L. D. (2002). Epidemiology of alcohol and other drug use among American college students. *Journal of Studies on Alcohol, 14,* 23–39.

O'Neill, S., & Sher, K. J. (2000). Physiological alcohol dependence symptoms in early adulthood: A longitudinal perspective. *Experimental and Clinical Psychopharmacology, 8,* 493–508.

Park, A., Sher, K. J., & Krull, J. (2006). Individual differences in the Greek effect on risky drinking: The role of self-consciousness. *Psychology of Addictive Behavior, 20,* 85–90.

Perrine, M. W., Mundt, J. C., Searles, J. S., & Lester, L. S. (1995). Validation of daily self-reported alcohol consumption using interactive voice response (IVR) technology. *Journal of Studies on Alcohol, 56,* 487–490.

Prentice, D. A., & Miller, D. T. (1993). Pluralistic ignorance and alcohol use on campus: Some consequences of misperceiving the social norm. *Journal of Personality & Social Psychology, 64,* 243–256.

Roberts, B.W., Caspi, A., & Moffitt, T. E. (2001). The kids are alright: Growth and stability in personality development from adolescence to adulthood. *Journal of Personality and Social Psychology, 81,* 670–683.

Roberts, B. W., Caspi, A., & Moffitt, T. E. (2003). Work experiences and personality development in young adulthood. *Journal of Personality and Social Psychology, 84,* 582–593.

Roberts, B. W., & Chapman, C. N. (2000). Change in the dispositional well-being and its relation to role quality: A 30-year longitudinal study. *Journal of Research in Personality, 34,* 26–41.

Roberts, B. W., Helson, R., & Klohnen, E. C. (2002). Personality development and growth in women across 30 years: Three perspectives. *Journal of Personality, 70,* 79–102.

Roberts, L. J., Neal, D. J., Kivlahan, D. R., Baer, J. S., & Marlatt, G. A. (2000). Individual drinking changes following a brief intervention among college students: Clinical significance in an indicated prevention context. *Journal of Consulting and Clinical Psychology, 68,* 500–505.

Roberts, B. W., Walton, K. E., & Viechtbauer, W. (2006). Patterns of mean-level change in personality traits across the life course: A meta-analysis of longitudinal studies. *Psychological Bulletin, 132,* 1–25.

Roberts, B. W., Wood, D., & Smith, J. L. (2005). Evaluating five factor theory and social investment perspectives on personality trait development. *Journal of Research in Personality, 39,* 166–184.

Robins, R. W., Caspi, A., & Moffitt, T. E. (2002). It's not just who you're with, it's who you are: Personality and relationship experiences across multiple relationships. *Journal of Personality, 70,* 925–964.

Robins, L. N., & Price, R. K. (1991). Adult disorders predicted by childhood conduct problems: Results from the NIMH Epidemiologic Catchment Area project. *Psychiatry: Journal for the Study of Interpersonal Processes, 54,* 116–132.

Romine, C. B., & Reynolds, C. R. (2005). A model of the development of frontal lobe functioning: Findings from a meta-analysis. *Applied Neuropsychology, 12,* 190–201.

Room, R., & Greenfield, T. (1993). Alcoholics anonymous, other 12-step movements and psychotherapy in the US population, 1990. *Addiction, 88,* 555–562.

Ross, L., Greene, D., & House, P. (1977). The false consensus effect: An egocentric bias in social perception and attribution processes. *Journal of Experimental Social Psychology, 13,* 279–301.

Rubio, G., Ponce, G., Rodriguez-Jiminez, R., Jiminez-Arriero, M. A., Hoenicka, J., & Palomo, T. (2005). Clinical predictors of response to naltrexone in alcoholic patients: who benefits most from treatment with naltrexone? *Alcohol and Alcoholism, 40,* 227–233.

Saha, T. D., Chou, S. P., & Grant, B. F. (2006). Toward an alcohol use disorder continuum using item response theory: results from the National Epidemiologic Survey on Alcohol and Related Conditions. *Psychological Medicine, 36,* 931–941.

Schulenberg, J. E., & Maggs, J. L. (2002). A developmental perspective of alcohol use and heavy drinking during adolescence and the transition to young adulthood. *Journal of Studies on Alcohol, 14,* 54–70.

Schulenberg, J., O'Malley, P. M., Bachman, J. G., Wadsworth, K. N., & Johnston, L. D. (1996). Getting drunk and growing up: Trajectories of frequent binge drinking during the transition to young adulthood. *Journal of Studies on Alcohol, 57*, 289–304.

Scollon, C. N., & Diener, E. (2006). Love, work, and changes in extraversion and neuroticism over time. *Journal of Personality and Social Psychology, 91*, 1152–1165.

Sharmer, L. (2001). Evaluation of alcohol education programs on attitude, knowledge, and self-reported behavior of college students. *Evaluation & the Health Professions, 24*, 336–357.

Sher, K. J., & Epler, A. (2004). Alcoholic denial: Self-awareness and beyond. In B. Beitman and J. Nair (Eds.), *Self-awareness deficits in psychiatric patients: Neurobiology, assessment, and treatment* (pp. 184–212). New York: W. W. Norton & Company.

Sher, K. J., & Gotham, H. J. (1999). Pathological alcohol involvement: A developmental disorder of young adulthood. *Development & Psychopathology, 11*, 933–956.

Sher, K. J., Gotham, H. J., & Watson, A. (2004). Trajectories of dynamic predictors of disorder: Their meanings and implications. *Development and Psychopathology, 16*, 825–856.

Slutske, W. S., Hunt-Carter, E. E., Nabors-Oberg, R. E., Sher, K. J., Bucholz, K. K., Madden, P. A., Anokhin, A., & Heath, A. C. (2004). Do college students drink more than their non-college attending peers? Evidence from a population-based longitudinal female twin study. *Journal of Abnormal Psychology, 113*, 530–540.

Sobell, L. C., Ellingstad, T. P., & Sobell, M. B. (2000). Natural recovery from alcohol and drug problems: Methodological review of the research with suggestions for future directions. *Addiction, 95*, 749–764.

Sobell, L. C., & Sobell, M. B. (2003). Alcohol consumption measures. In P. Allen & V. B. Wilson (Eds.), *Assessing alcohol problems: A guide for clinicians and researchers* (2nd ed., pp. 75–99). Bethesda, MD: National Institute on Alcohol Abuse and Alcoholism.

Tarter, R. E., Alterman, A. I., & Edwards, K. L. (1984). Alcoholic denial: A biopsychological interpretation. *Journal of Studies on Alcohol, 45*, 214–218.Vaillant, G. E. (1983). *The natural history of alcoholism.* Cambridge, MA: Harvard University Press.

Vaillant, G. E. (2005). Alcoholics Anonymous: cult or cure? *Australian and New Zealand Journal of Psychiatry, 39*, 431–436.

Volpicelli, J.R., Alterman, A.I., Hayashida, M., O'Brien, C.P. (1992). Naltrexone in the treatment of alcohol dependence. *Archives of General Psychiatry, 49*(11), 876–880.

Walters, S. T., Bennett, M. E., & Noto, J. V. (2000). Drinking on campus. What do we know about reducing alcohol use among college students? *Journal of Substance Abuse Treatment, 19*, 223–228.

Watson, A. L., & Sher, K. J. (1998). Resolution of alcohol problems without treatment: Methodological issues and future directions of natural recovery research. *Clinical Psychology: Science and Practice, 5*, 1–18.

Wechsler, H., & Austin, S. B. (1998). Binge drinking: The five/four measure. *Journal of Studies on Alcohol, 59*, 122–123.

Wechsler, H., Davenport, A., Dowdall, G., Moeykens, B., & Castillo, S. (1994). Health and behavioral consequences of binge drinking in college: A national survey of students at 140 campuses. *Journal of the American Medical Association, 272*, 1672–1677.

White, H. R., Labouvie, E. W., & Papadaratsakis, V. (2005). Changes in substance use during the transition to adulthood: A comparison of college students and their noncollege age peers. *Journal of Drug Issues, 35*, 281–306.

Wu, L.-T., Pilowsky, D. J., Schlenger, W. E., & Hasin, D. (2007). Alcohol use disorders and the use of treatment services among college-age young adults. *Psychiatric Services, 58*, 192–200.

Yamaguchi, K., & Kandel, D. (1985). On the resolution of role incompatibility: Life event history analysis of family roles and marijuana use. *American Journal of Sociology, 90*, 1284–1325.

Zucker, R. A. (1987). The four alcoholisms: A developmental account of the etiologic process. In P. C. Rivers (Ed.), *Alcohol and addictive behaviors: Nebraska Symposium on motivation* (pp. 27–83). Lincoln, NE: University of Nebraska Press.

Zucker, R. A. (1995). Pathways to alcohol problems and alcoholism: A developmental account of the evidence for multiple alcoholisms and for contextual contributions to risk. In R. A. Zucker, G. M Boyd, & J. Howard (Eds.), *The development of alcohol problems: Exploring the biopsychosocial matrix of risk* (NIAAA Research Monograph 26, pp. 255–289). Rockville, MD: Department of Health and Human Services.

Zucker R. A., Wong, M. M., Clark, D. B., Leonard, K. E., Schulenberg, J. E., Cornelius, J. R., Fitzgerald, H. E., Hornish, G. G., Merline, A., Nigg, J. T., O'Malley, P. M., & Puttler, L. I. (2006). Predicting risky drinking outcomes longitudinally: What kind of advance notice can we get? *Alcoholism, Clinical and Experimental Research, 30*, 243–252.

Chapter 19

Drug Use Disorders among Young Adults: Evaluation and Treatment

Edward V. Nunes

Daniel, a 20-year-old male, experimented with smoking marijuana and drinking alcohol with friends when he was 13 years of age. This behavior continued throughout high school without apparent problems. When he started college, Daniel began using prescription stimulants he had purchased from a friend. Stimulants allowed him to stay up late and complete his school work. They also improved concentration and helped his mood. Daniel had suffered from depression since childhood. Because friends were using stimulants as well, Daniel never felt they could cause problems for him.

For the past 2 years, Daniel has been using high doses of stimulants on a daily basis. He buys them from friends and has three physicians prescribing them. Always intending on stopping, Daniel's use has actually increased over time. His sleep has been erratic for months and he has problems relaxing. Although a bright young man, Daniel's school attendance has become sporadic and his school work has suffered. Due to increased irritability, Daniel's relationships with friends have also suffered. In addition, Daniel has begun isolating himself from friends and family because of his paranoia regarding their motives and his lack of trust.

Introduction

Substance experimentation is almost ubiquitous among adolescents, and a significant proportion of high school and college students use substances with some regularity. Alcohol and nicotine are the most frequently used substances among adolescents and are covered in other chapters in this volume. These are followed in order of prevalence by cannabis, stimulants (mainly cocaine, although methamphetamine and prescription stimulants are also significant), and opioids (heroin, and prescription opioids). Clinicians seeing adolescents and young adults also need to be aware of hallucinogens and club drugs such as methylenedioxymethamphetamine (MDMA or "ecstasy") and gamma-hydroxybutyrate (GHB, among others), which do not usually produce a dependence syndrome per se but carry significant health risks. Among athletes, anabolic steroids and other performance-enhancing drugs may be found.

In this chapter, I will seek to provide clinicians and researchers with an overview of the diagnosis and treatment of drug use disorders among young adults. This will hopefully provide a useful overview for clinicians working with young adults and highlight scientific issues in need of further research. Most clinical and epidemiological research on substance use disorders has focused on adults. There is also a considerable body of epidemiological work on children at risk and adolescents with substance use disorders. Research on treatment of drug use disorders among adolescents is limited, although more controlled studies are beginning to emerge. The young adult population per se has not often been a specific focus of study; thus, much of what will be presented here will be extrapolated from the adult or adolescent literature. Before launching into detailed coverage of diagnosis and treatment, there are several important themes that apply to all substance use problems and are important as background. These include the distinction between use versus abuse or dependence; addiction as a disorder of learning and memory; the stress-diathesis model as applied to substance use disorders; the gateway hypothesis that nicotine, alcohol, and cannabis lead in a causal pathway to other "harder" drugs; and the developmental perspective on substance use disorders.

Use, Abuse, and Dependence

Among adolescents and young adults, many will use substances, since alcohol and drugs are endemic in most high school or college settings, but only some will develop abuse or dependence. The task for the clinician is to detect use, determine what risks it poses, and ascertain if it represents abuse or dependence. As defined in DSM-IV (American Psychiatric Association, 1994), abuse represents a pattern of harmful use with adverse consequences to health or social functioning—for example, injury, drunk driving, and impact on school or work performance. Dependence is a regular pattern of use with loss of control, impairment, and tolerance and/or withdrawal. This will be covered in detail below. The point to make here is that in the case of alcohol, social drinking is well accepted and woven into the fabric of Western society. The occasional cigarette or cigar after a meal might be viewed similarly. However, in the case of drugs, the notion of non-problem or social use is less well accepted. In part, drug use is illegal, other than the use of specific controlled substances under the guidance and prescription of a physician. In part, the risks of use are generally higher. For example, fatal opioid overdose is a relatively common cause of death among adolescents and young adults who use opioids (De Angelis, Hickman, & Yang, 2004; Sherman, Cheng, & Kral, 2007), and this is most likely in those who have little experience using the drug and thus low tolerance. Cannabis use, on the other hand, presents less immediate danger, and many adolescents and young adults will use occasionally without apparent long-term harm, while a smaller proportion will go on to develop dependence. Drug use is also more deviant with respect to social norms, and as such should be viewed as a warning signal of a range of possible psychiatric problems.

The adolescent or young adult presenting for routine health screening, or for consultation about specific health or emotional problems, is likely to view his or her drug use as part of normal socializing and not problematic. The skilled clinician should be open to the patient's point of view, but mindful of the signs of risk or problem use and prepared to try to change the patient's perspective. Simple advice of a physician to quit substance use has been shown to have a useful impact (Fleming, Barry, Manwell, Johnson, & London, 1997). However, there should be follow-up, as many patients will resist such advice and require further attention and efforts to build motivation for change (Miller & Rollnick, 2002).

Addiction as a Disorder of Learning and Memory

Drugs as Positive Reinforcers—The Brain Reward System. In contrast to most other psychiatric disorders, where our understanding of pathophysiology remains incomplete and at a nascent stage despite much progress, the mechanisms of addictions are remarkably well understood. What sets alcohol, nicotine, and other addictive drugs apart from all other substances in nature is that they function as positive reinforcers within a behavioral paradigm. At the biological level, like other positive reinforcers, they lead to release of dopamine into the ventral striatum or nucleus accumbens from the terminals of the mesolimbic dopaminergic fibers originating in the ventral tegmental area that form the hub of the brain reward system (Gardner, 1997). Some addictive drugs like cocaine and the other psychostimulants are indirect acting sympathomimetics that promote dopamine release directly by blocking reuptake into nerve terminals or presynaptic vesicles. Others like alcohol, nicotine, opioids, or cannabinoids produce dopamine release and reinforcing effects through their inputs of other transmitter systems to the dopamine system. Thus, addiction can be viewed as a pattern of behaviors built up over time under control of the reinforcing properties of the drug.

Treatments, both behavioral and pharmacological, are focused on either substituting competing reinforcers or interfering with the reinforcing effects of the drug. This provides a powerful theoretical framework for treatment development and has yielded efficacious treatments ranging from cognitive-behavioral treatments, to treatments based on contingency management with incentives contingent upon abstinence, to pharmacological strategies involving agonists that substitute for the drug, or antagonists that block its reinforcing effects. It is also an important perspective for the clinician working with and trying to understand the problems of addicted patients, namely that the drugs are rewarding and pleasurable at some level—they feel good. This needs to be acknowledged and managed as part of the treatment.

Negative Reinforcement and "Self-Medication". Drugs may also serve to relieve aversive states, and as such addictive behavior may develop under a negative reinforcement mechanism. The most direct example of this phenomenon is drug use to relieve withdrawal symptoms. Use to relieve withdrawal is most prominent in opioid dependence and nicotine dependence. For those drugs, regular use followed by abrupt cessation usually produces unpleasant withdrawal, which is rapidly and gratifyingly relieved by reinstatement of use. Opioid- or nicotine-dependent patients will often describe relief of withdrawal as contributing significantly to their motivation for continued use. The regular use of alcohol, cannabis, stimulants, and other addictive drugs can also produce significant withdrawal syndromes, but with more variation. Some patients will report little or no withdrawal, while for others it becomes a significant drive to continued use. Thus, assessment of degree of withdrawal is an important aspect of the clinical evaluation.

A negative reinforcement mechanism may also be operating if a drug serves to relieve some other aversive state, such as physical pain, anxiety, or depression. This has often been described as the "self-medication" hypothesis (Khantzian, 1985; Quitkin, Rifkin, Kaplan, & Klein, 1972). This has been widely invoked to explain addiction as a response to other psychopathology, and it is in the popular awareness such that patients will often describe it in rationalizing their drug use. There is evidence to support this mechanism, although it is rarely the sole mechanism driving an addiction. Clinicians should take this rationale seriously and evaluate patients for co-occurring psychopathology or medical conditions (see sections on diagnosis and treatment below for more detail). However, evidence suggests that while treatment of co-occurring conditions may be helpful in treating an addiction, it is rarely a cure by itself (Nunes & Levin, 2004), suggesting other fundamental mechanisms are operating and other treatments directly targeting the addiction are generally needed.

Addiction and Classical Conditioning—Triggers and Craving. Addictive drugs function as unconditioned stimuli (UCS) producing unconditioned responses (UCR) of euphoria and other drug effects. Following the paradigm of classical conditioning, environmental stimuli with which drug use is paired come to function as conditioned stimuli (CS), which may produce conditioned drug-like effects (experienced and described by patients as resembling the drug high), or conditioned drug-opposite effects (described as resembling aversive withdrawal-like effects) (Childress, Ehrman, Robsenow, Robin, & O'Brien, 1992; Siegel & Ramos, 2002). These environmental stimuli or CSs often then function as cues or triggers to drug use. Emotional states, such as anger or sadness, that are paired with drug use can also come to function as triggers, and predictable patterns of physiological and brain activation in response to cues are observed (Childress et al., 1994). This process constitutes one of the most difficult aspects of addiction to address therapeutically since such classical conditioning can be resistant to extinction or may unexpectedly re-emerge after seemingly having been extinguished (Siegel & Ramos, 2002). A patient encounters a neighborhood or party scene, becomes angry or distraught, or meets someone with whom he/she has used in the past and suddenly feels a strong desire or "craving" to use. Craving itself has been a source of controversy, since it is a subjective state and has been somewhat elusive to measure as a target of treatment. However, the problem of drug use in response to environmental or internal emotional cues is very real and has been difficult to target therapeutically. Cognitive behavioral and other counseling strategies focus on helping patients to avoid such triggers and cope with them when they are encountered. Part of the problem is that the environmental cues are so ubiquitous—extinguish some with a behavioral treatment and others emerge (Childress et al., 1992). This is an important area of current research inquiry. Clinicians should help patients recognize their triggers to drug use and to cope with them.

The Stress-Diathesis Model and Substance Use Disorders

Genetics of Substance Use Disorders. Twin studies have shown that substance use disorders have a strong genetic component, with heritability estimates of 30% to 50% or more. Evidence suggests this may consist of a liability to substances in general, related in part to externalizing psychopathology (e.g., antisocial personality disorder syndrome) and genetic components that are specific to specific drugs of abuse (Fu et al., 2002; Tsuang, Bar, Harley, & Lyons, 2001). In short, individuals inherit different responses to substances of abuse. Some may have a neutral or even aversive response to a particular drug, and they will be relatively protected from developing abuse or dependence. Others may find a particularly drug more reinforcing, and it is they who may be particularly vulnerable to abuse and dependence. The drug may be either positively reinforcing—it feels good and the person wants more, or negatively reinforcing—the drug relieves an aversive feeling state. The important message to convey to young adult patients is that experimentation with drugs is a gamble. There is no way to know ahead of time who will find a drug too pleasant and be vulnerable to becoming addicted; and once the addiction takes hold it can be very destructive and difficult to reverse.

Stress, Trauma, and Substance Use. Environmental stress plays an important role in increasing the liability to substance abuse and dependence. In laboratory animal models, stress increases the propensity of animals to self-administer drugs and can prompt re-instatement of drug self-administration after it had been extinguished (Goeders, 2003). Thus, stress may alter the brain reward system such that it is more susceptible to the rewarding effects of drugs, or a negative reinforcement mechanism may come into play, where drugs relieve aversive states related to stress. Epidemiological studies in human populations have repeatedly shown an association between trauma and other forms of stress and drug abuse (Breslau, Davis, & Schultz, 2003), and posttraumatic stress disorder (PTSD) is a common co-occurring psychiatric disorder among substance-dependent patients. Stress among college students has been shown to be associated with increased levels of drinking (Park, Armeli, & Tennen, 2004). The stress–addiction connection represents a therapeutic opportunity and remains an important focus of treatment research. Clinicians should assess the history of trauma in patients, evaluate for PTSD, and attend to the general stress level impacting their patients.

The Gateway Hypothesis

The gateway hypothesis holds that initial experimentation with nicotine, alcohol or cannabis among adolescents leads in a causal sense to the development of more serious problems such as development of abuse and dependence, or progression to other drugs of abuse such as opioids or cocaine (Kandel, Yamaguchi, & Chen, 1992). This hypothesis is supported by epidemiological observations that early use is associated with increased risk of subsequent addictions. This finding has been a source of controversy, since there are two possible explanations. One is that early use reflects the presence of other risk factors (an inherited liability to addiction, stress, or other predisposing factors) that are directly responsible for the increased risk of progression to other drugs and drug problems. The other is that early substance use alters brain physiology in some way that increases subsequent risk or draws an individual into a deviant peer group that increases subsequent risk. This topic represents a fertile area for research. Clinically, early substance use is at the least a warning sign, if not a directly causal factor. For young adult patients, documenting the pattern of early use is an important part of the clinical evaluation. This evaluation should include documenting age of onset of drug use and progression in terms of frequency or use and drugs used.

Early Risk Factors for Substance Abuse and the Developmental Perspective

Developmental History. Substance use disorders can be viewed as developmental disorders with their roots in childhood, and with a characteristic progression through adolescence and young adulthood into later adulthood. Externalizing psychopathology, particularly conduct disorder, is an important risk factor for subsequent development of substance problems, and as noted above has been linked to the genetic diathesis to substance dependence. Internalizing psychopathology, particularly neuropsychological dysfunction and anxiety in childhood, also has been implicated (Kellam, Brown, Rubin, & Ensminger, 1983; Moss, Majumder, & Vanyukov, 1994). The developmental trajectory often begins with childhood school problems and may progress to school failure, association with deviant peer groups, and development of substance problems in adolescence. In evaluating a young adult, it is important to look for evidence of such a trajectory, bearing in mind that for higher functioning patients (e.g., those in college or early in careers) the trajectory may be less pronounced, consisting of failure to perform at a level consistent with the patient's high aptitudes, rather than outright failure. This may reveal problems that still need therapeutic attention, for example, a college student who struggles academically because of ongoing attentional, learning, mood, or antisocial problems.

Family History. A careful family history is an important component in the clinical evaluation of a patient with possible substance use problems. A positive family history of alcohol, nicotine, or drug problems may reflect inherited risk factors to addiction. Patients should be educated about this risk and encouraged to minimize it by not exposing themselves to addictive substances.

Diagnosis of Drug Use Disorders

DSM-IV Drug Abuse

In DSM-IV drug abuse is defined as "a pattern of maladaptive use leading to clinically significant impairment or distress" and then goes on to list four specific domains: *(1)* impairment of performance at work, home, or school; *(2)* hazardous drug use, that is, use in situations that results in physical danger such as driving while intoxicated; *(3)* legal problems related to drugs; and *(4)* interpersonal problems related to drug use, such as arguments or fights (American Psychiatric Association, 1994). During the clinical evaluation, it is important to query each of these areas of psychosocial functioning and look for potential impairment. The most important aspect of this syndrome is the danger it poses, either for physical danger or school, career, or relationship failure. Virtually any drug can produce significant impairment in each of the four domains listed in the DSM-IV criteria, and it is useful to review the listings of symptoms of intoxication on each of these drugs provided in DSM-IV. Particular features of intoxication syndromes of the various drugs that may be most likely to lead to impairment and physical danger are listed in Table 19-1.

Abuse Is Not Subsyndromal Dependence. Abuse is often thought of as a precursor to dependence or a subthreshold syndrome. However, the weight of the evidence suggests abuse and dependence are independent phenomena. Studies of community-based samples suggest that DSM-IV drug abuse is relatively common among adolescents and young adults, most commonly alcohol abuse, although this by itself does not convey an increased risk of progression to the syndrome of dependence (Hasin & Paykin, 1999). The most important clinical implication of this is that it is important to evaluate for both abuse and dependence, as either one or both may develop, and they each represent separate dimensions of substance-related problems. Abuse can be a more clinically obvious diagnosis due to the objective nature of the impairments (poor school or work performance, legal problems, relationship breakups, etc.). Detection of abuse both uncovers an important problem in itself and should serve as a warning flag to look for dependence and for other psychopathology.

DSM-IV Drug Dependence

Drug dependence is defined as a pattern of drug use, generally a pattern of regular use, leading to impairment and meeting at least three among seven specific criteria (see Table 19-2). The DSM-IV criteria are an outgrowth of the Edwards criteria

Table 19-1. Features of Drug Intoxication or Withdrawal Syndromes Likely to Contribute to Impairment of the Syndrome of Drug Abuse

Drug	Features of Intoxication Likely to Produce Impairment or Danger
Cannabis	Impaired coordination (accidents); impaired judgment; during withdrawal, irritability (fights and arguments)
Cocaine/stimulants	Hyperactivity; irritability (fights, arguments); excessive talkativeness; impaired judgment; paranoia and transient psychosis; depression and suicidal ideation during the "crash"; seizures; cardiovascular events
Opioids	Apathy; respiratory depression and sudden death from respiratory arrest; during withdrawal severe flu-like symptoms and obtundation
Hallucinogens	Paranoia; impaired judgment; impaired coordination
PCP	Agitation; aggressiveness; impaired judgment; impaired coordination; seizures; coma
Sedative hynpnotics	Impaired coordination; loss of inhibitions; aggressiveness; stupor or coma; respiratory depression and risk of fatal overdose when combined with other drugs/alcohol; during withdrawal, seizures, delirium
MDMA (Ecstacy)	Effects may resemble hallucinogens or stimulants; hyperthermia
GHB	Blackouts; date rape; stupor and coma

(Edwards & Gross, 1976) and include three domains of dependence symptoms: tolerance/withdrawal, loss of control, and impairment. (The criteria are organized according to these domains in Table 19-2.) DSM-IV does not officially recognize these domains as part of the criteria set, but they are included as a useful organizing principle. Semi-structured interviews such as the SCID (Spitzer, Williams, Gibbon, & First, 1992) or PRISM (Hasin et al., 2006) provide suggested leading and follow-up questions for judging each of the criteria, and practice with these instruments is to be encouraged as a way of developing diagnostic skill.

Opioid Dependence. Opioid dependence is virtually always associated with tolerance and

Table 19-2. DSM-IV Criteria for Substance Dependence

Symptom Domain	DSM-IV Criteria
	A maladaptive pattern of substance use, leading to clinically significant impairment or distress, as manifested by three (or more) of the following, occurring at any time in the same 12-month period
Physiological-tolerance/withdrawal	1. Tolerance, as defined by either of the following: a. need for markedly increased amounts of the substance to achieve intoxication or desired effect b. markedly diminished effect with continued use of the same amount of the substance
	2. Withdrawal, as manifested by either of the following: a. the characteristic withdrawal syndrome for the substance (refer to specific DSM-IV criteria for withdrawal for each substance) b. the same (or a closely related) substance is taken to relieve or avoid withdrawal symptoms
Loss of control	3. The substance is often taken in larger amounts or over a longer period than was intended 4. There is a persistent desire or unsuccessful efforts to cut down or control substance use 5. A great deal of time is spent in activities necessary to obtain the substance (e.g., visiting multiple doctors or driving long distances), use the substance (e.g., chain-smoking), or recover from its effects

Table 19-2. (Continued)

Symptom Domain	DSM-IV Criteria
Impairment	6. Important social, occupational, or recreational activities are given up or reduced because of substance use
	7. The substance use is continued despite knowledge of having a persistent or recurrent physical or psychological problem that is likely to have been caused or exacerbated by the substance (e.g., current cocaine use despite recognition of cocaine-induced depression, or continued drinking despite recognition that an ulcer was made worse by alcohol consumption

Note: The symptom domains (physiological, loss of control, impairment) are not part of the official criteria, but they stem from the original Edwards criteria and are useful as organizing principles. Reprinted with permission from the Diagnostic and Statistical Manual of Mental Disorders, Text Revision, Fourth Edition, (Copyright © 2000). American Psychiatric Association.

withdrawal, and the typical pattern of use consists of daily use, usually multiple times per day. Among adolescents, opioid use is often intermittent and part of a larger pattern of experimentation with multiple drugs, out of which those vulnerable to opioid dependence will emerge with the regular daily pattern of use. The typical history of an opioid-dependent patient consists of early onset of use of nicotine, alcohol, and other drugs, followed by experimentation with opioids and more or less rapid establishment of a daily pattern of use, usually by the mid or late teenage years. In addition to heroin, prescription opioids have emerged during the past decade as a substantial public health problem (Cicero, Inciardi, & Munoz, 2005). Opioid withdrawal is highly unpleasant, resembling a bad flu with nausea, diarrhea, muscle aches, fever and chills, and dysphoria (American Psychiatric Association, 1994) and will typically begin within 24 to 48 hours, depending upon whether the patient has been taking a short-acting opioid such as heroin or prescription painkillers such as oxycodone, or a longer acting agent such as methadone. Patients will usually describe avoidance or termination of withdrawal symptoms as a main drive to continued opioid use.

Cannabis Dependence. Cannabis dependence also is typically characterized by a daily pattern of use often multiple times per day, with both tolerance and withdrawal. Cannabis-dependent patients typically emerge from high school or college with a daily pattern of use, which is often described by the patient as pleasant or beneficial. Parents or significant others are more likely to complain about the patient's use, citing academic or work performance below expectations, or lack of attention to or interest in relationships or other previously valued activities. This impairment may become more problematic as patients pass from college into early career where the demands for performance are greater. Also, college is a setting where casual use of cannabis may be common, so that the daily user blends in. After college, the contrast between the daily user and his/her friends and peers may become more stark. Cannabis withdrawal is not recognized in DSM-IV, since up until the past decade it was largely believed not to exist. However, recent research has clearly delineated a withdrawal syndrome characterized among other symptoms by anxiety, disturbed sleep, reduced appetite, and often prominent irritability (Budney, Hughes, Moore, & Vandrey, 2004; Haney et al., 2004), and cannabis withdrawal will be included in DSM-V. Detection of withdrawal may be more difficult because the patient has rarely attempted to quit or run out of supplies of the drug, and patients tend to describe the pleasantness of the high as a reason to continue using. However, careful questioning will often reveal the occurrence of withdrawal when supplies have run out in the past. Patients, steeped in the belief that cannabis is a "safe" drug, are often unaware that they have been experiencing withdrawal, and describing the withdrawal symptoms to the patient is an important element of patient education.

Sedative/Hypnotic Dependence. Dependence on benzodiazepines or other sedative hypnotics is rarely observed in isolation. Rather, sedative use is more likely to be part of a larger pattern of drug use. Sedatives are often taken in conjunction with cocaine or stimulants to help "come down," or in conjunction with alcohol or opioids to combat the anxiety and insomnia of withdrawal. Sedative dependence may also be observed in patients with mood or anxiety disorders who derive relief of dysphoria or insomnia through sedative use, but then begin to experience tolerance and to escalate the daily dosage. Thus, a pattern of regular sedative use should prompt careful inquiry for the presence of mood or anxiety disorders. Most patients with mood or anxiety disorders who are prescribed sedatives use them safely, at recommended doses without tolerance or dose escalation. However, clinicians must be vigilant for the signs of dependence, including gradual escalation of the dose and drug-seeking behavior. A past history of alcohol or other drug dependence, or a positive family history, should prompt caution in regard to prescribing sedatives. Many other pharmacotherapies for anxiety or insomnia lack abuse potential, including buspirone or antidepressant medications for anxiety disorders and sedating antidepressants or low-dose atypical neuroleptics for sleep, and these should be considered as alternatives for vulnerable patients. Sedative withdrawal can usually be avoided by carrying out a gradual taper, although emergence of anxiety or insomnia may limit a patient's ability to effect the taper. Sedative withdrawal, following abrupt discontinuation of sedatives, resembles alcohol withdrawal, including such serious manifestations as convulsions and delirium. Therefore, sedatives should never be abruptly discontinued.

Cocaine/Stimulant Dependence. For cocaine and stimulant dependence, the pattern of use is often intermittent, with episodes of heavy use (binges), followed by days of abstinence, so that a patient may only use a few times in a week or even a month. The pattern often consists of a binge use lasting 1 or a few days, followed by a crash consisting of fatigue, hypersomnolence, and dysphoria lasting for several days during which cocaine is not used, followed by a variable period of abstinence and then another binge (Gawin & Kleber, 1986). With this pattern, tolerance and withdrawal are less likely to be observed, but the dependence syndrome will still be met, based on loss of control and impairment criteria. Cocaine and stimulant dependence may also present with a more regular, daily pattern of use with tolerance and withdrawal figuring more prominently. Alternatively, cocaine dependence may present.

Methamphatamine. Methamphetamine is an amphetamine that is present in the formulary in oral form (brand name Desoxyn) and is produced illicitly in laboratories for smoked or injected use. The prevalence of methamphetamine dependence varies markedly by geographic region, being more common on the West Coast and rural regions of the United States, and less common on the East Coast. It is also associated with the club scene and is prevalent among men who have sex with men.

Prescription Stimulants. Methylphenidate and dextro-amphetamine are stimulant medications that are highly effective and widely prescribed to children and adolescents for treatment of attention-deficit/hyperactivity disorder (ADHD). It is increasingly recognized that ADHD often persists into adulthood, and hence prescription of stimulants to young adults has become more common. Stimulants are also often used as adjunctive treatments for treatment-resistant mood disorders. As is the case with prescribed benzodiazepines, most patients use stimulants as prescribed and do not develop symptoms of abuse or dependence. Even when used to treat ADHD among cocaine-dependent patients, abuse of the medication was rarely observed (Levin et al., 2006; Levin, Evans, Brooks, & Garawi, 2007). However, clinicians need to remain vigilant for the development of a pattern of abuse or dependence, characterized by escalation of the dose, use to get a high, and drug seeking. Long-acting forms of prescribed stimulants (e.g. Ritalin-SR, Concerta, or Adderal XR) are preferable, as the slower absorption and elimination produce less euphoria.

College students and young adults may seek out stimulants to help them study or complete papers or other projects, usually borrowing or purchasing doses from friends who have prescriptions for ADHD. Stimulants enhance concentration and performance and reduce fatigue and the need for sleep. However, in addition to being illegal, excessive use of stimulants in this way carries the risks of stimulant intoxication or the development of dependence. Such patients should be counseled around time management (getting started on projects and studying earlier) such that last-minute cramming is not necessary. This pattern of use may also signal the presence of ADHD in young adults, which had previously gone unrecognized, and should thus prompt a careful review of the history for signs and symptoms of ADHD.

Club Drugs. While a variety of drugs, including cocaine, methamphetamine, and alcohol, are part of the bar and club scenes frequented by young adults, several others deserve specific mention: MDMA (a.k.a. Ecstasy), hallucinogens such as lysergic acid diethylamide (LSD), and GHB (Teter & Guthrie, 2001). Ecstasy is a stimulant-like drug with prominent serotonergic effects and is described as producing a prolonged state of elevated mood with a prominent sense of affiliation and connectedness to others; this may be followed by a crash resembling depression and lasting several days. Possible risks include damage to serotonergic neurons (Cowan, 2007) and hyperthermia and serotonin syndrome (Silins, Copeland, & Dillon, 2007). LSD and other hallucinogens (e.g., psilocybin mushrooms) can produce pleasant hallucinogenic experiences, but severe dysphoric reactions may also occur. GHB, also sometimes known as the "date rape drug," is a sedative-like drug that may produce amnesia, confusion, coma, respiratory depression, and abnormal involuntary movements. Among the many concerns with this class of drugs is that users do not really know whether what they are taking is what it is said to be, or its level or purity or adulterants.

Anabolic Steroids. Clinicians working with young adult patients need to remain alert to the possibility or use or abuse of anabolic steroids. These drugs are most commonly taken by athletes to enhance training or performance. A wide range of physical and psychiatric adverse events may occur, and a dependence syndrome may develop (Talih, Fattal, & Malone, 2007).

Approach to the Patient

Screening Questions and Therapeutic Stance. The essential point in approaching adolescent and young adult patients is to ask about use of drugs and to ask in an open, accepting, and nonjudgmental fashion. Patients may tend to minimize or hide their drug use and often need to be made to feel comfortable before opening up. If the clinician conveys disapproval or disinterest, drug use may not be revealed. Any use of drugs should lead to lines of questioning to establish whether abuse or dependence may be present along with other co-occurring psychopathology. In college, drugs may be widely available and somewhat normative, but as individuals progress into their 20s and early career development, continued drug use is more likely to be a sign of problems.

Clinical Course. After establishing the presence of a current drug abuse or dependence syndrome, the clinical history should include exploration of the history of drug and alcohol use, beginning with the age at first use and querying for the onset of first use and first regular use of each substance. Adolescent and young adult patients with a substance use disorder will often have used a number of substances and it is important to know which were used regularly and which progressed to an abuse or dependence syndrome in the past. If there is past dependence on a drug that is currently in remission, there is the risk that dependence will recur. Appropriate monitoring and patient education are warranted.

Family History. It is important to inquire about history among first-degree relatives with alcoholism, cigarette smoking, or other drug dependence. A positive family history is suggestive of greater genetic loading for addiction. It can also be used as a point to educate the patient, namely that he/she may carry this vulnerability and should incorporate this knowledge into decisions about abstaining from substance use.

Developmental History. It is useful to ask the patient, "What was elementary school like?" and then listen for the following: *(1)* problems with behavior such as inattention or disruptiveness that may be consistent with ADHD, conduct disorder, or oppositional defiant disorder; *(2)* learning problems, such as dyslexia, trouble learning to write, trouble learning math, or needing extra time to finish tasks; *(3)* anxiety, including excessive shyness, separation anxiety, or school phobia; and (4) stress and trauma, including physical or sexual abuse. Each of these, as noted previously, represents a potential risk factor for development of drug dependence, and each may continue to manifest into adolescence and early adulthood. It is important to identify these problems and incorporate interventions for each into the treatment plan.

Diagnosis of Co-occurring Psychiatric Disorders

Virtually all types of psychopathology common in young adults, including mood disorders (both unipolar and bipolar), all of the anxiety disorders, eating disorders, and schizophrenia, occur at elevated rates among patients with substance use disorders (Hasin, Nunes, & Meydan, 2004; Regier et al., 1990). Thus, detection of a substance use problem should prompt a thorough psychiatric history to uncover and initiate treatment for whatever other disorders may be operating, and vice versa.

DSM-IV Substance-Induced versus Independent Disorders. For some disorders, especially depression, bipolar II disorder, panic attacks, and generalized anxiety disorder, the symptoms of the disorder can be difficult to separate from the effects of drug intoxication, withdrawal, or chronic exposure to drugs. DSM-IV (American Psychiatric Association, 1994) recommends that a co-occurring psychiatric disorder can be considered independent of substance use disorders if the psychiatric disorder had its onset prior to the onset of substance use problems, or if it persists after a month or more of abstinence from the substance. Co-occurring syndromes for which this independence from substances cannot be established, but which nonetheless seem to exceed the usual intoxication and withdrawal effects of the substances the patient is concurrently taking, are classified in DSM-IV as substance-induced disorders. This does not necessarily mean the substance is causing the psychiatric disorder, and in fact longitudinal studies have shown that substance-induced major depression is often found to persist after abstinence during a follow-up period, converting to an independent disorder (Nunes, Liu, Samet, Matseoane, & Hasin, 2006).

Distinguishing independent psychiatric disorders from substance-induced disorders or the usual intoxicating or withdrawal effects of substances requires a careful longitudinal clinical history and consideration of whether each specific symptom of the psychiatric disorder (e.g., insomnia in the cases of major depression, or generalized anxiety disorder) might represent a usual effect of the substances concurrently being taken. The PRISM interview (Hasin et al., 2006) was designed to guide clinician-interviewers in taking such a history and making these distinctions, and readers are encouraged to practice interviewing with the PRISM as a way to sharpen their clinical diagnostic skills.

Making the distinction between independent and substance-induced disorder and the usual effects of substances is important, since evidence from a recent meta-analysis suggests co-occurring depressive disorders that persist after a period of abstinence are most likely to respond well to antidepressant medications (Nunes & Levin, 2004). In contrast, for a substance-induced disorder, the first therapeutic efforts should be to try to establish abstinence from drugs or alcohol and then to observe whether the psychiatric syndrome persists and calls for specific intervention.

Toward DSM-V

The framers of DSM-V have been asked to consider psychopathological classification based more upon pathophysiology and to consider alternative models such as dimensional classifications. The syndromes of abuse and dependence have a fairly strong basis in pathophysiology already and thus are likely to remain basically similar in DSM-V. However, serious consideration is being given to examining dependence as a dimensional phenomenon, for example, using quantity of use and/or degree of impairment as indicators. The Substance Dependence Severity Scale (Miele et al., 2000) quantifies each dependence criterion and then sums them to arrive at an overall severity score rather than simply generating a categorical classification. The exploration of the clinical utility of dimensional models of drug addiction is an important area for future research. The distinction of independent and substance-induced disorders is likely to be retained in DSM-V, but criteria for substance-induced disorders may be made more specific in an effort to delineate co-occurring psychiatric syndromes that are more likely to persist in abstinence or to require specific clinical intervention (Nunes & Rounsaville, 2006). Again, more research will be needed to help arrive at such refined criteria sets for substance-induced disorders.

Behavioral Treatment Modalities for Drug Dependence

Behavioral treatments form the foundation of treatment plans for drug dependence. In what follows, I first present a brief overview of each of the main types of behavioral treatment. Some of these modalities, such as family therapy or therapeutic communities, were developed from the outset with an emphasis on adolescents and young adults. Most of the others, including motivational interviewing, cognitive-behavioral approaches, contingency management, or 12-step methods, were developed mainly with adults, although in some cases studies with adolescents have also been performed. These treatments tend to apply across classes of drug, but instances where modalities have been applied to specific drugs will be noted. Table 19-3 provides an overview of the mechanisms of action and

Table 19-3. Overview of Behavioral Treatment Modalities for Drug Dependence

Modality	Hypothesized Mechanisms	Evidence for Effectiveness
Motivational interviewing (MI), motivational enhancement therapy (MET)	Increase motivation by eliciting discrepancy or dissonance between drug use consequences and patient's values, supporting self-efficacy to change, and avoiding confrontation	Extensive evidence for effectiveness from controlled trials, most regarding cigarettes or alcohol in adults. Effects sizes are modest. Nonauthoritarian stance well suited to adolescents or young adults, and some evidence from these populations as well
Cognitive-behavioral therapies (versions include Relapse Prevention, the Community Reinforcement Approach, and the Matrix Model)	Teaches skills for coping with cravings or desires to use drugs, avoiding situations where drug use is likely, coping with lapse or relapse if it does occur, and skills for fostering alternative sources of reinforcement (e.g., relationships, recreation)	Extensive evidence for effectiveness from controlled trials, mainly in adults, especially with cocaine or stimulant dependence. Effects are modest and tend to emerge after completion of treatment ("sleeper effect")
Contingency management with voucher incentives	Provides concrete alternative rewards in the form of monetary incentives contingent upon the target behavior, usually abstinence, or sometimes treatment plan adherence	Most extensively developed and tested for cocaine dependence in adults. Effect sizes can be moderate to large. Has been applied to adolescents with opioid or cannabis dependence
12-step approaches, manual-guided 12-step facilitation	Abstinence focus, spiritual focus, also imparts coping skills with some commonality with cognitive-behavioral methods	Alcoholics Anonymous and Narcotics Anonymous are time-honored rganizations. No direct evidence, but manual-guided 12-step facilitation guides clinicians in helping patients to attend groups like Alcoholics Anonymous (AA) or Narcotics Anoymous (NA), and enjoys evidence of efficacy, mainly in adults
Drug counseling (individual and group versions)	Emphasis on abstinence, coping skills, and attendance of 12-step meetings	A manual-guided distillation of the methods employed by experienced drug counselors; found effective for cocaine dependence in adults

(continued)

Table 19-3. (Continued)

Modality	Hypothesized Mechanisms	Evidence for Effectiveness
Residential treatment	Respite from drug-associated home environment, induce and protect initial abstinence, teach coping skills	Evidence for effectiveness derives from observational studies such as DATOS rather than controlled trials; clinically invaluable for patients with chaotic lifestyles and who cannot initiate abstinence as outpatients; relapse risk is high after discharge
Therapeutic community (TC)	Long-term residential approach that seeks to effect character and behavior change by engaging patients in a prosocial residential community; emphasis on confrontation	Evidence for effectiveness derives from observational studies, not controlled trials. Again, respite from chaotic or nonexistent home environment often seems clinically invaluable. Tends to engage younger populations.
Family therapy	Diagnose and correct dysfunctional family systems that evolve around drug using identified patient; with adolescents, restore parental authority and limit setting	Strongest evidence as a treatment for adolescents and young adults with support from multiple controlled trials

evidence for effectiveness of each of these modalities, and a brief discussion of each modality follows.

Motivational Interviewing. Motivational interviewing (MI) is a nonconfrontational persuasion technique that has been carefully characterized and extensively tested (Miller & Rollnick, 2002). It can be viewed as an essential clinical skill for approaching drug-dependent patients, from the outset of the evaluation through treatment planning and delivery, because it provides a way of talking to patients and engaging them. It may be particularly well suited to adolescents and young adults who are often struggling with establishing autonomy from parental authority and who may not respond well to the typical prescriptive or authoritative stance of clinicians (i.e., by being told what to do). Instead MI guides a clinician to be collaborative and to elicit and value the patient's point of view while helping the patient to find his or her own reasons for changing drug-using behavior. To give a concrete example, MI teaches clinicians a way to proceed when the patient asserts, "No doc, drug use is just social, no problems," other than just saying, "I think you're wrong." Thus, all clinicians working with adolescent and adult patients are strongly encouraged to obtain training in this technique.

Evidence suggests gaining skill in MI requires more than just attending a workshop (Miller & Mount, 2001), and clinicians are encouraged to follow-up a workshop with some form of supervised practice.

Cognitive-Behavioral Techniques. Versions of cognitive-behavioral therapies include relapse prevention (RP) (Carroll et al., 1994), the community reinforcement approach (CRA) (Miller, Meyers, & Hiller-Sturmhofel, 1999), and the matrix model (Rawson et al., 1995). Solid evidence from clinical trials supports the efficacy of these approaches. Interestingly, beneficial effects tend to emerge after treatment has ended, dubbed the "sleeper effect," suggesting that new skills have indeed been learned and continue to be practiced. These techniques assume a motivated patient, and combination with MI is often warranted. These techniques can also be cognitively demanding, requiring patients to master relatively complex concepts and skills and engage in considerable planning and self-monitoring. Thus, not surprisingly, subtle neurocognitive impairment in areas of attention and memory are associated with high dropout rates with this technique among adults (Aharonovich et al., 2006). As discussed in a previous section, neurocognitive impairment is common in drug-dependent patients, and cognitive-behavioral techniques may need to be modified for such patients, for example, with slower pace and more repetition in order to maintain engagement.

Contingency Management/Voucher Incentives. The first dramatic successes for voucher incentive treatments were demonstrated with cocaine-dependent patients in conjunction with the community reinforcement approach (Higgins et al., 1993). This technique depends upon the ability to measure the target behavior, mainly abstinence, objectively via urine toxicology, and has subsequently been extended to treatment of opioid dependence (Carroll et al., 2001; Preston et al., 1999) and to cannabis dependence among adolescents (Budney, Moore, Rocha, & Higgins, 2006). The effect size can be large, but it depends upon the value of the vouchers, which creates pragmatic concerns. Recently, a lower cost voucher incentive regimen based on a type of partial reinforcement schedule (Petry et al., 2005; Pierce et al., 2006) has been developed and found effective among adults.

12-Step Approaches. Alcoholics Anonymous, and subsequently Narcotics Anonymous and other similar self-help groups, grew out of the collective wisdom of alcohol- or drug-dependent patients gathering to help each other. The result is actually a rather structured program in which patients are encouraged to engage a sponsor (a group member with established sobriety) and work through the 12 therapeutic steps. In fact, much of the pragmatic advice conveyed in 12-step approaches resembles aspects of cognitive therapy approaches. One difference is that 12-step approaches have a strong emphasis on abstinence. These techniques have not been directly studied in clinical trials, but 12-step facilitation, a manual-guided approach which guides clinicians in steering patients toward 12-step groups, has evidence for effectiveness among adults (Project MATCH Research Group, 1998). Patients need to find a group or groups where they feel comfortable, as social anxiety may interfere with patients' participation. Especially when working with adolescents or young adults, clinicians should be aware of the risk that groups will backfire and engender drug use in a sort of contagion among group members (Dishion, Poulin, & Burraston, 2001).

Drug Counseling. Manual-guided drug counseling was developed for a clinical trial of behavioral therapies for adult cocaine abusers and was found, perhaps unexpectedly, to produce outcomes superior to professionally administered psychotherapies (Crits-Christoph et al., 1997). The emphasis is on abstinence, pragmatic strategies to maintain abstinence, and 12-step group attendance.

Residential Treatment and Therapeutic Communities. Like 12-step modalities, residential and therapeutic communities (TC) approaches evolved from grassroots efforts to help addicted patients and have not generally been studied in controlled trials, although their effectiveness is supported by observational studies (Hubbard, Craddock, & Anderson, 2003). In particular, the drug abuse treatment outcome study (DATOS) suggested residential treatment may be particularly effective for more severely addicted patients. On face value, the respite from a chaotic home and establishment of a more structured environment by virtue of seclusion may be extremely valuable. Many severely drug-dependent patients are homeless, and the long-term residence provides literally a stable living place, which can be most therapeutic. Nonetheless, dropout from these modalities is high and even for those who complete the residential program, relapse rates are high after return to outpatient status. Thus, the outpatient treatment plan that follows the residential phase is critically important.

Family Therapy. Family therapy is time consuming and can be difficult to perform skillfully; hence, it is often not the first modality chosen. However, family therapy is, ironically, the approach that has perhaps the most convincing evidence for effectiveness among adolescents (Liddle, Rowe, Dakof, Ungaro, & Henderson, 2004; Szapocznik & Williams, 2000). Among adolescents and young adults, drug abuse is often accompanied by distortion of the family system, where the young patient continues to depend on the parents for housing and financial support but the parents are unable to set limits and expectations. Family therapy in this circumstance coaches the parents to reprise authority and limit-setting while helping the young patient to move toward healthy autonomy without drug use. The family has leverage because of the young patient's material dependency, and effective exercise of that leverage can produce gratifying results.

Network Therapy. Network therapy is a treatment designed for office- or clinic-based use, and this approach is founded on the principle that a treatment for drug dependence can be assisted by inclusion of significant others (friends, family members, colleagues) who form a network around the patient to support the treatment plan (Galanter, 1993). This technique borrows from cognitive-behavioral approaches, contingency management, and family therapy approaches. Significant others may be engaged in delivering reinforcers contingent upon abstinence, helping the patient engage in activities that are alternatives to drug use, or monitoring the ingestion of medication such as buprenorphine or naltrexone.

Pharmacological Treatments

General pharmacological treatment strategies for drug dependence can be classified into agonist substitution, antagonist maintenance, high-affinity partial agonists, and indirect modulatory strategies, including treatment of co-occurring psychiatric disorders (see Table 19-4). Each mechanism is now briefly discussed in the context of specific drug problems.

Medication Treatment of Opioid Dependence

Agonist Substitution: Methadone. Methadone for opioid dependence (Dole & Nyswander, 1965) is the prototypical agonist substitution agent. It is taken orally, slowly absorbed, slowly metabolized, and prone to produce tolerance. With addictive drugs such as heroin, the euphoria

Table 19-4. Pharmacological Treatment Strategies for Drug Dependence

Pharmacological Strategy	Mechanism	Examples
Agonist substitution	—Substitutes for the addictive drug at its receptors but is slowly absorbed, and slowly metabolized, minimizing the euphoria and other agonist effects as well as the withdrawal associated; in contrast, typical addictive drug is rapidly absorbed and eliminated. —Sufficient receptor affinity to compete with the addictive drug to produce direct blockade and/or produce tolerance blockade; thus, effects of the addictive drug are blocked, and withdrawal is prevented. Overdose risk reduced. —Built-in reinforcement for adherence, since missed doses will result in development of withdrawal. —May be used to treat withdrawal, or as a long-term maintenance treatment to induce abstinence then prevent relapse.	—Nicotine replacement —Methadone for opioid dependence —Phenobarbitol or long-acting benzodiazepines (chlordiazepoxide or clonazepam are most often used) for alcohol or sedative withdrawal —Oral THC for cannabis dependence (investigational)
Antagonist maintenance	—Pharmacological antagonist with high receptor affinity blocks effects of the addictive drug. —Patient must first be detoxified; otherwise an antagonist will precipitate severe withdrawal.	—Mecamlyamine for nicotine dependence —Naltrexone for opioid dependence

Table 19-4. (Continued)

Pharmacological Strategy	Mechanism	Examples
High-affinity partial agonist	—Like an agonist, slowly absorbed and slowly eliminated. —High affinity, but only partially activates the receptor, producing blockade of effects of the addictive drug. —Maybe less abuse potential than full agonist, or easier to taper.	—Varenicline for nicotine dependence —Buprenorphine for opioid dependence
Indirect modulatory strategies	—Indirect agonist or antagonist. —Reduce cue or stress induced reinstatement of craving or drug seeking behavior by targeting modulatory inputs to the brain reward systems (e.g.glutamatergic, GABAergic, or serotonergic inputs). —Treat co-occurring psychiatric disorders (e.g. depression, bipolar disorder, anxiety disorders, ADHD)	—Clonidine to attenuate opioid withdrawal. —Various investigational approaches to cocaine dependence (e.g. oral amphetamine, topiramate, disulfiram) —Antidepressant medications, lithium or valproate for bipolar disorder, buspirone for generalized anxiety

and rewarding properties are partly related to the rate of rise in blood levels after administration, and the intravenous, smoked, or intranasal routes all produce spikes in blood level. In contrast, the slow absorption of methadone produces a relatively steady blood level without rapid rises. It competes with heroin or other opioids for receptors and also induces tolerance, such that the effects of other opioids are blocked, which leads to extinction of drug-seeking behavior and may protect against fatal overdose. The slow metabolism also eliminates rapid development of withdrawal, although patients will gradually go into withdrawal within 24 hours of missing the next day's dose. Methadone is a powerful treatment with a large effect size, and it represented a major breakthrough when it was first introduced in the 1960s and 1970s (Ball, Lange, & Myers, 1988). At least half of chronic opioid-dependent patients will have an excellent response with cessation of drug use and improvement in social functioning (e.g., return to work or home responsibilities). The dose is titrated gradually upward as tolerance develops and the usual effective dose is in the 60 mg to 100 mg per day range. Methadone is tightly regulated and can only be prescribed for the indication of methadone dependence out of specially licensed methadone clinics, and patients must attend frequently, generating a level of inconvenience that leads to a mixed reputation of this modality among addicts. Methadone can also be used in a gradual taper to effect detoxification from opioids, although the rates of relapse after completion of detoxification are very high, suggesting maintenance strategy is often warranted.

There is limited experience with methadone for treatment of opioid-dependent adolescence. Regulations restrict methadone use to opioid-dependent patients who have failed prior treatments or have some level of chronicity of illness. Adolescents and young adults are often at the early stages of experimentation with heroin or prescription opioids and thus do not qualify with specific exceptions, such as teenage pregnancies while opioid dependent. Limited clinical experience with methadone at specialized clinics for treatment of adolescents and young adults with opioid dependence suggests similar efficacy as for adults (Kellogg et al., 2006).

Antagonist Maintenance: Naltrexone. Naltrexone is the prototypical pharmacological antagonist. It binds opioid receptors with very high affinity, but it does not activate them. In fact, the parent compound, naltrexone, may be an inverse agonist, while the metabolite 6-beta-naltrexone is a more pure antagonist. It is effective in preventing relapse when taken regularly, but its use has been limited by poor adherence. Its use is also limited by the fact that a patient needs to be detoxified prior to initiating naltrexone in order to avoid precipitated withdrawal. Combination of naltrexone with behavioral treatments can improve adherence and outcome for oral naltrexone. Due to its long duration of action, naltrexone can be dosed as 50 mg daily, or alternatively with a three times per week schedule (e.g. 100 mg on Monday, 100 mg on Wednesday, and 150 mg on Friday); the latter schedule may lend itself better to ingestion supervised by clinic personnel or significant others. New long-acting injectable formulations of naltrexone circumvent the need for daily pill adherence and show considerable promise for treatment of opioid dependence (Comer et al., 2006). Vivitrol is a long-acting naltrexone injection now marketed for treatment of alcohol dependence, and this formulation produces naltrexone blood levels that should be sufficient to block opioid effects for a month (Dunbar, Turncliff, & Donq, 2006). It is not yet FDA approved for treatment of opioid dependence but might be considered for off-label use. Naltrexone may be a useful treatment option for preventing relapse and progression of opioid dependence among adolescents and young adults who are in the early stages of dependence. However, clinical research with naltrexone in adolescents is limited, although it has been used as a follow-up treatment after detoxification with buprenorphine (Marsch et al., 2005). Guidelines for its management of opioid-dependent patients, based on experience with adults, have been put forth (Sullivan, Comer, & Nunes, 2006).

High-Affinity Partial Agonist: Buprenorphine. Buprenorphine has a relatively short half-life in serum, but its affinity for opioid receptors is so high that its receptor binding is practically irreversible, leading to a very long duration of action. The combination of partial agonism (partial activation of receptors), high affinity, and long duration of effects results in a treatment for opioid dependence that produces little euphoria with less tolerance or abuse potential than a full agonist, blocks the effects of other opioids such as heroin or prescription agents, and generates fewer withdrawal symptoms if discontinued. Thus, it is an excellent choice for either detoxification or long-term maintenance treatment (Center for Substance Abuse Treatment, 2004; Fudala et al., 2003; McCance-Katz, 2004). A particularly tricky aspect of buprenorphine involves the induction of dosing. Other opioids should be largely off the receptors prior to initiation of buprenorphine; otherwise burprenorphine will displace agonist and precipitate withdrawal that may be atypical in its presentation. Clinically this circumstance can generally be ensured by waiting for the patient to clearly enter opioid withdrawal prior to giving the first dose, in which case buprenorphine's agonist properties usually lead to gratifying relief of withdrawal.

Buprenorphine is less tightly regulated than methadone and can be prescribed by any physician who has taken a brief course in its use. One clinical trial has found it to be safe and effective in adolescents for detoxification from opioids (Marsch et al., 2005), and a multisite trial in the NIDA Clinical Trials Network is completed with results due soon (G. Woody, personal communication). Relapse rates after buprenorphine cessation suggest longer-term maintenance may be needed. Thus, buprenorphine is probably the treatment of choice for adolescents and young adults with opioid dependence. Detoxification, if followed by sustained abstinence, can be followed with naltrexone to prevent relapse. Detoxification followed by relapse should prompt reinstitution of buprenorphine and a longer-term maintenance strategy.

Clonidine for Opioid Detoxification. The adrenergic alpha-2 agonist clonidine, indicated for treatment of hypertension, reduces norepinephrine release from presynaptic terminals by stimulating auto-receptors and it has been shown to reduce the severity of opioid withdrawal, which includes prominent noradrenergic activation. Clonidine is usually combined with other agents, including a benzodiazepine such as clonazepam for anxiety, an anti-emetic such as compazine or odansetron to reduce GI symptoms, and a nonsteroidal anti-inflammatory drug (NSAID) like ibuprofen to reduce muscle aches associated with withdrawal. The strategy may be moderately effective for some patients, but it has not compared favorably with the

Medication Treatment of Cannabis Dependence

Like for opioids, tetrahydrocannibinol (THC), the ingredient in cannabis thought to mediate its addictive potential, produces its euphorigenic and reinforcing effects by binding cannabinoid receptors in the brain. Thus, although as yet no medications have been approved for treatment of cannabis dependence, this drug problem should also lend itself to agonist and antagonist strategies. Oral THC (Marinol, Dronabinol) is currently approved and marketed for treatment of anorexia and wasting associated with HIV or cancer. Case reports suggest oral THC may be effective for detoxification of patients from marijuana smoking (Levin & Kleber, 2008) and placebo-controlled clinical trials are underway. As these results are awaited, off-label use may be entertained for treatment-resistant patients. Sativex is a combination of THC and cannabadiol, another component of cannabis, marketed in Canada for pain (Perez & Ribera, 2008). It represents another interesting candidate as an agonist treatment for cannabis dependence, and further research on this agent is needed.

The THC receptor antagonist rimonabant has been in clinical trials in Europe and the United States for treatment of obesity and cigarette smoking. However, serious psychiatric adverse events in U. S. trials have been reported, stalling its development here. It may be hoped that other antagonists or partial agonists may be developed and become clinically available.

Medication Treatment of Cocaine and Other Stimulant Dependence

Cocaine and amphetamines are indirectly acting sympathomimetics that increase release of dopamine and norepinephrine by blocking transmitter reuptake mechanisms on the synaptic membrane or vesicular membranes. This differs from the transmitter–receptor relationship that characterizes opioid and cannabis dependence, and development of agonists and antagonists has remained elusive. Oral dexedrine has been tested for cocaine dependence in adults and found to have some possible promise (Grabowki et al., 2004). Neuroleptics that block dopamine have been studied as an antagonist strategy, but results suggest poor tolerability and lack of effectiveness (Grabowski et al., 2004). Modafinil, which has stimulant-like properties, has also shown promise among cocaine-dependent adults (Dackis, Kampman, Lynch, Pettinati, and O'Brien, 2005).

Much interest has been focused on glutamatergic and GABAergic (GABA = gamma-aminobutyric acid) circuits, which have modulatory inputs to the dopamine nuclei and fibers in the brain reward system. Preclinical evidence suggests these modulatory inputs may have varied effects from triggering craving (Vorel, Liu, Hayes, Spector, & Gardner, 2001) to reducing dopamine output in response to cocaine-related stimuli (Peng et al., 2008). Thus, anticonvulsants with glutamatergic and/or GABAergic effects, including gabapentin (Bisaga et al., 2006) and topiramate (Kampman et al., 2004), have been tested for cocaine dependence in small placebo-controlled trials with data suggestive of efficacy. Noradrenergic antidepressants such as imipramine (Nunes et al., 1995), desipramine (Gawin et al., 1989), and bupropion (Poling et al., 2006) have shown some promise, although again results have been inconsistent. Of particular interest was a recent trial showing that bupropion was effective when combined with a behavioral treatment, namely contingency management with voucher incentives. Disulfiram is the medication with arguably the best-replicated evidence for efficacy for cocaine dependence (Carroll et al., 2004); interestingly, this effect does not seem to depend on co-occurring alcohol use and instead may operate through inhibition of the enzyme dopamine beta hyroxylase, which reduces conversion of dopamine to norepinephrine. None of these potential treatments for cocaine dependence has, as yet, FDA approval. Thus, cautious off-label use in treatment-resistant young adults may be considered. For treatment of adolescents, a higher threshold should be considered.

Treatment of Co-occurring Psychiatric and Substance Use Disorders

As noted previously, co-occurring psychiatric disorders are associated with substance use disorders and carry a worse prognosis (Hasin, Nunes, & Meydan, 2004). This suggests that identification and treatment of psychopathology has the potential to improve substance use outcome.

Major Depression. Depression is among the most common psychiatric disorders observed in drug-dependent patients. A meta-analysis of placebo-controlled trials of antidepressant medications for depressed substance-dependent patients (Nunes & Levin, 2004) suggests medication is effective, particularly if depression is diagnosed during a period of abstinence, although most of the positive studies concern alcohol dependence. Results of such studies among drug-dependent patients have been less consistent (Nunes, Sullivan, & Levin 2004). Recently a substantial placebo-controlled trial of fluoxetine among depressed adolescents with substance dependence has been reported (Riggs et al., 2007); all participants received CBT; results suggest modest efficacy of medication on one measure of depression, but not for self-reported substance use or measures of behavioral problems. An intensive follow-up of an open trial of fluoxetine in a small sample of substance-dependent adolescents similarly revealed considerable persistence of symptoms (Cornelius et al., 2005), suggesting the need for ongoing follow-up and treatment in these complex patients.

Bipolar Disorder. Bipolar disorder is more rare in the general population, but it is strongly associated with substance use disorders. Two studies in the literature, one with lithium treatment in adolescents (Geller et al., 1998) and one with valproate treatment in adults (Salloum et al., 2005), suggest that mood-stabilizer treatment improves both mood and substance use outcome among substance-abusing patients with bipolar illness.

Anxiety Disorders. One carefully conducted study suggests the efficacy of buspirone among adult alcoholics with generalized anxiety symptoms persisting after a period of inpatient detoxification (Kranzler et al., 1994). Studies of treatment of co-occurring PTSD and substance dependence are beginning to emerge, including one recent study suggesting the efficacy of the antidepressant sertraline among alcohol-dependent patients with prior-onset PTSD and later-onset drinking problems (Brady et al., 2005); patients with early-onset alcoholism actually had better drinking outcome on medication compared to placebo, reminiscent of the findings of several studies in nondepressed alcoholics.

Attention-Deficit/Hyperactivity Disorder. Clinical trials of methylphenidate and bupropion among adult drug-dependent patients have been largely negative (Levin et al., 2006, 2007). However, one placebo-controlled trial of pemoline among substance abusing adolescents was encouraging in showing medication superior to placebo on attention- deficit/hyperactivity disorder (ADHD) outcome, although not on substance use outcome (Riggs, Hall, Mikulich-Gilbertson, Lohman, & Kayser, 2004). This pattern of greater improvement in psychopathology as compared to substance abuse is fairly consistent across comorbidity studies and suggests that treatment of psychopathological symptoms is important in itself, but direct efforts to treat the substance problem should be continued and emphasized, as treatment of the comorbidity may have limited impact on the substance use. A multisite trial of long-acting methylphenidate for adolescents with ADHD and substance dependence is nearing completion in the NIDA Clinical Trials Network, and results of this study should emerge in the next several years (P. Riggs, personal communication).

Explosive Aggression. Anticonvulsants have been observed to have anti-aggressive properties. Donovan and colleagues have delineated a syndrome in children and teenagers of explosive temper that is distinct from mood disorder or conduct disorder and is associated with heavy cannabis use. Interestingly, these patients describe the cannabis as helpful to them in staying calm and curbing their anger. This syndrome appears to respond to valproate with marked improvement in irritability and some reduction in substance use (Donovan et al., 2000). More research is needed to determine what happens to this syndrome as patients pass from adolescence into young adulthood. The clinical impression is that some patients "age out" of this behavior, and patients who seem to have the syndrome as adults may not respond as readily to valproate. More treatment research in this area is needed, particularly research following children and adolescents with this diagnostic pattern into early adulthood.

Prevention Efforts in Young Adults

Prevention strategies in adolescents and young adults have shown mixed results. For example, the drug abuse resistance education (DARE) program, which seeks to educate school-aged individuals about the dangers of drug use, has largely been shown not to be effective (Clayton, Cattarello, & Johnstone, 1996). Other approaches have been associated with large-scale decrements in drug use. For example, raising the price of cigarettes has been associated with reductions in tobacco smoking, particularly among adolescents and young adults. College-based preventions have been more widely tested for alcohol use than for drug use (see Chapter 18). More research is needed to identify effective prevention strategies for drug use in young adults.

Conclusion

Drug dependence is a disorder influenced by genetic vulnerabilities, stress, and their interaction. It is best viewed as a developmental disorder with pre-existing risk factors in childhood, including conduct problems and anxiety, and a typical course of early-onset use during junior high school or the early high school years, giving way at some point to regular use and development of impairment. The transition from school into young adulthood and early career is a time when many individuals may "age out" of drug use, but some will persist and present with drug dependence. A variety of efficacious behavioral and pharmacological treatments are available for various drug dependencies. However, most of this treatment research, with a few exceptions, derives from adult rather than adolescent populations. Thus, more treatment research is needed to test promising treatments for drug dependence among adolescents and young adults. Research is also needed on preventive interventions to avert the development of drug abuse and dependence among college students and young adults. Future research into clinically relevant endophenotypes, dimensional as opposed to categorical divisions, and specific genetic and environmental contributions to drug dependence should aid significantly in the development of improved prevention and treatment strategies for drug dependence in young adults.

KEY POINTS

- Most adolescents and young adults are exposed to nicotine, alcohol, and other drugs, and many will try them, while only some will go on to develop a DSM-IV addictive disorder–substance abuse or dependence. That said, any episode of drug intoxication can be dangerous.
- Addiction is a disorder of learning and memory. Addictive drugs stimulate the brain reward system and function as positive reinforcers, engendering drug-seeking behavior. Drug-seeking may also follow a negative reinforcement model by which drug use may relieves aversive emotional states related to stress, other psychopathology, or drug withdrawal. Finally, internal stimuli (e.g., sadness, anger) and environmental stimuli (e.g., persons, places, and things) can become conditioned stimuli that trigger drug craving and use according to a Pavlovian conditioning model.
- Treatments for drug dependence seek to address these learning mechanisms. Medications seek to substitute for (e.g., buprenorphine for opioid dependence) or block the reinforcing effects of drugs (e.g., naltrexone for opioid dependence). Behavioral and cognitive

(Key Points continued)

techniques seek to bring behavioral under the control of healthy reinforcers that can compete with drug use (e.g., voucher incentives contingent on abstinence), or convey skills to manage situations or cravings that are linked to use (e.g., cognitive behavioral relapse prevention).

PRACTICE GUIDELINES

- Screening for alcohol and drug use should be part of routine health care for adolescents and young adults. It is important to take an open and accepting approach to questioning adolescents and young adults about drug use in order to get accurate information. A thorough clinical history is needed to establish diagnostic criteria, and to document risk factors in the psychiatric, developmental, and family histories. Drug testing is a useful adjunct to a good history.
- Young adults should be counseled about the potential dangers of intoxication, and about the risk of developing a drug use disorder (drug abuse or dependence). Motivational Interviewing is an effective method for questioning and helping motivate patients to reduce their risky behavior, by having the clinician take a collaborative rather than a confrontative or authoritative role. Training in Motivational Interviewing is recommended to clinicians working with young adults.
- For young adults with a drug use disorder, one or more evidence-based treatments should be initiated. Behavioral and psychosocial treatments are the mainstay of treatments for drug dependence. For opioid dependence, effective medications are available and should be considered (buprenorphine, methadone, naltrexone).

References

Aharonovich, E., Hasin, D. S., Brooks, A. C., Liu, X., Bisaga, A., & Nunes, E. V. (2006). Cognitive deficits predict low treatment retention in cocaine dependent patients. *Drug and Alcohol Dependence, 81*(3), 313–322.

Amass, L., Ling, W., Freese, T. E., Reiber, C., Annon, J. J., Cohen, A. J., McCarty, D., Reid, M. S., Brown, L. S., Clark, C., Ziedonis, D. M., Krejci, J., Stine, S., Winhusen, T., Brigham, G., Babcock, D., Muir, J. A., Buchan, B. J., & Horton, T. (2004). Bringing buprenorphine-naloxone detoxification to community treatment providers: the NIDA Clinical Trials Network field experience. *American Journal of Addiction, 13*(Suppl 1.), S42–S66.

American Psychiatric Association. (1994). *Diagnostic and statistical manual of mental disorders* (4 ed.). Washington, DC: Author.

Ball, J. C., Lange, W. R., & Myers, E. (1988). Reducing the risk of AIDS through methadone maintenance treatment. *Journal of Health and Social Behavior, 29*, 214–226.

Bisaga, A., Aharonovich, E., Garawi, F., Levin, F. R., Rubin, E., Raby, W. N., & Nunes, E. V. (2006). A randomized placebo-controlled trial of gabapentin for cocaine dependence. *Drug and Alcohol Dependence, 81*, 267–274.

Brady, K. T., Sonne, S., Anton, R. F., Randall, C. L., Back, S. E., & Simpson, K. (2005). Sertraline in the treatment of co-occurring alcohol dependence and posttraumatic stress disorder. *Alcoholism: Clinical and Experimental Research, 29*(3), 395–401.

Breslau, N., Davis, G. C., & Schultz, L. R. (2003). Posttraumatic stress disorder and the incidence of nicotine, alcohol, and other drug disorders in persons who have experienced trauma. *Archives of General Psychiatry, 60*(3), 289–294.

Budney, A. J., Hughes, J. R., Moore, B. A., & Vandrey, R. (2004). Review of the validity and significance of cannabis withdrawal syndrome. *American Journal of Psychiatry, 161*, 1967–1977.

Budney, A. J., Moore, B. A., Rocha, H. L., & Higgins, S. T. (2006). Clinical trial of abstinence-based vouchers and cognitive-behavioral therapy for cannabis dependence. *Journal of Consulting and Clinical Psychology, 74*(2), 307–316.

Carroll, K. M., Ball, S. A., Nich, C., O'Connor, P. G., Eagan, D. A., Frankforter, T. L., Triffleman, E. G., Shi, J., & Rounsaville, B. J. (2001). Targeting behavioral therapies to enhance naltrexone treatment of opioid dependence: Efficacy of contingency management and significant other involvement. *Archives of General Psychiatry, 58*(8), 755–761.

Carroll, K. M., Fenton, L. R., Ball, S. A., Nich, S. A., Frankforter, T. A., Shi, J., & Rounsaville, B. J. (2004). Efficacy of disulfiram and cognitive behavior therapy in cocaine-dependent outpatients. *Archives of General Psychiatry, 61*, 264–272.

Carroll, K. M., Rounsaville, B. J., Nich, C., Gordon, L. T., Wirtz, P. W., & Gawin, F. (1994). One-year follow-up of psychotherapy and pharmacotherapy for cocaine dependence. Delayed emergence of psychotherapy effects. *Archives of General Psychiatry, 51*(12), 989–997.

Center for Substance Abuse Treatment (2004). *Clinical guidelines for the use of buprenorphine in the treatment of opioid addiction.* TIP series no. 40. Rockville, MD: Author.

Childress, A. R., Ehrman, R. N., McLellan, A. T., MacRae, J., Natale, M., & O'Brien, C. P. (1994). Can induced moods trigger drug-related responses in opiate abuse patients? *Journal of Substance Abuse Treatment, 11*(1), 17–23.

Childress, A. R., Ehrman, R., Robsenow, D. J., Robin, S. J., & O'Brien, C. P. (1992). Classically conditioned factors in drug dependence. In J. H. Lowinson, R. Millman, & P. Ruiz (Eds.), *Substance abuse: A comprehensive textbook* (2nd ed., pp. 56–69). Baltimore: Williams & Wilkins.

Cicero, T. J., Inciardi, J. A., & Munoz, A. (2005). Trends in abuse of oxycontin and other opioid analgesics in the United States: 2002–2004. *Journal of Pain, 6*, 662–672.

Clayton, R., Cattarello, A. M, & Johnstone, B. M. (1996). The effectiveness of Drug Abuse Resistance Education (project DARE): 5-year follow-up results. *Prevention Medicine, 25*, 307–318.

Comer, S. D., Sullivan, M. A., Yu, E., Rothenberg, J. L., Kleber, H. D., Kampman, K., Dackis, C., & O'Brien, C. P. (2006). Injectable, sustained-release naltrexone for the treatment of opioid dependence: A randomized, placebo-controlled trial. *Archives of General Psychiatry, 63*(2), 210–218.

Cornelius, J. R., Clark, D. B., Bukstein, O. G., Birmaher, B., Salloum, I. M., & Brown, S. A. (2005). Acute phase and five-year follow-up study of fluoxetine in adolescents with major depression and a comorbid substance use disorder: A review. *Addictive Behavior, 30*(9), 1824–1833.

Cowan, R. L. (2007). Neuroimaging research in human MDMA users: A review. *Psychopharmacology (Berlin), 189*(4), 539–556.

Crits-Christoph, P., Siqueland, L., Blaine, J., Frank, A., Luborsky, L., Onken, L. S., Muenz, L., Thase, M. E., Weiss, R. D., Gastfriend, D. R., Woody, G., Barber, J. P., Butler, S. F., Daley, D., Bishop, S., Najavits, L. M., Lis, J., Mercer, D., Griffin, M. L., Moras, K., & Beck, A. T. (1997). The National Institute on Drug Abuse Collaborative Cocaine Treatment Study. Rationale and methods. *Archives of General Psychiatry, 54*(8), 721–726.

Dackis, C. A., Kampman, K. M., Lynch, K. G., Pettinati, H. M., & O'Brien, C. P. (2005). A double-blind, placebo-controlled trial of modafinil for cocaine dependence. *Neuropsychopharmacology, 30*(1), 205–211.

De Angelis, D., Hickman, M., & Yang, S. (2004). Estimating long-term trends in the incidence and prevalence of opiate use/injecting drug use and the number of former users: Back-calculation methods and opiate overdose deaths. *American Journal of Epidemiology, 160*(10), 994–1004.

Dishion, T. J., Poulin, F., & Burraston, B. (2001). Peer group dynamics associated with iatrogenic effects in group interventions with high-risk young adolescents. *New Directions in Child and Adolescent Development, 91*, 79–92.

Dole, V. P., & Nyswander, M. (1965). A medical treatment for diacetylmorphine (heroin) addiction. A clinical trial with methadone hydrochloride. *Journal of the American Medical Association, 193*, 646–650.

Donovan, S. J., Stewart, J. W., Nunes, E. V., Quitkin, F. M., Parides, M., Daniel, W., Susser, E., & Klein, D. F. (2000). Divalproex treatment for youth with explosive temper and mood lability: A double-blind, placebo-controlled crossover design. *American Journal of Psychiatry, 157*(5), 818–820.

Dunbar, J. L., Turncliff, R. Z., & Donq, Q. (2006). Single- and multiple-dose pharmacokinetics of long-acting injectable naltrexone. *Alcoholism:l Clinical and Experimental Research, 30*, 480–490.

Edwards, G., & Gross, M. M. (1976). Alcohol dependence: provisional description of a clinical syndrome. *British Medical Journal, 1*(6017), 1058–1061.

Fleming, M. F., Barry, K. L., Manwell, L. B., Johnson, K., & London, R. (1997). Brief physician advice for problem alcohol drinkers. A randomized controlled trial in community-based primary care practices. *Journal of the American Medical Association, 277*(13), 1039–1045.

Fu, Q., Heath, A. C., Bucholz, K. K., Nelson, E., Goldberg, J., Lyons, M. J., True, W. R., Jacob, T., Tsuang, M. T., & Eisen, S. A. (2002). Shared genetic risk of major depression, alcohol dependence, and marijuana dependence: Contribution of antisocial personality disorder in men. *Archives of General Psychiatry, 59*, 1125–1132.

Fudala, P. J., Bridge, T. P., Herbert, S., Williford, W. O., Chiang, C. N., Jones, K., Collins, J., Raisch, D., Casadonte, P., Goldsmith, R. J., Ling, W., Malkerneker, U., McNicholas, L., Renner, J., Stine, S., Tusel, D., & the Buprenorphine/Naloxone Collaborative Study Group. (2003). Office-based treatment of opiate addiction with a sublingual-tablet formulation of buprenorphine and naloxone. *New England Journal of Medicine, 349*, 949–958.

Galanter, M. (1993). *Network therapy for addictions: A new approach*. New York: Basic Books.

Gardner, E. L. (1997). Brain reward mechanisms. In J. H. Lowinson, P. Ruiz, R. B. Millman, & J. G. Langrod (Eds.) *Substance abuse: A comprehensive textbook* (pp. 51–85). Baltimore: Williams and Wilkins.

Gawin, F. H., & Kleber, H. D. (1986). Abstinence symptomatology and psychiatric diagnosis in cocaine abusers. Clinical observations. *Archives of General Psychiatry, 43*(2), 107–113.

Gawin, F. H., Kleber, H. D., Byck, R., Rounsaville, B. J., Kosten, T. R., Jatlow, P. I., & Morgan, C. (1989). Desipramine facilitation of initial cocaine abstinence. *Archives of General Psychiatry, 46*, 117–121.

Geller, B., Cooper, T. B., Sun, K., Zimerman, B., Frazier, J., Williams, M., & Heath, J. (1998). Double-blind and placebo-controlled study of lithium for adolescent bipolar disorders with secondary substance dependency. *Journal of the American Academy of Child and Adolescent Psychiatry, 37*(2), 171–178.

Goeders, N. E. (2003). The impact of stress on addiction. *European Neuropsychopharmacology, 13*(6), 435–441.

Grabowski, J., Rhoades, H., Stotts, A., Cowan, K., Kopecky, C., Dougherty, A., Moeller, F. G., Hassan, S., & Schmitz, J. (2004). Agonist-like or antagonist-like treatment for cocaine dependence with methadone for heroin dependence: Two double-blind randomized clinical trials. *Neuropsychopharmacology, 29*(5), 969–981.

Haney, M., Hart, C. L., Vosburg, S. K., Nasser, J., Bennett, A., Zubaran, C., & Foltin, R. W. (2004). Marijuana withdrawal in humans: Effects of oral THC or divalproex. *Neuropsychopharmacology, 29*, 158–170.

Hasin, D., Nunes, E., & Meydan, J. (2004). Comorbidity of alcohol, drug and psychiatric disorders: Epidemiology. In H. R. Kranzler & J. A. Tinsley (Eds.), *Dual diagnosis and treatment: Substance abuse and comorbid disorders*. New York: Marcel Dekker.

Hasin, D., & Paykin, A. (1999). Alcohol dependence and abuse diagnoses: Concurrent validity in a nationally representative sample. *Alcoholism: Clinical and Experimental Research, 23*(1), 144–150.

Hasin, D., Samet, S., Nunes, E., Meydan, J., Matseoane, K., & Waxman, R. (2006). Diagnosis of comorbid psychiatric disorders in substance users assessed with the Psychiatric Research Interview for Substance and Mental Disorders for DSM-IV. *American Journal of Psychiatry, 163*(4), 689–696.

Higgins, S. T., Budney, A. J., Bickel, W. K., Hughes, J. R., Foerg, F., & Badger, G. (1993). Achieving cocaine abstinence with a behavioral approach. *American Journal of Psychiatry, 150*, 763–769.

Hubbard, R. L., Craddock, S. G., & Anderson, J. (2003). Overview of 5-year follow-up outcomes in the drug abuse treatment outcome studies (DATOS). *Journal of Substance Abuse and Treatment, 25*(3), 125–134.

Kampman, K. M., Pettinati, H., Lynch, K. G., Dackis, C., Sparkman, T., Weigley, C., & O'Brien, C. P. (2004). A pilot trial of topiramate for the treatment of cocaine dependence. *Drug and Alcohol Dependence, 75*, 233–240.

Kandel, D. B., Yamaguchi, K., & Chen, K. (1992). Stages of progression in drug involvement from adolescence to adulthood: further evidence for the gateway theory. *Journal of Studies in Alcohol, 53*(5), 447–457.

Kellam, S. G., Brown, C. H., Rubin, B. R., & Ensminger, M. E. (1983). Paths leading to teenage psychiatric symptoms and substance use: Developmental epidemiological studies in Woodlawn. In S. B. Guze, F. J. Earls, & J. E. Barrett (Eds.), *Childhood psychopathology and development* (pp. 17–51). New York: Raven Press.

Kellogg, S., Melia, D., Khuri, E., Lin, A., Ho, A., & Kreek, M. J. (2006). Adolescent and young adult heroin patients: Drug use and success in methadone maintenance treatment. *Journal of Addictive Diseases, 25*(3), 15–25.

Khantzian, E. J. (1985). The self-medication hypothesis of addictive disorders: Focus on heroin and cocaine dependence. *American Journal of Psychiatry, 142*, 1259–1264.

Kranzler, H. R., Burleson, J. A., Del Boca, F. K., Babor, T. F., Korner, P., Brown, J., & Bohn, M. J. (1994). Buspirone treatment of anxious alcoholics. A placebo-controlled trial. *Archives of General Psychiatry, 51*, 720–731.

Levin, F. R., Evans, S. M., Brooks, D. J., & Garawi, F. (2007). Treatment of cocaine dependent treatment seekers with adult ADHD: Double-blind comparison of methylphenidate and placebo. *Drug and Alcohol Dependence, 87*, 20–29.

Levin, F. R., Evans, S. M., Brooks, D. J., Kalbag, A. S., Garawi, F., & Nunes, E. V. (2006). Treatment of methadone-maintained patients with adult ADHD: Double-blind comparison of methylphenidate, bupropion, and placebo. *Drug and Alcohol Dependence*, 81, 137–148.

Levin, F. R., & Kleber, H. D. (2008). Use of dronabinol for cannabis dependence: Two case reports and review. *American Journal of Addiction*, 17(2), 161–164.

Liddle, H. A., Rowe, C. L., Dakof, G. A., Ungaro, R. A., & Henderson, C. E. (2004). Early intervention for adolescent substance abuse: Pretreatment to posttreatment outcomes of a randomized clinical trial comparing multidimensional family therapy and peer group treatment. *Journal of Psychoactive Drugs*, 36(1), 49–63.

Ling, W., Amass, L., Shoptaw, S., Annon, J. J., Hillhouse, M., Babcock, D., Brigham, G., Harrer, J., Reid, M., Muir, J., Buchan, B., Orr, D., Woody, G., Krejci, J., Ziedonis, D., & Buprenorphine Study Protocol Group. (2005). A multi-center randomized trial of buprenorphine-naloxone versus clonidine for opioid detoxification: Findings from the National Institute on Drug Abuse Clinical Trials Network. *Addiction*, 100, 1090–1100.

Marsch, L. A., Bickel, W. K., Badger, G. J., Stothart, M. E., Quesnel, K. J., Stanger, C., & Brooklyn, J. (2005). Comparison of pharmacological treatments for opioid-dependent adolescents: A randomized controlled trial. *Archives of General Psychiatry*, 62(10), 1157–1164.

McCance-Katz, E. F. (2004). Office-based buprenorphine treatment for opioid-dependent patients. *Harvard Review of Psychiatry*, 12, 321–338.

Miele, G. M., Carpenter, K. M., Smith Cockerham, M., Dietz Trautman, K., Blaine, J., & Hasin, D. S. (2000). Concurrent and predictive validity of the Substance Dependence Severity Scale (SDSS). *Drug and Alcohol Dependence*, 59(1), 77–88.

Miller, W. R., Meyers, R. J., & Hiller-Sturmhöfel, S. (1999). The community-reinforcement approach. *Alcohol Research and Health*, 23(2), 116–121.

Miller, W. R., & Mount, K. A. (2001). A small study of training in motivational interviewing: Does one workshop change clinician and client behavior? *Behavioural and Cognitive Psychotherapy*, 29, 457–471.

Miller, W. R., & Rollnick, S. (2002). *Motivational interviewing: Preparing people for change* (2nd ed.). New York: Guilford Press.

Moss, H. B., Majumder, P. P., & Vanyukov, M. (1994). Familial resemblance for psychoactive substance use disorders: Behavioral profile of high risk boys. *Addictive Behaviors*, 19, 199–208.

Nunes, E. V., & Levin, F. R. (2004). Treatment of depression in patients with alcohol dependence or other drug dependence: A meta-analysis. *Journal of the American Medical Association*, 291, 1887–1896.

Nunes, E. V., Liu, X., Samet, S., Matseoane, K., & Hasin, D. (2006). Independent versus substance-induced major depressive disorder in substance-dependent patients: Observational study of course during follow-up. *Journal of Clinical Psychiatry*, 67(10), 1561–1567.

Nunes, E. V., McGrath, P. J., Quitkin, F. M., Ocepek-Welikson, K., Stewart, J. W., Koenig, T., Wagers, S., & Klein, D. F. (1995). Imipramine treatment of cocaine abuse: Possible boundaries of efficacy. *Drug and Alcohol Dependence*, 39, 185–195.

Nunes, E. V., & Rounsaville, B. J. (2006). Comorbidity of substance use with depression and other mental disorders: From Diagnostic and Statistical Manual of Mental Disorders, fourth edition (DSM-IV) to DSM-V. *Addiction*, 101(Suppl. 1), 89–96.

Nunes, E. V., Sullivan, M. A., & Levin, F. R. (2004). Treatment of depression in patients with opiate dependence. *Biological Psychiatry*, 56(10), 793–802.

Park, C. L., Armeli, S., & Tennen, H. (2004). The daily stress and coping process and alcohol use among college students. *Journal of Studies in Alcohol*, 65(1), 126–135.

Peng, X. Q., Li, X., Gilbert, J. G., Pak, A. C., Ashby, C. R. Jr, Brodie, J. D., Dewey, S. L., Gardner, E. L., & Xi, Z. X. (2008). Gamma-vinyl GABA inhibits cocaine-triggered reinstatement of drug-seeking behavior in rats by a non-dopaminergic mechanism. *Drug and Alcohol Dependence*, 97(3), 216–225.

Perez, J., & Ribera, M. V. (2008). Managing neuropathic pain with Sativex: A review of its pros and cons. *Expert Opinion in Pharmacotherapy*, 9(7), 1189–1195.

Petry, N. M., Peirce, J. M., Stitzer, M. L., Blaine, J., Roll, J. M., Cohen, A., Obert, J., Killeen, T., Saladin, M. E., Cowell, M., Kirby, K. C., Sterling, R., Royer-Malvestuto, C., Hamilton, J., Booth, R. E., Macdonald, M., Liebert, M., Rader, L., Burns, R., DiMaria, J., Copersino, M., Stabile, P. Q., Kolodner, K., & Li, R. (2005). Effect of prize-based incentives on outcomes in stimulant abusers in outpatient psychosocial treatment programs: A national drug abuse treatment clinical trials network study. *Archives of General Psychiatry*, 62(10), 1148–1156.

Pierce, J. M., Petry, N. M., Stitzer, M. L., Blaine, J., Kellogg, S., Satterfield, F., Schwartz, M., Kransky, J., Pencer, E., Silva-Vazquez, L., Kirby, K. C., Royer-Malvestuto, C., Roll, J. M., Cohen, A., Copersino, M. L., Kolodner, K., & Li, R. (2006). Effects of lower-cost incentives on stimulant abstinence in methadone maintenance treatment: A National Drug Abuse Treatment

Clinical Trials Network study. *Archives of General Psychiatry, 63*, 201–208.

Poling, J., Oliveto, A., Petry, N., Sofuoglu, M., Gonsai, K., Gonzalez, G., Martell, B., & Kosten, T. R. (2006). Six-month trial of bupropion with contingency management for cocaine dependence in a methadone-maintained population. *Archives of General Psychiatry, 63*, 219–228.

Preston, K. L., Silverman, K., Umbricht, A., DeJesus, A., Montoya, I. D., & Schuster, C. R. (1999). Improvement in naltrexone treatment compliance with contingency management. *Drug and Alcohol Dependence, 54*, 125–137.

Project MATCH Research Group. (1998). Matching alcoholism treatments to client heterogeneity: Treatment main effects and matching effects on drinking during treatment. *Journal of Studies in Alcohol, 59*(6), 631–639.

Quitkin, F. M., Rifkin, A., Kaplan, J., & Klein, D. F. (1972). Phobic anxiety syndrome complicated by drug dependence and addiction: A treatable form of drug dependence. *Archives of General Psychiatry, 27*, 159–162.

Rawson, R. A., Shoptaw, S. J., Obert, J. L., McCann, M. J., Hasson, A. L., Marinelli-Casey, P. J., Brethen, P. R., & Ling, W. (1995). An intensive outpatient approach for cocaine abuse treatment. The Matrix model. *Journal of Substance Abuse and Treatment, 12*(2), 117–127.

Regier, D. A., Farmer, M. E., Rae, D. S., Locke, B. Z., Keith, S. J., Judd, L. L., & Goodwin, F. K. (1990). Comorbidity of mental disorders with alcohol and other drug abuse—Results from the Epidemiological Catchment Area (ECA) Study. *Journal of the American Medical Association, 263*, 2511–2518.

Riggs, P. D., Hall, S. K., Mikulich-Gilbertson, S. K., Lohman, M., & Kayser, A. (2004). A randomized controlled trial of pemoline for attention-deficit/hyperactivity disorder in substance-abusing adolescents. *Journal of the American Academy of Child and Adolescent Psychiatry, 43*(4), 420–429.

Riggs, P. D., Mikulich-Gilbertson, S. K., Davies, R. D., Lohman, M., Klein, C., & Stover, S. K. (2007). A randomized controlled trial of fluoxetine and cognitive behavioral therapy in adolescents with major depression, behavior problems, and substance use disorders. *Archives of Pediatric and Adolescent Medicine, 161*(11), 1026–1034.

Salloum, I. M., Cornelius, J. R., Daley, D. C., Kirisci, L., Himmelhoch, J. M., Thase, M. E. (2005). Efficacy of valproate maintenance in patients with bipolar disorder and alcoholism: A double-blind placebo-controlled study. *Archives of General Psychiatry, 62*(1), 37–45.

Sherman, S. G., Cheng, Y., & Kral, A. H. (2007). Prevalence and correlates of opiate overdose among young injection drug users in a large U.S. city. *Alcohol Dependence, 88*(2–3), 182–187.

Siegel, S., & Ramos, B. M. (2002). Applying laboratory research: Drug anticipation and the treatment of drug addiction. *Experimental and Clinical Psychopharmacology, 10*(3), 162–183.

Silins, E., Copeland, J., & Dillon, P. (2007). Qualitative review of serotonin syndrome, ecstasy (MDMA) and the use of other serotonergic substances: Hierarchy of risk. *Australian and New Zealand Journal of Psychiatry, 41*(8), 649–655.

Spitzer, R. L., Williams, J. B., Gibbon, M., & First, M. B. (1992). The Structured Clinical Interview for DSM-III-R (SCID). I: History, rationale, and description. *Archives of General Psychiatry, 49*(8), 624–629.

Sullivan, M. A., Comer, S. D., & Nunes, E. V. (2006). Pharmacology and clinical use of naltrexone. In E. C. Strain & M. L. Stitzer, *The treatment of opioid dependence* (pp. 295–322). Baltimore: The Johns Hopkins University Press.

Szapocznik, J., & Williams, R. A. (2000). Brief strategic family therapy: Twenty-five years of interplay among theory, research and practice in adolescent behavior problems and drug abuse. *Clinical Child and Family Psychology Review, 3*(2), 117–134.

Talih, F., Fattal, O., & Malone, D., Jr. (2007). Anabolic steroid abuse: Psychiatric and physical costs. *Cleveland Clinical Journal of Medicine, 74*(5), 341–344, 346, 349–352.

Teter, C. J., & Guthrie, S. K. (2001). A comprehensive review of MDMA and GHB: Two common club drugs. *Pharmacotherapy, 21*(12), 1486–1513.

Tsuang, M. T., Bar, J. L., Harley, R. M., & Lyons, M. J. (2001). The Harvard Twin Study of Substance Abuse: What we have learned. *Harvard Review of Psychiatry, 9*(6), 267–279.

Vorel, S. R., Liu, X., Hayes, R. J., Spector, J. A., & Gardner, E. L. (2001). Relapse to cocaine-seeking after hippocampal theta burst stimulation. *Science, 292*(5519), 1175–1178.

Chapter 20

Impulse Control Disorders

Jon E. Grant and Marc N. Potenza

Brian, a 19-year-old male, started gambling on sporting events at 15 years of age with his father. By the time he started college, Brian was playing poker with friends for money on a regular basis. For the past 2 years, Brian was playing poker or gambling online approximately four evenings each week. Always intending on limiting the amount of time to only 2 or 3 hours, Brian would often play poker or gamble online for 8 to 10 hours each evening. In addition, he began gambling with larger amounts of money. Although a bright young man, Brian's school attendance became sporadic and his school work suffered as a result of his gambling.

Brian's relationships with family and friends also suffered. He often missed events with friends, choosing instead to gamble. In addition, Brian began lying to his family about his finances, asking more frequently for larger amounts of money and becoming angry when he was questioned about his spending or when he was denied the funds. Brian's lies to family members became more intricate, and the deception led to severe guilt.

Introduction

Impulse control disorders (ICDs) are characterized by an impaired ability to resist impulses to engage in ultimately self-destructive behaviors (or ones with deleterious long-term consequences). Although impulsivity may be a feature of many disorders (for example, bipolar disorder, substance use disorders, and attention-deficit/hyperactivity disorder), in DSM-IV-TR the category of Impulse Control Disorders Not Elsewhere Classified currently includes intermittent explosive disorder, kleptomania, pyromania, pathological gambling, and trichotillomania (American Psychiatric Association, 2000). In addition, diagnostic criteria for compulsive sexual behavior and compulsive buying have been proposed as preliminary data and suggest that these behaviors may be linked to ICDs currently operationalized in the DSM-IV-TR (Black et al., 1997; McElroy et al., 1994).

Data suggest that ICDs are relatively common among young adults, carry significant morbidity and mortality, and may be effectively treated with behavioral and pharmacological therapies (Grant & Potenza, 2004). Although as a group the ICDs generally have their age of onset in late adolescence or early adulthood, certain ICDs have their age of onset more commonly in childhood (trichotillomania) while others display a variable age of onset (pathological gambling). In addition, the clinical presentation of ICDs often differs depending on age, and interventions, both psychological and pharmacological, should be tailored for issues unique to young adults with ICDs. In this chapter, findings concerning how ICDs present in young adults are reviewed within a clinical context. The chapter also discusses how treatment of ICDs may be uniquely tailored for young adults as compared with other age groups.

Young Adult Development and a Predisposition toward Impulse Control Disorders

ICDs tend to start during adolescence or young adulthood and can be conceptualized as belonging to a larger constellation of developmental addictions. Data support a relationship between behavioral and drug addictions in both adults and adolescents. For example, high rates of both problem gambling and substance use disorders have been reported during adolescence (Chambers & Potenza, 2003; Wagner & Anthony, 2002), and gambling, substance use, and other risky behaviors frequently co-occur in adolescents (Proimos et al., 1998; Romer, 2003). More specifically, this co-occurrence of risky behaviors appears particularly strong in adolescent males (e.g., Gupta & Derevensky, 1998; Stinchfield, 2001; Wallisch, 1993), but recent research suggests that certain sensation-seeking behaviors may be as common or more common in adolescent females (e.g., pyromania and compulsive sexual behavior) (Grant et al., 2007) and may be particularly closely linked to depression in girls (Desai et al., 2005).

A growing body of data suggests the importance of environmental and genetic influences on brain function that lead to vulnerability to and expression of addictive disorders (Shah et al., 2005; Slutske et al., 2000; Tsuang et al., 2001). Both environmental and genetic factors are important influences on brain function and thus can contribute to addiction vulnerability in adolescence and young adulthood.

Motivated behavior involves integrating information about a person's internal state (e.g., hunger, sexual desire, pain), environmental factors (e.g., resource or reproductive opportunities, the presence of danger), and personal experiences (e.g., recollections of events deemed similar in nature). Specific brain regions and multiple neurotransmitters are involved in processing this information and guiding motivated behaviors.

The neurotransmitters that are arguably the best characterized that influence motivated behavior are dopamine and serotonin. Dopamine release into the nucleus accumbens has been associated with a wide array of experiences, including rewarding and reinforcing, novel and aversive or stressful stimuli (Chambers et al., 2003). Dopamine release into the nucleus accumbens seems maximal when reward probability is most uncertain, suggesting it plays a central role in guiding behavior during risk-taking situations (Fiorillo et al., 2003).

Diminished inhibitory mechanisms could also underlie risk-taking behaviors. Among the most well-studied inhibitory pathways is that involving serotonin function within the prefrontal cortex (Chambers et al., 2003). Decreased measures of serotonin have long been associated with a variety of adult risk-taking behaviors, including alcoholism, fire-setting, and pathological gambling (Potenza & Hollander, 2002).

The period from adolescence into young adulthood is a time of remarkable changes in brain structure and function, and developmental changes within primary motivational pathways may lead to increased novelty seeking and risk taking (Chambers et al., 2003). The transition period from adolescence into young adulthood may reflect a state of heightened dopaminergic activity in the setting of immature prefrontal cortical function. Vulnerability to addictive behaviors, particularly that observed during adolescence and young adulthood, might be increased by relative immaturity of cortico-limbic circuits, particularly in young males (Laucht et al., 2005).

Pathological Gambling

A range of prevalence estimates has been reported for pathological gambling depending upon the year and location of the study and the instruments used to diagnose the disorder. Surveys of community samples and a meta-analysis of 120 prevalence surveys have found lifetime prevalence rates for adults ranging from 0.42%–2.5% for pathological gambling, and 1.3%–3.85% for problematic gambling behavior (Cunningham-Williams et al., 2005; Gerstein et al., 1999; Petry et al., 2005; Shaffer et al., 1999; Welte et al., 2001). Studies specifically examining adolescents and young adults (i.e., college students) have reported similar or higher estimates of problematic gambling (ranging from 1% to 9%) (Blinn-Pike et al., 2007; Shaffer et al., 1994).

Clinical Characteristics

Of youth aged between 12 and 17 years, 50%–90% report gambling within the past year (Shaffer & Hall, 1996). As in the case of Brian, pathological gambling usually begins in adolescence or early adulthood, with males tending to start at an earlier age (Chambers & Potenza, 2003; Grant & Kim, 2001a). High estimates of pathological gambling in young adults suggest a similar natural history to that observed with substance use disorders (Chambers & Potenza, 2003).

Young adults with pathological gambling are more likely to be male and single (Petry, 2002). Although adolescents and young adults who gamble describe gambling as a social activity and less about winning money, young adult gamblers appear more likely to engage in strategic forms of gambling (e.g., blackjack), and this finding suggests that competitive risk-taking represents a particularly salient reason for gambling among this age group (Lynch et al., 2004). College students with gambling problems as compared to those without report less perceived social support (Weinstock & Petry, 2006) and more problems with food, alcohol, tobacco, and other drugs (Engwall et al., 2004).

Young adults with pathological gambling have more employment, social, and legal problems secondary to gambling than do older gamblers (Petry, 2002). Individuals who have pathological gambling in young adulthood are also more likely to have marital and financial (i.e., credit card debt, bankruptcy) problems due to gambling. Although many consequences of gambling appear to affect young adults more severely, many indicators of gambling severity (days spent gambling per week, percentage of monthly income spent gambling) suggest that young adults do not have a more severe form of pathological gambling compared to older adults (Petry, 2002).

Co-Occurring Disorders

Studies have repeatedly found that individuals with pathological gambling frequently suffer from lifetime mood (60%–76%) (Linden et al., 1986; McCormick et al., 1984; Roy et al., 1988), anxiety (16%–40%) (Crockford & el-Guebaly, 1998; Ibanez et al., 2001), and substance use (33%–63%) disorders (Black & Moyer, 1998; Grant, Kushner, & Kim, 2002). Young adult gamblers who started gambling as adolescents are more likely to have problems with alcohol and drug abuse, smoke tobacco, engage in sexual activity as adolescents, and report lifetime depression (Lynch et al., 2004).

Treatment

Pharmacotherapy. Various classes of medication have been studied in the treatment of pathological gambling. Studies using opioid antagonists, lithium, and selective serotonin reuptake inhibitors (SSRIs) (paroxetine, fluvoxamine) have all demonstrated efficacy in double-blind studies of pathological gambling (Grant & Potenza, 2004). Of the double-blind studies in the published literature (Black et al., 2007; Blanco et al., 2002; Grant et al., 2003, 2006; Grant, Kim, & Hartman, 2008; Grant & Potenza, 2006; Hollander et al., 1992, 2000, 2005; Kim et al., 2001, 2002; McElroy et al., 2008; Saiz-Ruiz et al., 2005), only one assessed whether young adults responded differently to treatment. In one trial of fluvoxamine, young male pathological gamblers appeared to respond preferentially to the medication (Blanco et al., 2002). However, the reported age and gender difference in treatment response should be viewed cautiously given the small number of subjects, and particularly the small group of young men completing the study. A separate study investigating pretreatment factors associated with clinical response to opioid antagonists or placebo found that a family history of alcoholism was most strongly associated with a positive clinical response to active drug, whereas younger age was the factor most closely associated with placebo response (Grant et al., in press).

Psychotherapy. Multiple behavioral treatments have been investigated with promising preliminary results (Hodgins & Petry, 2004; Petry, 2005). Cognitive therapy, which focuses on changing the patient's beliefs regarding perceived control over randomly determined events, has demonstrated success in small, randomized trials (Hodgins & Petry, 2004). Cognitive-behavioral therapy has also been used effectively to treat pathological gambling (Hodgins & Petry, 2004; Petry, 2005; Petry et al., 2006). Brief interventions in the form of motivational interventions and self-directed workbooks have led to significant reductions in gambling behavior (Hodgins, Currie, & el-Guebaly, 2001). Aversion therapy and imaginal desensitization have also resulted in improvement for pathological gamblers (McConaghy et al., 1983; McConaghy, Blaszczynski, & Frankova, 1991; Grant et al., in press).

Gamblers Anonymous and self-exclusion programs may also aid in reducing gambling behavior. Young adults with pathological gambling may be more likely than older gamblers to attend Gamblers Anonymous.

Of the various psychosocial interventions, however, none have assessed whether young adults respond differently than older individuals. The relatively small samples sizes studied in reports published to date have limited power in detecting age-related differences in treatment response. It is anticipated that future studies involving larger samples will provide additional insight into optimal treatments for young adults with pathological gambling.

A better understanding of treatment response in young adults may help in developing more prevention and treatment strategies. For example, one proposed intervention for college-aged gamblers that integrates alcohol prevention strategies with elements of gambling treatment has shown promise in reducing high-risk gambling among college students (Takushi et al., 2004). In addition, treatment for young adults may best tailor cognitive-behavioral therapy to sensation seeking, particularly for men.

Trichotillomania

Pathological hair pulling, trichotillomania, has been defined as repetitive, intentionally performed pulling that causes noticeable hair loss and results in clinically significant distress or functional impairment (APA, 2000). The prevalence of trichotillomania is difficult to estimate in the absence of a consensually agreed-upon definition of the problem (for example, 17% to 23% of people with clinically meaningful hair pulling fail to meet the DSM-IV criteria requiring either tension immediately before pulling or pleasure, gratification, or relief when pulling) (Christenson, MacKenzie, & Mitchell, 1991a). Current research, however, suggests that the severe, debilitating form of hair pulling has estimated prevalence rates of 1%–3% (Christenson, Pyle, & Mitchell, 1991b).

Hair pulling among young adults appears common. In studies of college students, 10% to 15% reported pulling their hair on a regular basis (Graber & Arndt, 1993; [a]Rothbaum et al., 1993). Studies have also found that although only 0.6% to 1% of college students meet all DSM-IV criteria for trichotillomania, 2% to 2.5% of college students pull their hair resulting in baldness or bald patches (Christenson et al., 1991b; Rothbaum et al., 1993).

Clinical Characteristics

Although hair pulling can begin at any age, for most young adults with trichotillomania, the disorder began in childhood (approximately 13 years of age) (Christenson et al., 1991b; Schlosser et al., 1994; Swedo & Leonard, 1992) and has been a chronic problem. Although no prospective study has documented associated events at the onset of trichotillomania, the genesis of hair pulling has been associated with scalp disease and stressful life events (Christenson & Mansueto, 1999). Hair pulling is subject to great fluctuations in severity with worsening of symptoms often related to stress.

Trichotillomania has traditionally been thought of as a disorder predominantly affecting females (Cohen et al., 1995; Graber & Arndt, 1993; Swedo & Leonard, 1992), but in children with trichotillomania, males are found in numbers nearly equal to females (Tay, Levy, & Metry, 2004). As children progress to adolescents and young adults, it has been believed that the ratio of females to males with trichotillomania increases (King et al., 1995; Reeve et al., 1992). One recent study of 791 college students, however, found equal estimates of trichotillomania in college men and women (Odlaug & Grant, 2008). A question exists whether trichotillomania is less common in young adult men or that men with trichotillomania avoid seeking professional help or blame hair loss on male pattern baldness (Christenson et al., 1994). Another theory posits that men may pull hair primarily from the beard and mustache and shaving may serve as a means by which men treat themselves (Christenson & Mansueto, 1999). When men do suffer from trichotillomania, however, the age of onset, severity, and related clinical features of the disorder appear similar to those found in women (Christenson et al., 1994; Cohen et al., 1995).

Co-occurring Disorders

Co-occurring psychiatric disorders are frequently reported by individuals with trichotillomania: depression (39%–65%), generalized anxiety disorder (27%–32%), and substance abuse (15%–20%) (Christenson & Mansueto, 1999; Swedo & Leonard, 1992). In addition, trichotillomania frequently co-occurs with compulsive nail biting and pathologic skin picking (Bohne et al., 2005). Co-occurring psychiatric disorders do not appear to differ between young adults with trichotillomania compared to older adults, although the numbers of subjects limit definitive statements on this issue.

Treatment

Pharmacological and behavioral treatments may be effective in the treatment of trichotillomania. Double-blind, controlled trials of different medications (e.g., serotonin reuptake inhibitors [clomipramine, fluoxetine], opioid antagonists [naltrexone], atypical antipsychotics [olanzapine]) have demonstrated some short-term efficacy in treating trichotillomania (O'Sullivan et al., 1999; van Ameringen et al., 2006). None of the studies assessed whether young adults responded differently than older individuals. Medications, however, are not effective with all sufferers and drugs may lose their efficacy over time.

Young adults with trichotillomania appear to respond to behavioral treatment. Only four controlled psychological treatment studies for trichotillomania have been published to date. Habit reversal training (HRT) (Azrin & Nunn, 1973) is a multicomponent treatment package that entails, among other techniques, self-monitoring of urges and behavior, incompatible response training, and coping skills training. Awareness of habit occurrence and training in the use of alternative coping responses are viewed as critical treatment steps. Azrin and colleagues randomized 34 subjects to either habit reversal therapy or negative practice (where subjects were instructed to stand in front of a mirror and act out motions of hair pulling without actually pulling) (Azrin et al., 1980). Habit reversal reduced hair pulling by more than 90% for 4 months, compared to 52%–68% reduction for negative practice at 3 months. A recent study compared acceptance and commitment therapy/habit reversal or wait list and found that those assigned to the therapy experienced significant reductions in hair pulling severity and impairment compared to those assigned to the wait list, and improvement was maintained at 3-month follow-up (Woods et al., 2006). Two studies using controlled designs to compare psychotherapy to medication found that cognitive-behavioral therapy was significantly more effective than clomipramine (Ninan et al., 2000) and that behavior therapy resulted in statistically significant reductions compared to fluoxetine (van Minnen et al., 2003).

Kleptomania

Kleptomania is characterized by repetitive, poorly controlled stealing of items not needed for their personal use: *(1)* a recurrent failure to resist an impulse to steal unneeded objects; *(2)* an increasing sense of tension before committing the theft; *(3)* an experience of pleasure, gratification, or release at the time of committing the theft; and *(4)* the stealing is not performed due to anger, vengeance, or psychotic symptomatology (APA, 2000).

No national epidemiological studies of kleptomania have been performed. A large community survey (n = 43,093) found that the overall lifetime prevalence of shoplifting in the general population was 11.3% (Blanco et al., 2008). A study of shoplifting and kleptomania in 791 college students found that 28.6% of the overall sample reported having stolen something in their lifetime, but that only 0.4% endorsed symptoms consistent with kleptomania (Odlaug & Grant, 2008).

Prevalence studies of kleptomania in clinical samples suggest that the disorder is not uncommon. A recent study of adolescent psychiatric inpatients (n = 102) found that 8.8% met criteria for kleptomania (Grant et al., 2007). A similar finding was reported in a study of adult psychiatric inpatients with multiple disorders (n = 204) (7.8% endorsed current kleptomania and 9.3% had lifetime kleptomania) (Grant et al., 2005). Other studies of specialized psychiatric populations have found similar estimates: 3.7% of depressed patients (Lejoyeux et al., 2002); 3.8% of patients with alcohol dependence (Lejoyeux et al., 1999); 5% of pathological gamblers (Specker et al., 1995); and 24% of those with bulimia (Hudson et al., 1983).

Clinical Characteristics

Although shoplifting usually begins first during adolescence, the age of onset for kleptomania appears to be approximately 28–30 years of age (Bayle et al., 2003). This suggests that for young adults with kleptomania, the prodrome period of episodic shoplifting begins during adolescence. Surveys of adolescents and adults in their early 20s, therefore, may underestimate the rates of kleptomania in the general population.

The course of illness is generally chronic with waxing and waning of symptoms. Individuals with kleptomania try unsuccessfully to stop. In one study, all participants reported increased urges to steal when trying to stop (Grant & Kim, 2002). The diminished ability to stop often leads to feelings of shame and guilt, reported in most (77.3%) subjects (Grant & Kim, 2002). Of married subjects, less than half had disclosed their behavior to their spouses due to shame and guilt (Grant & Kim, 2002). Patients may keep, hoard, discard, gift, or return stolen items (McElroy et al., 1991). Many (64% to 87%) have been apprehended at some time due to their behavior (McElroy et al., 1991), and 15% to 23% report having been incarcerated (Grant & Kim, 2002). No studies to date have systematically investigated for differences in younger as compared to older adults with kleptomania.

Co-occurring Disorders

Psychiatric disorders frequently co-occur with kleptomania. Estimates of lifetime co-occurring affective disorders range from 59% (Grant & Kim, 2002b) to 100% (McElroy et al., 1991). Estimates of co-occurring bipolar disorder have been reported as ranging from 9% (Grant & Kim, 2002) to 60% (McElroy et al., 1991). Studies have also found high lifetime estimates of co-occurring anxiety disorders (60% to 80%) (McElroy et al., 1991, 1992), impulse control disorders (20% to 46%) (Grant, 2003), substance use disorders (23% to 50%) (Grant & Kim, 2002a; McElroy et al., 1991), and eating disorders (60%) (McElroy et al., 1991).

Treatment

Rigorous studies examining treatment response in kleptomania are few. Various medications have been studied in case reports or case series, and several have suggestive efficacies: fluoxetine, nortriptyline, trazodone, clonazepam, valproate, lithium, fluvoxamine, paroxetine, and topiramate (Grant & Potenza, 2004; McElroy et al., 1991).

One formal medication trial involved 7 weeks of open-label escitalopram followed by having the responders randomized to either continue escitalopram or be switched to placebo for an additional 16 weeks. When the responders were randomized, 43% of those on escitalopram and 50% on placebo relapsed, thereby indicating no significant drug effect associated with treatment response (Koran et al., 2007). Another medication study was a 12-week, open-label study of naltrexone. Treatment resulted in a significant decline in the intensity of urges to steal, stealing thoughts, and stealing behavior (Grant & Kim, 2002c). This open-label study was followed by a double-blind examination of naltrexone which also demonstrated improvement in stealing behavior (Grant, Odlaug, & Kim, 2009). No study assessed whether age was associated with treatment response.

Multiple types of psychotherapies have been reported in the successful treatment of kleptomania, but no controlled trials exist in the literature. Case reports document the possible benefits of cognitive, behavioral, insight-oriented, and imaginal and covert sensitization (Goldman, 1991; McElroy et al., 1991). As no controlled trials of therapy for kleptomania have been published, the differential efficacies of these interventions in young adults or older individuals with kleptomania have not been adequately evaluated.

Intermittent Explosive Disorder

Intermittent explosive disorder is defined by recurrent, significant outbursts of aggression, often leading to assaultive acts against people or property, which are disproportionate to outside stressors and no better explained by another psychiatric diagnosis (APA, 2000). Although once considered relatively uncommon, recent research suggests intermittent explosive disorder may be relatively prevalent, with 5%–6% of community samples meeting criteria for lifetime intermittent explosive disorder (Coccaro et al., 2004, Kessler et al., 2006).

Clinical Characteristics

Intermittent explosive disorder appears as early as childhood (e.g., prepubertal) and peaks in mid-adolescence with a mean age of onset ranging from about 13 to 18 years (Coccaro et al., 2004). The average duration of symptomatic intermittent explosive disorder ranges from nearly 12 to 20 years to nearly the whole lifetime. While intermittent explosive disorder has been previously reported to occur much more commonly in males (i.e., 3:1), and its age of onset is earlier in males than females by about 6 years, recent data suggest the gender difference in prevalence of IED may be closer to 1:1 (Coccaro et al., 2004). Importantly, sociodemographic variables (e.g., sex, age, race, education, marital, occupational status, family income) do not seem to differ as a function of the presence or absence of intermittent explosive disorder.

Aggressive outbursts in intermittent explosive disorder have a rapid onset, often without a recognizable prodromal period. They are short lived (<30 minutes) and involve verbal assault, destructive and nondestructive property assault, or physical assault. Aggressive outbursts most commonly occur in response to a minor provocation by a close intimate or associate, and individuals with intermittent explosive disorder may have less severe episodes of verbal and nondestructive property assault in between more severe assaultive/destructive episodes. Episodes are associated with substantial distress and impairment in social and occupational functioning. Legal difficulties due to intermittent explosive disorder are common (McElroy et al., 1998).

Co-occurring Disorders

Intermittent explosive disorder has been associated with mood, substance use, impulse control, and anxiety disorders (Coccaro et al., 2004; McElroy et al., 1998; Olvera, 2002). Many individuals with intermittent explosive disorder report that their aggressive outbursts are secondary to changes in mood (McElroy et al., 1998). Although some studies suggest that intermittent explosive disorder and personality disorders frequently co-occur (Galovski et al., 2002), the estimates of borderline personality and antisocial personality disorders appear to be low (Coccaro et al., 2004). In most cases, the age of onset of intermittent explosive disorder precedes that of these other lifetime comorbid disorders, suggesting that intermittent explosive disorder is not a consequence of these other disorders.

Treatment

While there are no FDA-approved medications for the treatment of intermittent explosive disorder (or any other formal impulse control disorder), several psychopharmacologic agents appear to influence aggression. Classes of agents shown to have "anti-aggressive" effects in double-blind, placebo-controlled trials of individuals with "primary" aggression (i.e., not secondary to psychosis, severe mood disorder, or organic brain syndromes) include mood stabilizers (e.g., lithium), 5-HT uptake inhibitors (e.g., fluoxetine), and anticonvulsants (e.g., diphenydantoin, carbamazepine) (Coccaro & Danehy, 2006). While noradrenergic beta-blockers (e.g., propanolol, nadolol) have also been shown to reduce aggression, these agents have exclusively been tested in patient populations with "secondary" aggression (e.g., mental retardation, organic brain syndromes, etc.). Findings from double-blind, placebo-controlled, clinical trials suggest that anti-aggressive efficacy is specific to impulsive, rather than nonimpulsive, aggression.

Numerous studies and meta-analytic reviews suggest that relaxation training, skill training, cognitive therapy, and multicomponent treatments all have moderate to large effects in the treatment of anger, and that the anger-reducing effects of anger treatment remain at follow-up. Notably, however, the anger treatment literature does not discriminate between clinical anger problems without aggression and pathological aggression and so these findings may not generalize to more severely aggressive individuals with intermittent explosive disorder.

Pyromania

The DSM-IV describes pyromania as a preoccupation with fire setting and characterizes the behavior with the following diagnostic criteria: *(1)* deliberate and purposeful fire setting on more than one occasion; *(2)* tension or affective arousal before the act; *(3)* fascination with, interest in, curiosity about, or attraction to fire and its situational contexts; and *(4)* pleasure, gratification, or relief when setting fires or when witnessing or participating in their aftermath (APA, 2000).

There have been no epidemiological studies of pyromania in the community. One study of college students (n = 791), however, found that 1.0% met criteria for DSM-IV pyromania (Odlaug & Grant, 2008).

In one study suggesting the rare nature of pyromania, the authors found that only 3 (3.3%) of 90 arson recidivists had pure pyromania (Lindberg et al., 2005). Several studies of clinical, noncriminal samples, however, have found that pyromania may not be uncommon. One study of 107 patients with depression found that 3 (2.8%) met current DSM-IV criteria for pyromania (Lejoyeux et al., 2002). A recent study of 204 psychiatric inpatients revealed that 3.4% (n = 7) endorsed current symptoms and 5.9% (n = 12) had lifetime symptoms meeting DSM-IV criteria for pyromania (Grant et al., 2005). Although adolescent fire setting may be a symptom of various psychiatric disorders, a recent study of 102 adolescent psychiatric inpatients found that after excluding those patients who set fires due to conduct disorder, substance use disorders, bipolar disorder, psychotic disorders, or developmental disorders, 7 (6.9%) met criteria for current pyromania (Grant et al., 2007).

Clinical Characteristics

Although long thought to be a disorder primarily affecting men, recent research suggests that the gender ratio may be closer to 1:1 in adults and may be slightly higher among adolescent females than adolescent males (Odlaug & Grant, 2008; Grant et al., 2007). One study found that the mean age of onset is generally late adolescence (18 years of age), and the behavior appears chronic if left untreated (Grant & Kim, 2007). Urges to set fires are common in individuals with this behavior and the fire setting is almost always pleasurable. The behavior frequently intensifies in terms of frequency and intensity over time. Severe distress follows the fire setting, and individuals with pyromania report significant functional impairment (Grant & Kim, 2007).

Co-occurring Disorders

One study of comorbidity in pyromania found elevated estimates of mood disorders, substance use disorders, impulse control disorders, and anxiety disorders (Grant & Kim, 2007). In the majority of cases, the pyromania appears to have preceded the co-occurring disorders, suggesting that pyromania is not merely a consequence of these other disorders.

Treatment

There is no controlled pharmacological or psychological treatment data regarding pyromania. Case reports suggest that a variety of medications may be beneficial for the urges to set fires: topiramate, escitalopram, sertraline, fluoxetine, and lithium (Grant & Kim, 2007). Successful treatment using cognitive-behavioral therapy (using imaginal exposure and response prevention, cognitive restructuring, and relaxation training) has been reported in the case of one young adult with pyromania (Grant et al., 2006).

Compulsive Sexual Behavior

Compulsive sexual behavior is characterized by inappropriate or excessive sexual behaviors or thoughts that lead to subjective distress and/or impaired functioning (Black et al., 1997). Although not currently included in DSM-IV-TR, compulsive sexual behavior may be relatively common. No epidemiological studies of compulsive sexual behavior have been performed, but the prevalence of compulsive sexual behavior in adults is estimated to range from 3%–6% (Coleman, 1992). A recent study of 791 college students found that 3.7% reported symptoms consistent with compulsive sexual behavior (Odlaug & Grant, 2008). Although the disorder is believed to predominately affect men (Black et al., 1997; Kafka & Prentke, 1994; Raymond et al., 2003), a recent study of adolescent psychiatric inpatients (n = 102) found that compulsive sexual behavior was found exclusively among adolescent females (Grant et al., 2007).

Clinical Characteristics

Compulsive sexual behavior can involve a wide range of sexual behaviors, often including a mixture of paraphilic and nonparaphilic behaviors (Coleman, 1992; Kafka & Prentky, 1994). The sexual behavior may be intermittent or continuous. Although the compulsive sexual acts are gratifying, the behavior is followed by remorse or guilt (Barth & Kinder, 1987). The behavior is often driven by either pleasure seeking or anxiety reduction (Coleman, 1992). Individuals often report a feeling of being "out of control" with their sexual behavior and fear losing their jobs, friends, or family (Quadland, 1985). Although no clinical differences based on age have been reported, the samples of individuals with compulsive sexual behavior described in the literature are relatively small. Thus, little empirical data are available to describe how clinical features of compulsive sexual behavior might differ based on age.

Co-occurring Disorders

Comorbidity in compulsive sexual behavior is common with individuals frequently meeting criteria for mood, anxiety, and substance use disorders (Black et al., 1997; Kafka & Prentky, 1994; Raymond et al., 2003). One study of 36 subjects found that other impulse control disorders were also frequent in this population: compulsive buying (14%), kleptomania (14%), pathological gambling (11%), and pyromania (8%) (Black et al., 1997). Cluster B personality disorders are also commonly seen in individuals with compulsive sexual behavior (44%) (Black et al., 1997).

Treatment

Little published treatment research exists for compulsive sexual behavior. In the only double-blind study of compulsive sexual behavior published to date, those individuals assigned to citalopram demonstrated significant reductions in sexual desire, frequency of masturbation, and use of pornography compared to those on placebo. High-risk sexual behavior, however, did not differ between groups (Wainberg et al., 2006).

In addition, case series and open-label trials suggest that various other medications may be efficacious. Fluoxetine has demonstrated efficacy in reducing sexual urges and behavior in men with nonparaphilic sexual addiction (Kafka & Prentky, 1992). A smaller case series of five men with compulsive sexual behavior treated with fluoxetine, however, did not produce similarly robust effects (Stein et al., 1992). A retrospective study looking at men receiving nefazodone reported that 55% of the men improved with 45% achieving remission of symptoms (Coleman et al., 2000). Other medications with possible efficacy in treating compulsive sexual behavior include imipramine, lithium, buspirone, naltrexone, and naltrexone augmentation of an antidepressant (Grant & Kim, 2001b; Potenza & Hollander, 2002; Raymond et al., 2002). Hormonal treatments, including antiandrogens, estrogens, and gonadotropin-releasing hormone analogues, have also been reported to be helpful in men with compulsive sexual behavior (Potenza & Hollander, 2002).

Psychotherapy is commonly recommended for compulsive sexual behavior, and a variety of behavioral techniques, such as imaginal desensitization, aversion therapy, group therapy, and psychodynamic therapies, have been employed (Carnes, 1983; Goodman, 1993). A randomized trial found that imaginal desensitization was more effective at 1-year follow-up than covert sensitization in 20 men with compulsive sexual behavior (McConaghy et al., 1985). Another study examining the efficacy of group cognitive-behavioral therapy for gay and bisexual men with compulsive sexual behavior found that group therapy was effective in reducing targeted sexual behaviors (Quadland, 1985).

Compulsive Buying

Although not specifically recognized in the DSM-IV-TR, the following diagnostic criteria have been proposed: *(1)* maladaptive preoccupation with or engagement in buying (evidenced by frequent preoccupation with or irresistible impulses to buy; or frequent buying of items that are not needed or not affordable; or shopping for longer periods of time than intended); *(2)* preoccupations with the buying lead to significant distress or impairment; and *(3)* the buying does not occur exclusively during hypomanic or manic episodes (McElroy et al., 1994).

A recent random-sample study of 2,513 adults in the United States found that 5.8% of those surveyed screened positive for compulsive buying (Koran et al., 2006). In addition, a recent study of 791 college students found that 1.9% reported symptoms consistent with compulsive buying (Odlaug & Grant, 2008).

Clinical Characteristics

The onset of compulsive buying appears to occur during late adolescence or early adulthood, although the full disorder may take several years to develop (Black, 1996). Compulsive buying tends to be more common among females (Black, 1996; Christenson et al., 1994; McElroy et al., 1994). Individuals with compulsive buying report repetitive, intrusive urges to buy unneeded items. These urges may be triggered by being in stores and worsen during times of stress, emotional difficulties, or boredom. Compulsive buying regularly results in large amounts of financial debt, marital or family disruption, and even legal consequences (Christenson et al., 1994). Guilt, shame, and embarrassment typically follow the buying episodes. Most items are not used or even removed from the packaging, and hoarding of particular items is common (Christenson et al., 1994).

Co-occurring Disorders

Estimates of co-occurring mood disorders range from 28% to 95% (Christenson et al., 1994; McElroy et al., 1994; Schlosser et al., 1994), and the mood disorder usually precedes the compulsive buying (Christenson et al., 1994). Lifetime histories of anxiety (41% to 80%), substance use (30% to 46%), eating (17% to 35%), and impulse control (21% to 40%) disorders are common (Christenson et al., 1994; McElroy et al., 1994; Schlosser et al., 1994).

Treatment

Pharmacotherapy for compulsive buying has been examined in four double-blind, randomized, placebo-controlled trials. Two double-blind studies of fluvoxamine found that the proportion of respondents to medication did not differ from that to placebo (Black et al., 2000; Ninan et al., 2000). A third study found that citalopram demonstrated statistically significant decreases in the frequency of shopping and the intensity of thoughts and urges concerning shopping compared to placebo (Koran et al., 2003), but a study of escitalopram failed to demonstrate efficacy compared to placebo (Koran et al., 2007). In addition, case reports and open-label studies have suggested that the following agents may be beneficial: nortriptyline, fluoxetine, buprorion, lithium, clomipramine, naltrexone, and valproate (Black et al., 1997; Koran et al., 2002; McElroy et al., 1994).

Although cognitive-behavioral therapy has been discussed in uncontrolled reports, only one study has examined cognitive-behavioral therapy in compulsive buying. Mitchell and colleagues studied 39 subjects with compulsive buying (28 assigned to group cognitive-behavioral therapy and 11 assigned to wait list for 10 weeks [12 sessions]). Those assigned to group therapy were able to significantly reduce buying episodes and amount spent. In addition, the benefits were maintained for the 6 months of follow-up (Mitchell et al., 2006). Several case reports also suggest possible effective psychotherapeutic interventions might include exposure and response prevention, and supportive or insight-oriented psychotherapy (McElroy et al., 1994).

Conclusions

ICDs represent a clinically relevant group of disorders for young adults. ICDs generally have their onset in late adolescence or early adulthood. They appear relatively common and frequently go unrecognized. Treatments for these disorders are relatively poorly understood given a paucity of controlled trials for behavioral and pharmacological interventions. In addition, age-related differences in treatments and treatment responses have yet to be systematically investigated. Future research into how young adults with ICDs differ from similarly diagnosed adolescents or older adults should help advance prevention and treatment strategies for individuals from different age groups who suffer from these disorders.

KEY POINTS

- Although the onset of an ICD can occur at any age, the risk for developing an ICD is highest in late adolescence and early adulthood.
- The period from adolescence into young adulthood is a time of remarkable changes in brain structure and function, and developmental changes within primary motivational pathways may lead to increased novelty seeking and risk taking. This suggests that ICDs might be conceptualized as developmental disorders involving a combination of environmental, social, and biological contributions.
- ICDs can be conceptualized as belonging to a larger constellation of developmental addictions, and data support a relationship between behavioral and drug addictions in both adults and adolescents. This co-occurrence of addictive behaviors appears particularly strong in adolescent males.

PRACTICE GUIDELINES

- Although many young adults may not view risky behaviors as problematic, it is important to obtain clinical information about a range of ICDs in this population.
- Young adults may benefit from specific education and prevention strategies.
- Although treatment for most ICDs is relatively poorly understood given a paucity of controlled trials for behavioral and pharmacological interventions, young adults with certain ICDs (e.g., pathological gambling) may benefit from specific treatments (e.g., cognitive behavioral therapy, pharmacotherapies such as naltrexone). More work is needed to understand whether young adults with ICDs accept and adhere to treatment.

References[b]

American Psychiatric Association. (2000). *Diagnostic and statistical manual of mental disorders* (4th ed. Text revision.), Washington, DC: Author.

Azrin, N. H., & Nunn, R. G. (1973). Habit reversal: A method of eliminating nervous habits and tics. *Behavior Research and Therapy, 11,* 619–628.

Azrin, N. H., Nunn, R. G., & Frantz, S. E. (1980). Treatment of hairpulling (trichotillomania): a comparative study of habit reversal and negative practice training. *Journal of Behavior Therapy and Experimental Psychiatry, 11,* 13–20.

Barth, R. J., & Kinder, B. N. (1987). The mislabeling of sexual impulsivity. *Journal of Sex and Marital Therapy, 13,* 15–23.

Bayle, F. C., Caci, H., Millet, B., Richa, S., & Olié, J. P. (2003). Psychopathology and comorbidity of psychiatric disorders in patients with kleptomania. *American Journal of Psychiatry, 160,* 1509–1513.

Black, D.W. (1996). Compulsive buying: a review. *Journal of Clinical Psychiatry, 57* Suppl 8, 50–54.

Black, D. W. (2004). An open-label trial of bupropion in the treatment of pathologic gambling. *Journal of Clinical Psychopharmacology, 24,* 108–110.

Black, D. W., Gabel, J., Hansen, J., & Schlosser, S. (2000). A double-blind comparison of fluvoxamine versus placebo in the treatment of compulsive buying disorder. *Annals of Clinical Psychiatry, 12,* 205–211.

Black, D. W., Kehrberg, L. L. D., Flumerfelt, D. L., Schlosser, S. S. (1997). Characteristics of 36 subjects reporting compulsive sexual behavior. *American Journal of Psychiatry, 154,* 243–249.

Black, D. W., Monahan, P., & Gabel, J. (1997). Fluvoxamine in the treatment of compulsive buying. *Journal of Clinical Psychiatry, 58,* 159–163.

Black, D. W., & Moyer, T. (1998). Clinical features and psychiatric comorbidity of subjects with pathological gambling behavior. *Psychiatric Services, 49,* 1434–1439.

Black, D. W., Arndt, S., Coryell, W. H., Argo, T., Forbush, K. T., Shaw, M. C., Perry, P., & Allen, J. (2007). Bupropion in the treatment of pathological gambling: a randomized, double-blind, placebo-controlled, flexible-dose study. *Journal of Clinical Psychopharmacology, 27,* 143–150.

Blanco, C., Petkova, E., Ibanez, A., & Saiz-Ruiz, J. (2002). A pilot placebo-controlled study of fluvoxamine for pathological gambling. *Annals of Clinical Psychiatry, 14,* 9–15.

Blanco, C., Grant, J. E., Petry, N. M., Simpson, H. B., Alegria, A., Liu, S., & Hasin, D. (2008). Prevalence and correlates of shoplifting in the United States: results from the National Epidemiologic Survey on Alcohol and Related Conditions (NESARC). *American Journal of Psychiatry, 165*(7), 905–913.

Blinn-Pike, L., Worth, S. L., & Jonkman, J. N. (2007). Disordered gambling among college students: a meta-analytic synthesis. *Journal of Gambling Studies, 23*(2), 175–183.

Bohne, A., Wilhelm, S., & Keuthen, N. (2005). Grooming disorders: Pathologic hair pulling, skin picking, and nail biting. *Annals of Clinical Psychiatry, 17*(4), 227–232.

Carnes, P. (1983). *Out of the shadows: Understanding sexual addiction.* Minneapolis, MN: CompCare Publishers.

Chambers, R. A., & Potenza, M. N. (2003). Neurodevelopment, impulsivity, and adolescent gambling. *Journal of Gambling Studies, 19,* 53–84.

Chambers, R. A., Taylor, J. R., & Potenza, M. N. (2003). Developmental neurocircuitry of motivation in adolescence: A critical period of addiction vulnerability. *American Journal of Psychiatry, 160,* 1041–1052.

Christenson, G. A., Faber, R. J., de Zwaan, M., Raymond, N. C., Specker, S. M., Ekern, M. D., Mackenzie, T. B., Crosby, R. D., Crow, S. J., Eckert, E. D. (1994a). Compulsive buying: Descriptive characteristics and psychiatric comorbidity. *Journal of Clinical Psychiatry, 55,* 5–11.

Christenson, G. A., Mackenzie, T. B., & Mitchell, J. E. (1991a). Characteristics of 60 adult chronic hair pullers. *American Journal of Psychiatry, 148,* 365–370.

Christenson, G. A., Mackenzie, T. B., & Mitchell, J. E. (1994b). Adult men and women with trichotillomania. A comparison of male and female characteristics. *Psychosomatics, 35,* 142–149.

Christenson, G. A., & Mansueto, C. S. (1999). Trichotillomania: Descriptive characteristics and phenomenology. In D. J. Stein, G. A. Christenson, & E. Hollander (Eds.), *Trichotillomania* (pp. 1–42). Washington, DC: American Psychiatric Publishing.

Christenson, G. A., Pyle, R. L., & Mitchell, J. E. (1991b). Estimated lifetime prevalence of trichotillomania in college students. *Journal of Clinical Psychiatry, 52,* 415–417.

Coccaro, E. F., Schmidt, C. A., Samuels, J. F., Nestadt G. (2004). Lifetime and 1-month prevalence rates of intermittent explosive disorder in a community sample. *Journal of Clinical Psychiatry, 65,* 820–824.

Coccaro, E.F., Danehy, M. (2006). Intermittent explosive disorder. In E. Hollander, & D. J. Stein (Eds.), *Clinical Manual of Impulse Control Disorders* (pp. 19–37). Washington, DC: American Psychiatric Publishing.

Cohen, L. J., Stein, D. J., Simeon, D., Spadaccini, E., Rosen, J., Aronowitz, B., Hollander, E. (1995). Clinical profile, comorbidity, and treatment history in 123 hair pullers: A survey study. *Journal of Clinical Psychiatry, 56,* 319–326.

Coleman, E. (1992). Is your patient suffering from compulsive sexual behavior? *Psychiatry Annals, 22,* 320–325.

Coleman, E., Gratzer, T., Nesvacil, L., Raymond, N, C., (2000). Nefazodone and the treatment of nonparaphilic compulsive sexual behavior: a retrospective study. *Journal of Clinical Psychiatry, 61,* 282–284.

Crockford, D. N., & el-Guebaly, N. (1998). Psychiatric comorbidity in pathological gambling: A critical review. *Canadian Journal of Psychiatry, 43,* 43–50.

Cunningham-Williams, R. M., Cottler, L. B., Compton, W. M. 3rd, Spitznagel, E. L. (1998). Taking chances: Problem gamblers and mental health disorders—Results from the St. Louis Epidemiologic Catchment Area Study. *American Journal of Public Health, 88,* 1093–1096.

Cunningham-Williams, R. M., Grucza, R. A., Cottler, L. B., Womack, S. B., Books, S. J., Przybeck, T. R., Spitznagel, E. L., Cloninger, C. R. (2005). Prevalence and predictors of pathological gambling: results from the St. Louis personality, health and lifestyle (SLPHL) study. *Journal of Psychiatric Research, 39*(4), 377–390.

Desai, R. A., Maciejewski, P. K., Pantalon, M. V., Potenza, M. N. (2005). Gender differences in adolescent gambling. *Annals of Clinical Psychiatry, 17,* 249–258.

Engwall, D., Hunter, R., Steinberg, M. (2004).Gambling and other risk behaviors on university campuses. *Journal of American College Health, 52,* 245–255.

Fiorillo, C. D., Tobler, P. N., & Schultz, W. (2003). Discrete coding of reward probability and uncertainty by dopamine neurons. *Science, 299,* 1898–1902.

Galovski, T., Blanchard, E. B., & Veazey, C. (2002). Intermittent explosive disorder and other psychiatric comorbidity among court-referred and self-referred aggressive drivers. *Behavior Research and Therapy, 40,* 641–651.

Goldman, M. (1991). Kleptomania: Making sense of the nonsensical. *American Journal of Psychiatry, 148,* 986–996.

Goodman, A. (1993). What's in a name? Terminology for designating a syndrome of driven sexual behavior. *Sexual Addiction and Compulsivity, 8,* 191–213.

Graber, J., & Atndt, W. B. (1993). Trichotillomania. *Comprehensive Psychiatry, 34,* 340–346.

Grant, J. E. (2003). Family history and psychiatric comorbidity in persons with kleptomania. *Comprehensive Psychiatry, 44,* 437–441.

Grant, J. E., & Kim, S. W. (2001a). Demographic and clinical features of 131 adult pathological gamblers. *Journal of Clinical Psychiatry, 62,* 957–962.

Grant, J. E., & Kim, S. W. (2001b). A case of kleptomania and compulsive sexual behavior treated with naltrexone. *Annals of Clinical Psychiatry, 13,* 229–231.

Grant, J. E., & Kim, S. W. (2002a). Gender differences in pathological gamblers seeking medication treatment. *Comprehensive Psychiatry, 43,* 56–62.

Grant, J. E., & Kim, S. W. (2002b). Clinical characteristics and associated psychopathology of 22 patients with kleptomania. *Comprehensive Psychiatry, 43,* 378–384.

Grant, J. E., & Kim, S. W. (2002c). An open label study of naltrexone in the treatment of kleptomania. *Journal of Clinical Psychiatry, 63,* 349–356.

Grant, J. E., & Kim, S. W. (2003). Comorbidity of impulse control disorders in pathological gamblers. *Acta Psychiatrica Scandinavica, 108,* 207–213.

Grant, J. E., Kim, S. W., Hollander, E., & Potenza, M. N. (2008). Predicting response to opiate antagonists and placebo in the treatment of pathological gambling. *Psychopharmacology (Berl) 200*(4), 521–527.

Grant, J. E., Kim, S. W., Potenza, M. N., Blanco, C., Ibanez, A., Stevens, L., Hektner, J. M., & Zaninelli, R. (2003). Paroxetine treatment of pathological gambling: multi-center randomized controlled trial. *International Clinical Psychopharmacology, 18,* 243–249.

Grant, J. E., Kushner, M. G., & Kim, S. W. (2002). Pathological gambling and alcohol use disorder. *Alcohol Research and Health, 26,* 143–150.

Grant, J. E., Levine, L., Kim, D., et al. (2005). Impulse control disorders in adult psychiatric inpatients. *American Journal of Psychiatry, 162,* 2184–2188.

Grant, J. E., & Potenza, M. N. (2004). Impulse control disorders: Clinical characteristics and pharmacological management. *Annals of Clinical Psychiatry, 16,* 27–34.

Grant, J. E., & Potenza, M. N. (2006). Escitalopram in the treatment of pathological gambling with co-occurring anxiety: An open-label study with double-blind discontinuation. *International Clinical Psychopharmacology, 21,* 203–209.

Grant, J. E., Potenza, M. N., Hollander, E., Cunningham-Williams, R., Nurminen, T., Smits, G., & Kallio, A. (2006). A multicenter investigation of the opioid antagonist nalmefene in the treatment of pathological gambling. *American Journal of Psychiatry, 163,* 303–312.

Grant, J. E., & Kim, S. W. (2007). Clinical characteristics and psychiatric comorbidity of pyromania. *Journal of Clinical Psychiatry, 68,* 1717–1722.

Grant, J. E., Williams, K. A., & Potenza, M. N. (2007). Impulse control disorders in adolescent psychiatric inpatients: co-occurring disorders and sex differences. *Journal of Clinical Psychiatry, 68,* 1584–1592.

Grant, J. E., Kim S. W., & Hartman B. K. (2008). A double-blind, placebo-controlled study of the opiate antagonist naltrexone in the treatment of pathological gambling urges. *Journal of Clinical Psychiatry, 69*(5), 783–789.

Grant, J. E., Kim, S. W., Odlaug, B. L. (2009). A double-blind, placebo-controlled trial of the opioid antagonist, naltrexone, in the treatment of kleptomania. *Biological Psychiatry, 65*(7), 600–606.

Grant, J. E., Donahue, C. J., Odlaug, B. L., Kim, S. W., Miller, M. J., & Petry, N. M. Imaginal desensitization plus motivational interviewing in the treatment of pathological gambling: a randomized controlled trial. *British Journal of Psychiatry.* (in press).

Gupta, R., & Derevensky, J. L. (1998). Adolescent gambling behavior: A prevalence study and examination of the correlates associated with problem gambling. *Journal of Gambling Studies, 14,* 319–345.

Hodgins, D. C., Currie, S. R., & el-Guebaly, N. (2001). Motivational enhancement and self-help treatments for problem gambling. *Journal of Consulting and Clinical Psychology, 69,* 50–57.

Hodgins, D. C., & Petry, N. M. (2004). Cognitive and behavioral treatments. In J. E. Grant & M. N. Potenza (Eds.)., *Pathological gambling: A clinical guide to treatment.* Washington, DC: APPI.

Hollander, E., DeCaria, C. M., Finkell, J. N., Begaz, T., Wong, C. M., Cartwright, C. (2000). A randomized double-blind fluvoxamine/placebo crossover trial in pathological gambling. *Biological Psychiatry, 47,* 813–817.

Hollander, E., Frenkel, M., DeCaria, C., Trungold, S., Stein, D. J. (1992). Treatment of pathological gambling with clomipramine. *American Journal of Psychiatry, 149,* 710–711.

Hollander, E., Pallanti, S., Allen, A., Sood, E., Baldini Rossi, N. (2005). Does sustained-release lithium reduce impulsive gambling and affective instability versus placebo in pathological gamblers with bipolar spectrum disorders? *American Journal of Psychiatry, 162,* 137–145.

Hudson, J. I., Pope, H. G., Jr., Jonas, J. M., et al. (1983). Phenomenologic relationship of eating disorders to major affective disorder. *Psychiatry Research, 9,* 345–354.

Ibanez, A., Blanco, C., Donahue, E., Lesieur, H. R., Pérez de Castro, I., Fernández-Piqueras, J., Sáiz-Ruiz, J. (2001). Psychiatric comorbidity in pathological gamblers seeking treatment. *American Journal of Psychiatry, 158,* 1733–1735.

Kafka, M. P., & Prentky, R. (1992). Fluoxetine treatment of nonparaphilic sexual addictions and paraphilias in men. *Journal of Clinical Psychiatry, 53,* 351–358.

Kafka, M. P., & Prentky, R. (1994). Preliminary observations of DSM-III-R Axis I comorbidity in men with paraphilias and paraphilia-related disorders. *Journal of Clinical Psychiatry, 55,* 481–487.

Kessler, R. C., Coccaro, E. F., Fava, M., Jaeger, S., Jin, R., Walters, E. (2006). The prevalence and correlates of DSM-IV Intermittent Explosive Disorder in the National Comorbidity Survey Replication. *Archives of General Psychiatry, 63,* 669–678.

Kim, S. W., Grant, J. E., Adson, D. E., Shin, Y. C. (2001). Double-blind naltrexone and placebo comparison study in the treatment of pathological gambling. *Biological Psychiatry, 49,* 914–921.

Kim, S. W., Grant, J. E., Adson, D. E., Shin, Y. C., Zaninelli, R. (2002). A double-blind, placebo-controlled study of the efficacy and safety of paroxetine in the treatment of pathological gambling disorder. *Journal of Clinical Psychiatry, 63,* 501–507.

King, R. A., Scahill, L., Vitulano, L. A., Schwab-Stone, M., Tercyak, K. P., Jr., & Riddle, M. A. (1995). Childhood trichotillomania: clinical phenomenology, comorbidity, and family genetics. *Journal of the American Academy of Child and Adolescent Psychiatry, 34*(11), 1451–1459.

Koran, L. M., Bullock, K. D., Hartston, H. J., Elliott, M. A., D'Andrea, V. (2002). Citalopram treatment of compulsive shopping: an open-label study. *Journal of Clinical Psychiatry, 63,* 704–708.

Koran, L. M., Chuong, H. W., Bullock, K. D., Smith, S. C. (2003). Citalopram for compulsive shopping disorder: an open-label study followed by double-blind discontinuation. *Journal of Clinical Psychiatry, 64,* 793–798.

Koran, L.M., Faber, R. J., Aboujaoude, E., Large, M. D., Serpe, R. T. (2006). Estimated prevalence of compulsive buying behavior in the United States. *American Journal of Psychiatry, 163*(10), 1806–1812.

Koran, L. M., Aboujaoude, E. N., Gamel, N. N. (2007). Escitalopram treatment of kleptomania: an open-label trial followed by double-blind discontinuation. *Journal of Clinical Psychiatry, 68*(3), 422–427.

Koran, L. M., Aboujaoude, E. N., Solvason, B., Gamel, N. N., Smith, E. H. (2007). Escitalopram for compulsive buying disorder: a double-blind discontinuation study. *Journal of Clinical Psychopharmacology, 27*(2), 225–227.

Laucht, M., Becker, K., El-Faddagh, M., Hohm, E., Schmidt, M. H. (2005). Association of the DRD4 exon III polymorphism with smoking in fifteen-year-olds: A mediating role for novelty seeking? *Journal of the American Academy of Child and Adolescent Psychiatry, 44,* 477–484.

Lejoyeux, M., Arbaretaz, M., McLoughlin, M., Adès, J. (2002). Impulse control disorders and depression. *Journal of Nervous and Mental Disease, 190,* 310–314.

Lejoyeux, M., Feuche, N., Loi, S., Solomon, J., Adès, J. (1999). Study of impulse-control disorders among alcohol-dependent patients. *Journal of Clinical Psychiatry, 60,* 302–305.

Lindberg, N., Holi, M. M., Tani, P., Virkkunen, M. (2005). Looking for pyromania: characteristics of a consecutive sample of Finnish male criminals with histories of recidivist fire-setting between 1973 and 1993. *BMC Psychiatry 5,* 47 [letter]

Linden, R. D., Pope, H. G., & Jonas, J. M. (1986). Pathological gambling and major affective disorder:

Preliminary findings. *Journal of Clinical Psychiatry, 47,* 201–203.

Lynch, W. J., Maciejewski, P. K., & Potenza, M. N. (2004). Psychiatric correlates of gambling in adolescents and young adults grouped by age at gambling onset. *Archives of General Psychiatry, 61*(11), 1116–1122.

McConaghy, N., Armstrong, M. S., Blaszczynski, A., Allcock, C. (1983). Controlled comparison of aversive therapy and imaginal desensitization in compulsive gambling. *British Journal of Psychiatry, 142,* 366–372.

McConaghy, N., Armstrong, M. S., & Blaszczynski, A. (1985). Expectancy, covert sensitization and imaginal desensitization in compulsive sexuality. *Acta Psychiatrica Scandinavica, 72,* 176–187.

McConaghy, N., Blaszczynski, A., & Frankova, A. (1991). Comparison of imaginal desensitization with other behavioural treatments of pathological gambling: A two to nine year follow-up. *British Journal of Psychiatry, 159,* 390–393.

McCormick, R. A., Russo, A. M., Rameriz, L. F., Taber, J. I. (1984). Affective disorders among pathological gamblers seeking treatment. *American Journal of Psychiatry, 41,* 215–218.

McElroy, S. L., Hudson, J. I., Pope, H. G., Keck, P. E. Jr., Aizley, H. G. (1992). The DSM-III-R impulse control disorders not elsewhere classified: Clinical characteristics and relationship to other psychiatric disorders. *American Journal of Psychiatry, 149,* 318–327.

McElroy, S. L., Keck, P. E., Pope, H. G., Smith, J. M., Strakowski, S. M. (1994). Compulsive buying: A report of 20 cases. *Journal of Clinical Psychiatry, 55,* 242–248.

McElroy, S. L., Pope, H. G., Hudson, J. I., Keck, P. E. (1991). Kleptomania: A report of 20 cases. *American Journal of Psychiatry, 148,* 652–657.

McElroy, S. L., Soutullo, C. A., Beckman, D. A., Taylor, P. Jr., Keck, P. E. Jr. (1998). DSM-IV intermittent explosive disorder: A report of 27 cases. *Journal of Clinical Psychiatry, 59,* 203–210.

McElroy, S. L., Nelson, E. B., Welge, J. A., Kaehler, L., Keck, P. E. Jr. (2008). Olanzapine in the treatment of pathological gambling: a negative randomized placebo-controlled trial. *Journal of Clinical Psychiatry, 69*(3), 433–440.

Ninan, P. T., McElroy, S. L., Kane, C. P., Knight, B. T., Casuto, L. S., Rose, S.E., Marsteller, F. A., Nemeroff, C. B. (2000a). Placebo-controlled study of fluvoxamine in the treatment of patients with compulsive buying. *Journal of Clinical Psychopharmacology, 20,* 362–366.

Ninan, P. T., Rothbaum, B. O., Marsteller, F. A., Knight, B. T., Eccard, M. B. (2000b). A placebo-controlled trial of cognitive-behavioral therapy and clomipramine in trichotillomania. *Journal of Clinical Psychiatry, 61,* 47–50.

Odlaug, B. L., & Grant, J. E. (2008). Prevalence of impulse control disorders in a college sample. *New Research Program and Abstracts, 161st Annual Meeting of the American Psychiatric Association (NR2-069).* Washington, DC [poster].

Olvera, R. L. (2002). Intermittent explosive disorder: Epidemiology, diagnosis and management. *CNS Drugs, 16,* 517–526.

O'Sullivan, R. L., Christenson, G. A., & Stein, D. J. (1999). Pharmacotherapy of trichotillomania. In D. J. Stein, G. A. Christensen, & E. Hollander (Eds.), *Trichotillomania* (pp. 93–123). Washington, DC: American Psychiatric Publishing.

Petry, N. M. (2002). A comparison of young, middle-aged, and older adult treatment-seeking pathological gamblers. *The Gerontologist, 42,* 92–99.

Petry, N. M. (2005). *Pathological gambling: Etiology, comorbidity, and treatment.* Washington, DC: American Psychological Association.

Petry, N. M., Stinson, F. S., & Grant, B. F. (2005). Co-morbidity of DSM-IV pathological gambling and other psychiatric disorders: Results from the National Epidemiologic Survey on Alcohol and Related Conditions. *Journal of Clinical Psychiatry, 66,* 564–574.

Petry, N. M., Ammerman, Y., Bohl, J., Doersch, A., Gay, H., Kadden, R., Molina, C., & Steinberg, K. (2006). Cognitive-behavioral therapy for pathological gamblers. *Journal of Consulting and Clinical Psychology, 74*(3), 555–567.

Potenza, M. N., & Hollander, E. (2002). Pathological gambling and impulse control disorders. In J. T. Coyle, C. Nemeroff, D. Charney, & K. L. Davis (Eds.), *Neuropsychopharmacology: The fifth generation of progress* (pp. 1725–1741). Baltimore: Lippincott Williams and Wilkins.

Proimos, J., DuRant, R. H., Pierce, J. D., & Goodman E. (1998). Gambling and other risk behaviors among 8th- to 12th-grade students. *Journal of Pediatrics, 102,* e23.

Quadland, M. C. (1985). Compulsive sexual behavior: Definition of a problem and an approach to treatment. *Journal of Sex Marital Therapy, 11,* 121–132.

Raymond, N. C., Coleman, E., & Miner, M. H. (2003). Psychiatric comorbidity and compulsive/impulsive traits in compulsive sexual behavior. *Comprehensive Psychiatry, 44,* 370–380.

Raymond, N. C., Grant, J. E., Kim, S. W., Coleman, E. (2002). Treatment of compulsive sexual behavior with naltrexone and serotonin reuptake inhibitors. *International Clinical Psychopharmacology, 17,* 201–205.

Reeve, E. A., Bernstein, G. A., Christenson, G. A. (1992). Clinical characteristics and psychiatric comorbidity in children with trichotillomania. *Journal of the American Academy of Child and Adolescent Psychiatry 31*(1),132–138.

Romer, D. (Ed.) (2003). *Reducing adolescent risk: Toward an integrated approach.* Thousand Oaks, CA: Sage.

Rothbaum, B. O., Shaw, L., Morris, R., & Ninan, P. T. (1993). Prevalence of trichotillomania in a college freshman population. *Journal of Clinical Psychiatry, 54*(2), 72–73.

Roy, A., Ardinoff, B., Roehrich, L., Lamparski, D., Custer, R., Lorenz, V., Barbaccia, M., Guidotti, A., Costa, E., Linnoila, M. (1988). Pathological gambling: A psychobiological study. *Archives of General Psychiatry, 45,* 369–373.

Saiz-Ruiz, J., Blanco, C., Ibanez, A., Masramon, X., Gómez, M. M., Madrigal, M., Díez T. (2005). Sertraline treatment of pathological gambling: A pilot study. *Journal of Clinical Psychiatry, 66,* 28–33.

Schlosser, S., Black, D. W., Repertinger, S., Goldstein, R. B. (1994). Compulsive buying: Demography, phenomenology, and comorbidity in 46 subjects. *General Hospital Psychiatry, 16,* 205–212.

Shaffer, H. J., LaBrie, R., Scanlan, K. M., & Cummings, T. N. (1994). Pathological gambling among adolescents: Massachusetts gambling screen (MAGS). *Journal of Gambling Studies, 10*(4), 339–362.

Shaffer, H. J., & Hall, M. N. (1996). Estimating the prevalence of adolescent gambling disorders: A quantitative synthesis and guide toward standard gambling nomenclature. *Journal of Gambling Studies, 12*(2), 193–214.

Shaffer, H. J., Hall, M. N., & Vander B. ilt., J. (1999). Estimating the prevalence of disordered gambling behavior in the United States and Canada: A research synthesis. *American Journal of Public Health, 89,* 1369–1376.

Shah, K. R., Eisen, S. A., Xian, H., et al. (2005). Genetic studies of pathological gambling: A review of methodology and analyses of data from the Vietnam Era Twin (VET) Registery. *Journal of Gambling Studies, 21,* 179–203.

Slutske, W. S., Eisen, S., True, W. R., et al. (2000). Common genetic vulnerability for pathological gambling and alcohol dependence in men. *Archives of General Psychiatry, 57,* 666–673.

Specker, S. M., Carlson, G. A, Christenson, G. A., Marcotte, M. (1995). Impulse control disorders and attention deficit disorder in pathological gamblers. *Annals of Clinical Psychiatry, 7*(4), 175–179.

Stein, D. J., Hollander, E., Anthony, D. T., et al. (1992). Serotonergic medications for sexual obsessions, sexual addictions, and paraphilias. *Journal of Clinical Psychiatry, 53,* 267–271.

Stinchfield, R. (2001). A comparison of gambling among Minnesota public school students in 1992, 1995 and 1998. *Journal of Gambling Studies, 17,* 273–296.

Swedo, S. E., & Leonard, H. L. (1992). Trichotillomania: An obsessive compulsive spectrum disorder? *Psychiatric Clinics of North America, 15,* 777–790.

Takushi, R. Y., Neighbors, C., Larimer, M. E., Lostutter, T. W., Cronce, J. M., & Marlatt, G. A. (2004). Indicated prevention of problem gambling among college students. *Journal of Gambling Studies, 20*(1), 83–93.

Tay, Y. K., Levy, M. L., & Metry, D. W. (2004). Trichotillomania in childhood: Case series and review. *Pediatrics, 113,* e494–498.

Tsuang, M. T., Bar, J. L., Harley, R. M., et al. (2001). The Harvard Twin Study of Substance Abuse: What we have learned. *Harvard Review of Psychiatry, 9,* 267–279.

van Ameringen, M., Mancini, C., Patterson, B., Bennett, M., & Oakman, J. (2006). A randomized placebo controlled trial of olanzapine in trichotillomania. *European Neuropsychopharmacology, 16*(Suppl 4), p. S452. Papers of the 19th ECNP Congress, Paris, France: September 16–20, [poster].

van Minnen, A., Hoogduin, K. A., Keijsers, G. P., Hellenbrand, I., & Hendriks, G. J. (2003). Treatment of trichotillomania with behavioral therapy or fluoxetine: a randomized, waiting-list controlled study. *Archives of General Psychiatry, 60*(5), 517–522.

Wagner, F. A., & Anthony, J. C. (2002). From first drug use to drug dependence: Developmental periods of risk for dependence upon marijuana, cocaine, and alcohol. *Neuropsychopharmacology, 26,* 479–488.

Wainberg, M. L., Muench, F., Morgenstern, J., Hollander, E., Irwin, T. W., Parsons, J. T., Allen, A., & O'Leary, A. (2006). A double-blind study of citalopram versus placebo in the treatment of compulsive sexual behaviors in gay and bisexual men. *Journal of Clinical Psychiatry, 67*(12), 1968–1973.

Wallisch, L. (1993). *Gambling in Texas: 1992 Texas survey of adolescent gambling behavior.* Austin, TX: Texas Commission on Alcohol and Drug Abuse.

Weinstock, J., & Petry, N. M. (2006). Pathological gambling college students' perceived social support. *Journal of College Student Development, 49,* 625–632.

Welte, J., Barnes, G., Wieczorek, W., Tidwell, M. C., & Parker, J. (2001). Alcohol and gambling pathology among U.S. adults: prevalence, demographic patterns and comorbidity. *Journal of Studies on Alcohol, 62*(5), 706–712.

Woods, D. W., Wetterneck, C. T., & Flessner, C. A. (2006). A controlled evaluation of acceptance and commitment therapy plus habit reversal for trichotillomania. *Behaviour Research and Therapy, 44*(5), 639–656.

Chapter 21

Attention-Deficit/Hyperactivity Disorder in Young Adults

Joel V. Oberstar and George M. Realmuto

A 22-year-old college sophomore presents to the college health service for evaluation after having just broken up with a girlfriend of several months. He complains of being unable to maintain long-term relationships. He is feeling depressed and is in danger of flunking out of school because his grade point average is now below the college's acceptable standard.

A review of his depressive symptoms includes transient suicidal ideation with a lethal plan but neither intention nor means. The young man notes sleep disturbance with increased activity before bedtime and delayed bedtime but rapid sleep onset. He also has periods of sleepiness during the day and fatigue with high consumption of caffeinated beverages. Also noted are low energy and low productivity with failure to complete school reports and course requirements. Common behaviors include missed classes due to oversleeping, forgetting, or double-booking. He feels bored with some anhedonia. He has no difficulty with appetite, libido, or withdrawal/isolation.

On further questioning, it becomes clear that many of these symptoms have been chronic. For example, he always had difficulty setting a standard bedtime. He generally did well in school prior to college, especially in classes that utilized his considerable creativity and ingenuity. However, when teachers were very rigid and uninspiring, he became bored and either dropped out of the class or just barely got by. One of the ways he was most successful was by working with a study partner. His sister is a fraternal twin and they often studied together; he depended upon her to have the books necessary to do the assignments, as he would often forget them at school. She is attending a different college and this is the first time he has been without her assistance in school.

Prior to the present episode of illness, he did not have a history of depression. His peer relationships were unique in that his friends were risk takers, choosing sports like parachuting and bungee jumping. Many of his friends have been in chemical dependency treatment. After several episodes of binge drinking and marijuana use, his parents became quite concerned. With the use of strictly applied consequences for use, monitoring with home drug testing kits, expectation for change in friendships by excluding substance-abusing friends, and affiliating with his sister's more prosocial friends, he avoided the more severe problems associated with chemical abuse.

His family history is positive for depression on maternal side. He has a paternal uncle who died of circumstances that may have been related to a drug overdose. Another paternal uncle is characterized as being chronically underemployed; a paternal aunt is divorced and suffers from depression. The young man's father is a very successful salesman who is described as being "type A" and chronically overextended. His mother is a registered nurse who likes to read and was very successful in college but did not pursue a potential doctoral degree.

Further review of systems revealed a pattern of symptoms that included poor task completion, missed assignments, a history of multiple interests that were never pursued very far, and parents' frequent complaints about his messy room and uncompleted chores. In the time since obtaining his driver's license, he has had three automobile accidents, each described as fender benders related to carelessness. He has been criticized by his friends who claim he is too impatient but is also never on time, leaving them waiting often. He is always overcommitted and when given time to relax feels uncomfortable and chooses to do very active recreational activities like mountain biking. He recently had a fall while biking and sustained a broken wrist. This is his second such accident in the past 2 years.

Historical Perspective of Attention-Deficit/Hyperactivity Disorder

The concept of an adult manifestation of attention-deficit/hyperactivity disorder (ADHD) is over 35 years old. Its foremost proponent is Paul Wender, a pioneer researcher of the persistence of ADHD into adulthood. He published descriptions, proposed age-related symptom clusters, developed rating scales, and described the comorbid and psychosocial adversities of individuals with ADHD as they would appear in the adult age group. He was not proposing that ADHD was a late emerging disorder. Adults with ADHD would have shown typical symptoms in childhood true to the view that ADHD is a neurodevelopmental disorder. However, many children with ADHD are not diagnosed, requiring the clinician working with a young adult to make a retrospective diagnosis of the presence of the disorder at an early age. He also emphasized the presence of comorbid difficulties, including mood and irritability problems in adulthood that are different than and not related to mood disorders such as major depressive disorder (Wender, 2000).

Epidemiology and Etiology

ADHD is among the most common mental illnesses in children and adolescents, with prevalence estimates in this population ranging from 3%–6% (Sheehan, Hawi, Gill, & Kent, 2007). Males with ADHD tend to outnumber females. Symptoms of the illness typically appear early in life and often persist into adulthood. It was recently estimated that ADHD affects 2%–6% of adults (Weiss & Murray, 2003). The illness is marked by deficits in attention, hyperactivity, and impulsivity. While the precise etiology of the illness has yet to be elucidated, neuroimaging data suggest abnormal functioning in the prefrontal cortex and/or the frontostriatal networks of the brain (Durston, 2003). There is compelling evidence that both environmental and genetic factors contribute to ADHD. Indeed, family and twin studies have estimated heritability between 60% and 90% (Levy, Hay, McStephen, Wood, & Waldman, 1997; Thapar, Holmes, Poulton, & Harrington, 1999).

Recent research has sought to elucidate more precisely the genetic determinants of ADHD. Specific attention has been paid to the dopamine transporter (Mazei-Robinson & Blakely, 2006). Recent research (Lott, Kim, Cook, & de Wit, 2005) on the dopamine transporter gene (DAT1) demonstrated that of three genotypes studied, two carried with them a subjective response to acute amphetamine ingestion, while one of the three genotypes produced a subjective response similar to that generated with placebo ingestion (i.e., no response). A similar study, however, demonstrated no association with DAT1 and the response to or tolerability of methylphenidate (Mick, Biederman, Spencer, Faraone, & Sklar, 2006).

Additional studies have focused on other biochemical markers, including tryptophan hydroxylase 2 (Sheehan et al., 2007), the dopamine D_4 receptor (Mill et al., 2002), dopamine beta hydroxylase (Smith et al., 2003), serotonin transporter intron-2 (Banerjee et al., 2006), and the nicotinic-cholinergic system (Wilens, Verlinden, Adler, Wozniak, & West, 2006). Such studies will hopefully lead to an increased understanding of the biochemical underpinnings of ADHD and, perhaps, additional pharmacological treatment options for the illness.

Clinical Presentation and Impact of Illness

Adults suffering from ADHD present with many symptoms similar to those exhibited by children and adolescents with the condition, including inattention, distractibility, disorganization, and impulsivity. One study demonstrated that adults with ADHD had significantly less education than matched community controls (Murphy, Barkley, & Bush, 2002). Additionally, they were less likely to have graduated from college. Other researchers have demonstrated that adults with ADHD have deficits in executive functioning, including verbal fluency, inhibition, and set shifting (Boonstra, Oosterlaan, Sergeant, & Buitelaar, 2005). Researchers have also shown that adults with ADHD may exhibit deficits in nonexecutive function domains such as consistency of response, word reading, and color naming (Boonstra et al., 2005).

Adults with ADHD may also display impairments in driving similar to teens with the disorder. Barkley and colleagues showed that young adults were more likely than peers without ADHD to have had their driving licenses suspended or revoked, to have received repeated traffic violations (speeding in particular), and to be nearly four times more likely to have had an accident while driving (Barkley, Guevremont, Anastopoulos, DuPaul, & Shelton, 1993). Other functional and psychosocial impairments are common among adults with ADHD. Secnik and colleagues found that adults with ADHD tended to miss more days from work for "unofficial" absences; those with ADHD also had significantly higher utilization of outpatient and inpatient resources as well as prescription drug costs (Secnik, Swensen, & Lage, 2005). Adults with ADHD are more likely to be unemployed (Mulsow, O'Neal, & Murry, 2001; Seidman, Biederman, Weber, Hatch, & Faraone, 1998). Those that are employed are more likely to quit their jobs, to change employment, or to perform poorly at work when compared to matched controls (Murphy & Barkley, 1996; Selke, 2000). Gunter and colleagues found that ADHD conferred a risk for adult illegal behavior and arrest (Gunter, Arndt, Riggins-Caspers, Wenman, & Cadoret, 2006). Additionally, adults with ADHD have been found to test lower than non-ADHD adults on the Wechsler Adult Intelligence Scale, though the authors concluded that the difference was small and not thought to be clinically meaningful (Bridgett & Walker, 2006).

Attention-Deficit/Hyperactivity Disorder and Comorbid Conditions

Individuals with ADHD often suffer from one or more comorbid conditions. McGough and colleagues found that 87% of individuals with ADHD they studied had at least one additional psychiatric condition (as compared to 64% of non-ADHD subjects; McGough et al., 2005). In this same sample, 56% of the adults with ADHD had at least two additional psychiatric disorders, compared with only 27% of non-ADHD adults. In 2007, Frazier and colleagues found that adults with ADHD had higher rates of asthma, anxiety, bipolar disorder, depression, drug or alcohol abuse, antisocial personality, and oppositionality as compared to non-ADHD controls (Frazier, Youngstrom, Glutting, & Watkins, 2007). Similar results were observed by Shekim and colleagues, who assessed 51 clinically referred adults and found high rates of lifetime comorbidity: 51% had generalized anxiety disorder, 34% had alcohol abuse or dependence, 34% had other substance abuse or dependence, 25% had dysthymia, 18% had separation anxiety disorder, 13% had obsessive-compulsive disorder, and 10% had major depressive disorder (Shekim, Asarnow, Hess, Zaucha, & Wheeler, 1990).

A number of studies have explored the differences in comorbidity among the different ADHD subtypes (i.e., combined type, predominantly inattentive type, or predominantly hyperactive-impulsive type). Millstein and colleagues found higher rates of oppositional defiant disorder, bipolar disorder, and substance use disorders among patients with ADHD-combined type as compared with individuals with other subtypes of the illness (Millstein, Wilens, Biederman, & Spencer, 1997). Individuals with the hyperactive-impulsive type had higher rates of oppositional defiant disorder, OCD, and PTSD than those in with ADHD-inattentive type. Another study, however, failed to elucidate differences in anxiety, depression, or conduct disorder among types of ADHD (Murphy et al., 2002). Reimherr and colleagues found that adults with ADHD but without a comorbid anxiety/depressive diagnosis still exhibited features of emotional dysregulation (Reimherr et al., 2005). Interestingly, another study found that individuals without a formal diagnosis of ADHD but scoring positive on the Adult ADHD Self-Report Scale (ASRS) manifested higher rates of depression, problem drinking, lower educational attainment, and greater emotional and interpersonal difficulties than matched controls (no diagnosis of ADHD and scoring negative on the ASRS; Able, Johnston, Adler, & Swindle, 2007).

ADHD comorbid with substance use disorders also has been the focus of a variety of studies. A group of 101 hyperkinetic boys compared to nonhyperactive comparators exhibited higher rates of conduct disorder and nonalcoholic substance use disorders at early-adult follow-up (Mannuzza, Klein, Bessler, Malloy, & LaPadula, 1993). Overall, higher rates of antisocial behavior and substance use disorders appear to be relatively consistent findings among studies of youth with ADHD followed-up in adulthood (McGough et al., 2005). Interestingly, in evaluating a group of 435 parents of children with ADHD who had ADHD themselves, McGough and colleagues found that ADHD itself was not a significant risk factor for substance use disorders if male gender, disruptive behavior disorders, and socioeconomic status were controlled (McGough et al., 2005). Molina and colleagues found that childhood ADHD predicted heavy drinking, drunkenness, alcohol use disorder symptoms, and alcohol use disorders in 15- to 17-year-old adolescents but not for 11–14 year olds (Molina, Pelham, Gnagy, Thompson, & Marshal, 2007). Childhood ADHD did not predict young adult (18–25 year olds) drinking/alcohol use disorders. The authors note that heavy drinking in this age group was typical regardless of ADHD history. Conduct disorder and antisocial personality disorder were predictive of problem drinking for both adolescents and young adults.

Diagnosis of Attention-Deficit/Hyperactivity Disorder in Young Adults

As with many psychiatric conditions, the diagnosis of ADHD in a young adult remains a clinical diagnosis (McGough & Barkley, 2004). In making the diagnosis, the clinician must conduct a thorough psychiatric evaluation, focusing in particular on the core symptoms of ADHD (Greenhill et al., 2002). Collateral information from a parent, spouse or significant other, or alternate source is strongly recommended, as adults with ADHD may have poor insight into and/or underestimate the severity of their illness (Greenhill et al., 2002). Additionally, the patient may not be able to recall symptoms evident in childhood. There exists some controversy within the psychiatric community regarding the stringent application of DSM-IV-TR criterion B, which requires "some hyperactive-impulsive or inattentive symptoms [causing] impairment [be] present before age 7 years" (American Psychiatric Association, 2000). Patients may not be able to offer a clear history of symptoms at that age; some clinicians advocate broadening the age limit to consider symptoms presenting before age 12 years sufficient to meet this diagnostic criterion (McGough & Barkley, 2004).

The clinical interview should also include exploration of symptoms suggestive of disorders that might cause symptoms similar to ADHD and/or be comorbid with ADHD. Such illnesses include anxiety disorders, depressive or bipolar disorders, psychotic illnesses, and personality traits/disorders. Special attention should be paid to potential comorbid substance use disorders because of the potential for abuse/diversion of stimulants that might eventually be used to treat ADHD. Laboratory screening and a physical examination should be employed to help identify any organic/medical cause for the patient's symptoms.

While the clinical interview is undoubtedly a critical component of the diagnostic process, the clinician may make use of a variety of other techniques to help clarify the diagnosis. In particular, a variety of rating scales are commonly employed to help elucidate past and current symptoms of ADHD . In addition to such self-report measures, a computer-based Continuous Performance Test (CPT) can assist in diagnosis by measuring errors of omission and errors of commission (Solanto, Etefia, & Marks, 2004). The test does this by roughly evaluating the core symptom domain of inattention by counting the number of target stimuli among many stimuli missed because of failure to press a microswitch (errors of omission). The test can also calculate errors of commission; this is a rough estimate of impulsivity. The subject misidentifies nontargets as targets by pressing a microswitch even when the identified stimulus is not present. Some CPTs also measure reaction time, which may be more variable in ADHD then in non-ADHD.

Neuropsychological testing can also be employed to help clarify the presence or absence of ADHD; additionally, neuropsychological testing can help identify the presence of learning disorders as well as specific areas in which the patient experiences deficits. Adults with ADHD may show deficits in a number of neuropsychological functions, including "...sustained attention, signal detection, working memory, verbal fluency, motor and mental processing speed, and, to a less frequent extent, shifting and maintaining cognitive set" (Gallagher & Blader, 2001). A number of studies have demonstrated neuropsychological deficits that may be useful in differentiating adults with ADHD from adults without the condition as well as adults with ADHD from adults with other psychiatric illnesses (Gallagher & Blader, 2001). In addition to neuropsychological testing, some clinicians employ quantitative electroencephalograms (qEEGs) in assisting with diagnosis. A recent meta-analysis of qEEG power suggested that a "...theta/beta ratio increase is a commonly observed trait in ADHD relative to normal controls" (Snyder & Hall, 2006). The authors go on to acknowledge that other conditions can present with similar results and they suggest the need for a prospective study to help determine generalizability to clinical applications.

Treatment of Attention-Deficit/Hyperactivity Disorder in Young Adults

The treatment of ADHD in young adults typically involves the use of medication(s) and psychosocial interventions. Psychostimulants are often thought of as first-line medication treatment of ADHD in young adults. The psychostimulants include short- and long-acting preparations of methylphenidate, dexmethylphenidate, dextroamphetamine, and mixed amphetamine salts. A recent meta-analysis demonstrated strong support for methylphenidate's efficacy in treating ADHD in adults (Faraone, Spencer, Aleardi, Pagano, & Biederman, 2004). Turner and colleagues showed that methylphenidate resulted in an "...improvement in spatial working memory performance and sustained attention, together with a speeding in response time, in [adults with ADHD]" (Turner, Blackwell, Dowson, McLean, & Sahakian, 2005). Studies have shown that mixed amphetamine salts are also efficacious in the treatment of ADHD in adults (Spencer et al., 2001; Weisler, Chrisman, & Wilens, 2003; Weiss & Hechtman, 2006). Lisdexamfetamine is a pro-drug stimulant treatment recently approved for the treatment of ADHD.

Second-line medication treatments include bupropion, atomoxetine, and tricyclic antidepressants (Dodson, 2005). Though a study by Kuperman and colleagues (2001) did not show a sustained-release preparation of bupropion (Wellbutrin SR) to be superior to placebo, a more recent study showed that an extended-release preparation of bupropion (Wellbutrin XL) was an effective and well-tolerated treatment for ADHD in adults (Wilens et al., 2005). Atomoxetine has been shown in several studies to be efficacious in the treatment of ADHD in adults (Adler et al., 2006; Adler, Spencer, Milton, Moore, & Michelson, 2005; Michelson et al., 2003). Guanfacine, often used in the treatment of ADHD in children and adolescents, was not found to provide statistically significant improvement in cognitive measures in a study conducted by Muller and colleagues (2005). An extended-release formulation of guanfacine is currently under development. A phase I study demonstrated its tolerability (Swearingen, Pennick, Shojaei, Lyne, & Fiske, 2007), though efficacy data has not yet been published. Other medications, including modafinil, oxcarbazepine, and nicotine replacement therapy, have also been studied, though to a limited degree.

In addition to medications, psychosocial treatments for adult ADHD have also been studied and utilized. A study by Safren and colleagues showed that cognitive-behavioral therapy (CBT) in combination with pharmacotherapy resulted in a greater number of treatment responders as opposed to those not utilizing CBT (Safren et al., 2005). Recent studies by an Australian group utilized therapist-delivered and self-directed psychosocial treatments for adults suffering from ADHD (Stevenson, Stevenson, & Whitmont, 2003; Stevenson, Whitmont, Bornholt, Livesey, & Stevenson, 2002). The group found that therapist-delivered psychosocial interventions resulted in decreased ADHD symptoms, improved organizational skills, and fewer anger problems; many of the improvements were maintained at follow-up 1 year later. Self-directed interventions also led to reduced ADHD symptoms, fewer anger problems, and improvements in organizational skills and self-esteem.

Treatment of adults with ADHD and comorbid substance use disorders can be particularly challenging. In a small study of 25 adults with ADHD and concomitant substance use disorders, those treated with methylphenidate did not show beneficial improvements in symptom control as compared to those treated with placebo (Carpentier, de Jong, Dijkstra, Verbrugge, & Krabbe, 2005). Another group (Levin, Evans, Brooks, & Garawi, 2007) examined the treatment of cocaine-dependent adults with ADHD; both active treatment (methylphenidate) and placebo yielded improvements in ADHD symptoms (no difference between the two groups). However, methylphenidate (but not placebo) was associated with a reduction in cocaine use. Levin and colleagues studied a group of adults with opioid dependence in treatment with methadone maintenance; the randomized, double-blind study comparing sustained-release bupropion, methylphenidate, and placebo demonstrated no clear advantage for either active treatment over placebo (Levin et al., 2006).

Future Directions

While much about the etiology, clinical presentation, and treatment of ADHD in young adults is known, clearly there is much more left to discover. Shared genetic risk for disorders related to problems with impulses, risk taking, and sensation seeking may clarify the diverse pathways that individuals with ADHD follow as development unfolds. Identification of specific genetic markers may aid diagnosis and assist in matching choice of stimulant or other treatment option for a specific individual. New developments in pharmacotherapy have been remarkable in the proliferation of methods of delivery (i.e., patch, long-acting, and pro-drug formulations). Thus far, the field continues to be dominated with strategies for increasing dopamine or norepinephrine at key sites of the frontal cortex and nucleus accumbens. New mechanisms for treatment—for example, exploiting the nicotine or glutamate neurochemical systems to increase attention—have proved much less fruitful. Of particular interest might be nicotine receptor agonists, modafinil, and oxcarbazepine. Additionally, a recent study suggested that SPECT scanning might be useful in terms of predicting clinical response to medication (la Fougere et al., 2006). Such tools, if demonstrated to have practical and feasible clinical application, would be useful as a means of eliminating the current "hit and miss" approach to initiating therapy.

KEY POINTS

- A young adult with a substance use disorder and/or relationship or employment failure should increase the clinician's suspicion for previously undiagnosed ADHD.
- Poor management of health conditions such as diabetes mellitus, asthma, or hypertension may be due to the disorganizing effects of ADHD. Treatment of ADHD may improve compliance with medical management of other health conditions.

> *(Key Points continued)*
>
> - The use of stimulants in adults is a test of the doctor–patient relationship. Close monitoring, frequent office checks, and frank and frequent discussion about misuse of medication and strategies for harm reduction are consistent with good psychiatric care.

PRACTICE GUIDELINES

In any mental health assessment, the clinician should screen for ADHD, and the evaluation should consist of interviews with the parent to obtain information about the patient's school or day care functioning.

Evaluations should also assess comorbid psychiatric disorders, medical, social, and family histories, and may include psychological and neuropsychological testing if the history suggests low general cognitive ability or low achievement in language or mathematics relative to the patient's intellectual ability.

Initial psychopharmacological treatment of ADHD should be a trial of an agent approved by the Food and Drug Administration for the treatment of ADHD, and psychosocial treatment in conjunction with medication treatment is often beneficial

---

References

Able, S. L., Johnston, J. A., Adler, L. A., & Swindle, R. W. (2007). Functional and psychosocial impairment in adults with undiagnosed ADHD. *Psychological Medicine, 37*(1), 97–107.

Adler, L., Dietrich, A., Reimherr, F. W., Taylor, L. V., Sutton, V. K., Bakken, R., Allen A. J., & Kelsey D. (2006). Safety and tolerability of once versus twice daily atomoxetine in adults with ADHD. *Annals of Clinical Psychiatry, 18*(2), 107–113.

Adler, L. A., Spencer, T. J., Milton, D. R., Moore, R. J., & Michelson, D. (2005). Long-term, open-label study of the safety and efficacy of atomoxetine in adults with attention-deficit/hyperactivity disorder: An interim analysis. *Journal of Clinical Psychiatry, 66*(3), 294–299.

Adler, L. A., Sutton, V. K., Moore, R. J., Dietrich, A. P., Reimherr, F. W., Sangal, R. B., Saylor, K. E., Secnik, K., Kelsey, D. K., & Allen, A. J. (2006). Quality of life assessment in adult patients with attention-deficit/hyperactivity disorder treated with atomoxetine. *Journal of Clinical Psychopharmacology, 26*(6), 648–652.

American Psychiatric Association. (2000). *Diagnostic and statistical manual of mental disorders* (4th ed.). Washington, DC: Author.

Banerjee, E., Sinha, S., Chatterjee, A., Gangopadhyay, P. K., Singh, M., & Nandagopal, K. (2006). A family-based study of Indian subjects from Kolkata reveals allelic association of the serotonin transporter intron-2 (stin2) polymorphism and attention-deficit-hyperactivity disorder (ADHD). *American Journal of Medical Genetics B Neuropsychiatric Genetics, 141*(4), 361–366.

Barkley, R. A., Guevremont, D. C., Anastopoulos, A. D., DuPaul, G. J., & Shelton, T. L. (1993). Driving-related risks and outcomes of attention deficit hyperactivity disorder in adolescents and young adults: A 3- to 5-year follow-up survey. *Pediatrics, 92*(2), 212–218.

Boonstra, A. M., Oosterlaan, J., Sergeant, J. A., & Buitelaar, J. K. (2005). Executive functioning in adult ADHD: A meta-analytic review. *Psychological Medicine, 35*(8), 1097–1108.

Bridgett, D. J., & Walker, M. E. (2006). Intellectual functioning in adults with ADHD: A meta-analytic examination of full scale IQ differences between adults with and without ADHD. *Psychological Assessment, 18*(1), 1–14.

Carpentier, P. J., de Jong, C. A., Dijkstra, B. A., Verbrugge, C. A., & Krabbe, P. F. (2005). A controlled trial of methylphenidate in adults with attention deficit/hyperactivity disorder and substance use disorders. *Addiction, 100*(12), 1868–1874.

Dodson, W. W. (2005). Pharmacotherapy of adult ADHD. *Journal of Clinical Psychology, 61*(5), 589–606.

Durston, S. (2003). A review of the biological bases of ADHD: What have we learned from imaging studies? *Mental Retardation and Developmental Disabilities Research Review, 9*(3), 184–195.

Faraone, S. V., Spencer, T., Aleardi, M., Pagano, C., & Biederman, J. (2004). Meta-analysis of the efficacy of methylphenidate for treating adult attention-deficit/hyperactivity disorder. *Journal of Clinical Psychopharmacology, 24*(1), 24–29.

Frazier, T. W., Youngstrom, E. A., Glutting, J. J., & Watkins, M. W. (2007). ADHD and achievement: Meta-analysis of the child, adolescent, and adult literatures and a concomitant study with college students. *Journal of Learning Disabilities, 40*(1), 49–65.

Gallagher, R., & Blader, J. (2001). The diagnosis and neuropsychological assessment of adult attention deficit/hyperactivity disorder. Scientific study and practical guidelines. *Annals of the New York Academy of Sciences, 931*, 148–171.

Greenhill, L. L., Pliszka, S., Dulcan, M. K., Bernet, W., Arnold, V., Beitchman, J., Benson R. S., Bukstein O., Kinlan J., McClellan J., Rue D., Shaw J. A., & Stock S.; American Academy of Child and Adolescent Psychiatry. (2002). Practice parameter for the use of stimulant medications in the treatment of children, adolescents, and adults. *Journal of the American Academy of Child and Adolescent Psychiatry, 41*(Suppl. 2), 26S–49S.

Gunter, T. D., Arndt, S., Riggins-Caspers, K., Wenman, G., & Cadoret, R. J. (2006). Adult outcomes of attention deficit hyperactivity disorder and conduct disorder: Are the risks independent or additive? *Annals of Clinical Psychiatry, 18*(4), 233–237.

Kuperman, S., Perry, P. J., Gaffney, G. R., Lund, B. C., Bever-Stille, K. A., Arndt, S., Holman, T.L., Moser, D. J., & Paulsen J. S. (2001). Bupropion SR vs. methylphenidate vs. placebo for attention deficit hyperactivity disorder in adults. *Annals of Clinical Psychiatry, 13*(3), 129–134.

la Fougere, C., Krause, J., Krause, K. H., Josef Gildehaus, F., Hacker, M., Koch, W., Hahn, K., Tatsch, K., Dresel, S. (2006). Value of 99MTC-Trodat-1 SPECT to predict clinical response to methylphenidate treatment in adults with attention deficit hyperactivity disorder. *Nuclear Medicine Communications, 27*(9), 733–737.

Levin, F. R., Evans, S. M., Brooks, D. J., & Garawi, F. (2007). Treatment of cocaine dependent treatment seekers with adult ADHD: Double-blind comparison of methylphenidate and placebo. *Drug and Alcohol Dependence, 87*(1), 20–29.

Levin, F. R., Evans, S. M., Brooks, D. J., Kalbag, A. S., Garawi, F., & Nunes, E. V. (2006). Treatment of methadone-maintained patients with adult ADHD: Double-blind comparison of methylphenidate, bupropion and placebo. *Drug and Alcohol Dependence, 81*(2), 137–148.

Levy, F., Hay, D. A., McStephen, M., Wood, C., & Waldman, I. (1997). Attention-deficit hyperactivity disorder: A category or a continuum? Genetic analysis of a large-scale twin study. *Journal of the American Academy of Child and Adolescent Psychiatry, 36*(6), 737–744.

Lott, D. C., Kim, S. J., Cook, E. H., Jr., & de Wit, H. (2005). Dopamine transporter gene associated with diminished subjective response to amphetamine. *Neuropsychopharmacology, 30*(3), 602–609.

Mannuzza, S., Klein, R. G., Bessler, A., Malloy, P., & LaPadula, M. (1993). Adult outcome of hyperactive boys. Educational achievement, occupational rank, and psychiatric status. *Archives of General Psychiatry, 50*(7), 565–576.

Mazei-Robinson, M. S., & Blakely, R. D. (2006). ADHD and the dopamine transporter: Are there reasons to pay attention? *Handbook of Experimental Pharmacology, 175*, 373–415.

McGough, J. J., & Barkley, R. A. (2004). Diagnostic controversies in adult attention deficit hyperactivity disorder. *American Journal of Psychiatry, 161*(11), 1948–1956.

McGough, J. J., Smalley, S. L., McCracken, J. T., Yang, M., Del'Homme, M., Lynn, D. E., Loo S. (2005). Psychiatric comorbidity in adult attention deficit hyperactivity disorder: Findings from multiplex families. *American Journal of Psychiatry, 162*(9), 1621–1627.

Michelson, D., Adler, L., Spencer, T., Reimherr, F. W., West, S. A., Allen, A. J., Kelsey D., Wernicke J., Dietrich A., & Milton D. (2003). Atomoxetine in adults with ADHD: Two randomized, placebo-controlled studies. *Biological Psychiatry, 53*(2), 112–120.

Mick, E., Biederman, J., Spencer, T., Faraone, S. V., & Sklar, P. (2006). Absence of association with dat1 polymorphism and response to methylphenidate in a sample of adults with ADHD. *American Journal of Medical Genetics B Neuropsychiatric Genetics, 141*(8), 890–894.

Mill, J. S., Caspi, A., McClay, J., Sugden, K., Purcell, S., Asherson, P., Craig I., McGuffin P., Braithwaite A., Poulton R., & Moffitt T. E. (2002). The dopamine d4 receptor and the hyperactivity phenotype: A developmental-epidemiological study. *Molecular Psychiatry, 7*(4), 383–391.

Millstein, R., Wilens, T. E., Biederman, J., & Spencer, T. J. (1997). Presenting ADHD symptoms and subtypes in clinically referred adults with ADHD. *Journal of Attention Disorders, 2*, 159–166.

Molina, B. S., Pelham, W. E., Gnagy, E. M., Thompson, A. L., & Marshal, M. P. (2007). Attention-deficit/hyperactivity disorder risk for heavy drinking and alcohol use disorder is age specific. *Alcohol: Clinical and Experimental Research, 31*(4), 643–654.

Muller, U., Clark, L., Lam, M. L., Moore, R. M., Murphy, C. L., Richmond, N. K., Sandhu R. S., Wilkins I. A., Menon D. K., Sahakian B. J., & Robbins T. W. (2005). Lack of effects of guanfacine on executive and memory functions in healthy male volunteers. *Psychopharmacology (Berlin), 182*(2), 205–213.

Mulsow, M., O'Neal, K., & Murry, V. (2001). Adult attention deficit hyperactivity disorder, the family, and child maltreatment. *Trauma, Violence, & Abuse, 2*(1), 36–50.

Murphy, K., & Barkley, R. A. (1996). Attention deficit hyperactivity disorder adults: Comorbidities and adaptive impairments. *Comprehensive Psychiatry, 37*(6), 393–401.

Murphy, K. R., Barkley, R. A., & Bush, T. (2002). Young adults with attention deficit hyperactivity disorder: Subtype differences in comorbidity, educational, and clinical history. *Journal of Nervous and Mental Disease, 190*(3), 147–157.

Pliszka, S. (2007). AACAP Work Group on Quality Issues. Practice parameter for the assessment and treatment of children and adolescents with attention-deficit/hyperactivity disorder. *Journal of the American Academy of Child and Adolescent Psychiatry, 46*(7), 894–921.

Reimherr, F. W., Marchant, B. K., Strong, R. E., Hedges, D. W., Adler, L., Spencer, T. J., West S. A., & Soni P. (2005). Emotional dysregulation in adult ADHD and response to atomoxetine. *Biological Psychiatry, 58*(2), 125–131.

Safren, S. A., Otto, M. W., Sprich, S., Winett, C. L., Wilens, T. E., & Biederman, J. (2005). Cognitive-behavioral therapy for ADHD in medication-treated adults with continued symptoms. *Behavioral Research and Therapy, 43*(7), 831–842.

Secnik, K., Swensen, A., & Lage, M. J. (2005). Comorbidities and costs of adult patients diagnosed with attention-deficit hyperactivity disorder. *Pharmacoeconomics, 23*(1), 93–102.

Seidman, L. J., Biederman, J., Weber, W., Hatch, M., & Faraone, S. V. (1998). Neuropsychological function in adults with attention-deficit/hyperactivity disorder. *Biological Psychiatry, 44*(4), 260–268.

Selke, J. (2000). *Adults with ADHD in the workplace: A descriptive analysis and evaluation of the work place and job satisfaction.* Ph.D. dissertation. University of California, Berkeley, CA.

Sheehan, K., Hawi, Z., Gill, M., & Kent, L. (2007). No association between TPH2 gene polymorphisms and ADHD in a UK sample. *Neuroscience Letters, 412*(2), 105–107.

Shekim, W. O., Asarnow, R. F., Hess, E., Zaucha, K., & Wheeler, N. (1990). A clinical and demographic profile of a sample of adults with attention deficit hyperactivity disorder, residual state. *Comprehensive Psychiatry, 31*(5), 416–425.

Smith, K. M., Daly, M., Fischer, M., Yiannoutsos, C. T., Bauer, L., Barkley, R., Navia, B. A. (2003). Association of the dopamine beta hydroxylase gene with attention deficit hyperactivity disorder: Genetic analysis of the Milwaukee longitudinal study. *American Journal of Medical Genetics B Neuropsychiatric Genetics, 119*(1), 77–85.

Snyder, S. M., & Hall, J. R. (2006). A meta-analysis of quantitative EEG power associated with attention-deficit hyperactivity disorder. *Journal of Clinical Neurophysiology, 23*(5), 440–455.

Solanto, M. V., Etefia, K., & Marks, D. J. (2004). The utility of self-report measures and the continuous performance test in the diagnosis of ADHD in adults. *CNS Spectrum, 9*(9), 649–659.

Spencer, T., Biederman, J., Wilens, T., Faraone, S., Prince, J., Gerard, K., Doyle R., Parekh A., Kagan J., & Bearman S. K. (2001). Efficacy of a mixed amphetamine salts compound in adults with attention-deficit/hyperactivity disorder. *Archives of General Psychiatry, 58*(8), 775–782.

Stevenson, C. S., Stevenson, R. J., & Whitmont, S. (2003). A self-directed psychosocial intervention with minimal therapist contact for adults with attention deficit hyperactivity disorder. *Clinical Psychology and Psychotherapy, 10*, 93–101.

Stevenson, C. S., Whitmont, S., Bornholt, L., Livesey, D., & Stevenson, R. J. (2002). A cognitive remediation programme for adults with attention deficit hyperactivity disorder. *Australian and New Zealand Journal of Psychiatry, 36*(5), 610–616.

Swearingen, D., Pennick, M., Shojaei, A., Lyne, A., & Fiske, K. (2007). A phase I, randomized, open-label, crossover study of the single-dose pharmacokinetic properties of guanfacine extended-release 1-, 2-, and 4-mg tablets in healthy adults. *Clinical Therapeutics, 29*(4), 617–625.

Thapar, A., Holmes, J., Poulton, K., & Harrington, R. (1999). Genetic basis of attention deficit and hyperactivity. *British Journal of Psychiatry, 174*, 105–111.

Turner, D. C., Blackwell, A. D., Dowson, J. H., McLean, A., & Sahakian, B. J. (2005). Neurocognitive effects of methylphenidate in adult attention-deficit/hyperactivity disorder. *Psychopharmacology (Berlin), 178*(2–3), 286–295.

Weisler, R., Chrisman, A., & Wilens, T. (2003, October 20). *Adderall XR dosed once daily in adult patients with ADHD.* Paper presented at the Annual Meeting of the American Psychiatric Association, San Francisco, CA.

Weiss, M., & Hechtman, L. (2006). A randomized double-blind trial of paroxetine and/or dextroamphetamine and problem-focused therapy for attention-deficit/hyperactivity disorder in adults. *Journal of Clinical Psychiatry, 67*(4), 611–619.

Weiss, M., & Murray, C. (2003). Assessment and management of attention-deficit hyperactivity disorder in adults. *Canadian Medical Association Journal, 168*(6), 715–722.

Wender, P. (2000). *ADHD: Attentio- deficit/hyperactivity disorder in children, adolescents and adults.* New York: Oxford University Press.

Wilens, T. E., Haight, B. R., Horrigan, J. P., Hudziak, J. J., Rosenthal, N. E., Connor, D. F., Hampton K. D., Richard N. E., & Modell J. G. (2005). Bupropion xl in adults with attention-deficit/hyperactivity disorder: A randomized, placebo-controlled study. *Biological Psychiatry, 57*(7), 793–801.

Wilens, T. E., Verlinden, M. H., Adler, L. A., Wozniak, P. J., & West, S. A. (2006). Abt-089, a neuronal nicotinic receptor partial agonist, for the treatment of attention-deficit/hyperactivity disorder in adults: Results of a pilot study. *Biological Psychiatry, 59*(11), 1065–1070.

Chapter 22

Schizophrenia in Adolescents and Young Adults

Afshan Anjum, Priyanka Gait, Kathryn R. Cullen and Tonya White

In the early nineteenth century, German psychiatrist Emil Kraepelin used the term "dementia praecox" to define a constellation of symptoms that is presently called *schizophrenia*. Kraepelin's description defined an illness with a break from reality associated with a considerable decline in baseline functioning. Thus, by including the term "dementia" in his original description, he emphasized the impact on cognitive and social functioning, and the term "praecox" highlighted the early age of onset of the disorder in contrast to the dementias that occur later in life (McGrath et al., 2004).

Schizophrenia often considerably alters the developmental course for an individual. The age of onset of schizophrenia peaks during late adolescence and early adulthood, with most individuals developing the illness between the ages of 18 and 30 (Hafner, 1998), although a substantial minority develop the illness even earlier. The onset of schizophrenia during these early stages of life has a tremendous impact on the individual, their family, and society. The illness strikes during a time of development when young adults are gaining independence from their parents, moving away to college, and developing intimate relationships. It is not uncommon for young patients to postpone graduation from high school so as to receive services offered through various agencies up to the age of 21. Alternatively, many drop out of high school or college altogether, and some are alienated from their peers. Patients with schizophrenia often lose friends, change schools, and have an extended dependence on family. Families must often alter their expectations for their child and accommodate to the newfound disability and compromised function. It is not uncommon to see parents continuing as caretakers and decision makers for their children, sometimes well into later adulthood. Finally, there is a tremendous impact on society, based on the impact on productivity, downstream effects on family and relationships, and the health care burden that may extend into middle age and beyond. This chapter provides an overview of the epidemiology, neurobiology, diagnosis and differential diagnosis, course, and treatment of schizophrenia in older adolescents and young adults.

Epidemiology

The incidence of schizophrenia has been approximated at 1% for the general population irrespective of culture and gender. However, recent epidemiological estimates have challenged this, suggesting that this incidence in the general population is inflated (Perala et al., 2007). Factors such as sex, ethnicity, and location may account for some of the variability. For instance, results from the Three Center AESOP Study in London reported that incidence of schizophrenia was higher in males compared to females, in black and minority ethnic groups compared to the white population, and at the Southeast London study center when compared to Nottingham or Bristol centers (Kirkbride et al., 2006). These variations in incidence suggest the possibility of environmental interaction with genetic factors that may account for heterogeneity in the incidence of psychotic disorders.

Age of Onset

Although childhood-onset schizophrenia (COS) (onset of psychotic symptoms before age 13) is rare (McClellan & Werry, 1994), the incidence of schizophrenia rises sharply and steadily after the onset of puberty (Galdos, van Os, & Murray, 1993; Hafner & an der Heiden, 1997; Krausz & Muller-Thomsen, 1993). Since early-onset schizophrenia is associated with less-favorable outcomes, there has been considerable interest in exploring the impact of age of onset on the trajectory of symptom development and functioning in schizophrenia. These studies have found that the age of onset impacts a wide range of functioning in schizophrenia. Early onset negatively impacts a number of cognitive domains, including verbal learning and memory (Tuulio-Henriksson, Partonen, Suvisaari, Haukka, & Lonnqvist, 2004), executive function (Basso, Nasrallah, Olson, & Bornstein, 1997), performance IQ (Yang, Liu, Chiang, Chen, & Lin, 1995), abstraction (Jeste et al., 1998), overall academic performance (even before onset of psychosis) (Johnstone et al., 1989), and motor control (Manschreck, Maher, & Candela, 2004). Furthermore, patients with early-onset schizophrenia have been observed to have more severe symptoms (Johnstone et al., 1989) and higher levels of negative symptoms (Yang, Liu, Chiang, Chen, & Lin, 1995). These severe negative symptoms are associated with compromised cognition and inability to sustain attention and execute functions (Bellino et al., 2004).

Gender Differences

Although the lifetime risk for developing schizophrenia is similar for both sexes, the age of onset tends to be later for women (Hafner, 1998; Hafner, Maurer, Loffler, & Riecher-Rossler, 1993). Danish studies, including the OPUS trials, have pointed to the male sex as a significant risk factor for early onset of this illness. In the age range of 17–40 years, the risk for men seems to be the higher, but this is surpassed by women in the age range of 50–68 years (Thorup, Waltoft, Pedersen, Mortensen, & Nordentoft, 2007). This has been theorized to contribute to the better social adjustment and milder form of the illness in women (Thorup et al., 2007). Estrogen has been speculated to play a protective role in delaying the onset of psychotic symptoms (Hafner, Maurer, Loffler, & Riecher-Rossler, 1993). Similarly, some authors have reported the impact of gender on the duration of untreated psychosis (DUP), that is, the length of time experiencing psychotic symptoms before first contact with treatment services, suggesting that women may have a shorter DUP than men (Ho et al., 2003; Malla et al., 2002). Gender differences in phenomenology have also been observed. For instance, studies have suggested that men present with greater negative symptoms than women, whereas women tend to have higher positive symptoms. While men are likely to have a history of child abuse and neglect, women are more likely to have a history of suicide attempts despite having better social networks than men (Tang et al., 2007; Thorup et al., 2007).

Etiology

The underlying cause of schizophrenia has not been determined, but current research supports a multifactorial etiology. A multitude of risk factors, including genetic defects, obstetric complications, prenatal viral infections, and marijuana use during early adolescence, have been associated with the development of schizophrenia. Although touted as powerful risk factors for the development of schizophrenia, none of the above risk indicators seem to have consistently useful predictive value for the onset of schizophrenia. Recently, surmounting evidence has given credence for the neurodevelopmental hypothesis of schizophrenia that proposes both genetic and environmental factors processes culminate in a deviation from typical neurodevelopment that involves neurotransmitter dysfunction and aberrant neuronal connectivity. In this theoretical framework, early insults can impact neurodevelopment, resulting in aberrations that emerge during adolescence or young adulthood as the brain is undergoing further maturational processes.

In support of the neurodevelopmental hypothesis, a subgroup of patients with schizophrenia have a history of other neurodevelopmental disorders. For instance, in a British 1946 birth cohort the researchers found a lag in motor and speech development by 2 years in children who later manifested psychotic disorders (Jones, Rodgers, Murray, & Marmot, 1994). Also, motor delays in the northern Finland birth cohort were related to later manifestation of schizophrenia and other psychotic disorders. Infant motor development has been correlated with adolescent school performance and premorbid symptoms in schizophrenia patients (Isohanni et al., 2004).

Neuroimaging research in recent decades has pointed to some substantial changes that occur in brain structure that are supportive of a neurodevelopmental etiology of schizophrenia (Pantelis et al., 2005). Overall, neuroimaging studies in schizophrenia have consistently demonstrated structural brain abnormalities in patients such as decreased brain volume with a generalized loss of cortical thickness and enlargement of lateral and third ventricles (Shenton, Dickey, Frumin, & McCarley, 2001). In patients with child-onset schizophrenia, rates of gray matter reduction correlate highly with severe clinical symptoms at presentation and related premorbid impairment, but no correlation is seen with gender, ethnicity, or age at onset. Surprisingly, a higher rate of gray matter reduction in this group is also associated with greater clinical improvement, suggesting that these changes may in part represent a plastic response to illness (Sporn et al., 2003).

Genetic Risk

Twin, adoption, and family studies show that genes provide the greatest known contribution to the risk for development of schizophrenia. The concordance rate of developing schizophrenia approximates 50% in identical twins, whereas in fraternal twins it is around 15% (Gottesman & Shields, 1966; Kendler et al., 2000) For an offspring of two schizophrenic parents the risk of developing schizophrenia is between 30%–50%. These rates provide evidence that the etiology of schizophrenia is multifactorial, involving both genetic and environmental factors. Those with higher family loading for schizophrenia have an earlier age of onset.

Multiple chromosomes have been associated with the development of schizophrenia. Genetic linkage, while strong in some studies (LOD scores ranging between 3.5–8.7), has not proven to be consistently replicated. Several studies have supported the presence of susceptibility loci for schizophrenia on chromosomes 6 and 8 (Schultz & Andreasen, 1999). Chromosomes 1, 2, 3, 10, 11, 12, 17, and 22 have been implicated in the etiology of schizophrenia, but they are not supported as strongly (Bulayeva, Glatt, Bulayev, Pavlova, & Tsuang, 2007; Nicolson et al., 1999). It is likely that small alterations in multiple genes, coupled with interaction with the environment, result in the manifestation of the clinical phenotype associated with schizophrenia. Variability in presentation could be the result of the wide spectrum of genetic and environmental factors that may be interacting in any given individual. Individuals with stronger genetic loading may require less environmental influences to pass through the threshold of illness.

Environmental Risk

Environmental factors, through interaction with genetic predisposition, have been widely studied and are believed to precipitate the manifestation of psychosis. For instance, a genetic predisposition to the illness may not manifest if the environment is optimal. Environmental factors such as stressful events, urbanicity, immigration, family psychodynamics, and history of maltreatment during childhood have been shown to increase the risk for the onset of schizophrenia. An unfavorable intrauterine environment, whether a result of infection or hypoxia, may result in altered development of the fetal brain. Studies demonstrating increased rates of schizophrenia in children born during the winter months support the contribution of maternal infection to some individuals. Central nervous system infections, including bacterial and viral infections during the prenatal period, have been shown to increase the risk of schizophrenia in offspring (Brown et al., 2004), although other studies have not corroborated these findings (Isohanni et al., 2001; Koponen et al., 2004; Suvisaari, Haukka, & Lonnqvist, 2004). Viral infections may act by affecting cell functioning and also by imitating CNS neurotransmitters and receptors. Exposure to substances of abuse, such as PCP, cocaine, and methamphetamine, can sometimes cause symptoms similar to schizophrenia. In addition, cannabis use during early to mid adolescence is associated with a higher risk of developing schizophrenia in those with specific genetic liability (Caspi et al., 2005). Several studies have suggested that substance abuse may determine an earlier age of onset (Barnes, Mutsatsa, Hutton, Watt, & Joyce, 2006; Mauri et al., 2006). Although multiple environmental events contribute to the onset of schizophrenia, each may modulate neurodevelopmental trajectories in a common final pathway that results in the development of schizophrenia.

Neurotransmitter Hypothesis

With the discovery of typical antipsychotic medications nearly 50 years ago, there emerged the "dopamine hyperfunction" hypothesis of schizophrenia. This was based on the success rates of the D2 receptor antagonists' ability to treat the positive symptoms of schizophrenia. However, these medications have little effect on the negative symptoms and cognitive deficits associated with schizophrenia. Thus, the dopamine theory, although still providing clues to the etiology of schizophrenia, has fallen short of explaining the etiopathogenesis entirely.

The "glutamate hypofunction" hypothesis emerged from the propensity of certain drugs of abuse (i.e., phencyclidine) to mimic the positive, negative, and thought disorder symptoms of schizophrenia. PCP is a noncompetitive NMDA receptor antagonist. In patients with schizophrenia, PCP results in an exacerbation of symptoms. In addition, concentrations of glutamate in the cerebrospinal fluid of patients with schizophrenia are significantly lower compared with controls. The highest concentrations of NMDA receptors are in regions implicated in the pathophysiology of schizophrenia (i.e., the hippocampus, neocortex, nucleus accumbens, caudate, putamen, and the amygdala).

Connectivity Hypothesis

Finally, considerable work over the past decade supports the concept that schizophrenia involves a disruption in the orchestration of the multiple neural networks that participate in higher cognitive functions. The connectivity between neural networks arising during normal development is potentially disrupted, leading to the recruitment of either inappropriate regions for task execution, or alternatively, alters the processing requirements in expected regions. For example, studies utilizing both glucose metabolism (FDG-PET), SPECT, and Oxygen-15 PET have demonstrated hypofrontality in the dorslolateral prefrontal cortex (DLPFC) on tasks of executive function. Additionally, studies utilizing diffusion tensor imaging (DTI), which measures the coherence of neuronal fiber tracts, have shown a decrease in the coherence of white matter tracts in schizophrenia. This is presumed to be additional evidence for disrupted connectivity in schizophrenia. Altered connectivity is also supported by a global down-regulation of myelin-related genes in postmortem brains of individuals with schizophrenia (Hasak et al., 2001).

Diagnostic Criteria for Schizophrenia

The DSM-IV-TR criteria for diagnosis of schizophrenia are listed in Table 22-1. Whereas the criteria do not differ between the DSM-III, DSM-IV, and the DSM-IV-TR, they are different when compared to the current ICD 9 and 10 classifications. The ICD 9 does not lay down strict criteria for the duration of illness, whereas the DSM-IV-TR specifies 6-month duration of illness, including prodrome and/or residual symptoms with active phase symptoms lasting for at least 1 month.

Phases of Schizophrenia

The course of schizophrenia is often parsed into the prodromal, acute, recovery, and residual phases (Figure 22-1). Fifty percent of patients present with an insidious onset marked by extended prodromal and global delays. An insidious onset is more typical of an earlier age of onset. Acute onset of schizophrenia is possible, often with a clear precipitant or stressor. Those who have an abrupt onset typically have a better overall prognosis.

Prodromal Phase

It has long been reported that prior to onset of acute psychosis, a decline in functioning is

Table 22-1. DSM-IV-TR Diagnostic Criteria for Schizophrenia

A. Characteristic symptoms: Two (or more) of the following, each present for a significant portion of time during a 1-month period (or less if successfully treated):

   (1) Delusions
   (2) Hallucinations
   (3) Disorganized speech (e.g., frequent derailment or incoherence)
   (4) Grossly disorganized or catatonic behavior
   (5) Negative symptoms, i.e., affective flattening, alogia, or avolition

   Note: Only one Criterion A symptom is required if delusions are bizarre or hallucinations consist of a voice keeping up a running commentary on the person's behavior or thoughts, or two or more voices conversing with each other.

B. Social/occupational dysfunction: For a significant portion of the time since the onset of the disturbance, one or more major areas of functioning such as work, interpersonal relations, or self-care are markedly below the level achieved prior to the onset (or when the onset is in childhood or adolescence, failure to achieve expected level of interpersonal, academic, or occupational achievement).

C. Duration: Continuous signs of the disturbance persist for at least 6 months. This 6-month period must include at least 1 month of symptoms (or less if successfully treated) that meet Criterion A (i.e., active-phase symptoms) and may include periods of prodromal or residual symptoms. During these prodromal or residual periods, the signs of the disturbance may be manifested by only negative symptoms or two or more symptoms listed in Criterion A present in an attenuated form (e.g., odd beliefs, unusual perceptual experiences).

D. Schizoaffective and Mood Disorder exclusion: Schizoaffective Disorder and Mood Disorder With Psychotic Features have been ruled out because either (1) no Major Depressive, Manic, or Mixed Episodes have occurred concurrently with the active-phase symptoms; or (2) if mood episodes have occurred during active-phase symptoms, their total duration has been brief relative to the duration of the active and residual periods.

E. Substance/general medical condition exclusion: The disturbance is not due to the direct physiological effects of a substance (e.g., a drug of abuse, a medication) or a general medical condition.

F. Relationship to a Pervasive Developmental Disorder: If there is a history of Autistic Disorder or another Pervasive Developmental Disorder, the additional diagnosis of Schizophrenia is made only if prominent delusions or hallucinations are also present for at least a month (or less if successfully treated).

Reprinted with permission from the Diagnostic and Statistical Manual of Mental Disorders, Text Revision, Fourth Edition, (Copyright © 2000). American Psychiatric Association.

---

observed. The prodrome, defined as the nonspecific syndrome preceding the acute phase of schizophrenia, can last from a few days to several years and is characterized by social isolation, significant cognitive decline, and negative symptoms (Keshavan, Diwadkar, Montrose, Rajarethinam, & Sweeney, 2005). Premorbid symptoms may also include neurological symptoms, disruptive behaviors, attention problems, and developmental delays. One retrospective assessment of first-episode schizophrenia patients reported 40% had a history of a prodromal period (Hafner & Nowotny, 1995). Early symptoms are often difficult to recognize because they are nonspecific, and the presentation can vary widely across patient samples (Owens, Miller, Lawrie, & Johnstone, 2005). For instance, early presentations can mimic affective disorders, severe personality disorders, and pervasive developmental disorders, posing a huge diagnostic challenge (Masi, Mucci, & Pari, 2006). The prodrome is diagnosed retrospectively; since prodromal symptoms may resolve, they do not necessarily indicate a future

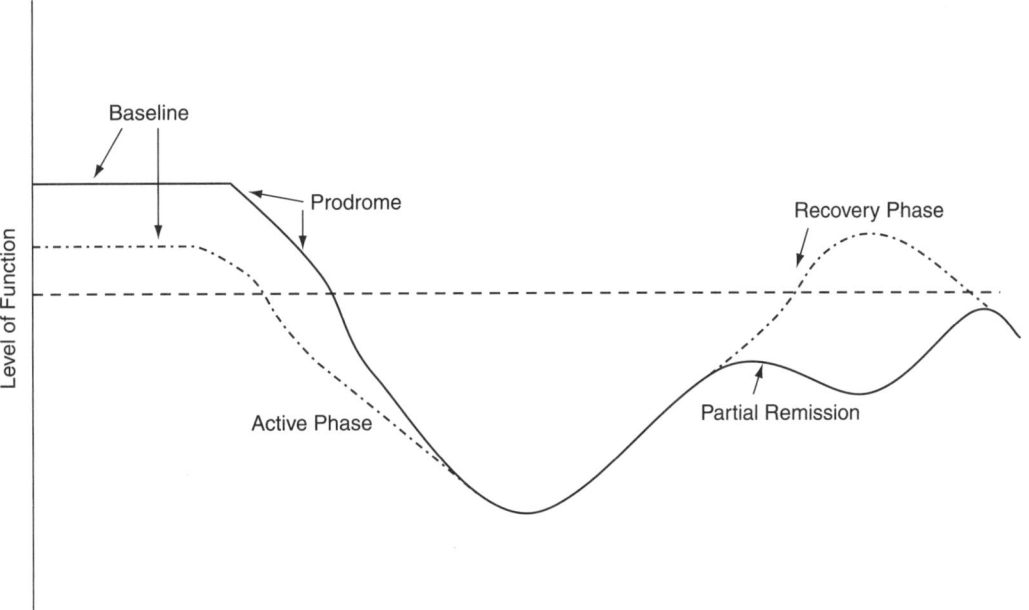

Figure 22-1. The phases of schizophrenia.

transition to a first psychotic episode. However, presence of symptoms that fit into the prodrome clinical picture indicates an increased risk for a future psychotic episode. Measures such as the Prodromal States Questionnaire (PSQ) (Loewy, Bearden, Johnson, Raine, & Cannon, 2005) and Comprehensive Assessment of At-Risk Mental States (CAARMS) (Yung et al., 2005) can be useful in identifying risk of psychosis in adolescents and young adults. For patients at high risk for developing schizophrenia, a few predictors of psychosis are poor functioning, long duration of symptoms, severely depressed state, and reduced attention (Yung, Phillips, Yuen, & McGorry, 2004). Problems with social adjustment and interpersonal relationships are associated with poor outcomes in schizophrenia (Asarnow & Ben-Meir, 1988; Werry, McClellan, & Chard, 1991).

Acute Phase

The acute phase is marked by positive symptoms of hallucinations, bizarre delusions, or a formal thought disorder evidenced by disorganized thinking or behavior. Auditory hallucinations occur in 70% of patients with schizophrenia, and visual hallucinations are reported by approximately 60%. Infrequently, patients may present with olfactory, gustatory, and kinesthetic misperceptions. Delusions may be grandiose, persecutory, nihilistic, and/or somatic in nature. Of note, delusions must be understood within the context of the individual's culture and religion, and family members or the community may help place nonbizarre delusions in context. Formal thought disorder, which includes tangential thinking, derailment, and circumstantiality is also a common presentation of acute schizophrenia. Thought disorder can also be manifested by bizarre behaviors, which can often be the reason that individuals come to the attention of the health care providers. Negative symptoms, such as alogia, apathy, amotivation, and blunted affect, can occur concurrently or may predate the onset of positive symptoms. The negative symptom phase may be prolonged in schizophrenia manifesting before the age of 20 (Hafner & Nowotny, 1995).

Recovery

During the recovery phase the illness may resolve completely or may continue in a low-level, chronic state of illness. While 49%–62% of patients go into remission after an acute episode following successful intervention, over 80% of the patients who have more than one psychotic episode do not recover completely and never reach their premorbid level of functioning (Ciompi, 1980).

Residual Phase

The residual phase is characterized by attenuated psychotic symptoms and, often times, prominent negative symptoms. Patients may continue in this phase for long periods of time, or they may cycle through acute, recovery, and residual phases.

Assessment

A careful diagnostic assessment, including physical and neurological examinations, neuropsychological tests, laboratory, and brain-imaging studies, is the first step in the evaluation of a young adult presenting with psychotic symptoms. The question of whether the patient's current presentation overlaps with a known physical or neurological disorder should be in the forefront of the clinician's mind. Progressive cognitive decline should raise the possibility of a degenerative brain condition. The differential diagnosis of schizophrenia covers a myriad of psychiatric and nonpsychiatric medical conditions. Because treatments are available for many of these nonpsychiatric illnesses, it is imperative that these conditions be ruled out first. Table 22-2 presents a list of conditions that should be considered in the differential diagnosis of schizophrenia. Most physical disorders with symptoms that overlap with schizophrenia can be ruled out with a thorough physical examination and laboratory assessment. Brain imaging or EEG studies should be obtained if clinically indicated (see below). Collateral history is also a crucial element in evaluating the course and current level of function of the patient.

Table 22-2. List of Nonpsychiatric Medical Conditions That Can Mimic Schizophrenia

Metabolic Conditions	*Substance-Related Disorders*	*Psychiatric Disorders*
Renal failure	Illicit substances, including alcohol, hallucinogens, heroin, inhalants, psychostimulants, and phencyclidine	Bipolar affective disorder
Hepatic failure		Major depressive disorder
Pancreatic disease		Borderline personality disorder
Hypercalcemia/ hypocalcemia	Prescription drugs, including steroids and stimulants	Posttraumatic stress disorder
Hypercalcemia/hypocalcemia		Substance use disorder
Hyperglycemia/hypoglycemia	Withdrawal syndromes associated with alcohol, hallucinogens, opiates, psychostimulants, or sedative-hypnotics	Brief psychotic disorder
Porphyria		Delusional disorder
Dehydration	Overdose with anticholinergics	*Neurologic Disorders*
Hyperosmolarity states	*Miscellaneous Conditions*	Wilson disease
Endocrine Conditions	Cerbrovascular accidents	Parkinson disease
Addison disease	Inborn errors of metabolism	Huntington disease
Cushing disease	Seizure (especially complex partial seizures)	Sydenham chorea
Hypothyroidism/ hyperthyroidism	Hydrocephalus	Idiopathic basal ganglia calcification
Hyperparathyroidism	Hypoxic encephalopathy	Spinocerebellar degeneration
Panhypopituitarism	Narcolepsy	Adrenoleukodystrophy
Nutritional Disorders	Carbon monoxide, or heavy metals poisoning	Metachromatic leukodystrophy
Thiamin deficiency	Trauma (especially to frontal and temporal regions)	Marchiafava-Bignami disease
Folate deficiency		Multiple sclerosis
B12 deficiency		*Infectious conditions*
Niacin deficiency		Herpes simplex
Autoimmune Conditions		HIV
Systemic lupus erythematosus		Syphilis
Temporal arteritis		Parasites

Source: From White, Anjum, & Schulz (2006).

Psychiatric Differential Diagnosis

Many psychiatric conditions present with psychotic features in addition to their core symptoms. Although replete with challenges, it is important that the clinician carefully discriminate these diagnostic groups since the prognosis and management of these patients can vary significantly by diagnosis. In addition, diagnosis has a tremendous impact on the services and the supports rendered to patients.

Affective Disorders

Depressive symptoms can be confused with negative symptoms of schizophrenia, and at times it is very difficult to tease these apart. Depressed patients frequently have greater insight and identify sad feelings and recognize a departure from their baseline. In contrast, schizophrenic patients with negative symptoms tend to have less insight and may have symptoms more characteristic of schizophrenia, such as disorganized speech or thought blocking. Acute phases of bipolar disorder and schizophrenia may be difficult to differentiate early on due to an overlap of symptoms, such as psychosis and irritability. Bipolar disorder can be distinguished in the presence of either an elated or irritable mood, increased energy, or increased goal-directed activity (McClellan & McCurry, 1999; Yung & McGorry, 1996).

Substance Use Disorders

Substance use has been documented in over 50% of young patients seen in psychiatric clinics (Martin, Milich, Martin, Hartung, & Haigler, 1997). It is essential to determine if the substance use is the cause for the psychotic symptoms or is the consequence of a psychotic illness. This determination can best be made by observing the patient during a period of abstinence from the drugs of abuse.

Pervasive Developmental Disorders

Historically, autism was believed to be the precursor of schizophrenia. The early presentation of schizophrenia in a subset of individuals and autism spectrum disorders may parallel each other. History of impaired development in the motor, language, and communication spheres; marked social withdrawal; and narrow interests may be common to both. Autism emerges early in life, almost always prior to the age of 3. These children show poor emotional reciprocity, stereotypies, and perseverative behaviors. Further, the presence of hallucinations and delusions and a period of typical early development may distinguish schizophrenia from autism.

Personality Disorders

Patients with certain personality disorders can sometimes masquerade as schizophrenia. A prodrome similar to that of schizophrenia has been observed in adolescent patients that are later diagnosed with borderline personality disorder or antisocial personality disorders (McClellan, Werry, & Ham, 1993). Past enduring patterns of dysfunctional interpersonal relationships distinguish a personality disorder from schizophrenia. Schizotypal personality disorder, which presents with attenuated psychotic symptoms, is not associated with a decline in premorbid function, as is typically seen in the schizophrenia prodrome (Handest & Parnas, 2005). Borderline personality disorder, which can present with brief psychotic symptoms, can be distinguished by a sense of emptiness and fear of abandonment, and it is not necessarily associated with the negative symptoms seen in schizophrenia.

Posttraumatic Stress Disorder

Psychotic symptoms such as auditory hallucinations, dissociative episodes, and delusions have been reported in children who have experienced considerable abuse and deprivation. Childhood trauma has long been associated with psychotic symptoms, specifically auditory hallucinations and delusions. A diagnosis of PTSD should be seriously considered in patients with history of trauma, although diagnosis of PTSD does not exclude the diagnosis of schizophrenia.

Laboratory and Imaging Findings

Laboratory studies should include a urine test for substances of abuse and blood tests to evaluate thyroid, renal, and liver function. In addition, serum electrolytes (including magnesium, phosphate, calcium, and glucose) and heavy metal screening should be performed. When abnormalities are found in the physical or neurological examination or in the initial laboratory studies, further testing is indicated. This may include serum ceruloplasmin, vitamin levels, HIV antibodies, cortisol levels, and serology (i.e., VDRL and Treponema pallidum hemagglutination assay). A family history of chromosomal abnormalities or mental retardation or the presence of dysmorphic features, relating to fragile X or chromosome 22q11 deletion syndrome, may indicate chromosomal analysis.

Imaging studies should be obtained when there is evidence of focal neurological symptoms, history of head injury, acute onset of symptoms, delirium, or evidence of a neurodegenerative disorder. While brain imaging studies are useful in ruling out nonpsychiatric medical conditions, they cannot yet be used for diagnosing schizophrenia; many of the findings in brain imaging studies demonstrate group changes, with considerable overlap between patients and controls.

Sleep-deprived EEG may be obtained to rule out seizures if there is a history of episodic loss of consciousness, repetitive movements or vocalizations, periodic staring spells, or ictal symptoms. The electrical activity in the electroencephalogram (EEG) and the event-related potentials extracted from the EEG provide additional temporal resolution for examining brain function (McCarley, Nakamura, Shenton, & Salisbury, 2008). Promising research is currently underway investigating the use of these techniques to obtain more information about brain functioning in schizophrenia (Roopan et al., 2008), but currently additional studies are needed to look for the possibility of spectral EEG as a diagnostic test for schizophrenia (Boutros et al., 2008).

Finally, IQ and psychological testing to evaluate general intelligence, attention, working memory, and processing speeds are recommended in patients presenting with psychosis. A large body of literature exists demonstrating that cognitive deficits exist upon diagnosis of schizophrenia (Fuller et al., 2002; Kenny et al., 1997; Kravariti, Morris, Rabe-Hesketh, Murray, & Frangou, 2003), and several studies of adults with schizophrenia have obtained retrospective data from childhood and adolescence showing premorbid cognitive dysfunction, including academic decline (Ang & Tan, 2004; Fuller et al., 2002). Since neurocognitive deficits are know to predict negative functional outcomes (Cervellione, Burdick, Cottone, Rhinewine, & Kumra, 2007), assessment of cognitive functioning will facilitate appropriate recommendations for school and vocational rehabilitation.

Treatment

Kraepelin (1919) described 59% of his patients as catatonic and 75% as seriously ill, reaching a terminal state of profound dementia. Complete recovery was reported only in 4.1% of the patients. Since the advent of effective treatments, subsequent studies have reported more favorable outcomes with remission rates ranging from 20% to 68% with the aid of biological and psychosocial interventions. Recent studies have shown that early intervention may result in improved outcomes (Perkins, Gu, Boteva, & Lieberman, 2005), which emphasizes the importance of early recognition of symptoms. The primary goals of treatment are as follows: *(1)* prevention of the onset of acute illness in at-risk populations, *(2)* control of acute psychotic symptoms, *(3)* prevention of relapses and hospitalization, *(4)* promotion of optimal functioning during periods of remission, *(5)* fostering of independent living for individuals in the chronic or the residual phases of the illness, and *(6)* education about the illness to the patient and the family.

Pharmacologic Treatments

The mainstay of the pharmacologic treatments includes the conventional antipsychotics (typical antipsychotics or first-generation antipsychotics [FGA]) and newer antipsychotic (atypical antipsychotics or second-generation antipsychotic [SGA]) medications. FGAs such as haloperidol, chlorpromazine, and fluphenazine have been used both in the acute and maintenance phases of schizophrenia. They are effective in controlling agitation and positive symptoms. FGAs target dopamine receptors (especially D2); within this class, higher potency is related to greater extrapyramidal neurologic side effects, whereas medium potency FGAs tend to cause hypotension and sedation.

The SGAs are known to be "multispectral," affecting dopamine, serotonin, acetylcholine, epinephrine, and histamine receptors. They differ from typical antipsychotics in possessing greater selectivity toward the mesolimbic and mesocortical dopamine receptors, presynaptic serotonin receptor blockade, and a greater balance in dopamine receptor D1 and D2 receptor blockade. The efficacy of these medications has been historically tied with dopamine (D2) receptor blockade. Recent studies have further strengthened this concept, showing that both efficacy and side effects are linked to dopamine receptor occupancy (Frankle et al., 2004; Medori, Mannaert, & Grunder, 2006; Zipursky et al., 2005). The SGAs seem to be more efficacious because of their action on both the dopamine and serotonergic receptors. Their unique side effect profile also stems from their differential affinities to both these receptors (Shapiro et al., 2003) (see Table 22-3). Recently there has been a surge in the use of SGAs because of their relative ease of use, efficacy in the treatment of positive and mood symptoms, and their low rate of neurological and motor side effects. The propensity of less neurological and motor side effects of the SGAs is secondary to greater selectivity toward the mesolimbic and mesocortical dopamine system, sparing the nigrostriatal dopamine pathways. As a class, however, SGAs can cause a metabolic syndrome that includes significant weight gain, dyslipidemias, and hyperglycemia. Despite this drawback, SGAs are currently the primary treatment for young adults with schizophrenia, and the following discussion will focus on the use of medications in this class.

For antipsychotic medications, there is an optimal occupancy of the receptors for efficacy; dosage leading to higher than optimal binding of the receptors may contribute toward side effects. For example, when risperidone was initially introduced, it was recommended in dosages of 12–16 mg/day to control positive symptoms. Later studies have shown the efficacy to be optimized with dosages between 4–6 mg/day (Marder, Conley, Ereshefsky, Kane, & Turner, 2003). The newer long-acting injectable form of risperidone is effective at doses of 25 or 50 mg injected i.m. every 2 weeks. This formulation causes minimal fluctuation in plasma levels and enables maintenance of D2-receptor occupancy at a level below the threshold for extrapyramidal side effects (EPS) (Medori, Mannaert, & Grunder, 2006). Of the SGAs, Risperidal is most associated with elevations in prolactin, which can sometimes lead to gynecomastia and galactorhhea.

The maximal recommended dosage for olanzapine is 20 mg for acute stages of the illness and around 10–15 mg for maintenance phases. In a randomized double-blind trial comparing olanzapine and haloperidol, both medications decreased symptom severity, but olanzapine treatment was associated with lower incidence of parkinsonian symptoms. However, weight gain in olanzapine-treated patients was substantial (Lieberman et al., 2003).

Table 22-3. Atypical Antipsychotics: Binding (Ki Values) at Neurotransmitter Receptors and Side Effects

Medication	5-HT$_2$ (nM)	D$_2$ (nM)	D$_1$ (nM)	Side Effects
Aripiprazole	3.4	3.4	265	Mild orthostasis
Clozapine	1.6	180	38	Sedation, weight gain, orthostasis, anti-cholinergic, metabolic syndrome/dyslipidemia
Olanzapine	4	11	31	Sedation, weight gain, metabolic syndrome/dyslipidemia
Quetiapine	294	160	455	Sedation
Risperidone	0.16	3.3	750	Hyper-prolactinemia, orthostasis
Ziprasidone	0.42	0.42	525	Mild orthostasis
Ziprasidone	0.42	4.79	339	Mild orthostasis

The recommended dosing for quetiapine is between 400–600 mg/day, although improvement with higher dosages has been reported (Small, Hirsch, Arvanitis, Miller, & Link, 1997).

Ziprasidone is most effective at doses of 100 mg/day and has shown to cause minimal weight gain. EKG monitoring has been advised to monitor QTc prolongation.

Aripiprazole has a unique mechanism of action as a dopamine D2 partial agonist, serotonin 5-HT(1A) partial agonist, and serotonin 5-HT(2A) antagonist. Treatment with aripirazole is associated with significant adverse effect on serum prolactin concentrations, or QTc prolongation, and minimal weight gain in both acute and long-term treatment trials (Keck & McElroy, 2003). A study comparing placebo and aripiprazole along with risperidone showed similar efficacy for both medications in reducing the positive symptoms. Aripiprazole treatment also resulted in improvement of negative symptoms with fewer extrapyramidal side effects. Prolactin levels were decreased in patients on aripiprazole when compared to those treated with risperidone (Potkin et al., 2003).

Patients seem to derive most benefit from clozapine at dosages of 300–600 mg/day. For treatment-resistant schizophrenia, clozapine has been effective in dosages of 500–900 mg/day with significant reduction in suicidality. Close monitoring for agranulocytosis, with weekly blood draws initially, extending to biweekly blood draws after 6 months is indicated. Risk for seizures is 2% per year at a dosage of 300 mg/day and increases to 6% per year at increased dosages of 900 mg/day. When dosages above the maximal are administered, it is recommended that an anticonvulsant be administered concomitantly. The side effects of excessive drooling, sedation, and weight gain have been observed with clozapine.

Patients suffering from chronic mental health problems are at increased risk for medical comorbidities, such as cardiovascular illness, obesity, and osteoarthritis. Prevalence of risk factors such as smoking, poverty, poor nutrition, sedentary lifestyles, and inadequate access to health care compound these risks. Medications can contribute to the risk factors by causing weight gain and metabolic abnormalities. Careful monitoring combined with recommendations for healthy living is advocated at the start of the medication. When unhealthy weight gain is apparent, a switch to a weight-neutral medication or addition of dietic or psychopharmacologic interventions is recommended.

Debate is ongoing regarding the merits and demerits of FGAs versus SGAs. It is abundantly clear that patients will not hesitate to discontinue medications that cause disabling side effects, even though the therapeutic benefits are apparent (Lieberman et al., 2005). Various head-to-head efficacy trials with FGAs, SGAs, and placebo have convincingly shown that although FGAs are just as effective as SGAs in positive symptom control, SGAs may be more efficacious in reducing the negative symptoms (Lieberman et al., 2003), although this has been challenged (Rosenheck et al., 2003).

While antipsychotics are the mainstay of treatment, other biological interventions are used to treat comorbid anxiety, depression, disruptive behaviors, and attention problems that can co-occur with schizophrenia. These include antidepressants, mood stabilizers, benzodiazepines, and in some cases stimulants. Caution must be exerted in prescribing stimulants because stimulants themselves can induce psychosis (Cornblatt, Lencz, & Obuchowski, 2002). Substance abuse is a significant comorbidity occurring in a majority of patients with schizophrenia. It also is a major determinant of treatment compliance. In addition to the above biological interventions, attention should be paid to address the substance abuse. Dual diagnoses (schizophrenia and substance use disorders) have also been associated with significantly higher scores on conceptual disorganization, depressed mood, hostility, hallucinations, and unusual thought content (Mauri et al., 2006).

A major caveat to the discussion about medication treatment for schizophrenia is that poor medication compliance is reportedly seen in about 80% of outpatients and is a significant determinant of outcome. To address this, psychoeducation is essential.

Psychosocial Treatments

Psychosocial treatments, including individual therapy, family psychoeducation, crisis management, and community services should be incorporated in the integrative supportive network for optimal outcome for patients with schizophrenia. Individual supportive therapy is helpful in the acute phase to limit hospital stay and decrease the severity of illness. Psychodynamic psychotherapy has not been successful in this population. Family psychoeducation geared toward educating families about the illness and treatment options, mitigating dysfunctional communication, and providing support to overwhelmed families has shown to decrease frequency of hospitalizations and improve compliance/ communication.

Cognitive-Behavioral Therapy

Cognitive-behavioral therapy (CBT) aims to positively influence emotions by modifying a person's automatic thoughts and behavior. The goal is to challenge and alter distorted beliefs and to replace them with more realistic thoughts. Interventions adding CBT to routine care has shown greater reductions on measures of overall schizophrenia symptoms, positive symptoms, disorganization, and social functioning; however, negative symptoms are slower to respond. CBT has also been found to reduce posttreatment and follow-up depression severity scores (Startup, Jackson, & Bendix, 2004). CBT interventions aimed at enhancing medication compliance may be helpful in the long-term adherence to treatment.

School and Vocational Interventions

School-based interventions, including social skills training, educational support, and vocational skills training, are indicated early in the course of the illness. The goal is to optimize the functioning of the young adults and to help them return as close as possible to their baseline level of function. Most adolescents and many young adults spend a significant portion of their day in a school setting and therefore school based interventions are highly relevant. Not only is the school environment demanding for patients suffering from an acute illness, but it can both create and perpetuate stress. It therefore becomes imperative for health care providers and caregivers to educate the school staff about schizophrenia and its typical presentation, including symptoms like inattention, aggression, and disruptive behaviors in order to create a collaborative effort toward fostering the well-being of these young people.

School interventions should be designed to meet individual needs of patients, comprehensively addressing their cognitive limitations, while carefully paying attention to avoid stigmatization. Ideally, these youth are better managed in smaller class settings with trained staff who can be attuned to their symptoms and early signs of relapse. Instructions need to be modified to meet the needs of the patient. Reinforcement of oral classes should be done with printed material. When the adolescent's illness precludes school attendance, home-based education and computer-based learning opportunities should be provided. Availability of mental health staff is helpful in the event that a crisis should arise. Opportunity should be provided to improve socialization and enhance participation in extracurricular activities when the individual is stable. Customized education or vocational plans should be drafted that take existing cognitive deficits into account. For those individuals who are unable to complete school/college, opportunities should be provided for vocational rehabilitation so that they can master activities of daily living and acquire some trade skills to enable independent living.

Prevention

There is effort underway in a number of academic centers to identify ultra high-risk adolescents and young adults manifesting subclinical psychotic symptoms or those who are at an increased genetic risk for developing psychosis ("prepsychotic" individuals) (McGlashan et al., 2007). These clinics are geared toward early identification and prevention of onset of acute psychotic illness with psychosocial and psychopharmacological interventions. Current evidence supports the view that early intervention in prodrome patients can delay the onset of illness (McGorry et al., 2002) and can decrease risk for suicidality (Melle et al., 2006).

Conclusion

Schizophrenia is a potentially devastating illness that has far-reaching effects for individuals, families, and the society at large. Recent strides in understanding schizophrenia have given credence to the biologic basis of the illness and to neurodevelopmental theories recognizing the combined contributions of genetic predisposition and environmental risk factors. Given recent evidence that early intervention may alter the trajectory of schizophrenia spectrum disorders and lead to improved outcomes (Schaffner & McGorry, 2001), early identification becomes vitally important. Newer medications have helped individuals suffering from schizophrenia optimize their functioning by minimizing the side effects and possibly improving cognition. Of prime importance is the realization that this illness affects a population during a critical period of development and thus impedes the ability of patients to reach their potential in various spheres. Interventions should be geared to optimize and support the individuals to restore normal developmental trajectories. In addition to medication management, psychoeducation and family support are deemed to be of vital importance in the treatment of these individuals. Increased awareness of the course of the illness in the younger individuals may help with early recognition and limit deterioration from the illness.

KEY POINTS

- Schizophrenia is a chronic illness that affects individuals during the early stages of life. As a result, it has a tremendous impact on not only the life of the individual, but also on the lives of their families and society at large.
- Schizophrenia is a multifactorial illness with a yet unknown etiology that involves both genetic and environmental factors.
- Recent research findings are supporting a biological diathesis which may pave way for better understanding of this illness and effective treatment interventions.
- Emerging treatements have been very effective for treating the positive symptoms of the illness. However, treating the negative symptoms and cognitive deficits has been more challenging.

PRACTICE GUIDELINES

- Effective psychopharmocological interventions will decrease the morbidity and modify the course of illness.
- Instituting preventive measures and closer monitoring can help alleviate adverse effects related to neuroleptics.
- Individual therapy and family psycho-education are important components of the treatment plan and may decrease the duration of hospitalization and improve compliance and outcome.

References

Ang, Y. G., & Tan, H. Y. (2004). Academic deterioration prior to first episode schizophrenia in young Singaporean males. *Psychiatry Research, 121*(3), 303–307.

Asarnow, J. R., & Ben-Meir, S. (1988). Children with schizophrenia spectrum and depressive disorders: A comparative study of premorbid adjustment, onset pattern and severity of impairment. *Journal of Child Psychology and Psychiatry, 29*(4), 477–488.

Barnes, T. R., Mutsatsa, S. H., Hutton, S. B., Watt, H. C., & Joyce, E. M. (2006). Comorbid substance use and age at onset of schizophrenia. *British Journal of Psychiatry, 188,* 237–242.

Basso, M. R., Nasrallah, H. A., Olson, S. C., & Bornstein, R. A. (1997). Cognitive deficits distinguish patients with adolescent- and adult-onset schizophrenia. *Neuropsychiatry, Neuropsychology, and Behavioral Neurology, 10*(2), 107–112.

Bellino, S., Rocca, P., Patria, L., Marchiaro, L., Rasetti, R., Di Lorenzo, R., Paradiso, E., & Bogetto, F. (2004). Relationships of age at onset with clinical features and cognitive functions in a sample of schizophrenia patients. *Journal of Clinical Psychiatry, 65*(7), 908–914.

Boutros, N. N., Arfken, C., Galderisi, S., Warrick, J., Pratt, G., & Iacono, W. (2008). The status of spectral EEG abnormality as a diagnostic test for schizophrenia. *Schizophrenia Research, 99*(1–3), 225–237.

Brown, A. S., Begg, M. D., Gravenstein, S., Schaefer, C. A., Wyatt, R. J., Bresnahan, M., Babulas, V. P., & Susser, E. S. (2004). Serologic evidence of prenatal influenza in the etiology of schizophrenia. *Archives of General Psychiatry, 61*(8), 774–780.

Bulayeva, K. B., Glatt, S. J., Bulayev, O. A., Pavlova, T. A., & Tsuang, M. T. (2007). Genome-wide linkage scan of schizophrenia: A cross-isolate study. *Genomics, 89*(2), 167–177.

Caspi, A., Moffitt, T. E., Cannon, M., McClay, J., Murray, R., Harrington, H., Taylor, A., Arseneault, L., Williams, B., Braithwaite, A., Poulton, R., & Craig, I. W. (2005). Moderation of the effect of adolescent-onset cannabis use on adult psychosis by a functional polymorphism in the catechol-O-methyltransferase gene: Longitudinal evidence of a gene X environment interaction. *Biological Psychiatry, 57*(10), 1117–1127.

Cervellione, K. L., Burdick, K. E., Cottone, J. G., Rhinewine, J. P., & Kumra, S. (2007). Neurocognitive deficits in adolescents with schizophrenia: Longitudinal stability and predictive utility for short-term functional outcome. *Journal of the American Academy of Child and Adolescent Psychiatry, 46*(7), 867–878.

Ciompi, L. (1980). The natural history of schizophrenia in the long term. *British Journal of Psychiatry, 136,* 413–420.

Cornblatt, B., Lencz, T., & Obuchowski, M. (2002). The schizophrenia prodrome: Treatment and high-risk perspectives. *Schizophrenia Research, 54*(1–2), 177–186.

Frankle, W. G., Gil, R., Hackett, E., Mawlawi, O., Zea-Ponce, Y., Zhu, Z., Kochan, L. D., Cangiano, C., Slifstein, M., Gorman, J. M., Laruelle, M., & Abi-Dargham, A. (2004). Occupancy of dopamine D2 receptors by the atypical antipsychotic drugs risperidone and olanzapine: Theoretical implications. *Psychopharmacology (Berlin), 175*(4), 473–480.

Fuller, R., Nopoulos, P., Arndt, S., O'Leary, D., Ho, B. C., & Andreasen, N. C. (2002). Longitudinal assessment of premorbid cognitive functioning in patients with schizophrenia through examination of standardized scholastic test performance. *American Journal of Psychiatry, 159*(7), 1183–1189.

Galdos, P., van Os, J., & Murray, R. (1993). Puberty and the onset of psychosis. *Schizophrenia Bulletin, 10*(1), 7–14.

Gottesman, II, & Shields, J. (1966). Schizophrenia in twins: 16 years' consecutive admissions to a psychiatric clinic. *British Journal of Psychiatry, 112*(489), 809–818.

Hafner, H. (1998). Onset and course of the first schizophrenic episode. *Kaohsiung Journal of Medical Science, 14*(7), 413–431.

Hafner, H., & an der Heiden, W. (1993). Epidemiology of schizophrenia. *Canadian Journal of Psychiatry, 42*(2), 139–151.

Hafner, H., Maurer, K., Loffler, W., & Riecher-Rossler, A. (1993). The influence of age and sex on the onset and early course of schizophrenia. *British Journal of Psychiatry, 162,* 80–86.

Hafner, H., & Nowotny, B. (1995). Epidemiology of early-onset schizophrenia. *European Archives of Psychiatry and Clinical Neuroscience, 245*(2), 80–92.

Hakak, Y., Walker, J. R., Li, C., Wong, W. H., Davis, K. L., Buxbaum, J. D., Haroutunian, V., & Fienberg, A. A. (2001). Genome-wide expression analysis reveals dysregulation of myelination-related genes in chronic schizophrenia. *Proceedings of the National Academy of Sciences USA, 98*(8), 4746–4751.

Handest, P., & Parnas, J. (2005). Clinical characteristics of first-admitted patients with ICD-10 schizotypal disorder. *British Journal of Psychiatry Supplement, 48,* s49–54.

Ho, B. C., Alicata, D., Ward, J., Moser, D. J., O'Leary, D. S., Arndt, S., & Andreasen, N. C. (2003). Untreated initial psychosis: Relation to cognitive deficits and brain morphology in first-episode schizophrenia. *American Journal of Psychiatry, 160*(1), 142–148.

Isohanni, M., Isohanni, I., Koponen, H., Koskinen, J., Laine, P., Lauronen, E., Miettunen, J., Maki, P., Riala, K., Rasanen, S., Saari, K., Tienari, P., Veijola, J., & Murray, G. (2004). Developmental precursors of psychosis. *Current Psychiatry Report, 6*(3), 168–175.

Isohanni, M., Jones, P. B., Moilanen, K., Rantakallio, P., Veijola, J., Oja, H., Koiranen, M., Jokelainen, J., Croudace, T., & Jarvelin, M. (2001). Early developmental milestones in adult schizophrenia and other psychoses. A 31-year follow-up of the Northern Finland 1966 Birth Cohort. *Schizophrenia Research, 52*(1–2), 1–19.

Jeste, D. V., McAdams, L. A., Palmer, B. W., Braff, D., Jernigan, T. L., Paulsen, J. S., Stout, J. C., Symonds,

L. L., Bailey, A., & Heaton, R. K. (1998). Relationship of neuropsychological and MRI measures to age of onset of schizophrenia. *Acta Psychiatrica Scandinavica, 98*(2), 156–164.

Johnstone, E. C., Owens, D. G., Bydder, G. M., Colter, N., Crow, T. J., & Frith, C. D. (1989). The spectrum of structural brain changes in schizophrenia: Age of onset as a predictor of cognitive and clinical impairments and their cerebral correlates. *Psychological Medicine, 19*(1), 91–103.

Jones, P., Rodgers, B., Murray, R., & Marmot, M. (1994). Child development risk factors for adult schizophrenia in the British 1946 birth cohort. *Lancet, 344*(8934), 1398–1402.

Keck, P. E., Jr., & McElroy, S. L. (2003). Aripiprazole: A partial dopamine D2 receptor agonist antipsychotic. *Expert Opinion on Investigational Drugs, 12*(4), 655–662.

Kendler, K. S., Myers, J. M., O'Neill, F. A., Martin, R., Murphy, B., MacLean, C. J., Walsh, D., & Straub, R. E. (2000). Clinical features of schizophrenia and linkage to chromosomes 5q, 6p, 8p, and 10p in the Irish Study of High-Density Schizophrenia Families. *American Journal of Psychiatry, 157*(3), 402–408.

Kenny, J. T., Friedman, L., Findling, R. L., Swales, T. P., Strauss, M. E., Jesberger, J. A., & Schulz, S. C. (1997). Cognitive impairment in adolescents with schizophrenia. *American Journal of Psychiatry, 154*(11), 1613–1615.

Keshavan, M. S., Diwadkar, V. A., Montrose, D. M., Rajarethinam, R., & Sweeney, J. A. (2005). Premorbid indicators and risk for schizophrenia: A selective review and update. *Schizophrenia Research, 79*(1), 45–57.

Kirkbride, J. B., Fearon, P., Morgan, C., Dazzan, P., Morgan, K., Tarrant, J., Lloyd, T., Holloway, J., Hutchinson, G., Leff, J. P., Mallett, R. M., Harrison, G. L., Murray, R. M., & Jones, P. B. (2006). Heterogeneity in incidence rates of schizophrenia and other psychotic syndromes: Findings from the 3-center AeSOP study. *Archives of General Psychiatry, 63*(3), 250–258.

Koponen, H., Rantakallio, P., Veijola, J., Jones, P., Jokelainen, J., & Isohanni, M. (2004). Childhood central nervous system infections and risk for schizophrenia. *European Archives of Psychiatry and Clinical Neuroscience, 254*(1), 9–13.

Kraepelin, E. *Dementia Praecox and Paraphrenia*. (1919). Translated and edited by R. M. Barclay and G. M. Robertson, Edinburgh, Scotland. E. % S. Livingstone, 1971.

Krausz, M., & Muller-Thomsen, T. (1993). Schizophrenia with onset in adolescence: An 11-year follow-up. *Schizophrenia Bulletin, 19*(4), 831–841.

Kravariti, E., Morris, R. G., Rabe-Hesketh, S., Murray, R. M., & Frangou, S. (2003). The Maudsley early onset schizophrenia study: Cognitive function in adolescents with recent onset schizophrenia. *Schizophrenia Research, 61*(2–3), 137–148.

Lieberman, J. A., Stroup, T. S., McEvoy, J. P., Swartz, M. S., Rosenheck, R. A., Perkins, D. O., Keefe, R. S., Davis, S. M., Davis, C. E., Lebowitz, B. D., Severe, J., & Hsiao, J. K. (2005). Effectiveness of antipsychotic drugs in patients with chronic schizophrenia. *New England Journal of Medicine, 353*(12), 1209–1223.

Lieberman, J. A., Tollefson, G., Tohen, M., Green, A. I., Gur, R. E., Kahn, R., McEvoy, J., Perkins, D., Sharma, T., Zipursky, R., Wei, H., & Hamer, R. M. (2003). Comparative efficacy and safety of atypical and conventional antipsychotic drugs in first-episode psychosis: A randomized, double-blind trial of olanzapine versus haloperidol. *American Journal of Psychiatry, 160*(8), 1396–1404.

Loewy, R. L., Bearden, C. E., Johnson, J. K., Raine, A., & Cannon, T. D. (2005). The prodromal questionnaire (PQ): Preliminary validation of a self-report screening measure for prodromal and psychotic syndromes. *Schizophrenia Research, 77*(2–3), 141–149.

Malla, A. K., Takhar, J. J., Norman, R. M., Manchanda, R., Cortese, L., Haricharan, R., Verdi, M., & Ahmed, R. (2002). Negative symptoms in first episode nonaffective psychosis. *Acta Psychiatrica Scandinavica, 105*(6), 431–439.

Manschreck, T. C., Maher, B. A., Candela, S. F. (2004). Earlier age of first diagnosis in schizophrenia is related to impaired motor control. *Schizophrenia Bulletin, 30*(2), 351–360.

Marder, S. R., Conley, R., Ereshefsky, L., Kane, J. M., & Turner, M. S. (2003). Clinical guidelines: Dosing and switching strategies for long-acting risperidone. *Journal of Clinical Psychiatry, 64*(Suppl. 16), 41–46.

Martin, C. A., Milich, R., Martin, W. R., Hartung, C. M., & Haigler, E. D. (1997). Gender differences in adolescent psychiatric outpatient substance use: Associated behaviors and feelings. *Journal of the American Academy of Child and Adolescent Psychiatry, 36*(4), 486–494.

Masi, G., Mucci, M., & Pari, C. (2006). Children with schizophrenia: Clinical picture and pharmacological treatment. *CNS Drugs, 20*(10), 841–866.

Mauri, M. C., Volonteri, L. S., De Gaspari, I. F., Colasanti, A., Brambilla, M. A., & Cerruti, L. (2006). Substance abuse in first-episode schizophrenic patients: A retrospective study. *Clinical Practice and Epidemiology in Mental Health, 2*, 4.

McCarley, R. W., Nakamura, M., Shenton, M. E., & Salisbury, D. F. (2008). Combining ERP and structural MRI information in first episode schizophrenia and bipolar disorder. *Clinical EEG Neuroscience, 39*(2), 57–60.

McClellan, J., & McCurry, C. (1999). Early onset psychotic disorders: Diagnostic stability and clinical characteristics. *European Child and Adolescent Psychiatry, 8*(Suppl. 1) 113–119.

McClellan, J., & Werry, J. (1994). Practice parameters for the assessment and treatment of children and adolescents with schizophrenia. *Journal of the American Academy of Child and Adolescent Psychiatry, 33*(5), 616–635.

McClellan, J. M., Werry, J. S., & Ham, M. (1993). A follow-up study of early onset psychosis: Comparison between outcome diagnoses of schizophrenia, mood disorders, and personality disorders. *Journal of Autism and Developmental Disorders, 23*(2), 243–262.

McGlashan, T. H., Addington, J., Cannon, T., Heinimaa, M., McGorry, P., O'Brien, M., Penn, D., Perkins, D., Salokangas, R. K., Walsh, B., Woods, S. W., & Yung, A. (2007). Recruitment and treatment practices for help-seeking "prodromal" patients. *Schizophrenia Bulletin, 33*(3), 715–726.

McGorry, P. D., Yung, A. R., Phillips, L. J., Yuen, H. P., Francey, S., Cosgrave, E. M., Germano, D., Bravin, J., McDonald, T., Blair, A., Adlard, S., & Jackson, H. (2002). Randomized controlled trial of interventions designed to reduce the risk of progression to first-episode psychosis in a clinical sample with subthreshold symptoms. *Archives of General Psychiatry, 59*(10), 921–928.

McGrath, J., Saha, S., Welham, J., El Saadi, O., MacCauley, C., & Chant, D. (2004). A systematic review of the incidence of schizophrenia: The distribution of rates and the influence of sex, urbanicity, migrant status and methodology. *BMC Medicine, 2*, 13.

Medori, R., Mannaert, E., & Grunder, G. (2006). Plasma antipsychotic concentration and receptor occupancy, with special focus on risperidone long-acting injectable. *European Neuropsychopharmacology, 16*(4), 233–240.

Melle, I., Johannesen, J. O., Friis, S., Haahr, U., Joa, I., Larsen, T. K., Opjordsmoen, S., Rund, B. R., Simonsen, E., Vaglum, P., & McGlashan, T. (2006). Early detection of the first episode of schizophrenia and suicidal behavior. *American Journal of Psychiatry, 163*(5), 800–804.

Nicolson, R., Giedd, J. N., Lenane, M., Hamburger, S., Singaracharlu, S., Bedwell, J., Fernandez, T., Thaker, G. K., Malaspina, D., & Rapoport, J. L. (1999). Clinical and neurobiological correlates of cytogenetic abnormalities in childhood-onset schizophrenia. *American Journal of Psychiatry, 156*(10), 1575–1579.

Owens, D. G., Miller, P., Lawrie, S. M., & Johnstone, E. C. (2005). Pathogenesis of schizophrenia: A psychopathological perspective. *British Journal of Psychiatry, 186*, 386–393.

Pantelis, C., Yucel, M., Wood, S. J., Velakoulis, D., Sun, D., Berger, G., Stuart, G. W., Yung, A., Phillips, L., & McGorry, P. D. (2005). Structural brain imaging evidence for multiple pathological processes at different stages of brain development in schizophrenia. *Schizophrenia Bulletin, 31*(3), 672–696.

Perala, J., Suvisaari, J., Saarni, S. I., Kuoppasalmi, K., Isometsa, E., Pirkola, S., Partonen, T., Tuulio-Henriksson, A., Hintikka, J., Kieseppa, T., Harkanen, T., Koskinen, S., & Lonnqvist, J. (2007). Lifetime prevalence of psychotic and bipolar I disorders in a general population. *Archives of General Psychiatry, 64*(1), 19–28.

Perkins, D. O., Gu, H., Boteva, K., & Lieberman, J. A. (2005). Relationship between duration of untreated psychosis and outcome in first-episode schizophrenia: A critical review and meta-analysis. *American Journal of Psychiatry, 162*(10), 1785–1804.

Potkin, S. G., Saha, A. R., Kujawa, M. J., Carson, W. H., Ali, M., Stock, E., Stringfellow, J., Ingenito, G., & Marder, S. R. (2003). Aripiprazole, an antipsychotic with a novel mechanism of action, and risperidone vs. placebo in patients with schizophrenia and schizoaffective disorder. *Archives of General Psychiatry, 60*(7), 681–690.

Roopun, A. K., Cunningham, M. O., Racca, C., Alter, K., Traub, R. D., & Whittington, M. A. (2008). Region-specific changes in gamma and beta2 rhythms in NMDA receptor dysfunction models of schizophrenia. *Schizophrenia Bulletin, 34*(5), 962–973.

Rosenheck, R., Perlick, D., Bingham, S., Liu-Mares, W., Collins, J., Warren, S., Leslie, D., Allan, E., Campbell, E. C., Caroff, S., Corwin, J., Davis, L., Douyon, R., Dunn, L., Evans, D., Frecska, E., Grabowski, J., Graeber, D., Herz, L., Kwon, K., Lawson, W., Mena, F., Sheikh, J., Smelson, D., & Smith-Gamble, V. (2003). Effectiveness and cost of olanzapine and haloperidol in the treatment of schizophrenia: A randomized controlled trial. *Journal of the American Medical Association, 290*(20), 2693–2702.

Schaffner, K. F., & McGorry, P. D. (2001). Preventing severe mental illnesses—New prospects and ethical challenges. *Schizophrenia Research, 51*(1), 3–15.

Schultz, S. K., & Andreasen, N. C. (1999). Schizophrenia. *Lancet, 353*(9162), 1425–1430.

Shapiro, D. A., Renock, S., Arrington, E., Chiodo, L. A., Liu, L. X., Sibley, D. R., Roth, B. L., & Mailman, R. (2003). Aripiprazole, a novel atypical antipsychotic drug with a unique and robust pharmacology. *Neuropsychopharmacology*, *28*(8), 1400–1411.

Shenton, M. E., Dickey, C. C., Frumin, M., & McCarley, R. W. (2001). A review of MRI findings in schizophrenia. *Schizophrenia Research*, *49*(1–2), 1–52.

Small, J. G., Hirsch, S. R., Arvanitis, L. A., Miller, B. G., & Link, C. G. (1997). Quetiapine in patients with schizophrenia. A high- and low-dose double-blind comparison with placebo. Seroquel Study Group. *Archives of General Psychiatry*, *54*(6), 549–557.

Sporn, A. L., Greenstein, D. K., Gogtay, N., Jeffries, N. O., Lenane, M., Gochman, P., Clasen, L. S., Blumenthal, J., Giedd, J. N., & Rapoport, J. L. (2003). Progressive brain volume loss during adolescence in childhood-onset schizophrenia. *American Journal of Psychiatry*, *160*(12), 2181–2189.

Startup, M., Jackson, M. C., & Bendix, S. (2004). North Wales randomized controlled trial of cognitive behaviour therapy for acute schizophrenia spectrum disorders: Outcomes at 6 and 12 months. *Psychological Medicine*, *34*(3), 413–422.

Suvisaari, J. M., Haukka, J. K., & Lonnqvist, J. K. (2004). No association between season of birth of patients with schizophrenia and risk of schizophrenia among their siblings. *Schizophrenia Research*, *66*(1), 1–6.

Tang, Y. L., Gillespie, C. F., Epstein, M. P., Mao, P. X., Jiang, F., Chen, Q., Cai, Z. J., & Mitchell, P. B. (2007). Gender differences in 542 Chinese inpatients with schizophrenia. *Schizophrenia Research*, *97*(1–3), 88–96.

Thorup, A., Petersen, L., Jeppesen, P., Ohlenschlaeger, J., Christensen, T., Krarup, G., Jorgensen, P., & Nordentoft, M. (2007). Gender differences in young adults with first-episode schizophrenia spectrum disorders at baseline in the Danish OPUS study. *Journal of Nervous and Mental Disease*, *195*(5), 396–405.

Thorup, A., Waltoft, B. L., Pedersen, C. B., Mortensen, P. B., & Nordentoft, M. (2007). Young males have a higher risk of developing schizophrenia: A Danish register study. *Psychological Medicine*, *37*(4), 479–484.

Tuulio-Henriksson, A., Partonen, T., Suvisaari, J., Haukka, J., & Lonnqvist, J. (2004). Age at onset and cognitive functioning in schizophrenia. *British Journal of Psychiatry*, *185*, 215–219.

Werry, J. S., McClellan, J. M., & Chard, L. (1991). Childhood and adolescent schizophrenic, bipolar, and schizoaffective disorders: A clinical and outcome study. *Journal of the American Academy of Child and Adolescent Psychiatry*, *30*(3), 457–465.

White, T., Anjum, A., & Schulz, S. C. (2006). The schizophrenia prodrome. *American Journal of Psychiatry*, *163*(3), 376–380.

Yang, P. C., Liu, C. Y., Chiang, S. Q., Chen, J. Y., & Lin, T. S. (1995). Comparison of adult manifestations of schizophrenia with onset before and after 15 years of age. *Acta Psychiatrica Scandinavica*, *91*(3), 209–212.

Yung, A. R., & McGorry, P. D. (1996). The initial prodrome in psychosis: Descriptive and qualitative aspects. *Australian and New Zealand Journal of Psychiatry*, *30*(5), 587–599.

Yung, A. R., Phillips, L. J., Yuen, H. P., & McGorry, P. D. (2004). Risk factors for psychosis in an ultra high-risk group: Psychopathology and clinical features. *Schizophrenia Research*, *67*(2–3), 131–142.

Yung, A. R., Yuen, H. P., McGorry, P. D., Phillips, L. J., Kelly, D., Dell'Olio, M., Francey, S. M., Cosgrave, E. M., Killackey, E., Stanford, C., Godfrey, K., & Buckby, J. (2005). Mapping the onset of psychosis: The Comprehensive Assessment of At-Risk Mental States. *Australian and New Zealand Journal of Psychiatry*, *39*(11–12), 964–971.

Zipursky, R. B., Christensen, B. K., Daskalakis, Z., Epstein, I., Roy, P., Furimsky, I., Sanger, T., & Kapur, S. (2005). Treatment response to olanzapine and haloperidol and its association with dopamine D receptor occupancy in first-episode psychosis. *Canadian Journal of Psychiatry*, *50*(8), 462–469.

Chapter 23

Bipolar Disorder in Early Adulthood: Clinical Challenges and Emerging Evidence

Alan C. Swann

Ms. Y is a 24-year-old woman, recently evaluated in outpatient clinic after relocating. Her chief complaint was "I have severe attention problems and can't hold down a job." She was currently taking a norepinephrine reuptake blocker commonly used to treat attention-deficit disorder. In brief, she had done well in elementary school, with good grades, and a few regular friends. During high school, she developed periods of being restless, with poor concentration, and severely variable mood. In her initial psychiatric evaluation she received the diagnosis of depressive disorder and was treated with an SSRI. Restlessness and agitation increased, and she received a second evaluation, diagnosed as attention-deficit disorder. She was treated first with methylphenidate, then with the norepinephrine reuptake blocker. She stated that these treatments improved her attention problem. Meanwhile, she graduated from high school and was able to complete an Associate's degree course at a local junior college. After graduating, she found work successfully, but she lost a succession of jobs due to sporadic attendance, inconsistent performance, and conflict with supervisors. She is currently unemployed and moved because her boyfriend was transferred. Further history revealed no problematic drug use or legal problems. Family history was positive for "hyperactivity" (her mother), depression, and substance use. On interview, she was casually dressed and cooperative. She was quite restless. She spoke rapidly and described racing thoughts. Her eyes were usually full of tears and she said she could cry at any moment. She was not currently suicidal but said she got no pleasure form her many activities, and that she must be an incompetent person and a misfit, because of her employment problems. Detailed history revealed that she had, in the past, met criteria for major depressive episodes and for hypomanic episodes, and she currently met criteria for both. She had never met criteria for attention-deficit/hyperactivity disorder.

Introduction

Bipolar disorder is a potentially devastating illness that afflicts from 1%–4% of the population (Judd & Akiskal, 2003; Swann, 2006b), depending on how the illness is defined (Judd et al., 2003). Defining bipolar disorder for epidemiological or genetic studies is not trivial, because there is no objective test to determine whether the illness is present. This leads to controversy over the existence and the incidence of the illness. The impact and clinical features of bipolar disorder vary across the life span. Early adulthood is a crucial time in the establishment of long-term occupational and social function. During early adulthood, individuals generally are completing their educations, entering the workforce, establishing their independent lives, and starting families. Bipolar disorder that is present at this stage of life can have a tremendous impact, usually had an earlier onset, and was likely to have been initially misdiagnosed. The onset of bipolar disorder is most commonly in adolescence, and there is, on average, a diagnostic delay of about 6 or 7 years with around one-third of patients requiring more than 10 years for accurate diagnosis (Hirschfeld, Lewis, & Vornik, 2003). Therefore, bipolar disorder with earlier onset is typically identified when it causes major problems during the crucial transitions of early adulthood.

Bipolar disorder appears to have cumulative effects on brain and health if it is not treated, and its clinical manifestations interfere with normal psychological, physical, and social development (Calabrese et al., 2003; Lish, Dime-Meenan, Whybrow, & Price, 1994). Untreated illness can end life, through suicide (Jamison, 2000) or increased all-cause mortality (Angst, Stassen, Clayton, & Angst, 2002), or can ruin it (Osby, Brandt, Correia, Ekbom, & Sparen, 2001). The potential for inappropriate labeling and treatment have hazards of their own (Healy, 2006), but prospective and retrospective studies converge to show that childhood-onset bipolar disorder continues into adulthood (Chang, 2007; Geller, Zimerman, Williams, Bolhofner, & Craney, 2001) and that early-onset illness is associated with severe impairment over the life span (Geller et al., 2000). In more severely ill patients, diagnostic delay can have severe consequences. For example, suicide is one of the three leading causes of death in young adults (Heuveline & Slap, 2002). Up to one-half of completed suicides in bipolar disorder occur during the first 6 years of illness, suggesting that for many patients suicide may occur before the illness has been accurately diagnosed or treated (Jamison, 2000).

In this chapter, we will attempt a practical focus on bipolar disorder in early adulthood. We will critically review and evaluate evidence for clinical pathways to early-onset bipolar disorder, mechanisms involved in the illness, and treatment strategies. In this way, we hope to be able to use science to foster a practical approach to this difficult illness.

Mechanisms of Recurrence and Chronicity in Bipolar Disorder

Recurrence and Sensitization

Bipolar disorder is an illness of recurrence and chronicity (Birmaher & Axelson, 2006). The course of illness varies widely, but it tends to fall into two patterns: *(1)* an episodic-stable course that emphasizes episodicity, with relative stability between episodes, and *(2)* an inherently unstable course that emphasizes progression toward chronicity, with more frequent episodes, susceptibility to depressive and manic features during the same episode, susceptibility to complications of bipolar disorder like substance-related and anxiety disorders, and persistent mood instability even between episodes (Masi, Perugi, Toni, et al., 2006). These courses of illness differ in treatment responsiveness, and they appear to run in families (Duffy et al., 2002; Duffy et al., 2007a). The inherently unstable course of illness appears to be associated with earlier onset of bipolar disorder and relative resistance to lithium treatment (Duffy et al., 2007a; Masi et al., 2000a, 2006b).

The course of illness in bipolar disorder resembles behavioral sensitization, a phenomenon described in animals (Cador et al., 1992) and in humans (Sax & Strakowski, 2001). Behavioral sensitization is characterized by a progressively increased response to repeated exposure to a stimulus, leading to a stable and persistently increased response. Classically the response is increased motor activity, and the stimulus is a central nervous stimulant drug (Robinson & Becker, 1986). Stimuli resembling stimulant drugs, whether endogenous or exogenous, can contribute to behavioral sensitization. Accordingly, cross-sensitization occurs among stimulants (Yang, Swann, & Dafny, 2003) and between stimulants and stressors (Barr, Hofmann, Weinberg, & Phillips, 2002; Covington & Miczek, 2001). In humans with bipolar disorder, frequency of episodes increases over time, exposure to so-called drugs of abuse accelerates the course of bipolar disorder (Post & Weiss, 1989), and exposure to severe stressors, especially early in life, is associated with more frequent episodes and a higher prevalence of substance abuse (Garno, Goldberg, Ramirez, & Ritzler, 2005).

There is substantial inter-individual variation in susceptibility to behavioral sensitization, in either humans or animals. In bipolar disorder, the course of illness runs in families. Relatives of patients with an episodic-stable course of illness tend to have that course pattern, while relatives of patients with an unstable course pattern have an unstable course pattern and are relatively resistant to lithium treatment (Duffy et al., 2007a).

Synthesis: Course of Illness

Bipolar disorder has general characteristics that must be kept in mind when interpreting psychiatric symptom presentations that may appear nonspecific. Table 23-1 summarizes characteristics of bipolar disorder in terms of its course of illness and clinical characteristics. In the evaluation of current problems or of histories of behavioral disturbance with early onset, these characteristics should be carefully considered in order to determine whether the disturbances are likely to be caused by bipolar disorder.

The presence of these characteristics in an individual with prominent psychiatric symptoms should raise the possibility that the individual has bipolar disorder—but does not prove that bipolar disorder is present (Swann et al., 2005).

The nature and timing of the first affective episode may determine lifetime illness characteristics. As noted above, early first episodes are associated with a greater likelihood of an unstable and complicated course (Masi et al., 2006a, 2006b). In addition, while on average depression is more common than mania across all patients with bipolar disorder, individuals with bipolar disorder tend to have a predominately depressive or manic course (Perlis et al., 2005). The first episode tends to predict characteristics of future episodes: a first manic episode is associated with a predominately manic course; a first depressive episode with a predominately depressive course, and with a substantially greater likelihood of initial misdiagnosis (Daban, Colom, Sanchez-Moreno, Garcia-Amador, & Vieta, 2006; Perlis et al., 2005; Perugi et al., 2000).

Clinical Pathways to Bipolar Disorder

When Does Bipolar Disorder Begin?

Bipolar disorder is defined in our nosological system in terms of depressive and manic episodes. During early adolescence, childhood, and even early adulthood, development of the brain is not complete, so the manifestations of these episodes, and the way in which these manifestations are expressed, are likely to differ across age groups. These considerations must be taken into account when obtaining the psychiatric history from patients in early adulthood. Bipolar disorder is not mania or depression, but an illness that predisposes to these nonspecific mood syndromes (Zis & Goodwin, 1979). It was almost certainly already present before a patient met criteria for a characteristic mood episode (Correll et al., 2007). Further, though the diagnosis of bipolar disorder requires mania, depression usually occurs first (Lish et al., 1994; Perugi et al., 2000). Other psychiatric syndromes can also precede mania. Therefore, we will review clinical pathways that lead to bipolar disorder.

Table 23-1. Characteristics of Bipolar Disorder

Genetic	Familial; multiple susceptibility genes; early onset associated with strong familiality (Chang, Steiner, & Ketter, 2000)
Onset	Usually adolescence (Leverich et al., 2007)
Course	Recurrent, sensitization-like course (Post & Weiss, 1989); more severe with early onset and/or severe early stressors (Post et al., 2003)
Basic behavioral disturbances	Motivation, reward, arousal, impulsivity (Carroll, 1983; Swann, Anderson, Dougherty, & Moeller, 2001); susceptible to activation by pharmacological or environmental stimuli (Post, Weiss, & Pert, 1988)
Comorbidities	Anxiety disorders (Masi et al., 2004), substance-use disorders (Borchardt & Bernstein, 1995), disruptive behavior disorders (Geller et al., 2006), ADHD (Geller et al., 2006; Masi et al., 2006a)
Characteristics associated with early onset	Chronicity/long symptomatic periods (Masi et al., 2006a); mixed states (Dilsaver, Benazzi, Rihmer, Akiskal, & Akiskal, 2005); high incidence of comorbidities (Masi et al., 2006)

Depression

Most episodes of bipolar disorder are depressive episodes (Lish et al., 1994), most lifetime morbidity is associated with depression (MacQueen et al., 2000; Swann, Bowden, Calabrese, Dilsaver, & Morris, 2000), and the first episode is usually a depressive episode rather than mania (Lish et al., 1994; Perugi et al., 2000). This leads to a diagnostic paradox where a clinician who saw a patient early enough and applied diagnostic criteria strictly would initially misdiagnose most patients. When depression is the first episode of bipolar disorder, the course of illness tends to be characterized by more depressive than manic episodes, more chronicity, and more severe suicidal behavior (Daban et al., 2006; Perlis et al., 2005; Perugi et al., 2000).

Early depressive episodes in bipolar disorder must be distinguished from major depressive illness, prodromes of schizophrenia, depression secondary to another medical or psychiatric illness, or demoralization (Akiskal et al., 1994; Geller et al., 2001; Winokur & Wesner, 1987). We will focus on the most difficult distinction: bipolar versus major depressive illness. Core depressive symptoms, like anhedonia, suicidal ideation, hopelessness, or a negative affect that may be experienced as extreme sadness or as being distinct from the patient's normal sadness, characterize childhood major depression of any cause. It should be remembered that the onset of bipolar disorder is, on average, earlier than major depressive illness (Strober et al., 1988), so as age decreases, the probability that a first depressive episode is bipolar disorder increases.

Clues that an early depressive episode may be bipolar are related to known characteristics of bipolar disorder summarized above and in Table 23-1. Geller studied a cohort of children whose average age was about 10 years old, who had major depressive episodes (average first episode at about 7 years). By 10 years later, during early adulthood, about half of the subjects had experienced manic or hypomanic episodes— even though patients with attention-deficit disorders or psychotic episodes had been excluded. The strongest predictor of bipolarity in this group was the presence of relatives with bipolar disorder (Geller et al., 2001).

The risk of bipolar disorder continues for patients with depressions in early adulthood. Goldberg and colleagues studied a group of 74 subjects who experienced major depressive episodes at a mean age of 23 years (Goldberg, Harrow, & Whiteside, 2001). At 15 years' follow-up, 27% of subjects had experienced at least one hypomanic episode, and another 19% had experienced at least one full manic episode. Psychotic features during the index depressive episode predicted eventual manic or hypomanic episode (recall that this was an exclusion criterion in the Geller study). Combined with the report by Geller and colleagues, for childhood-onset depression, the data suggest that bipolar disorder emerges with a half-life of about 10–15 years after an initial depressive episode.

Early depression can also be a prodrome of schizophrenia (Meyer et al., 2005), preceding psychotic symptoms by years in a substantial minority of patients with schizophrenia. Family history and social function are potentially useful clues for diagnosis.

Mania

As with depression, a manic first episode tends to predict a predominately manic course of illness (Yap, Covington, Gale, Datta, & Miczek, 2005). Similar to the case with depression, early-onset mania is characterized by core manic symptoms like grandiosity, pressured speech, racing thoughts, elation, hypersexuality, and reward-seeking behavior without regard for consequences (Geller et al., 2002). Also like depression, early-onset mania is more likely that later-onset mania to be chronic and to have mixed features (Craney & Geller, 2003). Finally, in interpreting these symptoms, it is vital to take developmental context into account. Pathological grandiosity differs, for example, between children and adults. Geller and colleagues published a useful comparison of symptoms in adult mania compared to childhood mania and normal childhood (Geller et al., 2002). When taking the history, it is important to take these considerations into account and to obtain data from multiple sources if possible.

A potential history of early mania must be differentiated from attention-deficit disorder with hyperactivity. This is exacerbated by the fact that almost all children experiencing manic episodes also have attention-deficit disorder, though the relationship appears to weaken with later onset (Biederman, Faraone, Keenan, & Tsuang, 1991; Biederman, Faraone, Wozniak, & Monuteaux, 2000; Luby, & Belden, 2006). Therefore, one must often determine whether a patient had attention-deficit disorder alone, or combined with bipolar disorder. There are, however, important differences between attention-deficit/hyperactivity disorder and mania. Both are characterized by hyperactivity, apparent inattention, and irritability (Biederman, Russell, Soriano, Wozniak, & Faraone, 1998). However, they can be differentiated by an observant clinician on the basis of the presence of the core motivation and reward-related mania symptoms, the frequent presence of core depressive symptoms, and positive family history for bipolar disorder (Craney & Geller, 2003; Geller et al., 2002).

Psychosis

Psychosis is a nonspecific syndrome that can occur in any phase of bipolar disorder but that also can be associated with many other illnesses, some of which are considered to be primary psychiatric illnesses, such as schizophrenia or affective disorders, while others, such as toxic psychoses, neoplasms, or consequences of brain trauma or infections, are not (Krauthammer & Klerman, 1978). Early psychotic episodes in patients with affective disorders are more likely than later episodes to have mood-incongruent features (Fennig, Bromet, Karant, Ram, & Jandorf, 1996). Mood-incongruent features, while not diagnostically useful, predict a course of illness with more severe psychosocial impairment (Strakowski et al., 2000).

The first manic episode is more likely to be psychotic, if it occurs in adolescence, than subsequent episodes (Ballenger, Reus, & Post, 1982; Conus & McGorry, 2002; Corkery, 1987; Weller, Weller, Tucker, & Fristad, 1986). Psychotic features can also occur in depressive or mixed episodes, especially as part of the highly variable and unstable symptom pattern that characterizes early-onset bipolar disorder. A first depressive episode with psychotic features may be associated with bipolar disorder (Goldberg et al., 2001). Unless prominent mood symptoms are also present, the diagnosis must be made using characteristics not directly related to the psychotic episode itself. Some features that are potentially useful are summarized in Table 23-2 (Ballenger et al., 1982; Corkery, 1987).

Premorbid social function and family history may be at least as useful as characteristics of the episode itself. Bipolar disorder and schizophrenia confer increased susceptibility to "secondary" symptomatic episodes associated with medical problems or pharmacological treatments (Krauthammer & Klerman, 1978).

Anxiety-Related Disorders

Bipolar disorder is strongly related to anxiety disorders throughout the life span, with a high rate of generalized anxiety disorder, panic disorder, and phobic disorders (Birmaher et al., 2002; Goodwin & Hamilton, 2002); as many as two-thirds of patients were reported to have met diagnostic criteria for a preexisting anxiety disorder when bipolar disorder was diagnosed (Masi et al., 2001). In addition, patients with bipolar disorder are more likely than those with other major psychiatric illnesses to have diagnoses of posttraumatic stress disorder (Cannon

Table 23-2. Diagnostic Clues in Psychotic Episodes

	Bipolar	Schizophrenia	Other (Substance-Induced or Medical Disorder)
Onset	Days–weeks	Insidious	Rapid
Premorbid social	Preserved	Impaired	Preserved
Family	Bipolar	Schizophrenia	Any
Mood symptoms	Usually present	Can be depressive	Variable
Orientation/cognition	"Confusion"	Orientation usually preserved	Variable

& Clarke, 2005) and obsessive-compulsive disorder (Chen & Dilsaver, 1995). Onset of illness was reported to be younger in patients with both bipolar disorder and obsessive-compulsive disorder than for either illness alone (Masi et al., 2004).

Anxiety- or stress-related disorders are also more likely to occur in children or adolescents who eventually develop bipolar disorder than in those who do not (DelBello & Geller, 2001). A family history of bipolar disorder predicts eventual diagnosis of bipolar disorder in children with anxiety- or stress-related disorders (Henin et al., 2005), and it is associated with increased prevalence of anxiety disorders in offspring who have not yet experienced depressive or manic episodes (Chang et al., 2000).

Prodromal Symptoms and Problems

Before the first prominent affective symptoms, individuals at high risk for bipolar disorder may experience problems related to the pathophysiology of the illness (Shaw, Egeland, Endicott, Allen, & Hostetter, 2005). Characteristics summarized in Table 23–1 may be signs of underlying bipolar disorder. Family history is always a useful diagnostic clue in bipolar disorder, but it is especially important in patients with early onset of illness (Pavuluri, Henry, Nadimpalli, O'Connor, & Sweeney, 2006). Children of parents with bipolar disorder may be at risk for prodromal signs of bipolar disorder and were reported to have an 11-fold greater risk of eventual bipolar disorder than children of non-bipolar parents (Singh et al., 2007). Among characteristics that differentiated bipolar offspring from offspring of parents with bipolar disorder were greater emotionality (Duffy et al., 2007b), increased hostility and irritability (Farchione et al., 2007), increased laboratory-measured disinhibition (Hirshfeld-Becker et al., 2006), coping and sleep disturbances (Jones, Tai, Evershed, Knowles, & Bentall, 2006), and increased anxiety, excitability, and attentional problems (Shaw et al., 2005).

Family history of bipolar disorder and perinatal complications are both associated with early-onset illness. A positive family history is associated with a 15-fold greater risk for developing bipolar disorder; each perinatal complication increased the likelihood 6-fold (Pavuluri et al., 2006). Children with early-onset bipolar disorder are more likely than their peers to have attention-deficit/hyperactivity disorder or disruptive behavior disorders (Masi et al., 2006a). Conversely, children with substance-use disorders (Simkin, 2002), conduct disorder (Sultzer, & Cummings, 1989) or attention-deficit disorder (Faraone, Biederman, Mennin, Wozniak, & Spencer, 1997), were likely to have an eventual diagnosis of bipolar disorder if they had positive family histories, but not in the absence of a positive family history.

Early Detection of Bipolar Disorder

The clinical presentation of bipolar disorder may differ according to age at onset. In young adults with prominent affective symptoms caused by bipolar disorder, onset of illness or its prodromes are likely to have occurred during earlier in life, during adolescence or childhood. Patients with early onset differed from those with later onset by having more chronic episodes, more mixed states and polyphasic episodes, and higher rates of other behavioral disturbances (Craney & Geller, 2003). The course of bipolar disorder is heterogeneous, however (Turvey et al., 1999). Adults with bipolar disorder may have a largely episodic course that is considered to be classic for bipolar disorder, but a substantial number have an inherently unstable course of illness associated with frequent, long symptomatic periods with mixed and polyphasic features and high rates of complicating disturbances including, substance-use and anxiety/stress-related disorders (Duffy et al., 2002). This more malignant form of adult bipolar disorder strongly resembles childhood-onset illness (Craney & Geller, 2003).

Potential Interaction of Genes and Environment in Bipolar Disorder

Genetic expression may by strongly influenced by environmental circumstances at specific times in development, referred to as gene by environment interaction (Caspi & Moffitt, 2006). Rutter and colleagues described four types of gene–environment interactions: *(1)* epigenetic mechanisms where environment altered gene effects, *(2)* variations in heredibility with environmental conditions, (3) gene–environment correlations, and (4) how specific identified genes interact with specific measured risks (Rutter, Moffitt, & Caspi, 2006). Several examples appear relevant to bipolar disorder, although they stem from other illnesses.

A classic example involves an abnormal allele of a gene coding for monoamine oxidase type A (MAO-A). Individuals who had experienced maltreatment during childhood were more likely than other children to develop antisocial behavior if they had the allele associated with lower levels of enzyme activity, but they appeared to be protected if they had the high-expression allele (Caspi et al., 2002). More generally, a study of 1,116 5-year-old British twin pairs and their families showed that maltreated children were more likely to develop conduct disorders if they were at high genetic risk (Jaffee et al., 2005). In another example, a functional polymorphism of the serotonin transporter gene, individuals with one or two copies of the short allele were more likely to experience depressive symptoms, depressive episodes, and suicidal behavior related to stressors (Caspi et al., 2003). Susceptibility to development of psychotic symptoms after marijuana use was associated with the catecholamine O-methyltransferase valine 158 allele, while individuals with the methionine allele appeared not to have this complication of marijuana use (Caspi et al., 2005).

Effects of early exposure to severe stressors may be examples of gene–environment interaction relevant to bipolar disorder. For example, early severe stressful events are associated with early onset of bipolar disorder (Duffy et al., 2007b) and with a more malignant course of bipolar disorder throughout the life span (Garno, Goldberg, Ramirez, & Ritzler, 2005; Post et al., 2003), with severe mood instability and susceptibility to substance-use disorders, suicidal behavior, and other behavioral problems (Leverich et al., 2007).

Treatment Considerations

Acute Psychopharmacological Treatments

We know of no large treatment studies that have focused on early adulthood. Most large controlled treatment studies covered a broad range (generally 18–65 years) of ages, with mean ages of 38–40 years (Bowden et al., 1994; Calabrese et al., 2005; Cookson, Keck, Ketter, & Macfadden, 2007; Goodwin et al., 2004; Hirshfeld-Becker et al., 2003; Keck et al., 2003, 2006; Tohen et al., 2000). A few studies have focused on treatment of bipolar disorder in adolescence, though the evidence is limited (Findling, 2005). Randomized treatment trials in adolescents are summarized in Table 23-3. Based on the limited amount of evidence available, it is not surprising that many young adults with bipolar disorder have histories of inadequate or inappropriate treatment, even if they received an accurate diagnosis.

Lithium is considered to be a relatively ineffective treatment in early-onset bipolar disorder. Yet Geller and colleagues showed that, in a group of early adolescent subjects with mania and a substance-use disorder, lithium improved manic symptoms and reduced substance abuse (Geller et al., 1998). Lithium, however, was not

Table 23-3. Randomized Treatment Trials in Adolescents with Bipolar Disorder

Reference	Drug	Composition	N	Age	Episode	Result
DelBello, Schwiers, Rosenberg, & Strakowski, 2002	QTP+DVP	PBO+DVP	30	12–18	Manic	QTP > PBO
Geller et al., 1998	Lithium	Placebo	25	16.3 ± 1.2	Manic + substance abuse	Li+ > PBO mania and substance use
Kafantaris et al., 2004	Lithium	PBO (DC)	40		Mania	Li+ = PBO
Tohen et al., 2007	Olanzapine	Placebo	107/54	13–17	Mania	OLZ > PBO

DC, discontinuation study; DVP, divalproex; OLZ, olanzapine; PBO, placebo; QTP, quetiapine.

more effective than placebo in a discontinuation study where subjects continued on lithium after 2 weeks and subjects switched to placebo had equally poor outcomes (52.6% relapse on lithium vs. 61.9% on placebo) (Kafantaris et al., 2004), or in an 18-month maintenance study (Findling et al., 2005). There are two positive studies of atypical antipsychotics in adolescents with mania (DelBello, Schwiers, Rosenberg, & Strakowski, 2002; Tohen et al., 2007).

Quetiapine and divalproex both appeared to improve impulsivity and reactive aggression in subjects with bipolar disorder combined with disruptive behavior (Barzman, DelBello, Adler, Stanford, & Strakowski, 2006). Divalproex was reported to be more effective than oxcarbazepine in patients with bipolar disorder and prominent aggressive behavior (MacMillan et al., 2006).

Many young adults with bipolar disorder were initially diagnosed with major depressive illness. Antidepressive agents may be associated with prominent mood instability in young patients. One study reported that 50% of patients receiving antidepressants experienced mania or hypomania, and 25% developed suicidal ideation (Baumer et al., 2006). Switch rates in antidepressants may be related to age, with SRIs having higher switch rates in younger patients, while switch rates were less related to age with tricyclics (Martin et al., 2004). One study comparing "prebipolar" depressed patients with unipolar patients of similar age found that outcomes were less favorable for "prebipolar" patients, with poorer antidepressive response and greater likelihood of treatment-emergent mixed states correlating with early age at onset (O'Donovan, Garnham, Hajek, & Alda, 2007). These results resemble a report in adults in which previously undiagnosed bipolar disorder was associated with loss of response to antidepressive treatments (Sharma, 2001).

Table 23-4 summarizes established treatments in bipolar disorder (Suppes et al., 2005; Swann, 2006a). As noted above, we know of no data differentiating response in young adults from other age groups. Young adults were prominently included in treatment trials with these agents, though mean ages were almost always 38–40 years. Several drugs and drug types have been found effective for treating acute manic episodes. Evidence for depression is less consistent; even when there have been placebo-controlled studies, results have been less consistent and quetiapine is the only FDA-approved monotherapy for depression in bipolar disorder. For maintenance treatment, there are even fewer alternatives.

Table 23-4. Pharmacological Treatments in Bipolar Disorder

Drug or class	Mania	Depression	Relapse prevention	FDA approval	Remarks
Lithium	P,C	P	P*,C	Mania, relapse	Family history, illness course
Valproate	P,C	P	P,C	Mania	
Carbamazepine; oxcarbazepine	P	P	C (M only)	Mania (ext release CBZ)	
Lamotrigine	—	P	P,C	Relapse	
A typical antipsychotics	P,C	P (QTP only)	P,C (Ari, 6 mo, M only); OLZ)	M; D (QTP only); relapse (OLZ, Ari)	
Antidepressive agents	—	P (as part of combination of fluoxetine-olanzapine)	None	None as monotherapy (D as part of combination)	

*Only treatment shown to prevent relapse in subjects not originally treated/stabilized with the same treatment.
Ari, aripiprazole; C, comparator-controlled; D, depression; CBZ, carbamazepine; M, mania; OLZ, olanzapine; P, placebo-controlled; QTP, quetiapine.
Sources: Suppes et al. (2005); Swann (2006).

There is relatively little information comparing the effectiveness of individual approved treatments. Lithium appears to be most effective in patients with family histories of lithium response and with a relatively stable course of illness (fewer or less frequent episodes, fewer mixed states) (Duffy et al., 1998, 2002; Swann, Bowden, Calabrese, Dilsaver, & Morris, 2000).

In general, treatments effective for acute episodes are potentially effective for preventing relapse. Essentially every positive maintenance study was in subjects who had initially responded to the study treatment (Swann, 2006a). An exception is with antidepressive treatments, where, despite some evidence for effectiveness in acute episodes, maintenance or continuation studies have been consistently negative (Ghaemi, Lenox, & Baldessarini, 2001), with the potential for worsening of the course of illness (Ghaemi, Hsu, Soldani, & Goodwin, 2003; Ghaemi et al., 2004). A critical aspect in the long-term treatment of bipolar disorder is the transition between treatment of an acute episode and the establishment of maintenance treatment. This phase of treatment establishes the eventual long-term strategy, so we will discuss it in more detail.

Transition between Acute Episode and Maintenance

Pharmacological Transitional Strategies. When acute symptoms have improved, functional impairment persists. It can take many months, or even years, for a patient to return to the level of function that preceded an episode of illness (Chengappa et al., 2005). The difficulty of this transitional period is compounded by the increase in responsibilities and reduction in structure and vigilance that tend to follow initial recovery. These considerations are especially crucial during young adulthood, when the individual is likely to still be establishing a social and occupational identity. The period directly after initial recovery is therefore a risky one for suicide (Sachs, Yan, Swann, & Allen, 2001), arrest (Quanbeck et al., 2004), substance abuse, and relapse (Perlis et al., 2006). Despite these considerations, the transitional period after an episode has not been extensively studied as an entity. There is indirect information, however, about treatment strategies for this period.

Manic episode. The period following a manic episode is associated with increased risk for behavioral problems including arrest and incarceration (Quanbeck et al., 2004). There is little information available about treatment during this period. Among subjects whose manic episodes had responded acutely to a combination of lithium or valproate with olanzapine were randomized to continuation of the combination or replacement of olanzapine with placebo (Tohen et al., 2004), half of those who were randomized to placebo relapsed during the first 3 months. The other half had outcome similar to that of subjects on combination treatment (survival curves were parallel). This result implies that treatments that were necessary to induce remission of a manic episode should be continued, at least for several months, after symptomatic improvement. If it is thought that part of a combination is not necessary for maintenance, a gradual taper (Faedda, Tondo, Baldessarini, Suppes, & Tohen, 1993) should not be undertaken until after at least several months, with the patient at or approaching the level of function that preceded the episode (Sachs, 1996).

Depressive episode. There is controversy over the continuation of antidepressants in a patient with bipolar disorder whose acute episode responded to these treatments. One contention is that antidepressive treatments should be discontinued as soon as possible, especially if a patient has experienced an unstable course of illness (Frye, Gitlin, & Altshuler, 2004). There is, however, the concern that hasty discontinuation of effective treatments could lead to increased mood instability, return of depressive symptoms, or increased suicide risk (already a feature of this recuperative period). In response to this dilemma, Altshuler and colleagues carried out two studies, one retrospective (Altshuler et al., 2001) and one prospective (Altshuler et al., 2003). The mean age of the subjects was about 42, though young adults were included. Both studies were naturalistic, without randomization. The patients in the study had required antidepressant treatment (therefore, they had not responded to mood-stabilizing agents that were generally given first) and had continued to tolerate antidepressant treatment after initial treatment. Among patients with these characteristics (about 20% of the total), patients in whom antidepressant were continued were compared to those whose antidepressants were discontinued. In both studies, patients whose antidepressants were discontinued experienced more relapses into depression than did those with continued antidepressant treatment, and they had no reduction in risk for mania. These results suggest strongly that, among that subgroup of patients who require, respond to, and tolerate antidepressive treatments, antidepressants should be continued for at least 6–12 months after recovery. It must be kept in mind that these results apply only to a minority of patients with bipolar depressive episodes, and that there was no information about reasons for discontinuation, so patients discontinuing antidepressants may have already been doing worse than those whose antidepressants were not discontinued, or they may have been more severely ill or had other differential clinical characteristics. Nevertheless, these studies are consistent with the results in mania in that, if part of a successful treatment combination is discontinued too early, risk of relapse is increased.

Nonpharmacological Transitional Strategies. Treatment during the transitional, recuperative period after an episode has many goals, including return to the pre-episode level of social and occupational function, establishing methods to monitor and proactively address symptoms, and addressing other potential problems like substance abuse and other complications of bipolar disorder. They include the following:

1. Identification of prodromes of episodes (Fava & Kellner, 1991), which can improve outcome (Lam, Wong, & Sham, 2001; Perry, Tarrier, Morriss, McCarthy, & Limb, 1999).
2. Use of life-charting methods to monitor symptoms, side effects, medicine, and events (Post, Roy Byrne, & Uhde, 1988); this can be applied to identification of prodromes.
3. Behavioral and cognitive strategies (Otto, Reilly-Harrington, & Sachs, 2003); these can have particular value for complications of bipolar disorder like substance abuse (Schmitz et al., 2002), mild depressive symptoms (DeRubeis et al., 2005), or anxiety disorders (Simon et al., 2004), which would otherwise require potentially mood-destabilizing treatments. Similar strategies have been adapted for protection of sleep, activity, and social rhythms (Frank et al., 1997, 2005). Cognitive-behavioral therapies can reduce relapse and improve occupational function and quality of life (Lam, Hayward, Watkins, Wright, & Sham, 2005).
4. Education and support of the patient and significant others. Participation in treatment is more strongly related to understanding of the illness more than any other single factor, even side effects; unfortunately, clinicians seem not to recognize this fact (Scott, & Pope (2002). Similarly, stress to caregivers depends more on understanding of illness than on severity of symptoms (Perlick et al., 1999) and was shown to predict poor treatment outcome at 9 and 15 months better than acute symptom severity did (Perlick, Rosenheck, Clarkin, Raue, & Sirey, 2001). Psychoeducation is a cost-effective strategy for improving outcome and quality of life (Michalak, Yatham, Wan, & Lam, 2005). Comprehensive educational materials have been developed, in collaboration with the National Alliance for the Mentally Ill and Depression Bipolar Support Alliance, by the Texas Medication Algorithm Project (TMAP) (Suppes et al., 2002).
5. Once the transitional period is over, medicines not considered essential may be discontinued (Sachs, 1996). This process should be gradual. Even a rapid reduction in lithium level can increase the probability of relapse (Perlis et al., 2002). Rapid discontinuation of antidepressants can precipitate mania (Goldstein et al., 1999).
6. Insight-oriented treatments or planned major life changes should be deferred, if at all possible, until after this transitional, recuperative stage of treatment, when pre-episode function has been restored (Sachs, 1996).

Conclusions

Young adulthood is a crucial stage of life that is overlooked in treatment studies. The processes of brain maturation that were active during adolescence reach completion during this period.

Individuals are establishing lifelong adaptive, social, and occupational patterns. In the context of the important transitions that occur during this period, bipolar disorder can be a challenging problem. Most patients with bipolar disorder have onset before adulthood, but early misdiagnosis and inaccurate treatment are common. Fortunately, there are clues that can be useful to us in determining whether severe psychiatric symptoms might have been related to early-onset bipolar disorder (Table 23-1). The strongest are syndromal depressive or manic symptoms that began in the developmental context of childhood, and behavioral or symptomatic disturbance consistent with underlying susceptibilities of bipolar disorder (like anxiety, impulsivity, or depression) combined with a family history of bipolar disorder. A range of treatments is available, as summarized in Table 23-4, but evidence for effectiveness against depression or in long-term treatment is still relatively weak. As recovery from an episode progresses, the transition to long-term treatment is a vital step in establishing long-term adaptive function and mood stability. Treatment decisions must balance the severity of current and projected future impairment and strength of supporting diagnostic evidence against the potential toxicities and still-preliminary evidence supporting treatments, must consider the possibility of synergistic effects of pharmacological and nonpharmacological treatments, and must address the illness in the context of the transitions that characterize this stage of life.

KEY POINTS

- Most young adults with bipolar disorder had onset of illness during adolescence or before.
- Bipolar disorder is usually misdiagnosed at first, and young adults with bipolar disorder are likely to have been diagnosed, and probably treated, for other illnesses.
- When there is a psychiatric history of depression, psychosis, anxiety, or of severe anxiety- or stress-related symptoms, it is necessary to determine whether these were manifestations of bipolar disorder by carefully investigating family history, developmental history, presence of mood symptoms that were missed, and patterns of treatment response.
- Effective pharmacological treatments are probably similar to those for older adults with bipolar disorder.

PRACTICE GUIDELINES

- In depressed patients, look for histories of early onset, frequent episodes, history of anxiety- or substance-related disorders, positive family history for bipolar disorder, and idiosyncratic or unsatisfactory responses to treatment.
- As with older adults, younger adults who have bipolar disorder combined with a substance-related disorder or with attention deficit-hyperactivity disorder need to be treated for both.
- Nonpharmacological treatments must address the transition to full adulthood and responsibility for health.

References

Akiskal, H. S., Maser, J. D., Zeller, P. J., Endicott, J., Coryell, W., Keller, M., Warshaw, M., Clayton, P., & Goodwin, F. (1994). Switching from 'unipolar' to bipolar II. An 11-year prospective study of clinical and temperamental predictors in 559 patients. *Archives of General Psychiatry, 52*, 114–123.

Altshuler, L., Kiriakos, L., Calcagno, J., Goodman, R., Gitlin, M., Frye, M., & Mintz, J. (2001). The impact of antidepressant discontinuation versus antidepressant continuation on 1-year risk for relapse of bipolar depression: A retrospective chart review. *Journal of Clinical Psychiatry, 62*(8), 612–616.

Altshuler, L., Suppes, T., Black, D., Nolen, W. A., Keck, P. E., Jr., Frye, M. A., McElroy, S., Kupka, R., Grunze, H., Walden, J., Leverich, G., Denicoff, K., Luckenbaugh, D., & Post, R. (2003). Impact of antidepressant discontinuation after acute bipolar depression remission on rates of depressive relapse at 1-year follow-up. *American Journal of Psychiatry, 160*(7), 1252–1262.

Angst, F., Stassen, H. H., Clayton, P. J., & Angst, J. (2002). Mortality of patients with mood disorders: Follow-up over 34–38 years. *Journal of Affective Disorders, 68*(2–3), 167–181.

Ballenger, J. C., Reus, V. I., & Post, R. M. (1982). The atypical clinical picture of adolescent mania. *American Journal of Psychiatry, 13*, 9602–9606.

Barr, A. M., Hofmann, B. A., Weinberg, J., & Phillips, A. G. (2002). Exposure to repeated, intermittent d-amphetamine induces sensitization of HPA axis to a subsequent stressor. *Neuropsychopharmacology, 26*(3), 286–294.

Barzman, D. H., DelBello, M. P., Adler, C. M., Stanford, K. E., & Strakowski, S. M. (2006). The efficacy and tolerability of quetiapine versus divalproex for the treatment of impulsivity and reactive aggression in adolescents with co-occurring bipolar disorder and disruptive behavior disorder(s). *Journal of Child and Adolescent Psychopharmacology, 16*(6), 665–670.

Baumer, F. M., Howe, M., Gallelli, K., Simeonova, D. I., Hallmayer, J., & Chang, K. D. (2006). A pilot study of antidepressant-induced mania in pediatric bipolar disorder: Characteristics, risk factors, and the serotonin transporter gene. *Biological Psychiatry, 60*(9), 1005–1012.

Biederman, J., Faraone, S. V., Keenan, K., & Tsuang, M. T. (1991). Evidence of familial association between attention deficit disorder and major affective disorders. *Archives of General Psychiatry, 48*, 633–642.

Biederman, J., Faraone, S. V., Wozniak, J., & Monuteaux, M.C. (2000). Parsing the association between bipolar, conduct, and substance use disorders: A familial risk analysis. *Biological Psychiatry, 48*(11), 1037–1044.

Biederman, J., Russell, R., Soriano, J., Wozniak, J., & Faraone, S. V. (1998). Clinical features of children with both ADHD and mania: Does ascertainment source make a difference? *Journal of Affective Disorders, 51*(2), 101–112.

Birmaher, B., & Axelson, D. (2006). Course and outcome of bipolar spectrum disorder in children and adolescents: A review of the existing literature. *Developmental Psychopathology, 18*(4), 1023–1035.

Birmaher, B., Kennah, A., Brent, D., Ehmann, M., Bridge, J., & Axelson, D. (2002). Is bipolar disorder specifically associated with panic disorder in youths? *Journal of Clinical Psychiatry, 63*(5), 414–419.

Borchardt, C. M., & Bernstein, G. A. (1995). Comorbid disorders in hospitalized bipolar adolescents compared with unipolar depressed adolescents. *Child Psychiatry and Human Development, 26*(1), 11–18.

Bowden, C. L., Brugger, A. M., Swann, A. C., Calabrese, J. R., Janicak, P. G., Petty, F., Dilsaver, S. C., Davis, J. M., Rush, A. J., Small, J. G., Garza Trevino, E. S., Risch, S. C., Goodnick, P. J., & Morris, D. D. (1994). Efficacy of divalproex vs lithium and placebo in the treatment of mania. *Journal of the American Medical Association, 27*, 1918–1924.

Cador, M., Dumas, S., Cole, B. J., Mallet, J., Koob, G. F., Le, M. M., & Stinus, L. (1992). Behavioral sensitization induced by psychostimulants or stress: Search for a molecular basis and evidence for a CRF-dependent phenomenon. *Annals of the New York Academy of Sciences, 65*, 4416–4420.

Calabrese, J. R., Hirschfeld, R. M., Reed, M., Davies, M. A., Frye, M. A., Keck, P. E., Lewis, L., McElroy, S. L., McNulty, J. P., & Wagner, K. D. (2003). Impact of bipolar disorder on a U.S. community sample. *Journal of Clinical Psychiatry, 64*(4), 425–432.

Calabrese, J. R., Keck, P. E., Jr., Macfadden, W., Minkwitz, M., Ketter, T. A., Weisler, R. H., Cutler, A. J., McCoy, R., Wilson, E., & Mullen, J. (2005). A randomized, double-blind, placebo-controlled trial of quetiapine in the treatment of bipolar I or II depression. *American Journal of Psychiatry, 162*(7), 1351–1360.

Cannon, M., & Clarke, M. C. (2005). Risk for schizophrenia—broadening the concepts, pushing back the boundaries. *Schizophrenia Research, 79*(1), 5–13.

Carroll, B. J. (1983). Neurobiologic dimensions in depression and mania. In J. Angst (Ed.), *The origins of depression* (pp. 163–186). Berlin: Springer-Verlag.

Caspi, A., McClay, J., Moffitt, T. E., Mill, J., Martin, J., Craig, I. W., Taylor, A., & Poulton, R. (2002). Role of genotype in the cycle of violence in maltreated children. *Science, 297*(5582), 851–854.

Caspi, A., & Moffitt, T. E. (2006). Gene-environment interactions in psychiatry: Joining forces with neuroscience. *Nature Reviews Neuroscience, 7*(7), 583–590.

Caspi, A., Moffitt, T. E., Cannon, M., McClay, J., Murray, R., Harrington, H., Taylor, A., Arseneault, L., Williams, B., Braithwaite, A., Poulton, R., & Craig, I. W. (2005). Moderation of the effect of adolescent-onset cannabis use on adult psychosis by a functional polymorphism in the catechol-O-methyltransferase gene: Longitudinal evidence of a gene X environment interaction. *Biological Psychiatry, 57*(10), 1117–1127.

Caspi, A., Sugden, K., Moffitt, T. E., Taylor, A., Craig, I. W., Harrington, H., McClay, J., Mill, J., Martin, J., Braithwaite, A., & Poulton, R. (2003). Influence of life stress on depression: Moderation by a polymorphism in the 5-HTT gene. *Science, 301*(5631), 386–389.

Chang, K. (2007). Adult bipolar disorder is continuous with pediatric bipolar disorder. *Canadian Journal of Psychiatry, 52*(7), 418–425.

Chang, K. D., Steiner, H., Ketter, T. A. (2000). Psychiatric phenomenology of child and adolescent bipolar offspring. *Journal of the American Academy of Child and Adolescent Psychiatry, 39*(4), 453–460.

Chen, Y. W., & Dilsaver, S. C. (1995). Comorbidity for obsessive-compulsive disorder in bipolar and unipolar disorders. *Psychiatry Research, 59*(1–2), 57–64.

Chengappa, K. N., Hennen, J., Baldessarini, R. J., Kupfer, D. J., Yatham, L. N., Gershon, S., Baker, R. W., & Tohen, M. (2005). Recovery and functional outcomes following olanzapine treatment for bipolar I mania. *Bipolar Disorder, 7*(1), 68–76.

Conus, P., & McGorry, P. D. (2002). First-episode mania: A neglected priority for early intervention. *Australian and New Zealand Journal of Psychiatry, 36*(2), 158–172.

Cookson, J., Keck, P. E., Jr., Ketter, T. A., & Macfadden, W. (2007). Number needed to treat and time to response/remission for quetiapine monotherapy efficacy in acute bipolar depression: Evidence from a large, randomized, placebo-controlled study. *International Clinical Psychopharmacology, 22*(2), 93–100.

Corkery, J. C. (1987). Recognition and treatment of depression. *American Family Physician, 35*, 197–200.

Correll, C. U., Penzner, J. B., Frederickson, A. M., Richter, J. J., Auther, A. M., Smith, C. W., Kane, J. M., & Cornblatt, B. A. (2007). Differentiation in the preonset phases of schizophrenia and mood disorders: Evidence in support of a bipolar mania prodrome. *Schizophrenia Bulletin, 33*(3), 703–714.

Covington, H. E., III, & Miczek, K. A. (2001). Repeated social-defeat stress, cocaine or morphine. Effects on behavioral sensitization and intravenous cocaine self-administration "binges." *Psychopharmacology (Berlin), 158*(4), 388–398.

Craney, J. L., & Geller, B. (2003). A prepubertal and early adolescent bipolar disorder-I phenotype: Review of phenomenology and longitudinal course. *Bipolar Disorders, 5*(4), 243–256.

Daban, C., Colom, F., Sanchez-Moreno, J., Garcia-Amador, M., & Vieta, E. (2006). Clinical correlates of first-episode polarity in bipolar disorder. *Comprehensive Psychiatry, 47*(6), 433–437.

DelBello, M. P., & Geller, B. (2001). Review of studies of child and adolescent offspring of bipolar parents. *Bipolar Disorder, 3*(6), 325–334.

DelBello, M. P., Schwiers, M. L., Rosenberg, H. L., & Strakowski, S. M. (2002). A double-blind, randomized, placebo-controlled study of quetiapine as adjunctive treatment for adolescent mania. *Journal of the American Academy of Child and Adolescent Psychiatry, 41*(10), 1216–1223.

DeRubeis, R. J., Hollon, S. D., Amsterdam, J. D., Shelton, R. C., Young, P. R., Salomon, R. M., O'Reardon, J. P., Lovett, M. L., Gladis, M. M., Brown, L. L., & Gallop, R. (2005). Cognitive therapy vs medications in the treatment of moderate to severe depression. *Archives of General Psychiatry, 62*(4), 409–416.

Dilsaver, S. C., Benazzi, F., Rihmer, Z., Akiskal, K. K., & Akiskal, H. S. (2005). Gender, suicidality and bipolar mixed states in adolescents. *Journal of Affective Disorders, 87*(1), 11–16.

Duffy, A., Alda, M., Kutcher, S., Cavazzoni, P., Robertson, C., Grof, E., & Grof, P. (2002). A prospective study of the offspring of bipolar parents responsive and nonresponsive to lithium treatment. *Journal of Clinical Psychiatry, 63*(12), 1171–1178.

Duffy, A., Alda, M., Kutcher, S., Fusee, C., & Grof, P. (1998). Psychiatric symptoms and syndromes among adolescent children of parents with lithium-responsive or lithium-nonresponsive bipolar disorder. *American Journal of Psychiatry, 155*(3), 431–433.

Duffy, A., Alda, M., Milin, R., & Grof, P. (2007a). A consecutive series of treated affected offspring of parents with bipolar disorder: Is response associated with the clinical profile? *Canadian Journal of Psychiatry, 52*(6), 369–376.

Duffy, A., Alda, M., Trinneer, A., Demidenko, N., Grof, P., & Goodyer, I. M. (2007b). Temperament, life events, and psychopathology among the offspring of bipolar parents. *European Child and Adolescent Psychiatry, 16*(4), 222–228.

Faedda, G. L., Tondo, L., Baldessarini, R. J., Suppes, T., & Tohen, M. (1993). Outcome after rapid vs gradual discontinuation of lithium treatment in bipolar disorders. *Archives of General Psychiatry, 50,* 448–455.

Faraone, S. V., Biederman, J., Mennin, D., Wozniak, J., & Spencer, T. (1997). Attention-deficit hyperactivity disorder with bipolar disorder: A familial subtype? *Journal of the American Academy of Child and Adolescent Psychiatry, 36*(10), 1378–1387.

Farchione, T. R., Birmaher, B., Axelson, D., Kalas, C., Monk, K., Ehmann, M., Iyengar, S., Kupfer, D., & Brent, D. (2007). Aggression, hostility, and irritability in children at risk for bipolar disorder. *Bipolar Disorder, 9*(5), 496–503.

Fava, G. A., & Kellner, R. (1991). Prodromal symptoms in affective disorders. *American Journal of Psychiatry, 14,* 8823–8830.

Fennig, S., Bromet, E. J., Karant, M. T., Ram, R., & Jandorf, L. (1996). Mood-congruent versus mood-incongruent psychotic symptoms in first-admission patients with affective disorder. *Journal of Affective Disorders, 37,* 23–29.

Findling, R. L. (2005). Update on the treatment of bipolar disorder in children and adolescents. *European Psychiatry, 20*(2), 87–91.

Findling, R. L., McNamara, N. K., Youngstrom, E. A., Stansbrey, R., Gracious, B. L., Reed, M. D., & Calabrese, J. R. (2005). Double-blind 18-month trial of lithium versus divalproex maintenance treatment in pediatric bipolar disorder. *Journal of the American Academy of Child and Adolescent Psychiatry, 44*(5), 409–417.

Frank, E., Hlastala, S., Ritenour, A., Houck, P., Tu, X. M., Monk, T. H., Mallinger, A. G., & Kupfer, D. J. (1997). Inducing lifestyle regularity in recovering bipolar disorder patients: Results from maintenance therapies in bipolar disorder protocol. *Biological Psychiatry, 41,* 1165–1173.

Frank, E., Kupfer, D. J., Thase, M. E., Mallinger, A. G., Swartz, H. A., Fagiolini, A. M., Grochocinski, V., Houck, P., Scott, J., Thompson, W., & Monk, T. (2005). Two-year outcomes for interpersonal and social rhythm therapy in individuals with bipolar I disorder. *Archives of General Psychiatry, 2*(9), 996–1004.

Frye, M. A., Gitlin, M. J., & Altshuler, L. L. (2004). Unmet needs in bipolar depression. *Depression and Anxiety, 19*(4), 199–208.

Garno, J. L., Goldberg, J. F., Ramirez, P. M., & Ritzler, B. A. (2005). Impact of childhood abuse on the clinical course of bipolar disorder. *British Journal of Psychiatry, 18,* 6121–6125.

Geller, B., Bolhofner, K., Craney, J. L., Williams, M., DelBello, M. P., & Gundersen, K. (2000). Psychosocial functioning in a prepubertal and early adolescent bipolar disorder phenotype. *Journal of the American Academy of Child and Adolescent Psychiatry, 39*(12), 1543–1548.

Geller, B., Cooper, T. B., Sun, K., Zimerman, B., Frazier, J., Williams, M., & Heath, J. (1998). Double-blind and placebo-controlled study of lithium for adolescent bipolar disorders with secondary substance dependency. *Journal of the American Academy of Child and Adolescent Psychiatry, 37*(2), 171–178.

Geller, B., Tillman, R., Bolhofner, K., Zimerman, B., Strauss, N. A., & Kaufmann, P. (2006). Controlled, blindly rated, direct-interview family study of a prepubertal and early-adolescent bipolar I disorder phenotype: Morbid risk, age at onset, and comorbidity. *Archives of General Psychiatry, 63*(10), 1130–1138.

Geller, B., Zimerman, B., Williams, M., Bolhofner, K., & Craney, J. L. (2001). Bipolar disorder at prospective follow-up of adults who had prepubertal major depressive disorder. *American Journal of Psychiatry, 158*(1), 125–127.

Geller, B., Zimerman, B., Williams, M., DelBello, M. P., Frazier, J., & Beringer, L. (2002). Phenomenology of prepubertal and early adolescent bipolar disorder: Examples of elated mood, grandiose behaviors, decreased need for sleep, racing thoughts and hypersexuality. *Journal of Child and Adolescent Psychopharmacology, 12*(1), 3–9.

Ghaemi, S. N., Hsu, D. J., Soldani, F., & Goodwin, F. K. (2003). Antidepressants in bipolar disorder: The case for caution. *Bipolar Disorder, 5*(6), 421–433.

Ghaemi, S. N., Lenox, M. S., & Baldessarini, R. J. (2001). Effectiveness and safety of long-term antidepressant treatment in bipolar disorder. *Journal of Clinical Psychiatry, 62*(7), 565–569.

Ghaemi, S. N., Rosenquist, K. J., Ko, J. Y., Baldassano, C. F., Kontos, N. J., & Baldessarini, R. J. (2004). Antidepressant treatment in bipolar versus unipolar depression. *American Journal of Psychiatry, 161*(1), 163–165.

Goldberg, J. F., Harrow, M., & Whiteside, J. E. (2001). Risk for bipolar illness in patients initially hospitalized for unipolar depression. *American Journal of Psychiatry, 158*(8), 1265–1270.

Goldstein, T. R., Frye, M. A., Denicoff, K. D., Smith-Jackson, E., Leverich, G. S., Bryan, A. L., Ali, S. O., & Post, R. M. (1999). Antidepressant discontinuation-related mania: Critical prospective observation and theoretical implications in bipolar disorder. *Journal of Clinical Psychiatry, 60*(8), 563–567.

Goodwin, G. M., Bowden, C. L., Calabrese, J. R., Grunze, H., Kasper, S., White, R., Greene, P., & Leadbetter, R. (2004). A pooled analysis of 2 placebo-controlled 18-month trials of lamotrigine and lithium maintenance in bipolar I disorder. *Journal of Clinical Psychiatry, 65*(3), 432–441.

Goodwin, R. D., & Hamilton, S. P. (2002). The early-onset fearful panic attack as a predictor of severe psychopathology. *Psychiatry Research, 109*(1), 71–79.

Healy, D. (2006). The latest mania: Selling bipolar disorder. *PLoS Medicine, 3*(4), e185.

Henin, A., Biederman, J., Mick, E., Sachs, G. S., Hirshfeld-Becker, D. R., Siegel, R. S., McMurrich, S., Grandin, L., & Nierenberg, A. A. (2005). Psychopathology in the offspring of parents with bipolar disorder: A controlled study. *Biological Psychiatry, 58*(7), 554–561.

Heuveline, P., & Slap, G. B. (2002). Adolescent and young adult mortality by cause: Age, gender, and country, 1955 to 1994. *Journal of Adolescent Health, 30*(1), 29–34.

Hirschfeld, R. M., Lewis, L., & Vornik, L. A. (2003). Perceptions and impact of bipolar disorder: How far have we really come? Results of the National Depressive and Manic-Depressive Association 2000 survey of individuals with bipolar disorder. *Journal of Clinical Psychiatry, 64*(2), 161–174.

Hirshfeld-Becker, D. R., Biederman, J., Calltharp, S., Rosenbaum, E. D., Faraone, S. V., & Rosenbaum, J. F. (2003). Behavioral inhibition and disinhibition as hypothesized precursors to psychopathology: Implications for pediatric bipolar disorder. *Biological Psychiatry, 53*(11), 985–999.

Hirshfeld-Becker, D. R., Biederman, J., Henin, A., Faraone, S. V., Cayton, G. A., & Rosenbaum, J. F. (2006). Laboratory-observed behavioral disinhibition in the young offspring of parents with bipolar disorder: A high-risk pilot study. *American Journal of Psychiatry, 163*(2), 265–271.

Jaffee, S. R., Caspi, A., Moffitt, T. E., Dodge, K. A., Rutter, M., Taylor, A., & Tully, L. A. (2005). Nature X nurture: Genetic vulnerabilities interact with physical maltreatment to promote conduct problems. *Developmental Psychopathology, 17*(1), 67–84.

Jamison, K. R. (2000). Suicide and bipolar disorder. *Journal of Clinical Psychiatry, 61*(Suppl.), 947–51.

Jones, S. H., Tai, S., Evershed, K., Knowles, R., & Bentall, R. (2006). Early detection of bipolar disorder: A pilot familial high-risk study of parents with bipolar disorder and their adolescent children. *Bipolar Disorder, 8*(4), 362–372.

Judd, L. L., & Akiskal, H. S. (2003). The prevalence and disability of bipolar spectrum disorders in the U.S. population: Re-analysis of the ECA database taking into account subthreshold cases. *Journal of Affective Disorders, 73*(1–2), 123–131.

Judd, L. L., Akiskal, H. S., Schettler, P. J., Coryell, W., Endicott, J., Maser, J. D., Solomon, D. A., Leon, A. C., & Keller, M. B. (2003). A prospective investigation of the natural history of the long-term weekly symptomatic status of bipolar II disorder. *Archives of General Psychiatry, 60*(3), 261–269.

Kafantaris, V., Coletti, D. J., Dicker, R., Padula, G., Pleak, R. R., & Alvir, J. M. (2004). Lithium treatment of acute mania in adolescents: A placebo-controlled discontinuation study. *Journal of the American Academy of Child and Adolescent Psychiatry, 43*(8), 984–993.

Keck, P. E., Jr., Calabrese, J. R., McQuade, R. D., Carson, W. H., Carlson, B. X., Rollin, L. M., Marcus, R. N., & Sanchez, R. (2006). A randomized, double-blind, placebo-controlled 26-week trial of aripiprazole in recently manic patients with bipolar I disorder. *Journal of Clinical Psychiatry, 67*(4), 626–637.

Keck, P. E., Jr., Marcus, R., Tourkodimitris, S., Ali, M., Liebeskind, A., Saha, A., & Ingenito, G. (2003). A placebo-controlled, double-blind study of the efficacy and safety of aripiprazole in patients with acute bipolar mania. *American Journal of Psychiatry, 160*(9), 1651–1658.

Krauthammer, C., & Klerman, G. L. (1978). Secondary mania: Manic syndromes associated with antecedent physical illnesses or drugs. *Archives of General Psychiatry, 35*, 1333–1339.

Lam, D., Wong, G., & Sham, P. (2001). Prodromes, coping strategies and course of illness in bipolar affective disorder–a naturalistic study. *Psychological Medicine, 31*(8), 1397–1402.

Lam, D. H., Hayward, P., Watkins, E. R., Wright, K., & Sham, P. (2005). Relapse prevention in patients with bipolar disorder: Cognitive therapy outcome after 2 years. *American Journal of Psychiatry, 162*(2), 324–329.

Leverich, G. S., Post, R. M., Keck, P. E., Jr., Altshuler, L. L., Frye, M. A., Kupka, R. W., Nolen, W. A., Suppes, T., McElroy, S. L., Grunze, H., Denicoff, K., Moravec, M. K., & Luckenbaugh, D. (2007). The poor prognosis of childhood-onset bipolar disorder. *Journal of Pediatrics, 150*(5), 485–490.

Lish, J. D., Dime-Meenan, S., Whybrow, P. C., & Price, R. A. (1994). The National Depressive and Manic-Depressive Association (DMDA) survey of bipolar members. *Journal of Affective Disorders, 31*, 281–294.

Luby, J., & Belden, A. (2006). Defining and validating bipolar disorder in the preschool period. *Developmental Psychopathology, 18*(4), 971–988.

MacMillan, C. M., Korndorfer, S. R., Rao, S., Fleisher, C. A., Mezzacappa, E., & Gonzalez-Heydrich, J. (2006). A comparison of divalproex and oxcarbazepine in aggressive youth with bipolar disorder. *Journal of Psychiatric Practice*, *12*(4), 214–222.

MacQueen, G. M., Young, L. T., Robb, J. C., Marriott, M., Cooke, R. G., & Joffe, R. T. (2000). Effect of number of episodes on wellbeing and functioning of patients with bipolar disorder. *Acta Psychiatrica Scandinavica*, *101*(5), 374–381.

Martin, A., Young, C., Leckman, J. F., Mukonoweshuro, C., Rosenheck, R., & Leslie, D. (2004). Age effects on antidepressant-induced manic conversion. *Archives of Pediatric and Adolescent Medicine*, *158*(8), 773–780.

Masi, G., Perugi, G., Millepiedi, S., Mucci, M., Toni, C., Bertini, N., Pfanner, C., Berloffa, S., & Pari, C. (2006a). Developmental differences according to age at onset in juvenile bipolar disorder. *Journal of Child and Adolescent Psychopharmacology*, *16*(6), 679–685.

Masi, G., Perugi, G., Toni, C., Millepiedi, S., Mucci, M., Bertini, N., & Akiskal, H. S. (2006b). The clinical phenotypes of juvenile bipolar disorder: Toward a validation of the episodic-chronic-distinction. *Biological Psychiatry*, *59*(7), 603–610.

Masi, G., Perugi, G., Toni, C., Millepiedi, S., Mucci, M., Bertini, N., & Akiskal, H. S. (2004). Obsessive-compulsive bipolar comorbidity: Focus on children and adolescents. *Journal of Affective Disorders*, *78*(3), 175–183.

Masi, G., Toni, C., Perugi, G., Mucci, M., Millepiedi, S., & Akiskal, H. S. (2001). Anxiety disorders in children and adolescents with bipolar disorder: A neglected comorbidity. *Canadian Journal of Psychiatry*, *46*(9), 797–802.

Meyer, S. E., Bearden, C. E., Lux, S. R., Gordon, J. L., Johnson, J. K., O'Brien, M. P., Niendam, T. A., Loewy, R. L., Ventura, J., & Cannon, T. D. (2005). The psychosis prodrome in adolescent patients viewed through the lens of DSM-IV. *Journal of Child and Adolescent Psychopharmacology*, *15*(3), 434–451.

Michalak, E. E., Yatham, L. N., Wan, D. D., & Lam, R. W. (2005). Perceived quality of life in patients with bipolar disorder. Does group psychoeducation have an impact? *Canadian Journal of Psychiatry*, *50*(2), 95–100.

O'Donovan, C., Garnham, J. S., Hajek, T., & Alda, M. (2007). Antidepressant monotherapy in pre-bipolar depression; Predictive value and inherent risk. *Journal of Affective Disorders*, *107*(1–3), 293–298.

Osby, U., Brandt, L., Correia, N., Ekbom, A., & Sparen, P. (2001). Excess mortality in bipolar and unipolar disorder in Sweden. *Archives of General Psychiatry*, *58*(9), 844–850.

Otto, M. W., Reilly-Harrington, N., & Sachs, G. S. (2003). Psychoeducational and cognitive-behavioral strategies in the management of bipolar disorder. *Journal of Affective Disorders*, *73*(1–2), 171–181.

Pavuluri, M. N., Henry, D. B., Nadimpalli, S. S., O'Connor, M. M., & Sweeney, J. A. (2006). Biological risk factors in pediatric bipolar disorder. *Biological Psychiatry*, *60*(9), 936–941.

Perlick, D., Clarkin, J. F., Sirey, J., Raue, P., Greenfield, S., Struening, E., & Rosenheck, R. (1999). Burden experienced by care-givers of persons with bipolar affective disorder. *British Journal of Psychiatry*, *175*, 56–62.

Perlick, D. A., Rosenheck, R. R., Clarkin, J. F., Raue, P., & Sirey, J. (2001). Impact of family burden and patient symptom status on clinical outcome in bipolar affective disorder. *Journal of Nervous and Mental Disease*, *189*(1), 31–37.

Perlis, R. H., DelBello, M. P., Miyahara, S., Wisniewski, S. R., Sachs, G. S., Nierenberg, A. A. (2005). Revisiting depressive-prone bipolar disorder: Polarity of initial mood episode and disease course among bipolar I systematic treatment enhancement program for bipolar disorder participants. *Biological Psychiatry*, *58*(7), 549–553.

Perlis, R. H., Ostacher, M. J., Patel, J. K., Marangell, L. B., Zhang, H., Wisniewski, S. R., Ketter, T. A., Miklowitz, D. J., Otto, M. W., Gyulai, L., Reilly-Harrington, N. A., Nierenberg, A. A., Sachs, G. S., & Thase, M. E. (2006). Predictors of recurrence in bipolar disorder: Primary outcomes from the Systematic Treatment Enhancement Program for Bipolar Disorder (STEP-BD). *American Journal of Psychiatry*, *163*(2), 217–224.

Perlis, R. H., Sachs, G. S., Lafer, B., Otto, M. W., Faraone, S. V., Kane, J. M., & Rosenbaum, J. F. (2002). Effect of abrupt change from standard to low serum levels of lithium: A reanalysis of double-blind lithium maintenance data. *American Journal of Psychiatry*, *159*(7), 1155–1159.

Perry, A., Tarrier, N., Morriss, R., McCarthy, E., & Limb, K. (1999). Randomised controlled trial of efficacy of teaching patients with bipolar disorder to identify early symptoms of relapse and obtain treatment [see comments]. *British Medical Journal*, *318*(7177), 149–153.

Perugi, G., Micheli, C., Akiskal, H. S., Madaro, D., Socci, C., Quilici, C., & Musetti, L. (2000). Polarity of the first episode, clinical characteristics, and course of manic depressive illness: A systematic retrospective investigation of 320 bipolar I patients. *Comprehensive Psychiatry*, *41*(1), 13–18.

Post, R. M., Leverich, G. S., Altshuler, L. L., Frye, M. A., Suppes, T. M., Keck, P. E., Jr., McElroy, S. L., Kupka, R., Nolen, W. A., Grunze, H., & Walden, J. (2003). An overview of recent findings of the Stanley Foundation Bipolar Network (Part I). *Bipolar Disorder*, *5*(5), 310–319.

Post, R. M., Roy Byrne, P. P., & Uhde, T. W. (1988). Graphic representation of the life course of illness in patients with affective disorder. *American Journal of Psychiatry, 145,* 844–848.

Post, R. M., & Weiss, S. R. (1989). Sensitization, kindling, and anticonvulsants in mania. *Journal of Clinical Psychiatry, 50,* 23–30.

Post, R. M., Weiss, S. R., & Pert, A. (1988). Implications of behavioral sensitization and kindling for stress-induced behavioral change. *Advances in Experimental Medicine & Biology, 245,* 441–463.

Quanbeck, C. D., Stone, D. C., Scott, C. L., McDermott, B. E., Altshuler, L. L., & Frye, M. A. (2004). Clinical and legal correlates of inmates with bipolar disorder at time of criminal arrest. *Journal of Clinical Psychiatry, 65*(2), 198–203.

Robinson, T. E., & Becker, J. B. (1986). Enduring changes in brain and behavior produced by chronic amphetamine administration: A review and evaluation of animal models of amphetamine psychosis. *Brain Research, 396*(2), 157–198.

Rutter, M., Moffitt, T. E., & Caspi, A. (2006). Gene-environment interplay and psychopathology: Multiple varieties but real effects. *Journal of Child Psychology and Psychiatry, 47*(3–4), 226–261.

Sachs, G. S. (1996). Bipolar mood disorder: Practical strategies for acute and maintenance phase treatment. *Journal of Clinical Psychopharmacology, 16*(2, Suppl. 1), 32S–47S.

Sachs, G. S., Yan, L. J., Swann, A. C., & Allen, M. H. (2001). Integration of suicide prevention into outpatient management of bipolar disorder. *Journal of Clinical Psychiatry, 62*(Suppl.), 25, 3–11.

Sax, K. W., & Strakowski, S. M. (2001). Behavioral sensitization in humans. *Journal of Addictive Disorders, 20*(3), 55–65.

Schmitz, J. M., Averill, P., Sayre, S. L., McCleary, P., Moeller, F. G., & Swann, A. C. (2002). Cognitive-behavioral treatment of bipolar disorder and substance abuse: A preliminary randomized study. *Addictive Disorders and Their Treatment, 1,* 17–24.

Scott, J., & Pope, M. (2002). Nonadherence with mood stabilizers: Prevalence and predictors. *Journal of Clinical Psychiatry, 63*(5), 384–390.

Sharma, V. (2001). Loss of response to antidepressants and subsequent refractoriness: Diagnostic issues in a retrospective case series. *Journal of Affective Disorders, 64*(1), 99–106.

Shaw, J. A., Egeland, J. A., Endicott, J., Allen, C. R., & Hostetter, A. M. (2005). A 10-year prospective study of prodromal patterns for bipolar disorder among Amish youth. *Journal of the American Academy of Child and Adolescent Psychiatry, 44*(11), 1104–1111.

Simkin, D. R. (2002). Adolescent substance use disorders and comorbidity. *Pediatric Clinics of North America, 49*(2), 463–477.

Simon, N. M., Otto, M. W., Wisniewski, S. R., Fossey, M., Sagduyu, K., Frank, E., Sachs, G. S., Nierenberg, A. A., Thase, M. E., & Pollack, M. H. (2004). Anxiety disorder comorbidity in bipolar disorder patients: Data from the first 500 participants in the Systematic Treatment Enhancement Program for Bipolar Disorder (STEP-BD). *American Journal of Psychiatry, 161*(12), 2222–2229.

Singh, M. K., DelBello, M. P., Stanford, K. E., Soutullo, C., Donough-Ryan, P., McElroy, S. L., & Strakowski, S. M. (2007). Psychopathology in children of bipolar parents. *Journal of Affective Disorders, 102*(1–3), 131–136.

Strakowski, S. M., Williams, J. R., Sax, K. W., Fleck, D. E., DelBello, M. P., & Bourne, M. L. (2000). Is impaired outcome following a first manic episode due to mood-incongruent psychosis? *Journal of Affective Disorders, 61*(1–2), 87–94.

Strober, M., Morrell, W., Burroughs, J., Lampert, C., Danforth, H., & Freeman, R. (1988). A family study of bipolar I disorder in adolescence: Early onset of symptoms linked to increased familial loading and lithium resistance. *Journal of Affective Disorders, 15,* 255–268.

Sultzer, D. L., & Cummings, J. L. (1989). Drug-induced mania—causative agents, clinical characteristics and management. A retrospective analysis of the literature. *Medical Toxicology and Adverse Drug Experience, 4,* 127–143.

Suppes, T., Dennehy, E. B., Hirschfeld, R. M., Altshuler, L. L., Bowden, C. L., Calabrese, J. R., Crismon, M. L., Ketter, T. A., Sachs, G. S., & Swann, A. C. (2005). The Texas implementation of medication algorithms: Update to the algorithms for treatment of bipolar I disorder. *Journal of Clinical Psychiatry, 66*(7), 870–886.

Suppes, T., Dennehy, E. B., Swann, A. C., Bowden, C. L., Calabrese, J. R., Hirschfeld, R. M., Keck, P. E., Jr., Sachs, G. S., Crismon, M. L., Toprac, M. G., & Shon, S. P. (2002). Report of the Texas Consensus Conference Panel on medication treatment of bipolar disorder 2000. *Journal of Clinical Psychiatry, 63*(4), 288–299.

Swann, A. C. (2006a). Treatment strategies for the management of bipolar disorder. In *Bipolar disorder disease management guide* (pp. 101–137). Montvale, NJ: Thomson PDR.

Swann, A. C. (2006b). What is bipolar disorder? *American Journal of Psychiatry, 163*(2), 177–179.

Swann, A. C., Anderson, J. C., Dougherty, D. M., & Moeller, F. G. (2001). Measurement of inter-episode impulsivity in bipolar disorder. *Psychiatry Research, 101*(2), 195–197.

Swann, A. C., Bowden, C. L., Calabrese, J. R., Dilsaver, S. C., & Morris, D. D. (1999). Differential effect of number of previous episodes of affective disorder on response to lithium or divalproex in acute mania. *American Journal of Psychiatry, 156,* 1264–1266.

Swann, A. C., Bowden, C. L., Calabrese, J. R., Dilsaver, S. C., & Morris, D. D. (2000). Mania: Differential effects of previous depressive and manic episodes on response to treatment. *Acta Psychiatrica Scandinavica, 101*(6), 444–451.

Swann, A. C., Geller, B., Post, R. M., Altshuler, L., Chang, K. D., DelBello, M. P., Reist, C., & Juster, I. A. (2005). Practical clues to early recognition of bipolar disorder: A primary care approach. *Primary Care Companion Journal of Clinical Psychiatry, 7*(1), 15–21.

Tohen, M., Chengappa, K. N., Suppes, T., Baker, R. W., Zarate, C. A., Bowden, C. L., Sachs, G. S., Kupfer, D. J., Ghaemi, S. N., Feldman, P. D., Risser, R. C., Evans, A. R., & Calabrese, J. R. (2004). Relapse prevention in bipolar I disorder: 18-month comparison of olanzapine plus mood stabiliser v. mood stabiliser alone. *British Journal of Psychiatry, 184,* 337–345.

Tohen, M., Jacobs, T. G., Grundy, S. L., McElroy, S. L., Banov, M. C., Janicak, P. G., Sanger, T., Risser, R., Zhang, F., Toma, V., Francis, J., Tollefson, G. D., & Breier, A. (2000). Efficacy of olanzapine in acute bipolar mania: A double-blind, placebo-controlled study. The Olanzipine HGGW Study Group. *Archives of General Psychiatry, 57*(9), 841–849.

Tohen, M., Kryzhanovskaya, L., Carlson, G., Delbello, M., Wozniak, J., Kowatch, R., Wagner, K., Findling, R., Lin, D., Robertson-Plouch, C., Xu, W., Dittmann, R. W., Biederman, J. (2007). Olanzapine versus placebo in the treatment of adolescents with bipolar mania. *American Journal of Psychiatry, 164*(10), 1547–1556.

Turvey, C. L., Coryell, W. H., Solomon, D. A., Leon, A. C., Endicott, J., Keller, M. B., & Akiskal, H. (1999). Long-term prognosis of bipolar I disorder. *Acta Psychiatrica Scandinavica, 99*(2), 110–119.

Weller, R. A., Weller, E. B., Tucker, S. G., & Fristad, M. A. (1986). Mania in prepubertal children: Has it been underdiagnosed. *Journal of Affective Disorders, 11,* 151–154.

Winokur, G., & Wesner, R. (1987). From unipolar depression to bipolar illness: 29 who changed. *Acta Psychiatrica Scandinavica, 76,* 59–63.

Yang, P. B., Swann, A. C., & Dafny, N. (2003). Chronic pretreatment with methylphenidate induces cross-sensitization with amphetamine. *Life Sciences, 73*(22), 2899–2911.

Yap, J. J., Covington, H. E., III, Gale, M. C., Datta, R., & Miczek, K. A. (2005). Behavioral sensitization due to social defeat stress in mice: Antagonism at mGluR5 and NMDA receptors. *Psychopharmacology (Berlin), 179*(1), 230–239.

Zis, A. P., & Goodwin, F. K. (1979). Major affective disorder as a recurrent illness. A critical review. *Archives of General Psychiatry, 36,* 835–839.

Chapter 24

Eating Disorders in Young Adults

Scott J. Crow

A 19-year-old woman presents for evaluation at a college mental health center. Her presenting complaint is depressed mood and she does endorse a number of agitated symptoms of depression; but in passing, she also describes feeling out of control of her eating. Further questioning reveals that, in her senior year of high school, she became increasingly worried about her weight and began dieting. Initially she cut back on the amount of food she ate, then began counting fat grams and avoiding sweets, and now avoids most carbohydrates. She lost some weight (though she started within the "normal" weight range) and received some compliments for this. However, after several months she began a pattern of eating large amounts of food and feeling out of control, and then began self-induced vomiting after eating. Recently, she briefly experimented with using laxatives but did not like those because they made her feel sick; and in high school, she briefly used over-the-counter diet pills. Currently, her height and weight reveal a BMI of 20.5; she denies using additional methods to control her weight. She states that her weight and shape account for 85% of her self-evaluation. She feels lightheaded at times and reports abdominal bloating and frequent sore throats.

Introduction

Eating disorders are common psychiatric disorders that, relative to their incidence and prevalence, receive little attention. Most recent estimates of the prevalence of eating disorders from the National Comorbidity Survey–Replication (Hudson, Hiripi, Pope, & Kessler, 2007) indicate a prevalence for eating disorders, taken as a whole, very similar to that seen for bipolar disorder and greater than that seen in NCS-R for obsessive-compulsive disorder (Kessler et al., 2005). Estimates of lifetime prevalence for anorexia nervosa (AN), bulimia nervosa (BN), and eating disorder not otherwise specified each exceeds typical estimates of the community prevalence of schizophrenia. Eating disorders are certainly pertinent to the topic of mental health in young adults. In fact, they may be unique among psychiatric disorders in the extent to which their onset, course, and treatment seeking is concentrated during the late adolescent/young adult period of life.

In this chapter, the current state of knowledge regarding the epidemiology of eating disorders and the currently employed diagnostic criteria are reviewed. The course and the complications will be discussed. The etiology will be examined with a particular eye to why these disorders may be so common among young adults. Finally, the current status of treatment will be examined.

Epidemiology

Classically, eating disorders (particularly AN) have been viewed as occurring primarily in young Caucasian women, perhaps particularly in those of high socioeconomic status. In the last two decades, the impression that these illnesses occur in Caucasians only and they occur only in certain socioeconomic strata has been repeatedly called into question. For example, carefully conducted community studies of eating disorder psychopathology find substantial risk for diagnosable eating disorders and for disordered eating more broadly among women of many, perhaps all ethnic groups (Striegel-Moore et al., 2003). While it is noteworthy that AN appears to occur at most very rarely among African Americans, the overall message of this line of research appears to be that women of widely varying ethnic backgrounds are at risk.

Eating disorders usually present in a fairly narrow age window. For example, in the National Co-Morbidity Survey, the mean age of onset was 18.9 years for AN, 19.7 years for BN, and 22.4 years for any binge eating (a relatively broadly defined phenotype examined in that study; Hudson, 2007). The standard errors for those mean ages were remarkably small, and inter-quartile ranges were also very small. Thus, in the NCS-R (as in clinical settings) the great majority of individuals with eating disorders have the onset of their illness between their early teens and about the age of 30.

Our understanding of the gender distribution of eating disorders may be changing. Historically, most texts have suggested ratios of women with eating disorders with men with eating disorders of around 10:1, to perhaps as much as 20:1 (one exception to this has been binge eating disorder, where traditionally the gender ratio has been closer to 3:1). In NCS-R, the female:male ratio for AN and BN was only 3:1, and for BED it was slightly less than 2:1. Reasons for this difference from prior work are somewhat unclear; while they could represent secular trends, it seems perhaps more likely that the widespread community nature of NCSR explains at least some of these findings. As with other psychiatric disorders, there may be gender disparities in help seeking, with women more likely to seek help for eating disorders than men (perhaps because of social acceptability factors, or because of preconceptions on the part of health care providers, which might diminish eating disorder case-finding among men).

Diagnostic Criteria

The currently used diagnostic criteria for AN and BN are found in Tables 24-1 and 24-2. The DSM also provides examples of disordered eating that would qualify for an EDNOS diagnosis. Generally these describe individuals lacking one AN or BN criterion or displaying AN or BN criteria for insufficient time or frequency. An additional set of diagnostic criteria for binge eating disorder (BED) are shown in Table 24-3. It is important to note that these BED criteria are provided in Appendix B of the DSM IV as a criterion set for further study. At present, with the publication of DSM V several years away, work is underway to better define criteria sets as well as to more clearly determine the diagnostic validity of BED. It appears likely that there will be some changes in DSM V. Most

Table 24-1. Anorexia Nervosa

A. Failure to maintain body weight at or above minimally normal weight (e.g., less than 85% of expected)
B. Intense fear of gaining weight or beginning fat, even though underweight
C. Disturbance in the way one's body weight or shape is experienced, undue influence of body weight or shape and self-evaluation, or denial of seriousness of current low body weight.
D. In postmenarchal females, amenorrhea.

Reprinted with permission from the Diagnostic and Statistical Manual of Mental Disorders, Text Revision, Fourth Edition, (Copyright © 2000). American Psychiatric Association.

Table 24-2. Bulimia Nervosa

A. Recurrent episodes of binge eating, defined as:
   1. Eating in a discrete period of time an amount of food that is definitely larger than most people would eat in a similar period of time and under similar circumstances.

   AND

   2. A sense of lack of control over eating during the episode.
B. Recurrent, inappropriate compensatory behavior in order to prevent weight gain, such as self-induced vomiting, misuse of laxatives, diuretics, enemas, other medications, fasting, or excessive exercise.
C. Binge eating and compensatory behaviors occurring at least twice a week for 3 months.
D. Self-evaluation is unduly influenced by shape or weight.
E. The disturbance does not occur exclusively during episodes of anorexia nervosa.

Reprinted with permission from the Diagnostic and Statistical Manual of Mental Disorders, Text Revision, Fourth Edition, (Copyright © 2000). American Psychiatric Association.

Table 24-3. Binge Eating Disorder

A. Recurrent episodes of binge eating:
1. Eating in a discrete period of time an amount of food definitely larger than most would eat in a similar period of time under similar circumstances.
2. A sense of lack of control over eating during the episode

B. Binge eating episodes are associated with three or more of the following:
1. Eating much more rapidly than normal
2. Eating until uncomfortably full
3. Eating large amounts of food when not feeling physically hungry
4. Eating alone because of binge, embarrassed by how much one is eating
5. Feeling disgusted with oneself, depressed, or very guilty after overeating

C. Marked distress regarding binge eating is present.
D. Binge eating occurs, on average, at least 2 days a week for 6 months.
E. Binge eating is not associated with the regular use of inappropriate compensatory behaviors and does not occur exclusively in the course of anorexia nervosa or bulimia nervosa.

Reprinted with permission from the Diagnostic and Statistical Manual of Mental Disorders, Text Revision, Fourth Edition, (Copyright © 2000). American Psychiatric Association.

likely among these potential changes is the elimination of amenorrhea as a required diagnostic criterion for AN. Numerous studies have failed to document significant differences between individuals who meet all AN criteria except for the absence of amenorrhea as compared to those who meet all the diagnostic criteria including amenorrhea. Additionally, while there is little literature to support its efficacy at present, it is common practice to provide hormonal replacement to women with anorexia symptoms and amenorrhea in hopes of protecting bone structure. This, too, complicates the use of amenorrhea as a diagnostic criterion.

Course and Complications

The course of AN and BN differs somewhat from that seen with other psychiatric illnesses: episode duration may be longer than that seen on the average, for example, with major depression, but the overall length of illness is not lifelong for most individuals (in contrast to conditions such as schizophrenia). Extensive work has now examined the course of AN. On average, AN lasts for a substantial number of years for most sufferers. Classically, over longer-term follow-up, about one-third of individuals appear to become free of eating disorder symptoms; one-third no longer meet diagnostic criteria for AN but still have some eating disorder symptoms; and about one-third at 5- to 10-year follow-up are still diagnosed with AN. A number of correlates of poor course have been identified; these include later age of onset, longer duration of illness at presentation, and longer treatment (Fichter, Quadflieg, & Hedlund, 2006).

An important aspect of anorexia nervosa outcome is mortality. Previous studies suggest that AN carries the highest suicide mortality rate (Harris & Barraclough, 1994) of any psychiatric illness, and all cause more mortality rates second only to opiate dependence (Harris & Barraclough, 1998). Studies directly examining mortality typically find standardized mortality ratios (the ratio of the observed mortality rate in the study population as compared to the expected mortality rate, given age, gender, ethnicity, and geographic location) of 5–10 or more. This translates into a crude mortality rate in most rigorously conducted studies of 10% or more (for example, see Crow, Praus, & Thuras, 1999b; Eckert, Halmi, Marchi, Grove, & Crosby, 1995), and one meta-analysis has estimated a yearly mortality rate of 0.59% (Sullivan, 1995).

The course for BN is somewhat more favorable. In the most rigorous and long-running study of outcome reported to date, Keel and colleagues (1999) showed that only about 11% of subjects with BN still had full diagnosable BN at 10- to 15-year follow-up. The majority (approximately two-thirds) of subjects were free from significant eating disorder symptoms at that interval. Studies examining mortality have consistently found lower mortality rates in subjects with BN, with little evidence to suggest mortality substantially above that seen in the general population, adjusted for age.

Eating disorders stand out among psychiatric illnesses for their strong association with medical complications (Mitchell & Crow, 2006). Because individuals with AN can display purging behaviors, and because those with BN can have periods of severe dietary restriction, it is probably more useful to consider the potential medical complications as associated with binge eating/purging and restricting behaviors, respectively, rather than breaking them out by diagnostic category. Thus, the commonly observed medical complications of binge eating/purging and severe restriction are shown in Tables 24-4 and 24-5. For young adults with BN, a significant minority come to attention based on hypokalemia identified at screening physical exams; low potassium is a relatively insensitive but highly specific marker for BN (Crow, Salisbury, Crosby, & Mitchell, 1997).

One particular complication of importance in young adults is the impact of eating disorder symptoms on fertility. While amenorrhea is not likely to remain a required feature for AN diagnosis, it is nonetheless very common; thus, fertility is clearly an issue for individuals actively ill with AN. Still, there are case reports and case series of patients actively ill with AN who become pregnant and clearly pregnancy can also occur later, after symptomatic improvement, in individuals with AN. More is known about fertility in BN, and the existing evidence suggests that fertility is preserved (Crow, Thuras, Keel, & Mitchell, 2002). There is also evidence to suggest that eating disorder symptoms improve with pregnancy, although for many individuals these symptoms tend to revert back to prepregnancy

Table 24-4. Complications of Binge Eating and Purging

Electrolyte disturbance (particularly hypokalemia)
Parotid gland hypertrophy
Dental enamel erosion
Menstrual irregularity
Esophagitis
Esophageal tear
Gastric rupture
Colonic dysfunction

Table 24-5. Complications of Restricting

Dry skin/hair
Lanugo
Osteoporosis
Hepatitis
Anemia/leukopenia
Electrolyte disturbance
Infertility
Hypothermia
Hypertension
Bradycardia

levels, following the conclusion of pregnancy (Crow, Agras, Crosby, Halmi, & Mitchell, 2008).

Psychiatric comorbidity can be considered another eating disorder complication, for cormordity is the rule, particularly in clinical samples. Most prominent are mood, anxiety, and substance use disorders (Bulik et al., 2004; Kaye, Bulik, Thornton, Barbarich, & Masters, 2004).

Etiology

Much is known about risk and maintenance factors that underlie the etiology of eating disorders (Stice, 2002). Eating disorders represent a striking interplay of preexisting and acquired biological factors interfacing with psychological factors, public health trends, and prevailing societal attitudes about weight and shape. Any understanding of the etiology of these illnesses must take into account several factors, including: *(1)* the seeming emergence of bulimia nervosa in the mid to late twentieth century, *(2)* evidence suggesting a substantially increased frequency of AN in the latter half of the twentieth century, *(3)* evidence suggesting a relatively flattening prevalence of AN and BN in the face of an obesity epidemic in the last two decades, *(4)* mounting evidence for a familial and genetic component for these conditions, and *(5)* the profound societal importance placed on thinness, weight, and shape in Western societies, particularly for women. A final factor to consider, in light of topic of this volume, is the strong predilection for young adult onset.

Historical references to behavior sounding very much like AN exist back to the Middle Ages (Keel & Klump, 2003). It appears, however, that this was quite rare and may have had a focus on other factors, such as religiosity (in contrast to recent times where themes regarding thinness have prevailed). In any event, AN and BN appear to be very strikingly more common in the latter half of the twentieth century. Mounting evidence suggests prominent familial and/or genetic components in the etiology of this illness. Numerous studies have now clearly demonstrated a familial component, for example (Strober, Freeman, Lampert, Diamond, & Kaye, 2000). Twin study designs clearly indicate that this familial component is primarily genetic (Culbert, Slane, & Klump, 2008). Recently, genome-wide association studies and candidate gene studies have increasingly identified candidate regions and genes that may play a role in the etiology of AN and BN.

How can one reconcile this strong evidence for a major genetic component with evidence of a markedly increasing frequency of illness over a time span much too short to allow substantial changes in the gene pool? In all likelihood, this situation represents an outstanding example of a gene-environment interaction (Keel & Klump, 2003). Powerful and (relatively) new societal messages about shape and weight interact with genes in susceptible individuals that either previously were not expressed behaviorally, or that in other environments were expressed as different kinds of psychopathology, or that in other environments were adaptive. Such genes seem likely to influence temperamental risk factors, rather than eating-related variables.

Why do so many present with eating disorder symptoms in early adulthood? Obviously, any genetic underpinnings for eating disorders are present lifelong, but there is abundant evidence available to even casual observation suggesting that societal messages about weight and shape are vigorously addressed to even young adolescents. Thus, in a gene–environment interaction model, the necessary components are present long before young adulthood. Several factors might help to explain this seeming contradiction. First, particularly in BN, it appears very common to develop substantial numbers of symptoms years prior to seeking treatment. In many instances, illness onset may pre-date young adulthood, even if help seeking does not. Second, the transition from high school to either college or working may present particular psychosocial and maturational stresses that could potentially make this a time of substantial risk.

Third, for many individuals, the transition from high school to college may represent a time of considerable change (usually a decrease) in physical activity level, which would likely predispose to weight gain and subsequently to both healthy and unhealthy weight control behaviors.

Treatment

Numerous treatments have been developed for eating disorders, but therapeutic approaches to eating disorders differ from most other areas of psychiatry in two main ways. First, nutritional rehabilitation and stabilization are absolutely essential to effective treatment. Second, unlike many other areas of psychiatry, psychotherapy plays a preeminent role with medication used, for the most part, only adjunctively. These various treatment approaches are considered below.

Nutritional Treatment

Nutritional stabilization is critical to integrate into the beginning of treatment; this is true regardless of treatment setting (i.e., inpatient vs. outpatient) and it is true regardless of whether psychotherapy, pharmacotherapy, or both are also used.

In individuals at low weight, nutritional treatment consists first and foremost of resuming a pattern of eating sufficient to support weight gain toward a goal weight within the "normal" weight range. Treatment centers currently use different criteria for this goal weight, with some aiming for body mass index (BMI) figures in the "normal" weight range, while others use height and weight tables to set initial treatment goals of somewhere between 90%–100% of ideal body weight. Treatment typically involves the reestablishment of consistent meals, often accompanied by 2–3 snacks per day. Extreme dietary restriction typically suppresses basal metabolic rate well below baseline levels; BMI typically climbs to well above baseline levels during refeeding (Salisbury, Levine, Crow, & Mitchell, 1995)and calories must be correspondingly increased in order to sustain necessary weight gain. Subsequently, once weight gain has been achieved, BMI typically drops, and calorie requirements do as well. The addition of snacks not only diminishes the amount of time between eating but also helps to distribute the number of calories required to be consumed throughout the day. During the process of refeeding, careful monitoring of serum phosphate is essential; early in refeeding, some patients may have normal serum phosphorus while still being total body phosphorus depleted, and they may become markedly (at times dangerously) hypophosphatemic.

In BN, nutritional rehabilitation typically consists of resuming a pattern of three meals per day, again usually with two or three snacks. This resumption is often very difficult for patients to undertake because they have markedly restricted their eating behavior in an attempt to lose weight, and many will come to treatment having eating binges late in the day but very little eating in other parts of the day. At the same time, patients typically report the experience of vomiting after binging, "until all the food is gone." Given this experience, the suggestion that they can resume consistent eating without having their weight go up markedly is highly counter-intuitive. Yet resumption of consistent eating without significant weight gain is typically what is seen. The reason appears to be that eating binges consist of consuming very large numbers of calories, and studies suggest that a significant number of binge calories are retained after purging (Kaye, Weltzin, Hsu, McConaha, & Bolton, 1993).

Nutritional approaches can play a prominent role in the treatment of BED. Given the common observation that the binge eating occurring in bulimia nervosa is often preceded by dieting, initial thinking suggested that dieting was to be avoided in individuals with BED. Subsequent work has shown that modest calorie-restricting dieting can lead to cessation of binge eating symptoms. In addition, a prominent goal of treatment for most individuals with BED is weight loss, and calorie-restrictive dieting can be associated with some (albeit modest) success in this regard (Wonderlich, de Zwaan, Mitchell, Peterson, & Crow, 2003).

Psychotherapy

Following or in conjunction with nutritional rehabilitation, psychotherapy is the second cornerstone of eating disorders treatment. A wide variety of treatments for BN have been studied, as reviewed elsewhere (Shapiro et al., 2007). An even wider variety is used in clinical practice, and research suggests that evidence-based treatments are infrequently used (Crow, Mussell, Peterson, Knopke, & Mitchell, 1999a). By far, the largest amount of empirical support exists for cognitive-behavioral therapy (CBT) specifically targeted at eating disorders (Agras et al., 2000a; Fairburn & Cooper, 1993). Cognitive-behavioral therapy for BN utilizes a conceptual model in which low self-esteem leads to extreme concerns about weight and shaping, resulting in the use of strict dieting. Eventually such strict attempts at diet cannot be maintained and lead to binge eating, which is typically followed by purging. This treatment has been shown to be effective in individual, group, and self-help formats. Group therapy often provides especially useful support for persons with BN; given the secretive nature of symptoms they have often had a strong sense of isolation prior to group work. In practice, the use of groups is largely contained to specialty clinical settings, simply because practitioners who see limited numbers of eating disorder patients rarely have enough potential participants to form a group at any given time. Interpersonal therapy (IPT) also has received considerable support, with some suggestion that initial response may be faster with CBT, but individuals receiving IPT could experience a "catch up" effect later (Agras, Walsh, Fairburn, Wilson, & Kraemer, 2000b).

Appropriate psychotherapy interventions for AN are less certain. A number of therapeutic approaches have been studied, and the main approach shown to be effective thus far is a specific form of family-based psychotherapy in which families are empowered early in treatment to take increased control over their adolescent's eating behavior (Eisler, Dare, Russell, Szmukler, le Grange, & Dodge, 1997; Eisler et al., 2000). This therapy has been shown to be highly effective for adolescents with AN who are still living at home; it has not been significantly tested in young adults; to this point, the components of young age and still living at home have both been viewed as critical. In this family-based treatment, parents are empowered to take charge of getting the patient adequate nutrition. This begins in the second session, a family meal where the entire family brings a meal to the therapist's office and eats it during the session. Parents play a central role in ensuring the child eats until adequate weight and stable eating are achieved. At this point responsibility for eating is gradually returned to the child.

Active work is currently examining CBT (Pike, Walsh, Vitousek, Wilson, & Bauer, 2003), specific supportive therapies aimed at restoring weight through facilitating eating (McIntosh et al., 2005), and novel psychotherapies targeting other symptoms. This work is particularly active in adults.

Psychotherapy interventions for BED very much follow on those used in bulimia nervosa with major emphasis on CBT and to a lesser extent IPT (Wonderlich et al., 2003). Overall decrements in target behaviors as well as overall abstinence rates tend to be higher than those seen with bulimia nervosa. However, as noted above, weight loss is a prominent goal for many individuals entering BED treatment, and psychotherapy interventions to date for BED have generally not been associated with significant weight loss.

Pharmacotherapy

Much as with psychotherapy, pharmacotherapy has received substantial attention and has generally been shown to be more useful in the treatment of BN than AN. For BN treatment, many medications have been studied with the great majority being antidepressants. In nearly all cases, antidepressive trials for BN have shown decreases in binge eating and purging. Where measured, they sometimes have shown improvements in eating disorder cognitions as well. Two caveats exist, however. First, in a bupropion trial (Horne et al., 1988), the drug was quite effective in reducing BN symptoms but was associated with a nearly 6% risk of seizures. For this reason, BN is viewed as a contraindication of bupropion use. Second, several studies have examined the use of MAOI inhibitors (Walsh et al., 1988). While these have typically done fairly well in BN trials, they are viewed as being roughly contraindicated in the treatment of BN because of concerns about dietary interactions with binges, as well as issues related to orthostatic symptoms in individuals with dehydration. At present, many would view the use of SSRIs as representing state-of-the-art pharmacologic treatment for BN. It is important to note that direct comparisons of low-dose vs. high-dose SSRI (specifically, 20 mg vs. 60 mg of fluoxetine; Fluoxetine Bulimia Nervosa Collaborative Study Group, 1992) have supported the use of high-dose SSRI.

For AN the picture is somewhat different. A very wide range of different types of medications has been studied. In particular, there have now been several short- or long-term, acute or relapse prevention trials of SSRIs. In very recent times, there has been increasing interest in the use of atypical antipsychotics (Powers, Santana, & Bannon, 2002). In the most recent SSRI trial, a recently published 1-year relapse prevention study (Walsh et al., 2006) clearly found no benefit for SSRI treatment in relapse prevention among individuals with AN who had achieved weight restoration and then received outpatient psychotherapy. Whether atypical antipsychotics can be of use in this group is unclear. A number of short-term open trials and case series suggest some potential benefit, but to this point, little in the way of placebo-controlled trials, either short or long term, are available.

Medications do play some role in the treatment of BED, and a somewhat wider range of agents have been examined. There is evidence to suggest that antidepressants of various sorts diminish binge eating, though again with limited effect on weight. A number of agents have been examined due to their weight loss potential, including both agents used primarily for weight loss (for example, Sibutramine) as well as agents causing weight loss or appetite suppression as a side effect (for example, Topirimate or Zonisimide). Some of these agents have been associated with more significant weight loss, but their efficacy in long-term treatment is as yet unproven.

Summary

In summary, eating disorders are very common, particularly among late adolescents and adults. Societal and genetic factors figure prominently in the etiology of these illnesses. The long-term course is favorable for BN, and more guarded for AN; relatively little is known about the course of ED NOS. Eating disorder treatment routinely focuses on nutritional restoration, and beyond nutrition, psychotherapy is the main mode of treatment. Medications may be very important adjuncts to treatment for BN, but effective pharmacotherapy for AN is as yet unclear.

> **KEY POINTS**
>
> - Eating disorders carry particularly high medical morbidity and suicide risk.
> - Eating disorders are most prevalent among young adults and adolescents, particularly (but not only) in women.
> - Nutritional stabilization plus psychotherapy is the cornerstone of eating disorder treatment.

> **PRACTICE GUIDELINES**
>
> - Careful assessment for medical risk, especially for those in need of weight gain, is a critical part of early treatment.
> - Cognitive-behavioral therapy for BN and family-based therapy for AN (in adolescents still at home) are empirically supported treatments.
> - Medications currently play an adjunctive role in ED treatment.

References

Agras, W. S., Crow, S. J., Halmi, K. A., Mitchell, J. E., Wilson, G. T., & Kraemer, H. C. (2000a). Outcome predictors for the cognitive behavior treatment of bulimia nervosa: Data from a multisite study. *American Journal of Psychiatry, 157*(8), 1302–1308.

Agras, W. S., Walsh, T., Fairburn, C. G., Wilson, G. T., & Kraemer, H. C. (2000b). A multicenter comparison of cognitive-behavioral therapy and interpersonal psychotherapy for bulimia nervosa. *Archives of General Psychiatry, 57*(5), 459–466.

American Psychiatric Association. (1994). *Diagnostic and statistical manual of mental disorders* (4th ed.). Washington, DC: Author.

Bulik, C. M., Klump, K. L., Thornton, L., Kaplan, A. S., Devlin, B., Fichter, M. M., Halmi, K. A., Strober, M., Woodside, D. B., Crow, S., Mitchell, J. E., Rotondo, A., Mauri, M., Cassano, G. B., Keel, P. K., Berrettini, W. H., Kaye, W. H. (2004). Alcohol use disorder comorbidity in eating disorders: A multicenter study. *Journal of Clinical Psychiatry, 65*(7), 1000–1006.

Crow, S., Mussell, M. P., Peterson, C., Knopke, A., & Mitchell, J. (1999a). Prior treatment received by patients with bulimia nervosa. *International Journal of Eating Disorders, 25*(1), 39–44.

Crow, S., Praus, B., & Thuras, P. (1999b). Mortality from eating disorders—a 5- to 10-year record linkage study. *International Journal of Eating Disorders, 26*(1), 97–101.

Crow, S. J., Agras, W. S., Crosby, R., Halmi, K., & Mitchell, J. E. (2008). Eating disorder symptoms in pregnancy: A prospective study. *International Journal of Eating Disorders. 41*(3), 277–279.

Crow, S. J., Salisbury, J. J., Crosby, R. D., & Mitchell, J. E. (1997). Serum electrolytes as markers of vomiting in bulimia nervosa. *International Journal of Eating Disorders, 21*(1), 95–98.

Crow, S. J., Thuras, P., Keel, P. K., & Mitchell, J. E. (2002). Long-term menstrual and reproductive function in patients with bulimia nervosa. *American Journal of Psychiatry, 159*(6), 1048–1050.

Culbert, K. M., Slane, J. D., & Klump, K. L. (2008). Genetics of eating disorders. In S. Wonderlich, J. Mitchell, M. De Zwaan & H. Steiger (Eds.), *Annual review of eating disorders part 2* (pp. 27–42). New York: Radcliffe Publishing.

Eckert, E. D., Halmi, K. A., Marchi, P., Grove, W., & Crosby, R. (1995). Ten-year follow-up of anorexia nervosa: Clinical course and outcome. *Psychological Medicine, 25*(1), 143–156.

Eisler, I., Dare, C., Hodes, M., Russell, G., Dodge, E., & Le Grange, D. (2000). Family therapy for adolescent anorexia nervosa: The results of a controlled comparison of two family interventions. *Journal of Child Psychology and Psychiatry, 41*(6), 727–736.

Eisler, I., Dare, C., Russell, G. F., Szmukler, G., le Grange, D., & Dodge, E. (1997). Family and individual therapy in anorexia nervosa: A 5-year follow-up. *Archives of General Psychiatry, 54*(11), 1025–1030.

Fairburn, C. G., & Cooper, Z. (1993). Cognitive behaviour therapy for binge eating and bulimia nervosa: A comprehensive treatment manual. In C. G. Fairburn & G. T. Wilson (Eds.), *Binge eating, nature, assessment and treatment* (pp. 361–404). New York: Guilford Press.

Fichter, M. M., Quadflieg, N., & Hedlund, S. (2006). Twelve-year course and outcome predictors of anorexia nervosa. *International Journal of Eating Disorders, 39*(2), 87–100.

Fluoxetine Bulimia Nervosa Collaborative Study Group. (1992). Fluoxetine in the treatment of bulimia nervosa. A multicenter, p.-c., double-blind trial. *Archives of General Psychiatry, 49*(2), 139–147.

Harris, E. C., & Barraclough, B. (1994). Suicide as an outcome for mental disorders. A meta-analysis. *British Journal of Psychiatry, 170*, 205–228.

Harris, E. C., & Barraclough, B. (1998). Excess mortality of mental disorder. *British Journal of Psychiatry, 173*, 11–53.

Horne, R. L., Ferguson, J. M., Pope, H. G., Jr., Hudson, J. I., Lineberry, C. G., Ascher, J., & Cato, A. (1988). Treatment of bulimia with bupropion: a multicenter controlled trial. *Journal of Clinical Psychiatry 49*(7), 262–266.

Hudson, J. I., Hiripi, E. Pope, H. G., Jr., & Kessler, R. C. (2007). The prevalence and correlates of eating disorders in the national comorbidity survey replication. *Biological Psychiatry, 61*(3), 348–358.

Kaye, W. H., Bulik, C. M., Thornton, L., Barbarich, N., & Masters, B. S. (2004). Comorbidity of anxiety disorders with anorexia and bulimia nervosa. *American Journal of Psychiatry, 161*, 2215–2221.

Kaye, W. H., Weltzin, T. E., Hsu, L. K., McConaha, C. W., & Bolton, B. (1993). Amount of calories retained after binge eating and vomiting. *American Journal of Psychiatry, 150*(6), 969–971.

Keel, P. K., & Klump, K. L. (2003). Are eating disorders culture-bound syndromes? Implications for conceptualizing their etiology. *Psychology Bulletin, 129*(5), 747–769.

Keel, P. K., Mitchell, J. E., Miller, K. B., Davis, T. L., & Crow, S. J. (1999). Long-term outcome of bulimia nervosa. *Archives of General Psychiatry, 56*(1), 63–69.

Kessler, R. C., Berglund, P., Demler, O., Jin, R., Merikangas, K. R., & Walters, E. E. (2005). Lifetime prevalence and age-of-onset distributions of DSM-IV disorders in the national comorbidity survey replication. *Archives of General Psychiatry, 62*(6), 593–602.

McIntosh, V. V., Jordan, J., Carter, F. A., Luty, S. E., McKenzie, J. M., Bulik, C. M., Frampton, C. M., & Joyce, P. R. (2005). Three psychotherapies for anorexia nervosa: A randomized, controlled trial. *American Journal of Psychiatry, 162*(4), 741–747.

Mitchell, J. E., & Crow, S. (2006). Medical complications of anorexia nervosa and bulimia nervosa. *Current Opinion in Psychiatry, 19*(4), 438–443.

Pike, K. M., Walsh, B. T., Vitousek, K., Wilson, G. T., & Bauer, J. (2003). Cognitive behavior therapy in the posthospitalization treatment of anorexia nervosa. *American Journal of Psychiatry, 160*(11), 2046–2049.

Powers, P. S., Santana, C. A., & Bannon, Y. S. (2002). Olanzapine in the treatment of anorexia nervosa: An open label trial. *International Journal of Eating Disorders, 32*(2), 146–154.

Salisbury, J. J., Levine, A. S., Crow, S. J., & Mitchell, J. E. (1995). Refeeding, metabolic rate, and weight gain in anorexia nervosa: A review. *International Journal of Eating Disorders, 17*(4), 337–345.

Shapiro, J. R., Berkman, N. D., Brownley, K. A., Sedway, J. A., Lohr, K. N., & Bulik, C. M. (2007). Bulimia nervosa treatment: A systematic review of randomized controlled trials. *International Journal of Eating Disorder, 40*, 321–336.

Stice, E. (2002). Risk and maintenance factors for eating pathology: A meta-analytic review. *Psychology Bulletin, 128*(5), 825–848.

Striegel-Moore, R. H., Dohm, F. A., Kraemer, H. C., Taylor, C. B., Daniels, S., Crawford, P. B., & Schreiber, G. B. (2003). Eating disorders in white and black women. *American Journal of Psychiatry, 160*(7), 1326–1331.

Strober, M., Freeman, R., Lampert, C., Diamond, J., & Kaye, W. (2000). Controlled family study of anorexia nervosa and bulimia nervosa: Evidence of shared liability and transmission of partial syndromes. *American Journal of Psychiatry, 157*(3), 393–401.

Sullivan, P. F. (1995). Mortality in anorexia nervosa. *American Journal of Psychiatry, 152*(7), 1073–1074.

Walsh, B. T., Gladis, M., Roose, S. P., Stewart, J. W., Stetner, F., & Glassman, A. H. (1988). Phenelzine vs placebo in 50 patients with bulimia. *Archives of General Psychiatry, 45*(5), 471–475.

Walsh, B. T., Kaplan, A. S., Attia, E., Olmsted, M., Parides, M., Carter, J. C., Pike, K. M., Devlin, M. J., Woodside, B., Roberto, C. A., & Rockert, W. (2006). Fluoxetine after weight restoration in anorexia nervosa: a randomized controlled trial. *Journal of the American Medical Association, 295*(22), 2605–2612.

Wonderlich, S. A., de Zwaan, M., Mitchell, J. E., Peterson, C., & Crow, S. (2003). Psychological and dietary treatments of binge eating disorder: Conceptual implications. *International Journal of Eating Disorders, 34*(Suppl), S58–73.

Chapter 25

Pervasive Developmental Disorders

Noha F. Minshawi, Naomi B. Swiezy, Stacie L. Pozdol, Melissa Stuart and Christopher J. McDougle

Case Vignette

Background

Sam is a 17-year-old male who was diagnosed with autistic disorder at the age of 4. In the area of communication, Sam uses verbal speech to express thoughts and ideas but has a marked impairment in his ability to engage in conversational language. If Sam initiates or maintains a conversation, it typically revolves around a single point of focus (i.e., cars). Sam also does not appear cognizant of others' level of interest or disinterest in a conversation and has difficulty understanding other peoples' perspective. Sam has difficulty maintaining relationships with same-age peers and prefers to be around younger children or adults. He also engages in repetitive play with cars (i.e., rolling back and forth repeatedly), and he has an excessive preoccupation with car-related items, including car keys, car magazines, and car parts.

Target Behaviors

Sam's parents presented for skill building and pharmacological and behavioral treatment for several target symptoms. Specifically, Sam is displaying social anxiety (trembling, sweating, and avoiding social situations), as well as deficits in self-help skills (i.e., personal hygiene and other daily living skills), and a lack of leisure skills (i.e., only interested in cars and refuses to participate in other activities). Sam is also currently engaging in both physical (i.e., hitting, kicking, throwing objects) and verbal aggression (i.e., name calling and threatening language when others do not comply with his desires). A comprehensive treatment plan was developed to address the need for skill development in the areas of socialization, communication, and adaptive skills. In addition, pharmacological and behavioral interventions were designed to reduce Sam's physical and verbal aggression.

Skill Building

Social and Communication Skills. Current treatment targets in the area of social and communication skills include teaching Sam appropriate greetings and topics of conversation, as well as developing reciprocal conversation skills. Sorting tasks to discriminate appropriate and inappropriate greetings as well as various social scripts were devised and rehearsed with Sam. These tools provide visual cues that Sam can be referred to prior to entering social situations where he will be expected to greet friends and/or strangers.

Adaptive Skills. Adaptive skill development has been addressed in the behavior intervention plan as well. Sam currently displays limited independence with personal hygiene and daily living tasks. To increase independence, task analyses (i.e., tasks broken down into various component steps) were conducted on several necessary activities (shaving, bathing, and doing laundry). The task analyses provided detailed step-by-step instructions for completing these tasks and the instructions were written into mini-schedules for Sam. These mini-schedules provide Sam with visual cues as to the order of steps in each activity, thereby providing a sense of structure, predictability, and stability. Sam uses these visual aides whenever engaging in these activities and his parents subsequently report increased independence and decreased resistance to completing the activities.

Pharmacological and Behavioral Interventions

Pharmacological and behavioral interventions are currently being employed to reduce Sam's target problem behaviors. Sam has been prescribed risperidone to address physical and verbal aggression. His parents report a reduction in these target behaviors since the introduction of risperidone. Side effects have included transient sedation and increased appetite. In conjunction with the risperidone, parent training was conducted to provide Sam's parents with strategies for managing problem behavior while increasing motivation. A first/then visual system was developed. Using this system, Sam's parents present him with pictures representing an undesirable task (such as taking a shower) followed by a desirable task (e.g., car magazines) and saying, "First you'll take a shower and then you can look at your car magazines." The use of a visual strategy assists in the realization that engaging in less preferred activities is followed by engaging in a highly preferred activity. In addition, a token economy was created in which Sam earns tokens for engaging in a predetermined schedule of activities and loses tokens for engaging in target problem behaviors. At the end of each day, Sam can exchange his tokens for a hierarchy of rewarding items and activities.

Transition Planning

In preparation for Sam's transition into adulthood, several concerns have arisen and are being addressed by home and school interventions. Sam is highly dependent on prompts in order to complete daily living skills and engage in social interactions. In addition, he has difficulty understanding social concepts and rules, which often result in him being taken advantage of, teased, or bullied. Visual schedules and social scripts are being utilized to increase Sam's independence and social appropriateness in these areas. Sam currently has limited interest in choices of vocations. His school and parents are encouraged to process and expose Sam to different vocational opportunities based on his very specific and individualized interests. In addition, plans for how the school system and family will begin to transition Sam away from school and into the community, as well as long-term care options, must also be explored.

Introduction

Of all of the psychopathological disorders of childhood and adolescence, one would be hard pressed to find a category that has recently received more public attention than the pervasive developmental disorders (PDD). PDD is the medical term used to refer to a number of developmental disabilities that share a similar symptom profile. The disorders included under the umbrella of PDD are autistic disorder, Asperger disorder, pervasive developmental disorder not otherwise specified (PDD-NOS), Rett disorder, and childhood disintegrative disorder. Another common term that is often used to describe the first three of these disorders is autism spectrum disorders (ASD). For the present chapter, the medical term PDD will be used.

The purpose of this chapter is to provide clinicians, researchers, and physicians with a broad overview of PDD in adolescents and young adults. Background information on the symptoms of PDD will be provided. This will be followed by a discussion of the etiology of PDD and the developmental trajectory of the disorders from childhood to adolescence. In addition, a discussion of skill development and an overview of behavioral and pharmacological treatments of the core and associated symptoms of PDD will be provided.

Diagnostic Criteria

When autism was initially described by Leo Kanner in 1943, it was believed to be a single disorder. However, in the past two decades this notion has been dismissed and it has become apparent that several different disorders with similar symptomatology may exist along a continuum. As discussed above, the three most common disorders that are subsumed under PDD are autistic disorder, Asperger disorder, and PDD-NOS.

These three disorders are based upon the same three core clinical criteria, but with some significant differences that are used for purposes of differential diagnosis. The triad of behaviors that overlap among the disorders are *(1)* challenges in social interaction; *(2)* difficulties in functional communication; and *(3)* repetitive or stereotyped patterns of behavior (Wing, 1997).

The challenges noted in social interaction of individuals with PDD are considered to be a defining feature of the disorders and unique from those observed in other developmental disorders (Rutter, 1978). Children, adolescents, and adults with PDD display difficulties in many areas of socialization, including both nonverbal and verbal interactions. Nonverbal social difficulties include challenges in developing appropriate eye-to-eye gaze (Volkmar & Mayes, 1990), demonstrating joint attention (McArthur & Adamson, 1996), and displaying imitation skills (Toth, Dawson, Meltzoff, Greenson, & Fein, 2007). Examples of impairments in verbal social interaction seen in PDD are unusual preverbal vocalizations (Sheinkopf, Mundy, Oller, & Steffens, 2000), limited interest in social interactions with others, which includes a preference to be alone, limited response to the initiations of others, and fewer attempts to initiate interaction with others (Carter, Davis, Klin, & Volkmar, 2005).

Language and communication skills in individuals with PDD are also markedly atypical and difficulties have been noted in both verbal and nonverbal communication. Individuals with PDD demonstrate challenges in language that range from a complete lack of expressive verbal language (Kanner, 1943) to difficulties in initiating and maintaining conversations (Adams, Green, Gilchrist, & Cox, 2002). Idiosyncratic language is also common and can include neologisms (Volden & Lord, 1991) and echolalia (Fay, 1969). Nonverbal communication deficits may include problems with distal pointing and coordination of eye gaze with language (Phillips, Baron-Cohen, & Rutter, 1992).

The final category of symptoms in PDD is restricted interests and repetitive or stereotyped patterns of behavior. This category subsumes many of the oddities and unusual behaviors demonstrated by individuals with PDD. Examples of some of these behaviors may include strict adherence to nonfunctional routines, engaging in ritualistic behavior, and unusual preoccupation with specific interests. In addition, stereotyped motor behaviors, such as rocking, hand flapping, and toe walking, are also common among individuals with PDD.

In addition to the triad of symptoms discussed, several other features are commonly associated with PDD. While individuals with PDD display a range of cognitive functioning, intellectual disability or mental retardation is comorbid in a large number of individuals with PDD, potentially as high as 45% to 50% (Chakrabarti & Fombonne, 2001). It is important to note, however, that current standardized measures of intelligence may not be appropriate for use with individuals with PDD (Edelson, 2006). In addition, individuals with PDD also may engage in a number of inappropriate or problem behaviors that are often the focus of intervention. These problem behaviors can range in severity from minimally disruptive behaviors, such as temper tantrums, impulsivity, or hyperactivity, to more severe behaviors such as aggression and self-injury.

Etiology

The study of the etiology of PDD has focused on the role of genetics, other biological variables, and environmental factors. While no one specific area has been identified as the sole cause of PDD, progress in understanding the role of each of these factors has begun to develop. In the area of genetics, researchers have shown a rate of concordance for autistic disorder of 60% among monozygotic twins and 4.5% among dizygotic twins (Veenstra-Vanderweele & Cook, 2003). These data have led researchers to further investigate the contribution of specific genes to the phenomenology of PDD. It has been reported that approximately 1.7% to 4.8% of individuals with autistic disorder exhibit some type of chromosomal abnormality (Reddy, 2005). The specific chromosomal abnormality most commonly reported as a cause of autism is maternally inherited duplication of chromosome 15q11–13 (Veenstra-Vanderweele & Cook, 2003). This specific abnormality is thought to account for 1% to 3% of cases of PDD. However, several other regions, including chromosomes 1q, 2q, 5q, 6q, 7q, and others, have also been highlighted in relation to PDD (Persico & Bourgeron, 2006). It is important to note that less than 10% of cases of PDD are the result of a known genetic disorder (Persico & Bourgeron, 2006). Therefore, further research into both genetics and other potential etiological factors is necessary.

While the evidence for genetic contributions to the etiology of autism is significant, abnormalities in this area clearly do not account for all cases of PDD. Therefore, other factors must be involved. Prenatal and neonatal biological and environmental factors have also been implicated in the development of PDD in some individuals. Specifically, exposure to several viral agents, including rubella and cytomegalovirus during the prenatal and perinatal periods, have been implicated in the development of PDD (Chess, Fernandez, & Korn, 1979; Sweeten, Posey, & McDougle, 2004). In addition, prenatal exposure to thalidomide and valproic acid have also been reported to result in PDD in some individuals (Christianson, Chesler, & Kromberg, 1994; Stromland, Nordin, Miller, & Akerstrom, 1994).

Developmental Trajectory of Pervasive Developmental Disorders

While autism was initially described by Kanner in 1943 as a childhood disorder, hence the name "infantile autism," researchers have demonstrated through follow-up and outcome studies that PDD are lifelong disorders. Most children with autism continue to meet criteria for a diagnosis in adolescence (McGovern & Sigman, 2005). A diagnosis of PDD is not "outgrown." However, individuals who fail to meet criteria for PDD in adolescence are usually those who were diagnosed with less severe disorders such as PDD-NOS or Asperger disorder in childhood.

Several factors have been associated with a more favorable outcome for adolescents and adults with PDD. As was previously mentioned, a childhood diagnosis of PDD-NOS or Asperger disorder has been associated with improvement in symptomatology later in life (McGovern & Sigman, 2005). This is most likely due to the fact that these two disorders are marked by less severe symptomatology than autistic disorder. Higher childhood cognitive functioning and the presence of some communicative language before age 6 years are also associated with improved outcome (Billstedt, Gillberg, & Gillberg, 2005). In addition, improvement in language skills in adolescence is predicted by functional play skills, response to joint attention attempts of others, and frequency of requesting behavior in early childhood (McGovern & Sigman, 2005). An important factor implicated in positive outcomes for individuals with PDD is early and ongoing intervention. Past researchers have shown that intervention beginning prior to age 5 years is a predictor of positive outcomes later in development (Fenske, Zalenski, Krantz, & McClannahan, 1985). As will be discussed in this chapter, effective behavioral and pharmacological treatments have been empirically derived to address many of the core and associated features of PDD. The implementation of these intervention strategies has been shown to improve many of the symptoms of PDD and the quality of life of these individuals.

For some individuals with PDD, however, the outcome in adolescence and adulthood can be less positive. In Billstedt et al.'s (2005) follow-up study of children with autistic disorder, 78% of the participants were classified as having a poor outcome (i.e., obvious severe handicap, no independent social progress, some clear verbal or nonverbal communication skills). Cognitive functioning has been shown to remain stable or decline through adolescence (McGovern & Sigman, 2005). Communication skills may improve somewhat with age, but the majority of adolescents and adults with PDD continue to display communication deficits (Seltzer, Shattuck, Abbeduto, & Greenberg, 2004). Socialization may also improve slightly, but to a lesser extent than communication (Seltzer et al., 2004). It is important to note that few studies have addressed the developmental trajectory of PDD through adolescence and adulthood. As a result, clear conclusions cannot be drawn at this time. More research identifying the factors that predict positive and negative outcomes for individuals with PDD is needed.

Intervention

The primary focus of treatment for individuals with PDD is the development, maintenance, and generalization of new skills. The core deficits of PDD persist across the life span and therefore interventions must be implemented to address these areas. The treatment of young adults with PDD should focus on three areas. The first area is the adaptations that should be made to the individual's environment in order to promote optimal success in academic, social, and adaptive functioning. The second area interventions must address is the teaching of new skills in the areas of social, communication, and adaptive functioning. Finally, interventions for adolescents with PDD may also require the use of behavioral reduction techniques such as applied behavior analysis (ABA) and/or pharmacotherapy to address behavior problems, such as aggression, self-injury, stereotypies, and other disruptive behaviors.

Environmental Adaptations

Adapting the environment so that an individual with PDD can learn and function optimally is often the first step to designing a treatment and maintaining treatment gains. Individuals with PDD often do not learn or process information in the same manner as typically developing individuals and may benefit from their environment being arranged to suit their own particular learning style. Researchers have demonstrated that children with PDD may not be able to learn effectively using social observation, imitation, and verbal instructions (Tsatsanis, 2004). These children do, however, exhibit facility at rote memorization, learn in gradual progressions, and are strong visual learners (e.g., O'Riordan, Plaisted, Driver, & Baron-Cohen, 2001; Williams, Goldstein, Carpenter, & Minshew, 2005). Therefore, these learning style differences must be addressed in order to effectively promote skill acquisition. Some common environmental adaptations include the use of visual strategies, adaptation of physical structure, and modification to work and curriculum.

Visual Strategies

Visual information has been shown to help individuals with PDD derive organization and provide a sense of structure, stability, and consistency in the environment (Janney & Snell, 2004a). The use of visual supports allows the individual to be less dependent on prompts and assistance from others (Schopler, Mesibov, & Hearsey, 1995). This point is especially important as prompt dependence is a common problem for children and adolescents with PDD (Odom & Watts, 1991). Visual strategies revolve around the use of pictures or written symbols intended to represent a specific activity or task. These picture symbols are arranged in the order that activities or tasks are to be performed. The use of visual representations of activities allows the individual with PDD to understand the order of events, which activities have been completed, as well as which activities are next. Visual strategies such as these can be used to cue a single response (e.g., ask for a break), organize an individual's entire day (e.g., activities from breakfast to bedtime), and can be used in combination with a task analysis to deconstruct a task (such as completing a chore) into its components (Kazdin, 2001). In addition, visual strategies can be used in combination with a reinforcement schedule or token economy as a visual representation of one's progress toward receiving reinforcement. Used effectively, visual supports have been shown by researchers to increase independence and motivation in children and young adults with PDD (Dettmer, Simpson, Myles, & Ganz, 2000).

Physical Supports

In addition to the use of visual strategies, arranging the physical environment has been shown to help individuals with PDD to perform more successfully (Heflin & Alberto, 2001). Physical supports can include the organization of activities, leisure items, and work tasks into separate bins or compartments that are each clearly labeled. Such supports can also include the arrangement of the physical environment in a manner that reduces distractions and provides order and clear physical boundaries for activities. For example, a specific area of a classroom could be designated for a particular task, such as leisure or group work. The segmentation of the physical environment can be accomplished through the use of items such as tape, carpet squares, or the use of actual pieces of furniture. This clear demarcation enables the individual to navigate his or her environment more comfortably and independently through an enhanced sense of organization and structure.

Curriculum and Work Adaptations

With the movement toward including children with PDD and other developmental disabilities into regular education classrooms and other inclusive environments, more attention has been paid to the modifications necessary to promote success for these students. Adaptations must therefore be made not only to the classroom environment but also to the work presented and the manner in which it is presented. Janney and Snell (2004a) recommend that modifications be made on an individual basis and that these modifications may include changes to curriculum goals, teaching materials, testing conditions, and teaching methods. Examples of these adaptations may include dividing assignments into discrete activities, providing the individual with all of the materials necessary to complete each task, providing models or examples, and using visual or picture cues in addition to oral instructions (Janney & Snell, 2004b). In addition to adaptations to curriculum or work tasks, visual supports (e.g., pictures, schedule) should also be used to provide the individual with all of the information needed to complete tasks (Schopler et al., 1995).

Social Skills Training

The social deficits seen in PDD were initially considered secondary to the cognitive deficits associated with these disorders (Rutter, 1978). Current thinking, in contrast, is that the social deficits are a characteristic and primary feature of PDD that requires instruction (Barry et al., 2003; Wolery & Garfinkle, 2002). Some areas of deficit are typically apparent as early as infancy. For example, parents report delayed social smiling (Chawarska et al., 2007) and other researchers have found differences in facial recognition (Chawarska & Volkmar, 2007) as compared to typically developing peers. Although early differences exist, the gap with same-age peers tends to widen in the adolescent years (Shea & Mesibov, 2005). Some of the social skills deficits that emerge in adolescence include difficulty in taking another person's perspective, understanding the emotions of others, and initiating and maintaining conversations (Rubin & Lennon, 2004).

An area that has received increased attention recently is the role of socialization difficulties in individuals with high functioning autism (HFA) and Asperger disorder. These individuals are characterized by typical language development and lack of significant cognitive delay. However, for individuals with HFA and Asperger disorder social skills can be greatly impaired despite adequate cognitive functioning and less severe symptomotology (Klin, Saulnier, Tsatsanis, & Volkmar, 2005). This point is further demonstrated by findings indicating that individuals with Asperger disorder and HFA are equally impaired in communication and social skills as individuals with autism (Saulnier & Klin, 2007). These findings and others illustrate that the severity of autistic symptomotology is not directly related to the presence of appropriate adaptive skills (Klin, Saulnier, Sparrow, Cicchetti, & Volkmar, 2007; Saulnier & Klin, 2007). Therefore, it is recommended that diagnosis (e.g., HFA, autism, Asperger disorder) be considered separate from an individual's communication and social skills (Saulnier & Klin, 2007).

Researchers have shown that having social deficits can lead individuals with PDD to feel ostracized or excluded (Barry et al., 2003). Further, these feelings of social isolation can lead to secondary feelings of depression and anxiety (APA, 2000). For these reasons, social skills training is a key component to any training program for young adults with PDD. Despite the importance of training individuals with PDD in social skills, many educational programs fail to include a social training component (White, Scahill, Klin, Koenig & Volkmar, 2007).

Some common areas of focus when teaching social skills include conversation skills and emotional understanding. Even individuals with strong verbal language skills often have difficulty with conversation skills (Barry et al., 2003).

Problems in emotion recognition range from difficulties in recognizing emotions (Bauminger, 2004; Heerey, Keltner, & Capps, 2003) to an inability to understand the thoughts and feelings of other people. (Bellini & Hopf, 2007; Parsons & Mitchell, 2002). Another broad area of difficulty for individuals with PDD is having an understanding of social cues and expectations (APA, 2000). Within this domain exists a range of skills central to most interactions in society, including taking turns, waiting in lines, and properly using eye contact (Wagner, 2002). As a result of the myriad social difficulties seen, individuals with PDD often have difficulty making friends and forming peer relationships (Barry et al., 2003).

When deciding how to teach social skills, a variety of training methods are available, including didactic instructions and the use of peer models. In general, didactic methods are led by the instructor and peer modeling is led by a typically developing peer. Another commonly used skill building procedure, incidental teaching, will be reviewed later in the discussion of functional communication skills.

If the goal is to teach skills related to appropriate behavior in common social situations, an instructor using didactic strategies may use role playing, virtual response training (VRT), social stories, or computer-based teaching, among other options. In role playing and modeling, the individual practices the difficult situation in pretend scenarios and specifically focuses on rehearsing appropriate responses. The modeling portion of the strategy involves having someone demonstrate the appropriate behavior first, and then the individual with PDD imitates that behavior. Another often-used strategy is video modeling, which has been used by a variety of researchers to teach social skills to individuals with PDD (see review by Ayers & Langone, 2005). In VRT, the role playing situation is carried out through virtual reality computer technology (Parsons & Mitchell, 2002). This technology allows the individual to rehearse the same situation repeatedly until he or she masters the scenario. VRT also permits slight variations of the situation to be practiced to help the individual learn how to generalize the skills learned. In addition, many different scenarios can be taught and rehearsed using VRT.

Social stories (i.e., written explanations of expected behavior in difficult situations) have also been used to teach social skills (Barry & Burlew, 2004; Delano & Snell, 2006; Sansosti & Powell-Smith, 2006). Social stories are written in first-person language and can be presented either to prepare an individual for a new situation (e.g., the first day of school) or to provide additional support for a commonly experienced and often difficult situation (e.g., waiting in line, responding to fire alarms).

Although many social skills lessons are focused on teaching skills related to specific social situations, lessons may also focus on emotional understanding or functional conversation skills. Emotions are taught through various strategies, including computer training (LaCava, Golan, Baron-Cohen, & Miles, 2007), live and video modeling (Gena, Couloura, & Kymissis, 2005), and by discussing emotions and providing information about them (Bauminger, 2002). Teaching conversational skills or appropriate verbal responses can often be done successfully through strategies such as scripts and visual prompts (Weiss & Harris, 2001). In these strategies, information is written down and presented to the individual with PDD to serve as a visual cue during the actual situation.

Peer models are often used in combination with the strategies stated above, or in separate situations, to help teach social skills to individuals with PDD. Although peers are used to teach social skills (Odom et al., 2003), simply putting individuals with PDD and typically developing peers in the same room does not constitute peer modeling. It is important to take time to train the peers, thus increasing their interactions with the children with PDD (Kamps et al., 2002) and making them more likely to impact the learning of the children with PDD.

There are a variety of skills to address and strategies available to teach social skills to individuals with PDD. Given the primacy of the social skills deficits in PDD, it is important to include some social skills training when working with individuals with PDD. Furthermore, no discussion of social skills would be complete without highlighting the importance of teaching and planning for generalization. It is important to teach generalization with any new skill because many people with PDD have difficulty generalizing skills from one situation to another (Weiss & Harris, 2001). When considering social skills, however, it can become even harder to learn to generalize because social expectations change according to the situation, as well as over the life span (Weiss & Harris, 2001). Because social expectations are so complex, it is especially important to highlight those skills that can be generalized.

Communication Skills

In addition to social skills impairments, the other core symptom of PDD that often serves as a primary focus of treatment is functional communication. Some of the communication deficits observed in young adults with PDD include asking inappropriate questions, nonliteral or abstract language use, and initiating and maintaining conversations (Landa, 2000; Marans, Rubin, & Laurent, 2005). These communication difficulties become more pronounced as the individual with PDD increases his or her interactions with peers and the community.

Communication difficulties are believed by many researchers and clinicians to be a causal factor in the development of behavior problems in individuals with PDD. Even those individuals with PDD who have adequate language often have difficulties in functionally communicating their basic wants and needs. Often such difficulties lead individuals to engage in maladaptive behaviors (Carr & Durand, 1985). Using this theoretical framework, a method of increasing communication skills, called functional communication training, is widely used in PDD. Functional communication training is based on teaching specific, discrete communication responses that serve the same function or purpose as the problem behavior. Functional communication utilizes a variety of different strategies for training the communicative responses. This can include the use of verbal expressive language, sign language, and picture exchange (Bondy & Frost, 1994a). Through the use of repetition and reinforcement, the individual with PDD is taught that engaging in a communication exchange with another person can result in positive events.

Several different methods have been developed for training functional communication skills to individuals with PDD. Three of the methods that are commonly used are verbal behavior, naturalistic training, and picture exchange. Verbal behavior is based on applied behavior analysis (ABA) principles and the early work of B. F. Skinner (1957). Skinner defined verbal behavior as behavior that is reinforced by another person's behavior (Skinner, 1957). With this method, language is functional and results in the individual being reinforced by the tangible item that he or she desires. In verbal behavior, responses are taught using discrete trial training whereby the individual is presented with items in a controlled setting and prompted to name the item. Upon emitting the appropriate verbal response, the individual is then reinforced through access to that item (Sundberg & Michael, 2001). Verbal behavior as a communication training approach is often criticized because language is taught in a contrived setting and therefore generalization to other settings is often difficult (Prizant & Wetherby, 2005).

In response to the criticisms of verbal behavior, more clinicians and researchers have begun to endorse more naturalistic forms of communication training. One such method is incidental teaching (Hart & Risley, 1975). Incidental teaching concentrates on teaching language in the natural environment at times when the individual is motivated to communicate (Charlop-Christy & Carpenter, 2000). Therefore, words taught are based on the items or activities that the individual is motivated to request in that specific teaching moment and the consequence for communication is access to that item or activity.

One naturalistic communication training technique that has become increasingly popular in PDD is the picture exchange communication system (PECS; Bondy & Frost, 1994a, 1994b). PECS was developed as a method for increasing communication in nonverbal children with PDD while capitalizing on the strong visual processing skills of this population (O'Riordan et al., 2001). A strength of PECS in this population is that it does not require any prerequisite language, attention, or imitation skills (Bondy & Frost, 1994a, 1994b).

With PECS, an individual with PDD is taught through behavioral strategies that handing the picture of a desired item to another individual results in receiving that desired item. Therefore, the function of communication is reinforced by the child receiving a discrete, salient reinforcer for engaging in a communicative response. Once an individual has been taught to seek out a communication partner and request a number of different items or activities, PECS training expands to include picture discrimination and constructing complete sentences (Frost & Bondy, 2002).

Researchers have noted the widespread use of PECS in classrooms and homes and have begun to empirically evaluate its efficacy. Two randomized clinical trials of PECS have recently been conducted. Howlin et al. (2007) reported that PECS training resulted in increased child communication attempts and use of picture symbols in a classroom setting. However, no increases in other areas of communication (i.e., verbal language, scores on language tests) were noted. In another randomized clinical trial, Yoder and Stone (2006) found that PECS training increased the number of requests made by nonverbal children with PDD, although improvements did not generalize to other areas of communication.

Reduction in Behavior Problems

In addition to the emphasis placed on the development of new skills, many young adults with PDD require additional intervention designed to address behavior problems, such as physical and verbal aggression, self-injury, impulsivity, and hyperactivity. Some behavior problems that are more commonly associated with adolescents and adults with PDD include inappropriate sexual behavior, compulsions, and temper outbursts (Shea & Mesibov, 2005). In addition, while some behavior problems, such as aggression and property destruction, may occur at the same frequency in adolescence as in childhood, the severity of these maladaptive behaviors increases as these individuals grow taller, heavier, and stronger (Shea & Mesibov, 2005). The two primary methods of intervening in these problem behaviors are behavioral (applied behavior analysis) and pharmacological.

Applied Behavior Analysis

Applied behavior analysis (ABA) is based on the operant conditioning work of B. F. Skinner (1938). The primary goals of ABA are to identify target problem behaviors, assess the environmental factors influencing the problem behaviors, and to design treatments that address these factors and reduce aberrant behaviors while increasing adaptive behaviors. At its core, ABA focuses on the antecedents (i.e., the environmental factors that precipitate the occurrence of a problem behavior) and consequences (i.e., the responses of others in the environment to the behavior) surrounding a specific problem behavior. The process of determining these variables is called a functional assessment (Kazdin, 2001).

Based upon the pattern of antecedents and consequences determined through the use of a functional assessment, a behavior is said to serve a specific function for the individual. The "function" of a behavior is the purpose it serves for the individual or what the individual is gaining by engaging in the behavior (Iwata, Dorsey, Slifer, Bauman, & Richman, 1982). Several functions of problem behavior have been well documented by researchers. These functions are based on the consequence surrounding a problem behavior and are presumed to be the individual's motivation for engaging in the problem behavior. The first function of behavior problems is attention from others. Many individuals gain social attention in the form of verbal language or physical contact from others after engaging in the target behavior. The second function of problem behaviors, "tangible," is said to occur when the individual engages in the behavior in order to gain access to a preferred item (e.g., food, toys, activities). The "escape" function is the label provided when an activity or event is terminated after the individual engages in the problem behavior. Finally, a "sensory" function is said to be occurring when the problem behavior itself elicits a pleasurable sensory experience or reduces the discomfort brought about by physical pain.

The function of a behavior problem is determined based on the results of several forms of behavioral assessment. These assessments can be direct in nature, such as the use of an experimental functional analysis (EFA). An EFA is usually conducted in a controlled, contrived environment where an individual is placed in several different situations designed to potentially illicit problem behaviors in each of the function areas (Iwata et al., 1982). The condition (i.e., attention, tangible, escape, sensory) in which the individual engages in the highest rate of problem behaviors is then said to be the primary function of the problem behavior for him or her. Another direct assessment of the function of problem behaviors is naturalistic observation. During a naturalistic functional assessment, the individual is observed in his or her natural environment. The observer records the antecedents and consequences for each instance of problem behavior and then inspects this data for patterns which may indicate the function of the problem behavior for that individual. In addition to the direct forms of functional assessment, indirect forms such as interviews (O'Neill et al., 1997) and checklists (Matson & Vollmer, 1995) are also commonly used.

Once the function of a problem behavior has been determined, behavioral interventions targeting those functions are designed and implemented. As previously discussed, interventions consisting of antecedent manipulations, such as the use of visual or physical supports, as well as skills acquisition strategies such as communication and social skills training, are often among the first interventions utilized for individuals with PDD. However, many behavior problems are of sufficient frequency or intensity that additional behavior reduction techniques must also be implemented. Positive reinforcement of appropriate adaptive behaviors is often used as a method of promoting appropriate behaviors. In addition, extinction (i.e., removing the reinforcement previously received as a consequence for the target behavior) is often used as a method for decreasing the reinforcement previously received for inappropriate behaviors (e.g., Richman, Wacker, Asmus, & Casey, 1998).

In addition to the use of positive reinforcement procedures, punishment techniques are also often necessary, especially for dangerous behaviors. ABA researchers have demonstrated that many punishment techniques are effective in reducing problem behaviors in children and young adults with PDD. For example, time-out from positive reinforcement has been used to decrease attention-maintained problem behaviors in adolescents with PDD and other developmental disabilities. Another commonly used procedure is overcorrection. In overcorrection, the consequence for engaging in problem behavior is the repeated practice of an appropriate replacement behavior (Kazdin, 2001).

Pharmacological Treatments

Research into the pharmacotherapy of PDD in children and adolescents has been increasing significantly over the past several years. This increase has lead to the understanding of the effects of several different classes of drugs on the symptoms of PDD. The classes of medications most commonly studied and prescribed in PDD are conventional antipsychotics, atypical antipsychotics, psychostimulants, and serotonin-reuptake inhibitors. A brief review of the research on each of these medication classes is provided.

Conventional Antipsychotics. Conventional antipsychotics were the class of drugs that received the most initial research in PDD (Posey & McDougle, 2000). Within the population of individuals with developmental disabilities, conventional antipsychotics have frequently been prescribed to address severe aggression (Aman & Singh, 1998). Haloperidol, a D-2 dopamine antagonist, has been highly studied in PDD. One of the first studies of haloperidol's effects in PDD was conducted by Campbell et al. in 1978. These researchers reported reductions in stereotypies and withdrawal in a sample of 40 children. In a later study, the same research group reported that the optimal dose of haloperidol was 1.11 mg daily and that this dosage resulted in improvements in stereotypies, hyperactivity, fidgetiness, and affect (Anderson et al., 1984). In addition, improvements in performance on discrimination learning tasks were also seen.

The safety of haloperidol has come into question due to a number of adverse side effects. Dose-dependent sedation was reported by Campbell, Anderson, & Meier (1978) and acute dystonic reactions by Anderson et al. (1984). Furthermore, Campbell et al. (1997) reported that 33.9% of a sample of 40 children developed withdrawal dyskinesias after haloperidol discontinuation. In a subgroup of 10 children who received higher doses of haloperidol, nine developed dyskinesias (Campbell et al., 1997). Based on the potential for severe and at times irreversible side effects from conventional antipsychotics, the use of these medications is now frequently reserved for individuals with PDD who exhibit severe, treatment-refractory symptomatology (Posey & McDougle, 2000).

Atypical Antipsychotics. Due to the adverse side effects often reported with conventional antipsychotics, attention has shifted toward the use of atypical antipsychotics in this population. Atypical antipsychotics, such as risperidone, are frequently utilized to manage severe behavior problems (i.e., aggression, self-injury) in individuals with PDD (McDougle et al., 2005). Results from a large-scale (n = 101) double-blind, placebo-controlled study of risperidone were reported by the Research Units on Pediatric Psychopharmacology Autism Network (RUPP) in 2002. During this 8-week trial with children and adolescents with autistic disorder, a 57% reduction was observed in irritability measures, and treatment response occurred in 69.4% of participants. Currently, risperidone is the only medication approved by the U.S. Food and Drug Administration (2006) for use in serious behavioral problems such as aggression, self-injury, and severe tantrumming in individuals with autistic disorder between the ages of 5 and 16 years. However, risperidone has not been approved to treat the core symptoms of PDD. Open-label studies of many of the other available atypical antipsychotics have been published. The most commonly reported side effects of atypical antipsychotics include weight gain, sedation, and hyperprolactinemia (Stigler et al., 2004).

Psychostimulants. Hyperactivity and inattention are two symptoms that are commonly reported in individuals with developmental disabilities (Expert Consensus Guideline Series, 2000), as well as in higher functioning individuals with PDD (Gilchrist et al., 2001). As a result, psychostimulant medications have been used in this population to address symptoms of hyperactivity, restlessness, impulsivity, and overactivity (Aman, Collier-Crespin, & Lindsay, 2000). While initial researchers studying psychostimulant use in individuals with PDD reported adverse side effects and lack of efficacy (Aman, 1982), more recent studies have been conducted. The RUPP Autism Network (2005) administered low, medium, or high doses of methylphenidate in a double-blind, crossover design to children with PDD and hyperactivity. The researchers reported that all three dose levels resulted in a significant positive effect when compared to placebo. Fifty percent of the children studied demonstrated a positive response to the methylphenidate. However, this result is significantly lower than that which is observed in 75% of typically developing children (Scahill & Pachler, 2007).

Posey et al. (2007) followed up the RUPP Autism Network (2005) study with an evaluation of secondary outcome measures in response to methylphenidate in children with PDD. They reported that hyperactivity and impulsivity improved significantly more than inattention, and that there were no significant effects on oppositionality or stereotyped and repetitive behavior.

The side effects of psychostimulant medications have been shown to occur more commonly in children with PDD than in typically developing children. Stigler et al. (2004) reported agitation, irritability, weight loss, and dysphoria as the most common side effects to stimulant medications in children with PDD. Other side effects observed include a higher rate of social withdrawal, tics, and stereotypies (Scahill & Martin, 2005).

Serotonin-Reuptake Inhibitors. The role of serotonin in autistic disorder and PDD has been evaluated in several studies. Researchers have found elevated whole-blood serotonin levels in individuals with autistic disorder compared to controls (McDougle et al., 2005). These observations, along with the widespread and successful use of serotonin-reuptake inhibitors (SRIs) as treatment for obsessive-compulsive disorder have led to serotonin being the most highly studied neurotransmitter in the field of PDD research (Anderson & Hoshino, 2005). Selective serotonin-reuptake inhibitors (SSRIs) have become widely used as a treatment for PDD. Importantly, however, to date only two double-blind, placebo-controlled studies have found SSRIs to be efficacious in the treatment of PDD. Fluvoxamine was investigated by McDougle et al. (1996) in a double-blind, placebo-controlled study of adults with autistic disorder and was found to improve repetitive thoughts and behaviors, and the repetitive use of language. McDougle, Kresch, & Posey (2000) described results from a study on the effects of fluvoxamine in children and adolescents with PDD that found that only 1 of 18 subjects responded positively to the drug.

Fluoxetine was investigated by Hollander et al. (2005) in children and adolescents with PDD. These researchers reported that participants treated with fluoxetine experienced a significant decrease in repetitive behaviors compared to placebo. In addition, no significant differences in side effects were reported between the drug and placebo groups. While the lack of side effects reported from this study is encouraging, case reports have included negative side effects, including extrapyramidal symptoms (Sokolski et al., 2004), hyperactivity (DeLong, Teague, & McSwain-Kamran, 1998), and aggressive behavior (DeLong et al., 1998), particularly in children and adolescents.

Transition from School to Community-Based Services

When discussing PDD in young adults, a primary concern is the transition from school-based to community-based services. This transition requires collaboration between the individual with PDD, the family, the school, and the agency responsible for service provision. According to the Individuals with Disabilities Education Improvement Act (IDEIA, 2004), when students with PDD graduate from school or turn 22 years of age, they move from an entitlement to a nonentitlement system. While in school, students receive services and supports mandated by state and federal law. As adults, these services are no longer guaranteed. Consequently, it is imperative that students, families, and schools understand the adult service system years before services will be needed (CCLC, 2006a). Transition planning, when effective, implemented gradually, and inclusive of students' skills and interests, can have a positive impact on outcomes for individuals with PDD transitioning to community-based services in the areas of independence, employment, and education.

Transition service is legally defined as a coordinated set of activities for a student with a disability designed to promote movement from school to postschool activities, including postsecondary education, vocational training, integrated employment (including supported employment), continuing and adult education, adult services, independent living, or community participation. The selection of these activities is based on the student's preferences, strengths, interests, and needs (CCLC, 2006b). Models that build upon the student's strengths have been shown to increase his or her self-esteem and hopefulness, which in turn leads to better outcomes in adulthood (Jonikas, Laris, & Cook, 2003; King, Baldwin, Currie, & Evans, 2005).

Beginning at age 16, a statement of transition services must be included in a student's individualized education plan (IEP). At this point, the IEP team must discuss and document the student's postschool goals in the areas of employment, independent living, recreation and leisure, community participation, and postsecondary education. Additionally, the IEP must include a general plan for achieving the goals such as relevant coursework or community experiences, as well as identify community-based service providers who will be responsible once the child exits the school system (CCLC, 2006b).

Several factors have been identified that mark successful transitions to adulthood for people with PDD: employment, independent living, economic self-sufficiency, postsecondary education, adult role taking, and social participation (Clegg, Sheard, & Cahill, 2001). Clegg et al. (2001) found that most individuals settled into their new services after 1 to 3 months. However, all smooth transitions involved a gradual introduction to the new services and providers; those who had more challenging transitions were those for whom the transition was abrupt.

Jonikas, Laris, and Cook (2003) found that a higher proportion of individuals with PDD were unemployed, and a much lower proportion attended postsecondary school or training. Individuals with Asperger disorder have demonstrated less positive employment experiences and show more preference for solitary activities in adulthood (Jennes-Coussens, Magill-Evans, & Koning, 2006; Renty & Roeyers, 2006). These individuals also tend to report lower social and physical quality of life compared to those without Asperger disorder or another disability (Jennes-Coussens, Magill-Evans, & Koning, 2006). Socially, individuals with Asperger disorder and high-functioning autism continue to have marked impairment (Jennes-Coussens et al., 2006). They also are less likely to marry and tend to have only social relationships with others based on special interests, as opposed to shared enjoyment.

Employment experiences may be particularly important for individuals with PDD because those experiences can provide a new outlet for demonstrating skills and competencies and for forming social networks. The likelihood of employment is influenced by the functional limitations of the person's disability, social skills, previous employment experience, and increasing age (Cameto, 2003). Individuals that received supported employment services were more likely to find work, have higher job levels, be in work for a greater percentage of the time, and receive higher wages (Mawhood, & Howlin, 1999).

Successful transition planning is thought to lead to better outcomes, including self-determination, higher rates of employment, higher success in postsecondary education, less poverty, greater happiness, and greater participation in the community. As a whole, transition plans that support informed choices by the student lead to more feelings of empowerment. The transition process is successful to the degree that the student is engaged in or able to adopt his or her desired adult role (King, Baldwin, Currie, & Evans, 2005). Transition planning, when done correctly, is gradual so that strong bonds made with the school staff can be unraveled and new bonds with adult service providers can be established at a pace that allows both parents and student to adjust (Clegg et al., 2001).

Conclusion

Our understanding of the presentation of PDD in young adults is still being developed. PDD is a category of lifelong disorders that affect an individual to varying degrees throughout his or her lifetime. This chapter provided an overview of the major areas of research in the field, although considerably more detail could be provided on any of these topics. The number of young children diagnosed with PDD has steadily increased; thus, it is reasonable to expect that over the next several decades, the number of adolescents and adults seeking treatment for PDD will also increase. More research is necessary to uncover the etiological factors that contribute to the symptom profiles. Clinicians and researchers who work with young adults with PDD must also be aware of the specific lifelong challenges faced by these individuals and their caregivers in the areas of adapting the environment, developing new skills, treating maladaptive and excessive behaviors, and transitioning into adulthood.

KEY POINTS

- Symptoms of PDD persist across the life span, although the degree of impairment may vary with age.
- Successful transition to adulthood for young adults with PDD requires that planning and training in the areas of employment, independent living, economic self-sufficiency, social skills, etc., begin at a young age.
- Behavior problems (e.g., aggression, self-injury, property destruction) are a significant issue for individuals with PDD that requires behavioral and/or pharmacological intervention.

> **PRACTICE GUIDELINES**
>
> - Social and communication deficits exist in individuals with PDD regardless of cognitive functioning; therefore, training in these areas is necessary.
> - Transition into adulthood should begin at an early age and families should be encouraged to begin thinking about these issues prior to and during adolescence.
> - Interventions should consist of antecedent manipulations, reduction of behavior problems, and teaching appropriate behavior (e.g., social skills training).

References

Adams, C., Green, J., Gilchrist, A., & Cox, A. (2002). Conversational behaviour of children with Asperger syndrome and conduct disorder. *Journal of Child Psychology and Psychiatry, 43,* 679–690.

Aman, M. G. (1982). Stimulant drug effects in developmental disorders and hyperactivity: Toward a resolution of disparate findings. *Journal of Autism and Developmental Disorders, 12,* 385–398.

Aman, M. G., Collier-Crespin, A., & Lindsay, R. L. (2000). Pharmacotherapy of disorders in mental retardation. *European Child and Adolescent Psychiatry, 9,* 98–107.

Aman, M. G., & Singh, N. N. (1988). Patterns of drug use, methodological considerations, measurement techniques, and future trends. In M. G. Aman & N. N. Singh (Eds.), *Psychopharmacology and the developmental disabilities* (pp. 1–28). New York: Springer.

American Psychiatric Association. (2000). *Diagnostic and statistical manual of mental disorders* (4th ed., Text revision), Washington, DC: Author.

Anderson, G. M., & Hoshino, Y. (2005). Neurochemical studies of autism. In F. R. Volkmar, R. Paul, A. Klin, & D. Cohen (Eds.), *Handbook of autism and pervasive developmental disorders* (3rd ed., pp. 453–472). Hoboken, NJ: John Wiley & Sons.

Anderson, L. T., Campbell, M., Grega, D. M., Perry, R., Small, A. M., & Green, W. H. (1984). Haloperidol in the treatment of infantile autism: Effects on learning and behavioral symptoms. *American Journal of Psychiatry, 141,* 1195–1202.

Ayers, K. M., & Langone, J. (2005). Intervention and instruction with video for students with autism: A review of the literature. *Education and Training in Developmental Disabilities, 40,* 183–196.

Barry, L. M., & Burlew, S. B. (2004). Using social stories to teach choice and play skills to children with autism. *Focus on Autism and Other Developmental Disabilities, 19,* 45–51.

Barry, T. D., Klinger, L. G., Lee, J. M., Palardy, N., Gilmore, T., & Bodin, S. D. (2003). Examining the effectiveness of an outpatient clinic-based social skills group for high-functioning children with autism. *Journal of Autism and Developmental Disorders, 33,* 685–701.

Bauminger, N. (2002). The facilitation of social-emotional understanding and social interaction in high functioning children with autism: Intervention outcomes. *Journal of Autism and Developmental Disorders, 32,* 283–298.

Bauminger, N. (2004). The expression and understanding of jealousy in children with autism. *Development and Psychopathology, 16,* 157–177.

Bellini, S., & Hopf, A. (2007). The development of the autism social skills profile: A preliminary analysis of psychometric properties. *Focus on Autism and Other Development Disabilities, 22,* 80–81.

Billstedt, E., Gillberg, C., & Gillberg, C. (2005). Autism after adolescence: Population-based 13- to 22-year follow-up study of 120 individuals with autism diagnosed in childhood. *Journal of Autism and Developmental Disorders, 35,* 351–360.

Bondy A. S., & Frost, L. A. (1994a). The picture exchange communication system. *Seminars in Speech and Language, 19,* 373–389.

Bondy A. S., & Frost, L. A. (1994b). The Delaware Autistic Program. In S. L. Harris & J. S. Handleman (Eds.), *Preschool education programs for children with autism* (pp. 37–54). Austin, TX: Pro-ed.

Cameto, R. (2003). Employment of youth with disabilities after high school. In M. Wagner, R. Cameto, & L. Newman (Eds.), *Youth with disabilities: A changing population. A report of findings from the National Longitudinal Transition Study (NLTS2),* (pp. 5.1–5.21). Menlo Park, CA: SRI International.

Campbell, M., Anderson, L., & Meier, M. (1978). A comparison of haloperidol and behavior therapy and their interactions in autistic children. *Journal of the American Academy of Child Psychiatry, 17,* 227–239.

Campbell, M., Armenteros, J. L., Malone, R. P., Adams, P. B., Eisenberg, Z. W., Overall, J. E. (1997). Neuroleptic-related dyskinesias in autistic children: A prospective, longitudinal study. *Journal of the American Academy of Child Psychiatry, 36,* 835–843.

Carr, E., & Durand, V. M. (1985). Reducing behavior problems through functional communication training. *Journal of Applied Behavior Analysis, 18,* 111–126.

Carter, A. S., Davis, N. O., Klin, A., & Volkmar, F. R. (2005). Social development in autism. In F. R. Volkmar, R. Paul, A. Klin, & D. Cohen (Eds.), *Handbook of autism and pervasive developmental disorders* (3rd ed., pp. 312–334). Hoboken, NJ: John Wiley & Sons.

Center on Community Living and Careers (CCLC). (2006a). *Implementing transition services for youth with disabilities.* Indianapolis, IN: Indiana Institute on Disability and Community.

Center on Community Living and Careers (CCLC). (2006b). *Transitions from school to adult life: A shared responsibility.* Indianapolis, IN: Indiana Institute on Disability and Community.

Chakrabarti, S., & Fombonne, E. (2001). Pervasive developmental disorders in preschool children. *Journal of the American Medical Association, 285,* 3093–3099.

Charlop-Christy, M. H., & Carpenter, M. H. (2000). Modified incidental teaching sessions: A procedure for parents to increase spontaneous speech in their children with autism. *Journal of Positive Behavior Interventions, 2,* 98–112.

Chawarska, K., Paul, R., Klin, A., Hannigen, S., Dichtel, L. E., & Volkmar, F. (2007). Parental recognition of developmental problems in toddlers with autism spectrum disorders. *Journal of Autism and Developmental Disorders, 37,* 62–72.

Chawarska, K., & Volkmar, F. (2007). Impairments in monkey and human face recognition in 2-year-old toddlers with autism spectrum disorder and developmental delay. *Developmental Science, 10,* 266–279.

Chess, S., Fernandez, P., & Korn, S. (1979). Behavioral consequences of congenital rubella. *Annual Progress in Child Psychiatry and Child Development, 1979,* 467–475.

Christianson, A. L., Chesler, N., & Kromberg, J. G. R. (1994). Fetal valproate syndrome: Clinical and neurodevelopmental features in two sibling pairs. *Developmental Medicine and Child Neurology, 36,* 361–369.

Clegg, J., Sheard, C., & Cahill, J. (2001). Severe intellectual disability and transition to adulthood. *British Journal of Medical Psychology, 74,* 151–166.

Delano, M., & Snell, M.E. (2006). The effects of social stories on the social engagement of children with autism. *Journal of Positive Behavior Interventions, 8,* 29–42.

DeLong, G. R., Teague, L. A., & McSwain-Kamran, M. (1998). Effects of fluoxetine treatment in young children with idiopathic autism. *Developmental Medicine and Child Neurology, 40,* 551–562.

Dettmer, S., Simpson, R. L., Myles, B. S., & Ganz, J. B. (2000). The use of visual supports to facilitate transitions of students with autism. *Focus on Autism and Other Developmental Disabilities, 15,* 163–169.

Edelson, M. G. (2006). Are the majority of children with autism mentally retarded? A systematic evaluation of the data. *Focus on Autism and Other Developmental Disabilities, 21,* 66–83.

Expert Consensus Guideline Series. (2000). Expert Consensus Guideline Series: Treatment of psychiatric and behavioral problems in mental retardation. *American Journal of Mental Retardation, 105,* 159–226.

Fay, W. (1969). On the basis of autistic echolalia. *Journal of Communication Disorders, 2,* 38–47.

Fenske, E., Zalenski, S., Krantz, P., & McClannahan, L. (1985). Age at intervention and treatment outcome for autistic children in a comprehensive intervention program. *Analysis and Intervention in Developmental Disabilities, 5,* 7–31.

Frost, L. A., & Bondy, A. S. (2002). *The Picture Exchange Communication System training manual* (2nd ed.). Newark, NJ: Pyramid Education Products, Inc.

Gena, A., Couloura, S., & Kymisis, E. (2005). Modifying the affective behavior of preschoolers with autism using in-vivo or video modeling and reinforcement contingencies. *Journal of Autism and Developmental Disorders, 35,* 545–556.

Gilchrist, A., Green, J., Cox, A., Burton, D., Rutter, M., & Le Couteur, A. (2001). Development and current functioning in adolescents with Asperger syndrome: A comparative study. *Journal of Child Psychology and Psychiatry, 42,* 227–240.

Hart, B. M., & Risley, T. R. (1975). Incidental teaching of language in the preschool. *Journal of Applied Behavior Analysis, 8,* 411–420.

Heerey, E. A., Keltner, D., & Capps, L. M. (2003). Making sense of self-conscious emotion: Linking theory of mind and emotion in children with autism. *Emotion, 3,* 394–400.

Heflin, L. J., & Alberto, P. A. (2001). Establishing a behavioral context for learning for students with autism. *Focus on Autism and Other Developmental Disabilities, 16,* 93–101.

Hollander, E., Phillips, A., Chaplin, W., Zagursky, K., Novotny, S., Wasserman, S., & Iyengar, R. (2005). A placebo-controlled crossover trial of liquid fluoxetine on repetitive behaviors in childhood and adolescent autism. *Neuropsychopharmacology, 30,* 582–589.

Howlin, P., Gordon, R. K., Pasco, G., Wade, A., & Charman, T. (2007). The effectiveness of Picture Exchange Communication System (PECS) training for teachers of children with autism: A pragmatic group randomized controlled trial. *Journal of Child Psychology and Psychiatry, 48,* 473–481.

Iwata, B. A., Dorsey, M. F., Slifer, K. J., Bauman, K. E., & Richman, G. S. (1982). Toward a functional analysis of self-injury. *Journal of Applied Behavior Analysis, 27,* 197–209.

Janney, R. E., & Snell, M. E. (2004a). *Teachers' guides to inclusive practices: Modifying schoolwork* (2nd ed.). Baltimore: Brookes.

Janney, R. E., & Snell, M. E. (2004b). Modifying schoolwork in inclusive classrooms. *Theory into Practice, 45,* 215–223.

Jennes-Coussens, M., Magill-Evans, J., & Koning, C. (2006). The quality of life of young men with Asperger syndrome. *Autism, 10*(4), 403–414.

Jonikas, J. A., Laris, A., & Cook, J. A. (2003). The passage to adulthood: Psychiatric rehabilitation service and transition-related needs of young adult women with emotional and psychiatric disorders. *Psychiatric Rehabilitation Journal, 27*(2), 114–121.

Kamps, D., Royer, J., Dugan, E. Kravits, T., Gonzalez-Lopez, A., Garcia, J., Carnazzo, K., Morrison, L., & Kane, L. G. (2002). Peer training to facilitate social interaction for elementary students with autism and their peers. *Exceptional Children, 68,* 173–187.

Kanner, L. (1943). Autistic disturbances of affective contact. *Nervous Child, 2,* 217–250.

Kazdin, A. E. (2001). *Behavior modification in applied settings* (6th ed.). Belmont, CA: Wadsworth/Thomson Learning.

King, G. A., Baldwin, P. J., Currie, M., Evans, J. (2005). Planning successful transitions from school to adult roles for youth with disabilities. *Children's Health Care, 34*(3), 195–216.

Klin, A., Saulnier, C. A., Sparrow, S. S., Cicchetti, D. V., & Volkmar, F. R. (2007). Social and communication abilities and disabilities in higher functioning individuals with autism spectrum disorders: The Vineland and the ADOS. *Journal of Autism and Developmental Disorders, 37,* 748–759.

Klin, A., Saulnier, C. A., Tsatsanis, K., & Volkmar, F. R. (2005). Clinical evaluation in autism spectrum disorders: Psychological assessment within a transdisciplinary framework. In F. R. Volkmar, A. Klin, R. Paul, & D. Cohen (Eds.), *Handbook of autism and developmental disorders* (3rd ed., pp. 772–798). New York: Wiley.

LaCava, P. G., Golan, O., Baron-Cohen, S., & Myles, B. S. (2007). Using assistive technology to teach emotion recognition to students with Asperger syndrome. *Remedial and Special Education, 28,* 174–181.

Landa, R. (2000). Social language use in Asperger syndrome and high-functioning autism. In A. Klin, F. R. Volkmar, & S. S. Sparrow (Eds.), *Asperger syndrome* (pp. 125–155). New York: Guilford Press.

Marans, W. D., Rubin, E., & Laurent, A. (2005). Addressing social communication skills in individuals with high-functioning autism and Asperger syndrome: Critical priorities in educational programming. In F. R. Volkmar, R. Paul, A. Klin, & D. Cohen (Eds.), *Handbook of autism and pervasive developmental disorders* (3rd ed., pp. 977–1002). Hoboken, NJ: John Wiley & Sons.

Matson, J. L. & Vollmer, T. (1995). *Questions about behavioral function (QABF).* Baton Rouge, LA: Disability Consultants, LLC.

Mawhood, L., & Howlin, P. (1999). The outcome of a supported employment scheme for high-functioning adults with autism or Asperger syndrome. *Autism, 3*(3), 229–254.

McArthur, D., & Adamson, L. (1996). Joint attention in preverbal children: Autism and developmental language disorder. *Journal of Autism and Developmental Disorder, 26,* 481–496.

McDougle, C. J., Kresch, L. E., & Posey, D. J. (2000). Repetitive thoughts and behavior in pervasive developmental disorders: Treatment with serotonin reuptake inhibitors. *Journal of Autism and Developmental Disorders, 30,* 427–435.

McDougle, C. J., Naylor, S. T., Cohen, D. J., Volkmar, F. R., Heninger, G. R., & Price, L. H. (1996). A double-blind, placebo-controlled study of fluvoxamine in adults with autistic disorder. *Archives of General Psychiatry, 53,* 1001–1008.

McDougle, C. J., Scahill, L., Aman, M. G., McCracken, J. T., Tierney, E., Davies, M., Arnold, L. E., Posey, D. J., Martin, A., Ghuman, J. K., Shah, B., Chuang, S. Z., Swiezy, N. B., Gonzalez, N. M., Hollway, J., Koenig, K., McGough, J. J., Ritz, L., & Vitiello, B. (2005). Risperidone for the core symptom domains of autism: Results from the study by the Autism Network of the Research Units on Pediatric Psychopharmacology. *American Journal of Psychiatry, 162,* 1142–1148.

McGovern, C. W., & Sigman, M. (2005). Continuity and change from early childhood to adolescence in autism. *Journal of Child Psychology and Psychiatry, 46,* 401–408.

Odom, S. L., Brown, W. H., Frey, T., Karasu, N., Smith-Canter, L. L., & Strain, P. S. (2003). Evidence-based practice for young children with autism: Contributions for single-subject design research. *Focus on Autism and Other Developmental Disabilities, 18,* 166–175.

Odom, S. L., & Watts, E. (1991). Reducing teacher prompts in peer-mediated interventions for young children with autism. *The Journal of Special Education, 25,* 26–43.

O'Neill, R. E., Horner, R. H., Albin, R. W., Sprague, J. R., Storey, K., & Newton, J. S. (1997). *Functional assessment and program development for problem behavior.* Pacific Grove, CA: Brooks/Cole Publishing.

O'Riordan, M. A., Plaisted, K. C., Driver, J., & Baron-Cohen, S. (2001). Superior visual search in autism. *Journal of Experimental Psychology: Human Perception and Performance, 27,* 719–730.

Parsons, S., & Mitchell, P. (2002). The potential of virtual reality in social skills training for people with autistic spectrum disorders. *Journal of Intellectual Disability Research, 46,* 430–443.

Perisco, A. M., & Bourgeron, T. (2006). Searching for a way out of the autism maze: Genetic, epigenetic and environmental clues. *Trends in Neuroscience, 29,* 349–358.

Phillips, W., Baron-Cohen, S., & Rutter, M. (1992). The role of eye contact in goal detection: Evidence from normal infants and children with autism or mental handicap. *Development and Psychopathology, 4,* 375–383.

Posey, D. J., Aman, M. G., McCracken, J. T., Scahill, L., Tierney, E., Arnold, L. E., Vitiello, B., Chuang, S. Z., Davies, M., Ramadan, Y., Witwer, A. N., Swiezy, N. B., Cronin, P., Shah, B., Carroll, D. H., Young, C., Wheeler, C., McDougle, C. J. (2007). Positive effects of methylphenidate on inattention and hyperactivity in pervasive developmental disorders: An analysis of secondary measures. *Biological Psychiatry, 61,* 538–544.

Posey, D. J., & McDougle, C. J. (2000). The pharmacotherapy of target symptoms associated with autistic disorder and other pervasive developmental disorders. *Harvard Review of Psychiatry, 8,* 45–63.

Prizant, B. M., & Wetherby, A. M. (2005). Critical issues in enhancing communication abilities for persons with autism spectrum disorders. In F. R. Volkmar, R. Paul, A. Klin, & D. Cohen (Eds.), *Handbook of autism and pervasive developmental disorders* (3rd ed., pp. 925–976). Hoboken, NJ: John Wiley & Sons.

Reddy, K. S. (2005). Cytogenetic abnormalities and fragile X-syndrome in autism spectrum disorders. *BMC Medical Genetics, 6,* 3.

Renty, J., & Roeyers, H. (2006). Quality of life in high-functioning adults with autism spectrum disorder. *Autism, 10*(5), 511–524.

Research Units on Pediatric Psychopharmacology Autism Network. (2002). Risperidone in children with autism and serious behavioral problems. *New England Journal of Medicine, 347,* 314–321.

Research Units on Pediatric Psychopharmacology Autism Network. (2005). A randomized controlled crossover trial of methylphenidate in pervasive developmental disorders with hyperactivity, *Archives of General Psychiatry, 62,* 1266–1274.

Richman, D. M., Wacker, D. P., Asmus, J. M., & Casey, S. D. (1998). Functional analysis and extinction of different behavior problems exhibited by the same individual. *Journal of Applied Behavior Analysis, 31,* 475–478.

Rubin, E., & Lennon, L. (2004). Challenges in social communication in Asperger syndrome and high-functioning autism. *Topics in Language Disorders, 24,* 271–285.

Rutter, M. (1978). Diagnosis and definition of childhood autism. *Journal of Autism and Childhood Schizophrenia, 8,* 139–161.

Sansosti, F. J., & Powell-Smith, K. A. (2006). Using social stories to improve the social behavior of children with Asperger syndrome. *Journal of Positive Behavior Interventions, 8,* 43–57.

Saulnier, C. A., & Klin, A. (2007). Brief report: Social and communication abilities and disabilities in higher functioning individuals with autism and Asperger syndrome. *Journal of Autism and Developmental Disorders, 37,* 788–793.

Scahill, L., & Martin, A. (2005). Psychopharmacology. In F. R. Volkmar, R. Paul, A. Klin, & D. Cohen (Eds.), *Handbook of autism and pervasive developmental disorders* (3rd ed., pp. 1102–1117). Hoboken, NJ: John Wiley & Sons.

Scahill, L., & Pachler, M. (2007). Treatment of hyperactivity in children with pervasive developmental disorders. *Journal of Child and Adolescent Psychiatric Nursing, 20,* 59–62.

Schopler, E., Mesibov, G. B., & Hearsey, K. (1995). Structured teaching in the TEACCH system. In E. Schopler & G. Mesibov (Eds.), *Learning and cognition in autism* (pp. 243–267). New York: Plenum Press.

Seltzer, M. M., Shattuck, P., Abbeduto, L., & Greenberg, J. S. (2004). Trajectory of development in adolescents and adults with autism. *Mental Retardation and Developmental Disabilities Research Reviews, 10,* 234–247.

Shea, V., & Mesibov, G. B. (2005). Adolescents and adults with autism. In F. R. Volkmar, R. Paul, A. Klin, & D. Cohen (Eds.), *Handbook of autism and pervasive developmental disorders* (3rd ed., pp. 288–311). Hoboken, NJ: John Wiley & Sons.

Sheinkopf, S. J., Mundy, P., Oller, D., & Steffens, M. (2000). Vocal atypicalities of preverbal autistic children. *Journal of Autism and Developmental Disorders, 30,* 345–354.

Skinner, B. F. (1938). *The behavior of organisms: An experimental analysis.* Oxford, England: Appleton-Century.

Skinner, B. F. (1957). *Verbal behavior.* Englewood Cliffs, NJ: Prentice Hall.

Sokolski, K., Chicz-Demet, A., Demet, E. M. (2004). Selective serotonin reuptake inhibitor-related extrapyramidal symptoms in autistic children: A case series. *Journal of Child and Adolescent Psychopharmacology, 14,* 143–147.

Stigler, K. A., Desmond, L. A., Posey, D. J., Wiegand, R. E., & McDougle, C. J. (2004). A naturalistic retrospective analysis of psychostimulants in pervasive developmental disorders. *Journal of Child and Adolescent Psychopharmacology, 14,* 49–56.

Stromland, K., Nordin, V., Miller, M., & Akerstrom, B. (1994). Autism in thalidomide embryopathy: A population study. *Developmental Medicine and Child Neurology, 36,* 351–356.

Sundberg, M. L., & Michael, J. (2001). The benefits of Skinner's analysis of verbal behavior for children with autism. *Behavior Modification, 25,* 698–724.

Sweeten, T. L., Posey, D. J., & McDougle, C. J. (2004). Brief report: Autistic disorder in three children with cytomegalovirus infection. *Journal of Autism and Developmental Disorders, 34,* 583–586.

Toth, K., Dawson, G., Meltzoff, A. N., Greenson, J., & Fein, D. (2007). Early social imitation, play, and language abilities of young non-autistic siblings of children with autism. *Journal of Autism and Developmental Disorder, 37,* 145–157.

Tsatsanis, K. D. (2004). Heterogeneity in learning style in Asperger syndrome and high-functioning autism. *Topics in Language Disorders, 24,* 260–270.

U.S. Food and Drug Administration (2006). *New indication for risperidone.* Retrieved March 1, 2007, from http//www.fda.gov/cder/foi/lab

Veenstra-Vanderweele, J., & Cook, E. H. (2003). Genetics of childhood disorders: XLVI. Autism, Part 5: Genetics of autism. *Journal of the American Academy of Child and Adolescent Psychiatry, 42,* 116–118.

Volden, J., & Lord, C. (1991). Neologisms and idiosyncratic language in autistic speakers. *Journal of Autism and Developmental Disorder, 21,* 109–130.

Volkmar, F. R., & Mayes, L. C. (1990). Gaze behavior in autism. *Development and Psychopathology, 2,* 61–69.

Wagner, S. (2002). *Inclusive programming for middle school students with autism/Asperger's syndrome.* Arlington, TX: Future Horizons.

Weiss, M. J., & Harris, S. L. (2001). *Topics in autism: Reaching out, joining in—Teaching social skills to young children with autism.* Bethesda, MD: Woodbine House.

White, S. W., Scahill, L., Klin, A., Koenig, K., & Volkmar, F. R. (2007). Educational placements and service use patterns of individuals with autism spectrum disorders. *Journal of Autism and Developmental Disorders, 37,* 1403–1412.

Williams, D. L., Goldstein, G., Carpenter, P. A., & Minshew, N. J. (2005). Verbal and spatial working memory in autism. *Journal of Autism and Other Developmental Disorders, 35,* 747–756.

Wing, L. (1997). The history of ideas on autism. *Autism, 1,* 13–23.

Wolery, M., & Garfinkle, A. N. (2002). Measures in intervention research with young children who have autism. *Journal of Autism and Developmental Disorders, 32,* 463–478.

Yoder, P. J., & Stone, W. L. (2006). Randomized comparison of two communication interventions for preschoolers with autism spectrum disorders. *Journal of Consulting and Clinical Psychology, 74,* 426–435.

Chapter 26

Personality Disorders

Donald W. Black and Nancee Blum

Douglas was interviewed for a follow-up study of persons with antisocial personality disorder (ASPD). He had a chaotic and abusive childhood. Because his mother was unable to care for him, he was placed in foster care and was later adopted. Douglas had a criminal streak from early childhood. He lied, cheated, and shoplifted; he burglarized a church and, when older, stole an automobile. Because of continued lawbreaking, he was sent to a juvenile reformatory at age 16. At 18 he was diagnosed with ASPD. Douglas was reinterviewed at age 48. He was living in an impoverished area of a small Midwestern town and was using an alias; he appeared ill and gaunt. Douglas admitted to having more than 20 arrests and 5 felony convictions on charges ranging from attempted murder and armed robbery to driving while intoxicated. He had spent more than 17 years in prison. Douglas had never held a full-time job, and he was currently unemployed. He had lived in six different states and in the last 10 years had moved more than 20 times. Nine persons lived in his home, including his four children and common-law wife. He admitted to excessive drinking and several admissions for detoxification. He sometimes attended Alcoholics Anonymous but otherwise did not socialize outside his family. Douglas admitted that he had not yet "settled down;" he still spent money foolishly, was reckless, and had frequent fights.

Personality disorders (PDs) are found in persons at all stages of life, from childhood through senescence. They represent an enduring pattern of inner experience and behavior that "deviates markedly from the expectations of the individual's culture, is pervasive and inflexible, has an onset in adulthood, is stable over time, and leads to distress or impairment" (American Psychiatric Association, 1994, p. 685). As a general rule, PDs are representative of long-term functioning and are not limited to episodes of illness. A personality disorder is not diagnosed, for instance, in a person who develops transient personality changes during an episode of major depression. Nor is PD diagnosed in persons with chronic psychotic disorders. Schizophrenia, for example, is so devastating to the personality that the concept of PD becomes meaningless. In these cases, when the psychotic disorder is preceded by a preexisting PD, the PD is recorded on Axis II followed by the word "premorbid" in parentheses.

Personality disorders are widely considered disorders of adulthood, but they often have their onset in childhood or adolescence or are rooted in childhood symptoms that are precursors to an adult disorder, as evident in Douglas from the case study above. The best example is the child with a conduct disorder who meets criteria for antisocial personality disorder (ASPD) at age 18. Yet, as Paris (2003) points out, the restriction on diagnosing ASPD is a matter of terminology: a 17-year-old boy with a severe conduct disorder is "no less antisocial than he will be when he reaches his eighteenth birthday" (p. 27).

Classification of Personality Disorders

The classification of PDs has evolved over the past 60 years. DSM-I, published in 1952, listed seven different types of personality disturbances, a list expanded to 10 PDs in DSM-II (American Psychiatric Association, 1952, 1968), and 11 PDs in DSM-III (American Psychiatric Association, 1980). The publication of DSM-III was a watershed moment for PDs, because these disorders were accorded new status on a separate axis in the multiaxial diagnostic system that was developed. Several new PDs were created in response to clinical and research observations, including the avoidant, schizotypal, and borderline types. The list of PDs was pared to 10 in DSM-IV, published in 1994 (American Psychiatric Association, 1994) (see Table 26-1). A committee is now developing recommendations on PDs for DSM-V (Widiger, Simonsen, Krueger, Livesley, & Verheul, 2005).

The purpose of creating a separate axis for PDs was to separate them from the major (Axis I) mental disorders, but this decision has led to ongoing criticism and debate among clinicians and researchers (Skodol, 1997). To some, coding PDs on Axis II devalues their importance and contributes to the impression that PDs are lesser disorders that a clinician can choose to ignore in favor of the "major disorder." Yet, for many patients, the preponderant problem is their PD, not the dysthymia, panic disorder, or adjustment disorder comorbid on Axis I. These false debates have the effect of trivializing and stigmatizing attempts to understand and treat PDs. The present classification scheme has been criticized by clinicians and researchers across a spectrum of theoretical backgrounds and orientations (Livesley & Jang, 2000). The validity of the current system has been questioned, particularly by investigators interested in dimensional approaches to diagnosis. They point out that while the DSM approach offers more rigorously defined PDs than were available before, they remain artificial constructs often irrelevant to clinical practice and are not especially helpful in treating patients. Along these lines, Westen and Arkowitz-Westen (1998) showed that when presented with prototypical descriptions of the various PDs, most clinicians were unable to identify patients in their practice who fit.

There is growing consensus among personality theorists that the major share of differences in personality among individuals can be described with four or five traits. For example, schemes have been developed by McCrae and Costa (1987) involving five factors (extroversion, neuroticism, openness to experience, conscientiousness, and agreeableness), and Cloninger et al. (1993) who described the temperamental dimensions of novelty seeking, reward dependence, harm avoidance, and persistence. Using factor analysis, Livesley, Jang, & Vernon (1998) identified four factors: emotional dysregulation, dissocial behavior, inhibitedness, and compulsivity. All competing schemes are fairly similar with the same characteristics clustering together. In a dimensional diagnostic system, a person could be scored along a continuum (low, medium, or high) for a particular trait.

Epidemiology of Personality Disorders

Epidemiologic surveys have confirmed the high prevalence of PDs, with figures ranging from 9%–16% of the general population meeting criteria for one or more PD (Coid, Yang, Tyrer, Roberts, & Ullrich, 2006; Grant et al., 2004a, 2004b; Lenzenweger, Loranger, Korfine, & Neff, 1997; Reich et al., 1989; Samuels et al., 2002). Prevalence is far greater in psychiatric samples, where in some studies from 30% to 50% of outpatients have a PD, though the frequency and types differ among the Axis I disorders. For example, Zimmerman, Rothschild, and Chelminski (2005) found that 51% of persons with major depression, 64% of persons with generalized anxiety disorder, and 56% of persons with panic disorder had a PD. Incarcerated

Table 26-1. DSM-IV-TR Personality Disorders

Cluster A (the eccentric disorders)
    Paranoid
    Schizoid
    Schizotypal
Cluster B (the dramatic disorders)
    Antisocial
    Borderline
    Histrionic
    Narcissistic
Cluster C (the anxious disorders)
    Avoidant
    Dependent
    Obsessive-compulsive

persons have an even higher frequency of PD (Rotter, Way, Steinbacher, Sawyer, & Smith, 2002).

The frequency of specific PDs differs by gender (Grant et al., 2004a). Antisocial personality disorder occurs more frequently in men, whereas borderline PD, avoidant PD, and dependent PD are more frequent in women (Grant et al., 2004a; Zimmerman & Coryell, 1989). Others have a fairly equal gender distribution (schizoid PD, schizotypal PD, obsessive-compulsive PD). Younger persons are at greater risk for a PD than older individuals, as its prevalence diminishes with advancing age (Coid et al., 2006; Grant et al., 2004a; Moran, Coffey, Mann, Carlin, & Patton, 2006). Other general risk factors for PD include lower levels of education and lower socioeconomic status (Coid et al., 2006; Grant et al., 2004a). Both substance misuse (alcohol and drugs) and cigarette smoking are more frequent among those with a PD that those without (Black, Zimmerman, & Coryell, 1999; Grant et al., 2004b).

Personality disorders tend to have an onset in adolescence and are established by young adulthood. Personality changes that appear later in life strongly suggest the presence of a major mental illness (e.g., early schizophrenia), a brain disorder, or a disorder caused by medical illness or the effects of a substance. DSM-IV requires that maladaptive personality features be present for at least 1 year if a PD is to be diagnosed in a person under age 18. The exception is ASPD in which an age requirement is specified (18 years), as is the requirement that certain childhood behaviors be present along with the adult traits. While no other PDs have child or adolescent criteria, research suggests that behavioral precursors such as affective lability or impulsivity can sometimes be traced back to childhood (Rey, Morrie-Yates, Singh, Andrews, & Stewart, 1995; Rey, Singh, Morris-Yates, & Andrews, 1997). Further, personality pathology in childhood or adolescence is predictive of adult maladjustment and both Axis I and II disorders (Johnson et al., 1999b). For example, Lewinsohn, Rhode, Seeley, & Klein (1997) reported that children with a history of major depressive disorder were at elevated risk for PD in adulthood. Personality disorders occur in adolescents with a frequency similar to that found in young adults, suggesting that the disorders present in adolescents are valid forms of most adult PDs (Grilo et al., 1998).

Personality disorders cause enormous problems for individuals and society, and they are frequently associated with impaired social, interpersonal, and occupational adjustment (Nakao et al., 1992). Family life, marriages, and academic and work performance suffer. Rates of unemployment, homelessness, divorce and separation, domestic violence, and substance misuse are excessive. These disorders also are associated with increased rates of health care utilization and high rates of traumatic accidents (e.g., motor vehicle accidents), emergency room visits, and psychiatric hospitalization (Bender et al., 2001; Moran, Rendu, Jenkins, Tylee, & Mann, 2001). As a group, individuals with PDs are at risk for early death from suicide or accidents (Black, Warrack, & Winokur, 1985).

Personality disorders are generally thought to be stable and enduring, yet several recent follow-up studies reveal a more subtle and complex picture (Grilo et al., 2004; Shea et al., 2004; Zanarini, Frankenburg, Hennen, Reich, & Silk, 2005). Over varying lengths of follow-up, fewer people will meet criteria for a PD, yet most remain impaired in interpersonal, occupational, and other domains of life. For example, in the Collaborative Longitudinal Personality Disorders Study (CLPS), 668 patients at five sites were followed. In an initial analysis following 2 years around 40% of persons initially assessed to meet criteria for the schizotypal, borderline, avoidant, or obsessive-compulsive types still met criteria for the PD. This study determined that affective instability, anger, and impulsivity were the most stable traits underlying PD. Persons with the poorest functioning initially tended to have the poorest functioning at follow-up. These studies tend to confirm what psychiatrists have long held to be true, that is, that many persons with PD tend to improve as the patient ages, and while some may experience remission, most continue to have impaired functioning in important life domains. With regard to ASPD and borderline PD, this phenomenon has been called "burnout." This term implies that the disturbance diminishes over time like a light bulb dimming until its glow fades (Black, 1999). Which symptoms burn out is a matter of conjecture, but at least for BPD, diminished impulsivity is one such symptom (Blum et al., 2008). Follow-up studies also suggest that PDs tend to wax and wane in severity over time often in response to significant life events (Grilo, McGlashan, & Skodol, 2000).

Psychiatric comorbidity is the rule and not the exception (Zanarini et al., 1998). Nearly all persons with PD have comorbid Axis I disorders—major depression being the most frequent. Other mood, anxiety, substance use, and eating disorders are all commonly diagnosed in persons with a PD. Comorbidity among the PDs is also very common, as persons with one PD frequently meet criteria for another (Pfohl, Coryell, Zimmerman, & Stangl, 1986). Few persons have a "pure" case in which they meet criteria for only one PD. The relationship between the PD and comorbid disorder is important to understand because of the many differences between persons with a PD and those without. For example, depressed patients with PDs are younger, are more likely to be female, are more likely to have a history of marital instability, are more likely to report precipitating stressors for the depression, and are more likely to have a history of nonserious suicide attempts. These findings suggest that depressed patients with PDs may form an important subgroup that differs biologically from depressed patients with primary depressive illness (Schiavone et al., 2006). Importantly, the presence of a PD is often associated with a poorer response to treatment, as has been shown for several Axis I disorders, including major depression, panic disorder, and obsessive-compulsive disorder (Baer, Jenike, Black, Treece, & Greist, 1992; Black, Bell, Hulbert, & Nasrallah, 1988; Reich & Green, 1991).

Etiology and Pathophysiology of Personality Disorders

The cause of PDs is unknown, though speculation includes developmental, genetic, neurobiologic, and cultural influences. Psychoanalysts have long suggested that early life events were causative factors, and in fact childhood maltreatment is associated with increased risk for PD, particularly the borderline and antisocial types (Coid, 1999; Johnson et al., 1999a). The psychological trauma resulting from abuse is thought to cause difficulty in developing trust and intimacy. An early home environment in which domestic abuse, divorce, separation, or parental absence occurred contributes to the risk of developing a PD. The risk from childhood adversity is relative because most persons with PD do not have a history of abuse.

Genetic factors help to explain the development of PD as well as personality traits (e.g., callousness, intimacy problems) (Livesley, Jaang, Jackson, & Vernon, 1993). Early studies confirmed that several PDs (antisocial, borderline, schizotypal) were familial, and twin studies suggested that PDs are likely genetic as well. A large twin study from Norway (Torgerson et al., 2000) showed that PDs as a whole have a heritability coefficient of 0.60 (0.37 for cluster A, 0.60 for cluster B, and 0.62 for cluster C). Surprisingly, borderline PD, often thought to primarily result from adverse childhood experiences, had a heritability coefficient of 0.69. Another important research paradigm, the adoption study, has been used to show that offspring of antisocial parents adopted in childhood are more likely to develop ASPD than are adoptees without an antisocial parent (Cadoret, Yates, Troughton, & Woodworth, 1995). The value of adoption studies is that they enable researchers to tease apart genetic from environmental influences. Molecular genetic approaches are now being applied to psychiatric disorders, including PD, and while no "personality" genes have been identified, Caspi et al. (2002) found that one particular gene (the low-activity MAO-A genotype) was associated with aggressiveness and symptoms of ASPD in adult men, when combined with a history of severe childhood maltreatment. This study points to the difficulty in linking genes to personality traits without taking environment into account.

The neurobiology of PDs is being actively pursued, particularly for the borderline, antisocial, and schizotypal types. Schizotypal PD has been associated with impaired smooth pursuit eye movement, impaired performance on tests of executive function, and increased ventricular-brain ratio on computed tomography (Trestman et al., 1995; Wei, Silverman, & Siever, 1997). Aberrant serotonin neurotransmission has been linked to impulsive and aggressive behaviors typical of both borderline and antisocial PDs (Coccaro, Kavoussi, Sheline, Lish, & Csernansky, 1996). As a group, antisocial persons have low resting pulse rates, low skin conductance, and increased amplitude on event-related potentials. These findings suggest that these individuals are chronically underaroused; perhaps such persons seek out potentially dangerous or risky situations to raise their arousal to more optimal levels to satisfy their craving for excitement (Scarpa & Raine, 1997).

Abnormal brain structure and function have been associated with borderline PD and ASPD. With the former, positron emission tomography has shown altered metabolism in prefrontal regions, including the anterior cingulate cortex, and reduced frontal and orbitofrontal volume has been reported (Lieb, Zanarini, Schmahl, Linehan, & Bohus, 2004). Raine, Lencz, Bihrle, LaCasse, & Colletti (2000) found that antisocial persons have reduced prefrontal gray matter, while Kiehl et al. (2001) identified specific abnormalities in the processing of emotions in psychopathic criminals. On functional magnetic resonance imaging scans, the criminals showed less affect-related activity in important limbic structures and increased activity in the fronto-temporal cortex. Because these brain regions help regulate mood and behavior, impulsive aggression or emotional instability could stem from functional abnormalities in these areas.

Cultural factors may affect the development and expression of a PD. The best evidence for this comes from cross-cultural research showing very low rates of ASPD in Taiwan, China, and Japan. Paris (2003) points out that family structure in these East Asian cultures maintain high levels of cohesion. Similarly low rates of ASPD occur in Jewish families, presumably because of their strong family structures. Yet, as Paris points out, the repressive style seen in these same families may have an association with cluster C disorders.

Assessment and Diagnosis of Personality Disorders

Persons with a PD often have little insight into the difficulties their maladaptive traits create, and so they are prone to view others as the source of their problems. For that reason, the presence of a PD disorder itself rarely leads the person to seek help. More likely it is ongoing troubles, such as chronic depression, poor work performance, and interpersonal problems that lead the person to seek help. At that point, the clinician's task is to help the person understand how his or her maladaptive personality traits contribute to their difficulties. The clinician can then assist the patient in developing tools to modify the maladaptive traits that contribute to their difficult life situations.

Table 26-2 shows the general diagnostic criteria for a PD. The essential elements are *(1)* an enduring pattern; *(2)* pervasiveness across domains of functioning; *(3)* inflexibility and maladaptive nature; *(4)* stability and duration;

Table 26-2. DSM-IV-TR General Diagnostic Criteria for a Personality Disorder

A. An enduring pattern of inner experience and behavior that deviates markedly fro the expectations of the individual's culture. This patter is manifested in two or more of the following areas:
  (1) cognition (i.e., ways of perceiving and interpreting self, other people, and events)
  (2) affectivity (i.e., the range, intensity, lability, and appropriateness of emotional response)
  (3) interpersonal functioning
  (4) impulse control

B. The enduring pattern is inflexible and pervasive across a broad range of personal and social situations.
C. The enduring pattern leads to clinically significant distress or impairment in social, occupational, or other important areas of functioning.
D. The pattern is stable and of long duration and its onset can be traced back at least to adolescence or early adulthood.
E. The enduring pattern is not better accounted for as a manifestation or consequence of another mental disorder.
F. The enduring pattern is not due to the direct physiological effects of a substance (e.g., a drug of abuse, a medication) or a general medical condition (e.g., head trauma).

Reprinted with permission from the Diagnostic and Statistical Manual of Mental Disorders, Text Revision, Fourth Edition, (Copyright © 2000). American Psychiatric Association.

and (5) independence from other mental and physical disorders.

The diagnosis of a PD requires a thorough personal and social history and a careful mental status examination. Several structured interviews and self-report instruments are available to help with diagnosis, but they are mainly used in research. These include the Structured Interview for DSM-IV Personality (Pfohl et al., 1997), the Structured Clinical Interview for DSM-IV Personality Disorders (First et al., 1995), and the Personality Diagnostic Examination (Loranger, Sussman, Oldham, & Russakoff, 1987). Self-report measures include the Schedule for Nonadaptive and Adaptive Personality (Clark, 1996), the Personality Diagnostic Questionnaire–4 (Hyler, 1994), and the Millon Clinical Multiaxial Inventory–III (Millon, Davis, & Million, 1997). Research has shown that while these instruments may be reliable and valid, they frequently correspond poorly to one another (Zimmerman, 1994).

More informally, a clinician's inquiries will lead to the conclusion that a PD may be present. When a PD is suspected the clinician should inquire about the kinds of symptoms found in these patients (Table 26-3). The author has observed that one clue to the presence of a PD is that the patient's immediate problem and social history intertwine. Like other psychiatric or behavioral disorders, the patient's history forms the most important basis for diagnosing a PD. The clinician's initial goal is to define the extent of the disorder through relatively nonintrusive inquiries, and then to move on to more specific behaviors and use patterns. For general screening purposes, a clinician might ask about problems in the following domains: interpersonal relationships, sense of self, work, affects, impulse control, and reality testing. For example, the following six questions are from a questionnaire (Langbehn et al., 1999) that yields an 80% chance or better that a PD is present when two or more items are endorsed:

- How often do you have days when your mood is constantly changing?
- How do you feel when you are not the center of attention?
- Do you frequently insist on having what you want right now?
- Are you concerned that certain friends or coworkers are not really loyal or trustworthy?
- Are you concerned about saying the wrong things in front of other people?
- How often do you avoid getting to know someone because you are worried he or she may not like you?

After the clinician is able to form initial impressions about the patient and his or her personality, disorder-specific inquiries can be made guided by the core features of the suspected disorder. Because there is great overlap among the different PDs, inquires may need to be fairly broadly based.

Table 26-3. Core Features of DSM-IV Personality Disorders

Disorder	Features
Cluster A	
Paranoid	Distrust, suspiciousness
Schizoid	Social detachment, restricted emotions
Schizotypal	Interpersonal deficits, cognitive distortions, eccentricities
Cluster B	
Antisocial	Disregard for rights of others, irresponsibility
Borderline	Emotional instability, impulsivity
Histrionic	Attention seeking, shallow emotions
Narcissistic	Grandiosity, need for admiration
Cluster C	
Avoidant	Social inhibition, inadequacy
Dependent	Need to be taken care of
Obsessive-compulsive	Orderliness, perfectionism, control

Care should be taken when considering a diagnosis of PD in a child or adolescent. In that age range, a PD diagnosis should be uncommon and apply to persons in whom the maladaptive traits are pervasive and persistent, and not likely due to an Axis I disorder or a particular developmental stage. These caveats aside, Paris (2003) believes that restrictions against diagnosing PD in young persons reflect a "sentimental" prejudice that may prevent some from getting needed help. Nonetheless, for many children with maladaptive personality traits, the traits recede or disappear as the child matures.

Collateral information is important to obtain when a PD is suspected, but the patient is unaware of his or her maladaptive traits (or denies them) and tends to boost the reliability of the assessment (Zimmerman, Pfohl, Stangl, & Corenthal, 1986). For example, a person with ASPD may deny criminal activity or minimize its significance (Black, Baumgard, & Bell, 1995). Information from friends, relatives, or a parole officer can be helpful in confirming its severity and extent. An informant also can be helpful in determining whether an observed behavior is characteristic of the patient's long-term functioning, or if the trait has been sufficiently severe to cause recurrent problems in how the person interacts with others. Of course, confidentiality has to be protected, so informants can be interviewed only with the patient's consent.

It is important that a PD diagnosis not be made prematurely. Patients with major depression are often socially anxious and dependent on others, and while these traits might suggest the presence of an anxious cluster PD, the traits may recede when the depression resolves. For that reason, caution needs to be exercised in making the diagnosis, particularly when the patient has an Axis I disorder like major depression that can distort one's normal personality or exaggerate preexisting personality traits. If the maladaptive traits persist after a depression has remitted, at that point a case could be made for the presence of a PD.

Long-term observation may be necessary with some patients to confirm a PD diagnosis. Sometimes a clinician will defer the diagnosis of a PD—even when it is suspected—until he or she has seen the patient several times and has had the opportunity to gather additional information.

Personality disorder also needs to be separated from normal personality. Most persons have minor personality quirks or idiosyncrasies, but these rarely rise to the level of a disorder. A key distinction is that the trait in question is inflexible and maladaptive, and leads to distress or impairment in one or more domain of life. Most people learn to adapt to changing circumstances and learn from experience. People with a PD often persist with their maladaptive behaviors regardless of their consequences. The clinician should also be aware of cultural issues that may affect a PD diagnosis because certain traits may be considered normal in some societies (i.e., magical thinking), but not others.

Treatment of Personality Disorders

It is difficult to generalize about the treatment of PDs. First, few of the 10 PDs have been studied sufficiently to recommend specific treatments. For this reason, recommendations made below are often based on clinical experience, not empirical evidence. Second, the disorders are sufficiently different that treatment recommendations for one PD may not apply to another. For example, the person with avoidant PD may be extremely anxious and inhibited, whereas the person with borderline PD is angry, moody, and impulsive. That said, contrary to assumptions that persons with PD cannot benefit from treatment, reviews of outcome studies show that treatment results are largely positive (Sanislow & McGlashan, 1998).

Treatment of PDs can be divided into pharmacologic or psychological interventions. Though many drug treatment studies of PD have been conducted over the past few decades, the pace of progress has been slow compared with the major mental disorders such as major depression or schizophrenia. There are currently no medications approved by the U. S. Food and Drug Administration (FDA) for *any* PD. Further, some disorders have been studied intensively (e.g., borderline PD) and others not at all (e.g., histrionic PD). The same is true for psychotherapy (mainly individual and group treatments): borderline PD has been actively studied, and several evidence-based psychotherapies now exist, while schizoid PD, for example, has been virtually ignored. Other forms of psychological treatment for PD, including family therapy and marital (or couples) therapy, have such a small data base that no recommendations can be made for these forms of treatment.

The DSM-IV Personality Disorders

Presently, 10 PDs are described in DSM-IV. They are divided among three clusters, each cluster characterized by PDs that are similar in phenomenology or PDs that substantially overlap. It should be kept in mind that while the clusters are a useful tool for thinking about and learning the PDs, research suggests that the actual distribution of diagnoses provides only weak support for the clusters (Fabrega, Ulrich, Pilkonis, & Mezzich, 1991).

The clusters include the following:

- Cluster A consists of the eccentric disorders—paranoid, schizoid, and schizotypal PDs. They are characterized by a pervasive pattern of abnormal cognition, self-expression, or of relating to others.
- Cluster B consists of the dramatic disorders—borderline, antisocial, histrionic, and narcissistic PDs. They are characterized by a pervasive pattern of violating social norms, impulsivity, excessive emotionality, grandiosity, or "acting out" through tantrums, self-abusive behavior, or angry outbursts.
- Cluster C consists of the anxious disorders—avoidant, dependent, and obsessive-compulsive PDs. They are characterized by a pervasive pattern of abnormal fears involving social relationships, separation, and need for control.

A residual category exists for individuals with mixed or atypical traits that do not fit into the better-defined categories (personality disorder not otherwise specified, or PDNOS). This category is one of the most frequently diagnosed PDs (Verheul, Bartak, & Widiger, 2007), which suggests that for many persons with a PD, the clinician has limited information regarding its extent or severity, or a disorder is present but does not meet more specific criteria.

A description of the DSM-IV PDs follows.

Paranoid Personality Disorder

Paranoid PD is characterized by chronic suspiciousness and a pervasive and unwarranted distrust of others, though frank delusions are absent. Persons with paranoid PD assume that others will exploit, harm, or deceive them. They rarely seek treatment, most likely because of their general mistrust of others, including psychiatrists and therapists. Paranoid PD is relatively common and has a prevalence estimated to range from 1%–4.5% (Torgerson, Kringlen, & Cramer, 2001).

People with paranoid PD are rarely motivated to seek treatment because they see the "trouble" as originating with others, not themselves (Stone, 2006). Thus, the disorder tends to be recognized when the patient seeks treatment for an associated mood or anxiety disorder. Apart from diagnosing and managing the patient's main complaint, the clinician should take care to be supportive and to listen patiently to their accusations and complaints, while being open, honest, and respectful. Once rapport has been established, alternative explanations for the patients' misperceptions can be suggested. Group therapy should be avoided because patients with paranoid PD tend to misinterpret statements and situations that arise in the course of the therapy. Antipsychotic medications may help to reduce suspiciousness, but these drugs have not been studied specifically in these patients.

Schizoid Personality Disorder

Patients with schizoid PD have no close relationships and choose solitary activities. They rarely experience strong emotions, express little desire for sexual experiences with another person, are indifferent to praise or criticism, and display a constricted affect. The disorder is not diagnosed in persons with schizophrenia or other psychotic disorders because these conditions are typically accompanied by a schizoid adjustment.

Schizoid PD is found in less than 1% of adults in the general population (Torgerson et al., 2001) but is also uncommon in clinical settings because persons with this disorder rarely seek psychiatric help. Like the person with paranoid PD, when they come to clinical attention it is usually because of an associated problem such as depression, anxiety, or substance abuse (Stone, 2006). Schizoid persons lack the insight and motivation necessary for individual psychotherapy and would likely find the intimacy of therapy threatening. Although few schizoid individuals would tolerate group therapy, it could foster the development of social skills and relationships. If the patient expresses a strong desire for social contact, avoidant PD may be the more appropriate diagnosis.

Schizotypal Personality Disorder

Schizotypal PD is characterized by a pattern of peculiar behavior, odd speech and thinking, and unusual perceptual experiences. Schizotypal patients frequently are socially isolated and have "magical" beliefs, mild paranoia, inappropriate or constricted affect, and social anxiety. Schizotypal PD has a prevalence of between 1% and 2% (Samuels et al., 2002; Torgerson et al., 2001). Associated mood, substance use, and anxiety disorders are common, and the gender distribution is equal.

The disorder was created in the development of DSM-III. Research had shown that relatives of schizophrenic patients often had a cluster of schizophrenic-like traits, a fact noted earlier by Kraepelin and Bleuler (Siever & Gunderson, 1983). Schizotypal PD is considered part of the schizophrenia spectrum, along with schizophreniform disorder, schizoaffective disorder, and perhaps psychotic mood disorders (Tienari et al., 2003).

The treatment of schizotypal PD often centers on issues that led the person to seek treatment, such as feelings of alienation or isolation, paranoia, or suspiciousness. Exploratory and group psychotherapies are overly threatening to these patients, but social skills training can be helpful. The goal is to help the individual to develop an awareness of what behaviors others may consider odd or eccentric and to develop a repertoire of social skills that will help make social interactions more productive and satisfying. Antipsychotics may help reduce the intense anxiety, paranoia, and odd perceptual experiences that can cause significant distress (Konigsberg et al., 2003).

Antisocial Personality Disorder

Antisocial personality disorder consists of recurrent misbehavior starting early in life. The diagnosis requires that patients have a history of conduct disorder before age 15 and a history of adult antisocial behavior since age 18. Childhood misconduct includes behaviors such as fighting with peers, conflicts with adults, lying, cheating, and stealing. A history of fire setting and cruelty to animals and other children is particularly worrisome. In adulthood, other problems develop such as uneven job performance, domestic abuse, unreliability, and reckless behavior. Criminal behavior, pathological lying, and the use of aliases are also common.

Antisocial behavior has been recognized since the nineteenth century when the terms *manie sans delire* ("mania without delirium") and *moral insanity* were used to describe immoral or guiltless behavior in the absence of impaired reasoning. In DSM-I, the disorder was called *sociopathic personality disorder* and was renamed ASPD in DSM-III.

The disorder has prevalence between 2.5% and 3.6%, and it is more frequent in men and young persons (Compton et al., 2005; Samuels et al., 2002; Torgerson et al., 2001). Prevalence is higher in psychiatric hospitals and clinics, in prisons, in homeless persons, and in alcohol- and drug-addicted persons. Alcohol or drug use disorders, mood disorders, anxiety disorders, attention-deficit/hyperactivity disorder, pathological gambling, and other PDs are common (Compton et al., 2005). ASPD is worse early in its course, and antisocial symptoms tend to recede with advancing age (Black et al., 1995). Antisocial persons frequently attempt suicide, and mortality studies show high rates of death from natural causes as well as accidents, suicides, and homicides (Black, Baumgard, Bell, & Kao, 1996).

There are no standard treatments for ASPD. Antisocial persons are difficult patients because of their tendency to blame others, their low frustration tolerance, and their impulsivity. Cognitive-behavioral therapy has been used with antisocial persons and involves challenging their distorted beliefs and attitudes (Davidson & Tyrer, 1996).

Several drugs, such as lithium carbonate, have been shown to reduce aggression, the chief problem of many antisocial persons (Davis, Janicak, & Ayd, 1995). Other drugs, including serotonin-reuptake inhibitor antidepressants, atypical antipsychotics, and mood stabilizers, have also been used but have not been formally studied. Treatment of comorbid psychiatric disorders may result in overall syndromal improvement.

Borderline Personality Disorder

Borderline PD represents a pervasive pattern of mood instability, unstable and intense interpersonal relationships, impulsivity, inappropriate or intense anger, lack of control of anger, recurrent suicidal threats and gestures, self-mutilating behavior, marked and persistent identity disturbance, chronic feelings of emptiness or boredom, and frantic efforts to avoid real or imagined abandonment. Patients also may experience transient paranoid ideation or dissociation.

Introduced in DSM-III, borderline PD has long been of interest to psychoanalysts. Kernberg (1984), for example, uses the term *borderline personality organization* to describe a broad range of problems, including the presence of identity diffusion, the use of primitive defense mechanisms such as splitting (e.g., exaggerated dichotomies of good and evil, or black and white thinking), and the maintenance of reality testing except in the perception of self and others.

One of the more common PDs in clinical settings, borderline PD has a frequency in the general population from 1% to 2% (Torgerson et al., 2001). Nearly three-quarters of these patients deliberately hurt themselves (e.g., cutting, burning, overdoses), and about 10% commit suicide (Black, Blum, Pfohl, & Hale, 2004). These patients frequently have comorbid major depression, dysthymia, anxiety disorders, and substance use disorders (Zanarini et al., 1998). Borderline PD also overlaps with schizotypal, histrionic, and antisocial PDs.

There is little agreement on the appropriate treatment of borderline PD, yet this is the only disorder for which official treatment guidelines exist (American Psychiatric Association, 2001). There are now evidence-based psychological treatments that reduce its symptoms and overall severity, several of which employ cognitive-behavioral techniques to help correct maladaptive thoughts, beliefs, and behaviors. Dialectical behavior therapy (DBT), the best known of these programs, involves an intensive year-long program including both individual and group therapy (Linehan et al., 2006). The 20-week Systems Training for Emotional Predictability and Problem Solving (STEPPS) program combines psychoeducation and skills training, and through weekly sessions patients learn to recognize symptoms, self-monitor changes in mental state, and make more skillful use of their social support network (Blum et al., 2008). A partial hospital program employing a psychoanalytic approach also appears to be effective (Bateman & Fonagy, 1999).

Pharmacotherapy tends to focus on the patients' target symptoms (Zanarini, 2004). Selective serotonin-reuptake inhibitors may be helpful in reducing depressive symptoms and suicidal ideations and behaviors. Antipsychotics can help treat perceptual distortions, anger dyscontrol, suicidal behaviors, and mood instability. Benzodiazepine tranquillizers should be avoided because they can cause behavioral disinhibition (Cowdry & Gardner, 1988).

Histrionic Personality Disorder

Persons with histrionic PD show a pattern of excessive emotionality and attention-seeking behavior. Typical symptoms include excessive concern with appearance and desire to be the center of attention. Histrionic persons are often gregarious and superficially charming but can be manipulative, vain, and demanding.

The disorder has a prevalence of nearly 2% in the general population; histrionic persons tend to seek out medical attention and to make frequent use of available health services (Nestadt et al., 1990). Some experts suggest that histrionic PD is a gender-biased diagnosis that merely describes a caricature of stereotypic femininity because it is frequently diagnosed among women in clinical samples (Slavney & McHugh, 1974). This contrasts with the results of community studies using structured diagnostic assessments that find virtually equal rates of histrionic PD in men and women (Grant et al., 2004a; Nestadt et al., 1990). Histrionic PD has been linked to somatization disorder and ASPD in family studies (Lilienfeld, Van Valkenberg, Larntz, & Akiskal, 1986).

The treatment of histrionic PD is not well understood. Some experts recommend a supportive, problem-solving approach or cognitive-behavioral therapy to help patients counter their distorted thinking, such as the inflated self-image that many histrionic patients have. With interpersonal psychotherapy, the patient can focus on conscious (or unconscious) motivations for seeking out disappointing lovers and being unable to commit oneself to a stable, meaningful relationship. Group therapy may be useful in addressing provocative and attention-seeking behavior. Patients may not be aware of their annoying behaviors, and it may be helpful to have others point them out.

Narcissistic Personality Disorder

Narcissistic PD is characterized by grandiosity, lack of empathy, and hypersensitivity to evaluation by others. Narcissistic persons are egotistical, inflate their accomplishments, and often manipulate or exploit those around them to achieve their own aims. They have an exaggerated sense of entitlement and believe that they deserve special treatment. Narcissistic individuals are often irritating, haughty, or difficult; although they appear outwardly charming, relationships tend to be superficial and cold. They tend to have little insight into their narcissism.

Narcissistic PD is named after Narcissus from Greek mythology, who fell in love with his own reflection. Freud used the term to describe persons who were self-absorbed; the term was later expanded to describe the more general concept of excessive self-love and grandiosity. Little is known about the neurobiologic factors underlying this disorder, though in the twin study of Torgerson et al. (2000) narcissistic PD had a heritability coefficient of 0.77.

Narcissistic PD is relatively uncommon (Coid et al., 2006; Torgerson et al., 2001). The disorder has been criticized as not being distinctive because narcissistic traits are common in most individuals with a PD. Like other Axis II disorders, narcissistic PD is viewed as stable over time, although research suggests that it may vary under the influence of significant life events, such as achievement and new relationships (Ronningstam, Gundersen, & Lyons, 1995).

There are few data on the treatment of narcissistic PD, though because of their poor insight, it is doubtful that many seek help, unless it is for the anger or depression they feel when deprived of something they felt entitled to, such as a promotion. This is sometimes referred to as a "narcissistic injury." Paris (2003) observes that these individuals are difficult to treat because their narcissistic traits directly interfere with the process of psychotherapy. For example, grandiosity can lead them to resist admitting personal responsibility for their problems, while their sense of entitlement can lead them to make unreasonable demands on the therapist.

Avoidant Personality Disorder

Persons with avoidant PD are inhibited, introverted, and anxious. They tend to have low self-esteem, are hypersensitive to rejection, and are apprehensive, mistrustful, and socially awkward. They are also shy, timid, uncomfortable, and self-conscious, and they fear being embarrassed in public. Some investigators have questioned the independence of avoidant PD, which they believe lies along a spectrum with the anxiety disorders (Rettew, 2000). Many features of avoidant PD are indistinguishable from those of social phobia, and the two disorders frequently overlap. Avoidant PD may involve a genetic predisposition to chronic anxiety.

Several psychotherapeutic strategies have evolved for the treatment of avoidant PD. Group therapy may help the person to overcome social anxiety and to develop interpersonal trust. Assertiveness and social skills training may be helpful, as might systematic desensitization to treat anxiety symptoms, shyness, and introversion. Cognitive-behavioral therapy has been recommended to help correct dysfunctional attitudes (e.g., "I had better not open my mouth because I'll probably say something stupid."). A recent randomized controlled trial found that cognitive-behavioral therapy was superior to a wait list or brief dynamic therapy in reducing avoidance and social distress (Emmelkamp et al., 2006). Benzodiazepines can be useful while the patient is attempting to reverse previously avoided behavior. It is best to limit the use of these drugs to short periods, although some patients will benefit from long-term use. Selective serotonin-reuptake inhibitors also may be helpful because they are effective in treating social phobia (Kapfhammer & Hippius, 1998).

Dependent Personality Disorder

Dependent PD is characterized by a pattern of relying excessively on others for emotional support. While there has been considerable research on the psychology of dependency, there are few empirical studies of dependent PD. One criticism of the disorder is that it is not sufficiently distinctive to stand alone and that dependency on others is common in other PDs; it is also common in persons with chronic medical or psychiatric disorders. Persons with dependent PD are more likely to be female and to be older than patients with other types of PDs (Loranger, 1995; Reich, 1996). Comorbid psychiatric disorders are common, particularly mood and anxiety disorders. Persons with dependent PD have poor social and family ties, in part because their dependency on others accentuates and promotes interpersonal conflicts.

There is little consensus on the treatment of dependent PD. Cognitive-behavioral psychotherapy is recommended as a way to encourage emotional growth, assertiveness, effective decision making, and independence. The therapist might have the patient set goals for each session and challenge his or her assumptions related to dependency (e.g., "I won't be able to make up my mind without mother's input."). Some patients benefit from more focused assertiveness training or social skills training. Marital counseling is indicated when the patient's dependence on his or her spouse is adversely affecting their relationship.

Obsessive-Compulsive Personality Disorder

Obsessive-compulsive PD represents a lifelong pattern of perfectionism and inflexibility typically associated with overconscientiousness and constricted emotions. It is one of the more frequent PDs, with an estimated prevalence of 1%–2% (Samuels et al., 2002). Unlike most PDs, this disorder appears to be more common in those with higher levels of education, and those in higher income brackets (Grant et al., 2004a). Comorbidity with mood and anxiety disorders is frequent. While it was long thought that obsessive-compulsive PD led to the development of axis I obsessive-compulsive disorder (OCD), obsessive-compulsive PD and OCD do not have a one-to-one relationship (Eisen et al., 2006; Pollack, 1987). Individuals with OCD are generally more willing to identify their symptoms as pathologic, whereas individuals with obsessive-compulsive PD tend to view many of their traits as desirable, such as hoarding (or saving) and perfectionism (Pfohl & Blum, 1991).

Obsessive-compulsive PD is relatively difficult to treat. Some experts recommend psychodynamic psychotherapy; however, while these patients tend to intellectualize and may be insightful, they develop little feeling or emotion. Cognitive-behavioral therapy may help these individuals develop a greater tolerance to the notion that the world is mostly made up of gray and not clearly defined black and white lines of rigidly held beliefs. Serotonin-reuptake inhibitor antidepressants may be helpful in reducing the need for perfectionism and the unnecessary ritualizing that sometimes develop (Feinberg, Sharma, Sivakumaran, Sahakian, & Chamberlain, 2007).

KEY POINTS

1. Patients with PDs have enduring, long-term problems that are not easily understood or treated.
2. PDs are common, but are often underappreciated and underdiagnosed.
3. Patients with PDs often experience considerable pain and suffering, and are deserving of empathy and support.

> **PRACTICE GUIDELINES**
>
> 1. The presence of a PD can adversely impact the treatment of comorbid Axis I disorders.
> 2. There are no FDA-approved medications for any PD.
> 3. Refer patients with borderline personality disorder to evidence-based psychosocial treatment programs such as DBT or STEPPS.

References

American Psychiatric Association. (1952). *Diagnostic and statistical manual of mental disorders* (1st ed.). Washington, DC: Author.

American Psychiatric Association. (1968). *Diagnostic and statistical manual of mental disorders* (2nd ed.). Washington, DC: Author.

American Psychiatric Association. (1980). *Diagnostic and statistical manual of mental disorders* (3rd ed.). Washington, DC: Author.

American Psychiatric Association. (1994). *Diagnostic and statistical manual of mental disorders* (4th ed.). Washington, DC: Author.

American Psychiatric Asssociation. (2001). Practice guidelines for the treatment of patients with borderline personality disorder. *American Journal of Psychiatry, 158*(Suppl. 10), 1–52.

Baer, L., Jenike, M. A., Black, D. W., Treece, C., & Greist, J. (1992). Effect of axis II diagnosis on treatment outcome with clomipramine in 55 patients with obsessive-compulsive disorder. *Archives of General Psychiatry, 49,* 862–866.

Bateman, A., & Fonagy, P. (1999). Effectiveness of partial hospitalization in the treatment of borderline personality disorder—A randomized controlled trial. *American Journal of Psychiatry, 156,* 1563–1569.

Bender, D. S., Dolan, R. T., Skodol, A. E., Sanislow, C. A., Dyck, I. R., McGlashan, T. H., Shea, M. T., Zanarini, M. C., Oldham, J. M., & Gunderson, J. G. (2001). Treatment utilization by patients with personality disorders. *American Journal of Psychiatry, 158,* 295–302.

Black, D. W. (1999). *Bad boys, Bad men: Confronting antisocial personality disorder.* New York: Oxford University Press.

Black, D. W., Baumgard, C. H., & Bell, S. E. (1995). A 16- to 45-year follow-up of 71 men with antisocial personality disorder. *Comprehensive Psychiatry, 36,* 130–140.

Black, D. W., Baumgard, C. H., Bell, S. E., & Kao, C. (1996). Death rates in 71 subjects with antisocial personality disorder compared with general population mortality. *Psychosomatics, 37,* 131–136.

Black, D. W., Bell, S., Hulbert, J., & Nasrallah, A. (1988). The importance of Axis II in patients with major depression: A controlled study. *Journal of Affective Disorders, 14,* 115–122.

Black, D. W., Blum, N., Pfohl, B., & Hale, N. (2004). Suicidal behavior in borderline personality disorder: prevalence, risk factors, prediction, and prevention. *Journal of Personality Disorder, 18,* 226–239.

Black, D. W., Warrack, G., & Winokur, G. (1985). The Iowa Record-Linkage Study III. Excess mortality among patients with 'functional disorders'. *Archives of General Psychiatry, 42,* 82–88.

Black, D. W., Zimmerman, M., & Coryell, W. H. (1999). Cigarette smoking and psychiatric disorder in a community sample. *Annals of Clinical Psychiatry, 11,* 129–136.

Blum, N., McCormick, B., Franklin, J., Hansel, R., Pfohl, B., St. John, D., Allen, J., & Black, D. W. (2008). Relationship of age to symptom severity, psychiatric comorbidity, and health care utilization in subjects with borderline personality disorder. *Personality and Mental Health.*

Blum, N., Pfohl, B., St. John, D., Stuart, S., McCormick, B., Allen, J., Arndt, S., & Black, D. W. (2008). Systems Training for Emotional Predictability and Problem Solving (STEPPS) for outpatients with borderline personality disorder: A randomized controlled trial and 1-year follow up. *American Journal of Psychiatry, 165*(4), 468–478.

Cadoret, R. J., Yates, W. R., Troughton, E., & Woodworth, G. (1995). Genetic-environment interaction in the genesis of aggressivity and conduct disorders. *Archives of General Psychiatry, 52,* 916–924.

Caspi, A., McClay, J., Moffitt, T. E., Mill, J., Martin, J., Craig, I. W., Taylor, A., & Poulton, R. (2002). Role of genotype in the cycle of violence in maltreated children. *Science, 297,* 851–854.

Clark, L. (1996). *Schedule for Nonadaptive and Adaptive Personality (SNAP): Manual for administration scoring, and interpretation.* Minneapolis: University of Minneapolis Press.

Cloninger, C. R., Svrakic, D. M., & Przybeck, T. R. (1993). A psychobiological model of temperament and character. *Archives of General Psychiatry, 50*(12), 975–990.

Coccaro, E. F., Kavoussi, R. J., Sheline, Y. I., Lish, J. D., & Csernansky, J. D. (1996). Impulsive aggression in personality disorder correlates wtih tritiated paroxetine binding in the platelet. *Archives of General Psychiatry, 53,* 531–536.

Coid, J. W. (1999). Aetiological risk factors for personality disorders. *British Journal of Psychiatry, 174,* 530–538.

Coid, J., Yang, M., Tyrer, P., Roberts, A., & Ullrich, S. (2006). Prevalence and correlates of personality disorder in Great Britain. *British Journal of Psychiatry, 188,* 423–431.

Compton, W. M., Conway, K. P., Stinson, F. S., Colliver, J. D., & Grant, B. F. (2005). Prevalence, correlates, and comorbidity of DSM-IV antisocial personality syndromes and specific drug use disorders in the United States: results from the National Epidemiologic Survey on Alcohol and Related Conditions. *Journal of Clinical Psychiatry, 66,* 677–685.

Cowdry, R. W., & Gardner, D. (1988). Pharmacotherapy of borderline personality disorder. *Archives of General Psychiatry, 45,* 111–119.

Davidson, K. M., & Tyrer, P. (1996). Cognitive therapy for antisocial and borderline personality disorders: single case study series. *British Journal of Clinical Psychology, 35,* 413–429.

Davis, J. M., Janicak, P. G., & Ayd, F. J. (1995). Psychopharmacology of the personality disordered patient. *Psychiatry Annals, 25,* 614–620.

Eisen, J. L., Coles, M. E., Shea, M. T., Pagano, M. E., Stout, R. L., Yen, S., Grilo, C., & Rasmussen, S. A. (2006). Clarifying the convergence between obsessive compulsive personality disorder and obsessive compulsive disorder. *Journal of Personality Disorders, 20,* 294–305.

Emmelkamp, P. M., Benner, A., Kuipers, A., Feiertag, G. A., Koster, H. C., & van Apeldoorn, F. J. (2006). Comparison of brief dynamic and cognitive-behavioural therapies in avoidant personality disorder. *British Journal of Psychiatry, 189,* 60–64.

Fabrega, H., Ulrich, R., Pilkonis, P., & Mezzich, J. (1991). On the homogeneity of personality disorder clusters. *Comprehensive Psychiatry, 32,* 373–386.

Feinberg, N., Sharma, P., Sivakumaran, T., Sahakian, B., & Chamberlain, S. (2007). Does obsessive-compulsive personality disorder belong within the obsessive compulsive spectrum? *CNS Spectrums, 12,* 476–482.

First, M. B., Spitzer, R. L., Gibbon, M., Williams, J. B. W., Davies, M., Borus, J., Howes, M., Kane, J., Pope, H. G., & Rounsaville, B. (1995). The Structured Clinical Interview for DSM-III-R Personality Disorders (SCID-II). Part II: Multi-site test-retest reliability study. *Journal of Personality Disorders, 9,* 92–104.

Grant, B. F., Hasin, D. S., Stinson, F. S., Dawaon, D. A., Chou, S. P., Ruan, W. J., & Pickering, R. P. (2004a). Prevalence, correlates, and disability of personality disorders in the United States: Results from the National Epidemiologic Survey on Alcohol and Related Conditions. *Journal of Clinical Psychiatry, 65,* 948–958.

Grant, B. F., Stinson, F. S., Dawson, D. A., Chou, S. P., Ruan, W. J., & Pickering, R. P. (2004b). Co-occurrence of 12-month alcohol and drug use disorders and personality disorders in the United States – results from the National Epidemiological Survey on Alcohol and Related Conditions. *Archives of General Psychiatry, 61,* 361–368.

Grilo, C. M., McGlashan, T. H., Quinlan, D. M., Walker, M. L., Greenfeld, D., & Edell, W. S. (1998). Frequency of personality disorders in two age cohorts of psychiatric inpatients. *American Journal of Psychiatry, 155,* 140–142.

Grilo, C. M., McGlashan, T. H., & Skodol, A. E. (2000). Stability and course of personality disorders. *Psychiatry Quarterly, 71,* 291–307.

Grilo, C. M., Sanislow, C. A., Gunderson, J. G., Pagano, M. E., Yen, S., Zanarini, M. C., Shea, M. T., Skodol, A. E., Stout, R. L., Morey, L. C., & McGlashan, T. H. (2004). Two-year stability and change of schizotypal, borderline, avoidant, and obsessive-compulsive personality disorders. *Journal of Consulting and Clinical Psychology, 72,* 767–775.

Hyler, S. (1994). *Personality Diagnostic Questionnaire 4.* New York: New York Psychiatric Institute.

Johnson, J. G., Cohen, P., Brown, J., Smailes, E. M., & Bernstein, D. P. (1999a). Childhood maltreatment increases risk for personality disorders during young adulthood. *Archives of General Psychiatry, 56,* 600–606.

Johnson, J. G., Cohen, P., Skodol, A. E., Oldham, J. M., Kasen, S., & Brook, J. S. (1999b). Personality disorders in adolescence and risk of major mental disorders and suicidality during adulthood. *Archives of General Psychiatry, 56,* 805–811.

Kapfhammer, H. P., & Hippius, H. (1998). Pharmacotherapy in personality disorders. *Journal of Personality Disorders, 12,* 277–288.

Kernberg, O. (1984). *Severe personality disorders.* New Haven, CT: Yale University Press.

Kiehl, K. A., Smith, A. M., Hare, R. D., Mendrek, A., Forster, B. B., Brink, J., Liddle, P. F. (2001). Limbic abnormalities in affective processing in criminal psychopaths as revealed by functional magnetic resonance imaging. *Biological Psychiatry, 50,* 677–684.

Koenigsberg, H. W., Reynolds, D., Goodman, M., New, A. S., Mitropoulou, V., Trestman, R. L., Silverman, J., & Siever, L. J. (2003). Risperidone in the treatment of schizotypal personality disorder. *Journal of Clinical Psychiatry, 64,* 628–634.

Langbehn, D. R., Pfohl, B. M., Reynolds, S., Clark, L. A., Battaglia, M., Bellodi, L., Cadoret, R., Grove, W., Pilkonis, P., & Links, P. (1999). The Iowa Personality Disorders Screen: Development and preliminary validation of a brief screening interview. *Journal of Personality Disorders, 13,* 75–89.

Lenzenweger, M. F., Loranger, A. W., Korfine, L., & Neff, C. (1997). Detecting personality disorders in a nonclinical population: Application of a 2-stage procedure for case identification. *Archives of General Psychiatry, 52,* 345–351.

Lewinsohn, P. M., Rohde, P., Seeley, J. R., & Klein, D. N. (1997). Axis II psychopathology as a function of axis I disorders in childhood and adolescence. *Journal of the American Academy of Child and Adolescent Psychiatry, 36,* 1752–1759.

Lieb, K., Zanarini, M. C., Schmahl, C., Linehan, M. M., & Bohus, M. (2004). Borderline personality disorder. *Lancet, 364,* 453–461.

Lilienfeld, S. O., Van Valkenberg, C., Larntz, K., & Akiskal, H. S. (1986). The relationship of histrionic personality disorder to antisocial personality and somatization disorder. *American Journal of Psychiatry, 143,* 718–722.

Linehan, M. M., Comtois, K. A., Murray, A. M., Brown, M. Z., Gallop, R. J., Heard, H. L., Korslund, K. E., Tutek, D. A., Reynolds, S. K., & Lindenboim, N. (2006). Two-year randomized controlled trial and follow-up of dialectical behavior therapy vs. therapy by experts for suicidal behaviors and borderline personality disorder. *Archives of General Psychiatry, 63,* 757–766.

Livesley, W. J., & Jang, K. L. (2000). Toward an empirically based classification of personality disorder. *Journal of Personality Disorder, 14,* 137–151.

Livesley, W. J., Jang, K. L., Jackson, D. N., & Vernon, P. A. (1993). Genetic and environmental contributions to dimensions of personality disorder. *American Journal of Psychiatry, 150,* 1826–1831.

Livesley, W. J., Jang, K. L., & Vernon, P. A. (1998). Phenotypic and genetic structure of traits delineating personality disorder. *Archives of General Psychiatry, 55,* 941–948.

Loranger, A. (1995). Dependent personality disorder—age, sex, and axis I comorbidity. *Journal of Nervous and Mental Disease, 184,* 17–21.

Loranger, A. W., Sussman, V. L., Oldham, J. M., & Russakoff, L. M. (1987). The Personality Disorder Examination: A preliminary study. *Journal of Personality Disorder, 1,* 1–13.

McCrae, R., & Costa, T. (1987). Validation of the five-factor model of personality across instruments and observers. *Journal of Personality and Social Psychology, 52,* 81–90.

Million, T., Davis, C., & Million, C. (1997). *MCMI-III manual* (2nd ed.). Minneapolis, MN: National Computer Systems.

Moran, P., Coffey, C., Mann, A., Carlin, J. B., & Patton, G. C. (2006). Personality and substance use disorders in young adults. *British Journal of Psychiatry, 188,* 374–379.

Moran, P., Rendu, A., Jenkins, R., Tylee, A., & Mann, A. (2001). The impact of personality disorder in UK primary care: A 1-year follow-up of attendees. *Psychological Medicine, 31,* 1447–1454.

Nakao, K., Gunderson, J. G., Phillips, K. A., Tanaka, N., Yorifuji, K., Takaishi, J., & Nishimura, T. (1992). Functional impairment in personality disorders. *Journal of Personality Disorders, 6,* 24–31.

Nestadt, G., Romanoski, A. J., Chahal, R., Merchant, A., Folstein, M. F., Gruenberg, E., & McHugh, P. R. (1990). An epidemiological study of histrionic personality disorder. *Psychological Medicine, 20,* 413–422.

Paris, J. (2003). *Personality disorders over time–Precursors, course, and outcome.* Washington, DC: American Psychiatric Publishing, Inc.

Pfohl, B., Coryell, W., Zimmerman, M., & Stangl, D. (1986). DSM-III personality disorders: Diagnostic overlap and internal consistency of individual DSM-III criteria. *Comprehensive Psychiatry, 27,* 21–34.

Pfohl, B., & Blum, N. (1991). Obsessive-compulsive personality disorder: A review of available data and recommendations for DSM-IV. *Journal of Personality Disorders, 5,* 363–375.

Pfohl, B., Blum, N., & Zimmerman, M. (1997). Structured Interview for DSM-IV Personality. American Psychiatric Publishing, Inc. Washington, DC.

Pollack, J. (1987). Obsessive-compulsive personality. *Journal of Personality Disorders, 1,* 248–262.

Raine, A., Lencz, T., Bihrle, S., LaCasse, L., & Colletti, P. (2000). Reduced prefrontal gray matter volume and reduced autonomic activity in antisocial personality disorder. *Archives of General Psychiatry, 57,* 119–127.

Reich, J. (1996). The morbidity of DSM-III-R dependent personality disorder. *Journal of Nervous and Mental Disease, 84,* 22–26.

Reich, J., Yates, W., & Nduaguba, M. (1989). Prevalence of DSM-III personality disorders in the community. *Social Psychiatry and Psychiatric Epidemiology, 24*(1), 12–16.

Reich, J. H., & Green, A. I. (1991). Effect of personality disorders on outcome of treatment. *Journal of Nervous and Mental Disease, 179,* 74–82.

Rettew, D. C. (2000). Avoidant personality disorder, generalized social phobia, and shyness: putting the personality back into personality disorders. *Harvard Review of Psychiatry, 8,* 283–297.

Rey, J. M., Morris-Yates, A., Singh, M., Andrews, G., & Stewart, G. W. (1995). Continuities between psychiatric disorders in adolescents and personality disorders in young adults. *American Journal of Psychiatry, 152,* 895–900.

Rey, J. M., Singh, M., Morris-Yates, A., & Andrews, G. (1997). Referred adolescents as young adults: The relationship between psychosocial functioning and personality disorder. *Australian and New Zealand Journal of Psychiatry, 31,* 219–226.

Ronningstam, E., Gundersen, J., & Lyons, M. (1995). Changes in pathological narcissism. *American Journal of Psychiatry, 152,* 253–257.

Rotter, M., Way, B., Steinbacher, M., Sawyer, D., & Smith, H. (2002). Personality disorders in prison: Aren't they all antisocial? *Psychiatry Quarterly, 73,* 337–349.

Samuels, J., Eaton, W. W., Bienvenu, O. J. III, Brown, C. H., Costa, P. T., & Nestadt, G. (2002). Prevalence and correlates of personality disorders in a community sample. *British Journal of Psychiatry, 180,* 536–542.

Sanislow, C. A., & McGlashan, T. H. (1998). Treatment outcome of personality disorders. *Canadian Journal of Psychiatry, 43,* 237–250.

Scarpa, A., & Raine, A. (1997). Psychophysiology of anger and violent behavior. *Psychiatric Clinics of North America, 20,* 375–403.

Schiavone, P., Dorz, S., Conforti, D., Scarso, C., Borgherini, G. (2006). The clinical implications of DSM-IV personality disorder comorbidity in depressed inpatients: a replication study in an Italian setting. *Journal of Personality Disorders, 20*(1), 1–8.

Shea, M. T., Stout, R., Gunderson, J. G., Morey, L. C., Grilo, C. M., McGlashan, T., Skodol, A. E., Dolan-Sewell, R., Dyck, I., Zanarini, M. C., & Keller, M. B. (2004). Short-term diagnostic stability of schizotypal, borderline, avoidant, and obsessive-compulsive personality disorders. *American Journal of Psychiatry, 159,* 2036–2041.

Siever, L. J., & Gunderson, J. G. (1983). The search for a schizotypal personality: Historical origins and current status. *Comprehensive Psychiatry, 24,* 199–212.

Skodol, A. E. (1997). Classification, assessment, and differential diagnosis of personality disorders. *Journal of Practical Psychiatry and Behavioral Health, 3,* 261–274.

Slavney, P. R., & McHugh, P. R. (1974). The hysterical personality: A controlled study. *Archives of General Psychiatry, 30,* 325–329.

Stone, M. (2006). *Personality disordered patient – Treatable and untreatable.* Washington, DC: American Psychiatric Publishing, Inc.

Tienari, P., Wynne, L., Laksy, K., Mohring, J., Nieminen, P., Sorri, A., Lahti, I., & Wahlberg, K. E. (2003). Genetic boundaries of the schizophrenia spectrum: Evidence from the Finnish adoptive family study of schizophrenia. *American Journal of Psychiatry, 160,* 1587–1594.

Torgerson, S., Kringlen, E., & Cramer, V. (2001). The prevalence of personality disorders in a community sample. *Archives of General Psychiatry, 58,* 590–596.

Torgerson, S., Lygren, S., Oien, P. A., Skre, I., Onstad, S., Edvardsen, J., Tambs, K., & Kringlen, E. (2000). A twin study of personality disorders. *Comprehensive Psychiatry, 41,* 416–425.

Trestman, R. L., Keefe, R. S. E., Mitropoulou, V., Harvey, P. D., deVegvar, M. L., Lees-Roitman, S., Davidson, M., Aronson, A., Silverman, J., & Siever, L. J. (1995). Cognitive function and biologic correlates of cognitive performance in schizotypal personality disorder. *Psychiatry Research, 59,* 127–136.

Verheul, R., Bartak, A., & Widiger, T. (2007). Prevalence and construct validity of personality disorder not otherwise specified (PDNOS). *Journal of Personality Disorders, 21,* 359–370.

Wei, T., Silverman, J., & Siever, L. J. (1997). Ventricular volume and asymmetry in schizotypal personality disorder and schizophrenia assessed with magnetic resonance imaging. *Schizophrenia Research, 27,* 45–53.

Westen, D., & Arkowitz-Westen, L. (1998). Limitations of axis II in diagnosing personality pathology in clinical practice. *American Journal of Psychiatry, 155,* 1767–1771.

Widiger, T. A., Simonsen, E., Krueger, R., Livesley, J., & Verheul, R. (2005). Personality disorder research agenda for the DSM-V. *Journal of Personality Disorders, 19,* 315–338.

Zanarini, M. C. (2004). Update on pharmacotherapy of borderline personality disorder. *Current Psychiatry Reports, 6,* 66–70.

Zanarini, M. C., Frankenburg, R., Hennen, J., Reich, B., & Silk, K. R. (2005). The McLean study of adult development (MSAD): Overview and implications of the first six years of prospective follow-up. *Journal of Personality Disorders, 19,* 505–523.

Zanarini, M. C., Frankenburg, F. R., Hennen, J., & Silk, K. R. (2003). The longitudinal course of borderline psychopathology: 6-year prospective follow-up of the phenomenology of borderline personality disorder. *American Journal of Psychiatry, 160,* 274–283.

Zimmerman, M. (1994). Diagnosing personality disorders: A review of issues and research methods. *Archives of General Psychiatry, 51,* 225–245.

Zimmerman, M., & Coryell, W. (1989). DSM-III personality disorder diagnosis in a non-patient sample. *Archives of General Psychiatry, 46,* 682–689.

Zimmerman, M., Pfohl, B., Stangl, D., & Corenthal, C. (1986). Assessment of DSM-III personality disorders: The importance of interviewing an informant. *Journal of Clinical Psychiatry, 47,* 261–263.

Zimmerman, M., Rothschild, L., & Chelminski, I. (2005). The prevalence of DSM-IV personality disorders in psychiatric outpatients. *American Journal of Psychiatry, 162,* 1911–1918.

Index

Note: Page numbers followed by *t* indicate a table; page numbers followed by *f* indicate a figure.

A

"Abandonment" depression, 98
Academic/occupational stress, 6, 84–85
Acculturation factor, 118–119
Acquired immune deficiency syndrome (AIDS), 43, 52, 160
Acute phase of schizophrenia, 366, 367*f*
Addictions
   development trajectories in, 73
   with drug use disorders, 312–314
   genetic influences on, 45, 46, 51, 319, 336
   reward process for, 28, 275, 280
   sexual, 343
   withdrawal cravings from, 279
   See also Alcohol use/abuse; Drug use/abuse; Smoking/tobacco use; Substance use/abuse
ADHD. *see* Attention-deficit hyperactivity disorder
Adolescent issues
   amygdala activity, 31
   body image, 128
   introduction to, 19–21
   life events, 210–211
   major depressive disorder, 212, 215–216
   pathological gambling, 336–337
   romantic relationships, 163
   sexual behavior, 164
   violence, 102
Adult issues
   amygdala activity, 31
   attention deficit disorder, 354–356
   developmental trauma, 147–148
   emotional influences, 104
Adverse life events, 210–211
Affective disorders, 48–49, 88, 369
Affiliation issues, 112, 119–120, 159, 319
   See also Peer pressure
African American youth
   atypical antipsychotic medication for, 115–116
   incarceration rates, 97
   psychiatric disorders, 116–117
   substance abuse rates, 45
   as uninsured, 200
"Age-crime curve", 13
Age-group classification, 111–112
Aggression issues, 25, 64, 328–329
Agonist substitution/maintenance treatment, 324–326, 324*t*–325*t*
Alcohol use/abuse
   binge drinking, 14, 41, 97, 299
   during college, 80, 89
   conduct disorder and, 48
   genetic factors in, 45, 212
   during marriage, 175
   peer influence on, 50
   prevalence rates, 41–42
   tobacco use and, 278
   treatment and, 195
   with work-related stress, 143–144
Alcohol use disorder (AUD)
   "alcohol denial", 302
   alcohol involvement, 292–293
   college students *vs.* non, 298–299
   epidemiology of, 294–295, 295*f*
   "maturing out" effect, 296, 300–301
   medications for, 303–304
   qualitative differences in, 295–298, 296*f*, 297*f*
   risk-taking behavior and, 48
   treatment of, 301–304
   understanding, 293–294
Alcohol Use Disorders Identification Test (AUDIT), 52
Alcoholics Anonymous (AA), 302, 323
Amenorrhea, 134, 398*t*, 399, 400
American Indian or Alaska Native (AIAN), 113, 114, 273
American Indian Service Utilization, Psychiatric Epidemiology, Risk and Protective Factors Project (AI-SUPERPFP), 114
Amphetamines
   addiction treatments for, 327
   for ADHD, 356
   behavioral responses to, 22
   dextroamphetamine addiction, 356
   methamphetamine addiction, 318, 319, 364
   toxicology of, 217, 353
Amygdala
   of adolescents *vs.* adults, 31
   anatomy and connectivity of, 23–24, 23*f*, 29
   in anxiety disorders, 232
   basolateral nuclear group and, 24
   circuits of, 20, 22, 25
   in fractal triadic model, 30–32, 32*f*
   in major depressive disorder, 213
   ontogeny of, 24–26
Anabolic steroids, 129, 311, 319
Anjum, Afshan, 362–378
Anorexia nervosa (AN)
   characterizations of, 134–135
   complications with, 132, 214, 399–400
   diagnostic criteria, 398–399, 398*t*
   epidemiology of, 397–398
   etiology of, 400–401
   nutritional treatment for, 401–402
   pharmacotherapy for, 327, 403
   psychotherapy for, 402–403
   suicide rates with, 399
Antidepressant therapy
   for anxiety disorders, 234–235, 238, 240–245
   for bipolar disorder, 387–388
   electroconvulsive therapy and, 222
   light therapy and, 222
   maintenance of, 221–222
   medication as, 218–220, 219*t*
   monotherapy *vs.* augmentation, 221
   prescription guidelines, 220
   psychological treatment, 222–223
   special considerations, 221
   suicide ideation and, 386
   switching, 221
Antipsychotic medications, 371–372, 415–416
Antisocial personality disorder (ASPD), 72–73, 341, 424, 426–428, 432–433
Anxiety disorders
   with bipolar disorder, 383–384
   development trajectories in, 70–71
   drug use disorders and, 315, 328
   generalized, 110, 231, 239–242
   non-trauma-related, 70–71
   not otherwise specified, 231
   panic disorder, 231, 236–239
   personality disorder and, 431
   severe mood dysregulation, 72
   social anxiety disorder, 215, 231–235
   See also Obsessive-compulsive disorder; Posttraumatic stress disorder
Applied behavior analysis (ABA), 410, 412, 413–415

Applied relaxation (AR) therapy, 233, 238, 240
Approach/reward behavior, 21–22
Aripiprazole treatment, 371t, 372
Asian American and Pacific Islander (AAPI), 114, 118
Asian Americans, 116–117, 119
Asperger disorder, 411, 418
Assault recovery, 8–9
Atomoxetine treatment, 356
Attachment parenting style, 159–160, 185, 188–190
Attention-deficit hyperactivity disorder (ADHD), 71–72, 354–355
　clinical presentation of, 353–354
　conductive disorder and, 73
　development trajectories in, 73–74
　diagnosis of, 355–356
　drug use disorders and, 328
　mania and, 382–383
　OCD and, 261
　prescription stimulant addiction, 318–319
　risk-taking behaviors with, 40–41, 47–48
　severe mood dysregulation and, 72
　SSRIs for, 64
　tobacco use and, 278
　treatment of, 19, 356–357
Atypical antipsychotics, 115–116, 416, 433
Auslander, Beth A., 158–168, 159–168
Autistic disorder, 64–65, 369, 407, 411, 416–417
Avoidance/withdrawal behavior, 21–22
Avoidant attachment style, 160, 187–189
Avoidant personality disorder, 434–435
Axis I/Axis II disorders, 110, 299, 425–427, 430

B

Barry, Declan T., 110–125
Basolateral nuclear group (BLNG), 24, 29
Behavior factors in adolescence, 112–113, 130, 263, 407
Behavior therapy for smoking, 281
Behavioral marital therapy (BMT), 176
Behavioral sensitization, 380
Beitel, Mark, 110–125
Benzodiazepines, 238, 317–318, 434–435
Binge drinking, 14, 41, 97, 299
Binge eating disorder (BED), 398, 399t, 400t, 402
Bipolar disorder
　characteristics of, 381, 381t
　clinical pathways to, 381–384, 383t
　depression and, 382, 387–388
　development trajectories in, 71–72
　in drug use disorders, 328
　genetic influences in, 384–385

introduction to, 379–380
　kleptomania with, 340
　mania and, 382–383, 387
　pharmacological treatments, 385–387, 385t, 386t
　recurrence mechanisms, 380–381
Black, Donald W., 424–440
Blum, Nancee, 424–440
Body dysmorphic disorder (BDD), 126, 129, 133–134, 256
Body image
　cultural differences, 131–132
　developmental course, 128
　eating disorders, 134–135
　gender differences, 128–129
　during marriage, 175–176
　media influences on, 129–130
　neurobiology disturbance of, 132–133
　peer teasing and, 130–131
　prevention programs, 136–137
　significance of, 127–128
　treatment programs, 135–136
Body mass index (BMI), 127, 128, 401
Borderline personality disorder, 341, 433
Bowlby, John, 66
"Boy code", 102–103, 104
Brain-derived neurotrophic factor (BDNF), 69
Brain development changes
　during adolescence, 7, 9–10, 14
　environment impact on, 336
　genetic impact on, 336
　in personality disorders, 428
　pre-adult, 68
　risk-taking behaviors and, 46–47
　with trauma exposure, 69
　in young males, 104
Brown Longitudinal OCD study (BLOCS), 258, 259, 261, 261f
Buhlmann, Ulrike, 126–142
Bulimia nervosa (BN)
　characterizations of, 134–135
　complications with, 399–400
　epidemiology of, 397–398, 398t
　etiology of, 400–401
　nutritional treatment for, 401–402
　pharmacotherapy for, 403
　psychotherapy for, 402–403
Bupropion, 220, 282, 356
Burt, Keith B., 5–18

C

Cannabis use. see Marijuana use
Career stress. see College and/or career stressors
Causation perspective of marriage, 172–173
Chambers, R. Andrew, 64–79
Chantix treatment, 282–283
Child abuse, 49, 69, 385
Child mental health problems
　ADHD in, 355
　autistic disorder, 64–65
　bipolar disorder onset, 380, 384

developmental trajectories of, 65–66, 70–74
　disruptive behavior disorders, 72–74
　fragile X syndrome, 64
　models of, 66–68
　neurological derailment, 68–70
　OCD onset, 256, 265
　personality disorders onset, 424, 428
　PTSD, 70
Childhood-onset schizophrenia (COS), 363
Children/childhood issues, 49, 69, 128, 136–137, 159–160, 174, 380, 384, 385
　See also Parenting/parenthood
Chinese Americans, 115
Cigarette smoking. see Smoking/tobacco use
Clonidine treatment, 326–327
Clozapine, 371t, 372
Club drugs, 319
Cocaine addiction, 312, 327
Cognitive-behavioral therapy (CBT)
　for ADHD, 356–357
　for anxiety disorders, 235, 237, 238, 240
　for compulsive buying, 344
　cultural considerations in, 111
　definition of, 222
　for drug use disorders, 314, 321, 322–323
　for eating disorders, 134, 135–136
　for OCD, 256, 262, 264, 435
　for pathological gambling, 337
　for personality disorders, 432, 434
　for PTSD, 244
　for pyromania, 342
　for schizophrenia, 373
　for social anxiety disorder, 233
　stress and, 151, 152
　for trichotillomania, 339
Cognitive development, 19, 20, 21–22, 23–30, 263–264
Cognitive therapy (CT), 233
Collaborative Longitudinal Personality Disorders Study (CLPS), 426
College and/or career stressors
　academic vs. occupational, 6, 82–83, 84–85, 88
　alcohol abuse, 80, 298–299
　anxiety disorders, 231–232, 236, 242
　buffers for, 90–91, 150
　exercise buffer for, 89, 91–92
　finances, 87–88, 200
　grades, 110
　impulse control disorders, 335
　intra/interpersonal stress, 85–87
　management approaches to, 89–92
　mental health challenges, 88–89
　procrastination, 86–87
　secondary sexual characteristics, 80
　young vs. emerging adulthood, 81–82
Communication issues, 119, 162, 411–412, 414
Comorbidity of major depressive disorder, 215

Index

Competence development, 6, 8–9, 10–12, 13
Comprehensive Assessment of At-Risk Mental States (CAARMS), 367
Compulsive buying, 343–344
Compulsive sexual behavior, 342–343
Conditioned stimuli (CS), 313
Conduct disorder, 47–48, 72–73, 355
Connectivity hypothesis in schizophrenia, 365
Contingency management (CM), 281–282, 323
Continuous Performance Test (CPT), 355–356
Conventional antipsychotics, 415–416
Corbin, William R., 80–95
"Cravings", 313–314
Credit card debt, 87–88
Criminal behavior, 43, 47, 73, 146
  See also Antisocial personality disorder
Cronce, Jessica M., 80–95
Crow, Scott J., 397–405
Cullen, Kathryn, 362–378
Cultural/ethnic considerations
  American Indian or Alaska Native, 114, 116–117
  Asians, 114, 116–117
  in body image, 131–132
  Chinese Americans, 115
  classification of, 111–112
  factors in, 118–120
  Japanese immigrants, 110–111, 115
  Korean Americans, 85, 115
  mental health and, 112–117, 120
  Native Hawaiians, 114
  sociocultural features of young adults, 81
  in substance use/abuse disorders, 117–118
  See also African American youth

D

Dahl, Ronald, 104
Delinsky, Sherrie S., 126–142
Department of Health and Human Services (DHHS), 112
Dependant personality disorder, 435
Depression
  "abandonment", 98
  with bipolar disorder, 382, 387–388
  drug use/abuse and, 48, 328
  exercise and, 91–92
  with mood disorders, 207–208, 214
  tobacco use and, 277
  treatment and, 195
  in undergraduates, 84–85, 89
  unipolar depression, 71
  See also Antidepressant therapy; Major depressive disorder
Depressive disorder not otherwise specified, 208
Developmental issues
  in drug use disorders, 319–320
  in emerging adults, 183–184

examples of, 7f
  in pervasive developmental disorders, 409–410
  in risk-taking behavior, 47–48
  transitional development and, 6–8
Developmental psychopathology, 5, 7, 14–15, 65, 67–68
Developmental trajectories in mental health, 65–66, 70–74
Dexamethasone suppression test (DST), 217
Dexedrine treatment, 327
Dextroamphetamine, 318, 356
Diagnostic Statistical Manual of Mental Disorders, Fourth Edition (DSM-IV)
  alcohol abuse, 42, 52
  alcohol use disorder, 293–294
  anxiety disorders, 234, 235
  Axis I/Axis II disorders, 110
  drug dependence/abuse, 315–319, 316t–317t
  drug use disorders, 312, 320–321
  impulse control disorders, 335
  major depressive disorder, 208t, 212, 218
  mood disorders, 207
  obsessive-compulsive disorders, 256, 257t
  personality disorders, 424–425, 425t, 428t, 429, 429t, 431–435
  pyromania, 342
  schizophrenia, 365, 366t
  somatoform disorder, 133
Diffusion tensor imaging (DTI), 365
Disruptive behavior disorders, 72–73
Disulfiram treatment, 327
Divorce rates, 170–171, 171f
Dopamine
  ADHD and, 353
  in cocaine addiction, 327
  in drug use disorders, 312
  in impulse control disorders, 336
  lesions and, 22
  nicotine dependence and, 274
  receptor polymorphism link and, 45
  risk-taking behaviors and, 46–47
  in schizophrenia, 371
  as striatal mediator, 28
Dopamine receptor gene (DRD2), 276
Dorsolateral prefrontal cortex (DLPFC), 365
Dramatic disorders, 431
"Dropout" stressors, 87
Drug use/abuse
  counseling services for, 323
  depression and, 48, 328
  genetic factors in, 45
  neurobehavioral contributors to, 46–47
  peer influence on, 49
  prevalence of, 42
  resistance education (DARE), 329
Drug use disorders
  addiction issues, 312–314
  ADHD and, 328
  anxiety disorders and, 315, 328
  approaches for, 319–320

DSM-IV classification, 315–319, 316t–317t, 320–321
  gateway hypothesis of, 314
  introduction to, 311–312
  pharmacological treatments in, 324–327, 324t–325t
  prevention efforts, 329
  psychiatric disorders and, 320–321, 327–329
  PTSD and, 314, 328
  risk factors for, 315
  subsyndromal dependence in, 315
  treatment modalities for, 321–324, 321t–322t
Drug Use Disorders Identification Test (DUDIT), 52
DSM-IV. *see Diagnostic Statistical Manual of Mental Disorders, Fourth Edition*
Duration of untreated psychosis (DUP), 363
Dysthymic disorder, 207–208

E

Early Developmental States of Psychopathology (EDSP) study, 212
Eating disorder not otherwise specified (ED-NOS), 134
Eating disorders
  diagnostic criteria for, 398–399, 399t
  epidemiology of, 397–398
  genetic influences on, 401
  introduction to, 397
  restrictive eating, 400, 400t
  types, 134–135
Eccentric disorders, 431
Ecstasy (methylenedioxy methamphetamine), 311, 319
Educational support for disorders, 245, 273, 388, 417
Eisen, Jane, 255–271
Electrocardiogram (ECG), 217
Electroconvulsive therapy (ECT), 222
Electroencephalogram (EEG), 370
Elliott, Sinikka, 169–180
Emerging adulthood
  alcohol use disorder during, 300
  developmental norms, 183–184
  environmental factors and, 50–51
  intimate relationships during, 181–182
  parenthood and, 183
  stress of, 145–146
  substance use during, 148–149
  theory and support of, 9–10
  vulnerability in, 13–14, 146–147
  vs. young adulthood, 81–82
Emotional balance issues
  "boy code", 102–103, 104
  "psychic separation", 98
  shame, 101–102
  "shame-free zones", 104–105
  in young adult males, 97–98, 101
Emotionally focused therapy (EFT), 176
Employment issues. *see* Job/workplace issues

Environmental influences
   on alcohol use disorders, 299
   on bipolar disorder, 385
   on brain functioning, 336
   for developing children, 103
   genetics and, 51
   genotype-environment interactions, 211
   Internet, 50
   on major depressive disorder, 210–211
   on pervasive developmental disorder, 410
   on risk-taking behaviors, 49–51
   on schizophrenia, 364–365
   on smoking, 280
Epidemiologic Catchment Area (ECA) Survey, 294
Erickson, Craig A., 64–79
Erickson, Eric, 66
Erikson's life cycle theory, 6
Ernst, Monique, 19–39
Ethnic considerations. *see* Cultural/ethnic considerations
Exercise benefits, 89, 91, 152, 175–176
Experimental functional analysis (EFA), 414
Exposure and response (ritual) prevention (E/RP), 264
Extended amygdala, 24
Extrapyramidal side effects (EPS), 371
Eye movement desensitization and reprocessing (EMDR), 241

F

Family history benefits, 315, 319, 352, 384
Family support needs, 110, 209, 210, 223, 323–324
Fear responses, 25, 196f, 198–199, 237
Female mental health issues
   amenorrhea and, 134, 398t, 399, 400
   body-dissatisfied women, 130
   body image, 127–128
   early parenthood, 184
   male friends, 105–106
   OCD and, 263
   See also Eating disorders; Gender issues/differences
Financial stressors, 87–88, 196f, 199–200, 200, 344
Finnish Health Care Survey, 215, 218
First-generation antipsychotics (FGA), 370–371, 372
Fluoxetine, 417
Fractal triadic model, 30–32, 32f
Fragile X syndrome, 64
Friends' support needs, 105–106, 111, 146, 161
Fudge, Julie, 19–39

G

Gait, Priyanka, 362–378
Gamblers Anonymous, 338

Gambling behavior
   genetic factors in, 45–46
   Internet influence on, 50
   pathological, 336–338
   risk of, 43–44
   See also Impulse control disorders
Gateway hypothesis, 314
Gender issues/differences
   attachment parenting styles, 189
   biological proclivities, 103
   body image, 128–129
   dating violence, 165
   emotional balance, 97–98, 101
   homophobic stereotyping, 103
   intimacy development, 162
   "male-friendly" treatment approach, 98–101
   in marriage, 173–174
   modern models for mental health, 105–106
   with OCD, 259
   with personality disorders, 426
   with PTSD, 243
   risk-taking behaviors, 43
   in romantic relationships, 163
   with schizophrenia, 363
   in sexual behavior, 164
   substance abuse and, 96, 97, 199
   with trichotillomania disorder, 338–339
   See also Emotional balance
"Gender straitjackets", 106
General Educational Development (GED) credential, 82–83, 92
Generalized anxiety disorder (GAD), 110, 146, 215, 220, 239–242
Generalized social anxiety disorder (GSAD), 232–233
Genetic influences
   on addiction, 45, 46, 51, 319, 336
   on alcohol abuse, 45, 212
   bipolar disorder, 384–385
   on brain functioning, 336
   drug use disorders, 314
   eating disorders, 401
   vs. environmental, 51
   genotype-environment interactions, 211
   major depressive disorder, 209–210
   on neurological derailment, 69
   OCD and, 262–263
   personality disorders, 427
   pervasive developmental disorders, 408–409
   on puberty, 190–191
   on risk-taking behavior, 44–46
   on tobacco use, 276–277
GenomeLinkage Scan, 210
Genotype–environment interactions, 211
Global Burden of Disease study, 206
Goddard, Andrew, 231–254
Gold, Steven N., 143–157
Grant, Jon E., 3–4, 231–254, 335–351
Greenberg, Jennifer L., 126–142

Group cognitive behavioral therapy (GCBT), 233
Group therapy, 244, 434

H

Habit reversal training (HRT), 339
Hair pulling disorder (trichotillomania), 338–339
Harm-reduction treatments, 303
High functioning autism (HFA), 411
Hispanic youths, 44, 115–117, 200
Histrionic personality disorder, 433–434
Hoarding behavior, 340
Hofstein, Yariv, 195–205
Homophobic gender stereotyping, 103
Homosexual-committed relationships, 163
HPA axis. *see* Hypothalamic-pituitary-adrenal system
Hulvershorn, Leslie A., 64–79
Human immunodeficiency virus (HIV), 43, 44, 52, 160, 327
Humanistic/experiential therapy, 111
Hyman, Scott M., 143–157
Hypnotic dependence, 317–318
Hypothalamic-pituitary-adrenal system (HPA axis), 48–49, 51

I

"Image concerns" factor, 197
Impulse control disorders (ICDs)
   compulsive buying, 343–344
   compulsive sexual behavior, 342–343
   intermittent explosive disorder, 340–342
   introduction to, 335
   kleptomania, 339–340
   pathological gambling, 336–338
   pyromania, 342
   trichotillomania, 338–339
   young adult predisposition, 335–336
   See also Gambling behavior
Incentive salience theory, 28
Individual cognitive behavioral therapy (ICBT), 233
Individualized education plan (IEP), 417
Individuals with Disabilities Education Improvement Act (IDEIA), 417
Intermittent explosive disorder (IED), 335, 340–342
Internet-based therapy (IBT), 234
Internet issues, 41, 50, 103, 281
Intimacy issues, 112
Intimacy process model, 162
Intimate romantic relationships
   attachment theory, 159–160
   delaying, 183
   during emerging adulthood, 181–182
   neurobiological basis of, 158–159
   quality and conflict, 164–165
   romantic *vs.* sexual, 162–165

Index

sexual maturation, 20, 160
social cognitive theory, 160–161
theories of, 161–162
See also Pregnancy issues; Sexual transmitted diseases
Isolation issues, 112, 119, 146

J

Japanese culture, 110–111, 115, 132
Jewish young adults, 144
Job/workplace issues, 89, 146, 150, 337
Juvenile delinquency, 13, 14

K

Kanner, Leo, 407, 409
Klein, Melanie, 66
Kleptomania, 339–340
Korean Americans, 85, 115
Kraeplin, Emil, 362
Krishnan-Sarin, Suchitra, 272–291

L

Lejuez, Carl W., 40–63
Life history theory, 184–185
Light therapy, 222
Limbic system dysfunctions, 243
Listening to Boys Voices Project, 105
Lithium treatment, 385–386, 385*t*, 386*t*, 433
Littlefield, Andrew K., 292–310
Liu, Hui, 169–180
Long-term reproductive strategy, 186
Lysergic acid diethylamide (LSD), 319

M

Maddaus, Michael, 5, 14
Magidson, Jessica, 40–63
Magnetic resonance imaging (MRI), 25, 27–28, 30, 69, 133, 213, 217, 232–233, 240, 243, 428
Mahler, Margaret, 66
Mahmud, Waqar, 231–254
Major depressive disorder (MDD), 116, 206–208, 210–211, 215–216
 alcohol use and, 212
 biological studies of, 213–214
 cognitive behavior therapy for, 222
 diagnosis/clinical features of, 216–218
 environmental factors and, 210–211
 epidemiology of, 208, 208*t*
 genetic influences, 209–210
 genotype-environment interactions, 211
 psychological studies of, 214–215
 substance abuse disorders and, 211–212
 suicide factors, 212
 treatment of, 218–223, 219*t*
See also Antidepressant therapy
Major depressive episode (MDE), 196

"Male-friendly" treatment approach, 98–101
Male mental health issues, 98–101, 105–106, 184. *See also* Gender issues/differences
Mancebo, Maria C., 255–271
Mania with bipolar disorder, 382–383, 387
Marijuana use
 aggression and, 328
 on college campuses, 42
 dependence on, 45, 49, 278, 311–312, 317, 323
 gateway hypothesis and, 314
 marriage and, 176
 OCD and, 256
 schizophrenia and, 363
 social/academic competence, 13
 symptoms of, 73, 211–212, 385
 toxicology of, 217, 283, 313, 364–365
 treatment of, 327
Marriage, 51, 160–161, 169–170, 171–174, 300
 counseling for, 435
 delay of, 169, 170*f*, 183
 depression and, 210
 dissolution of, 170–171
 health behaviors and, 175–176
 perceptions of, 160–161
 problem treatments in, 176
 same-sex, 170
Masten, Ann S., 5–18
"Mating effort" in parenting, 185
"Maturing out" effect, 296, 300–301
"Maturity principle", 301
Mayes, Linda, 40–63
McDougle, Christopher J., 406–423
McMahon, Thomas J., 181–194
Media influences in body image, 129–130, 136
Memory problems, 213–214, 312–314
Mental health challenges. *See also* Emotional balance
 cultural/ethnic and, 112–117, 120
 marriage, 171–174
 modern models for, 105–106, 120
 of undergraduates, 88–89
Mental health service utilization
 barriers to, 196–202, 196*f*
 constraints with, 201
 logistical barriers to, 199–202
 for major depressive disorder, 218
 nonresponsive services, 201–202
 normative influences, 196–197, 196*f*
 recognition/skepticism/fear and, 196*f*, 198–199
 stigma concerns, 196*f*, 197–198
 substance use/abuse and, 196*f*, 199
 use data on, 196
Mental illness stigma, 197–198
Mesolimbic dopamine systems, 46
Methadone treatment, 324–325, 357
Methamphetamine addiction, 318, 319, 364
Methylenedioxymethamphetamine (MDMA/ecstasy), 311, 319
Methylphenidate, 318, 357

Mexican Americans, 116–117
Michael, Lesley A., 195–205
Mindfulness-based stress reduction (MBSR), 151, 233–234
Minnesota Heart Health program, 282
Minshawi, Noha F., 406–423
Mirror retraining, 136
Mirtazapine (Remeron), 220, 221
"Model minority myth", 114–115
Monitoring the Future Study, 44
Monoamine oxidase inhibitors (MAOIs), 219–220, 234, 245, 403
Monoamine oxidase (MAO), 46–47, 385, 427
Monotherapy *vs.* augmentation, antidepressants, 221
Montgomery-Asberg Depression Rating Scale (MADRS), 206
Mood Disorder Questionnaire (MDQ), 217
Mood disorders, 72, 207–208, 214, 341
Mood states, 48, 275–276
Mortality/morbidity rates
 in adolescents, 20
 in major depressive disorder, 206–207
 racial demographics of, 113–114
 in young adults, 97
Motivational interviewing (MI), 281, 322
Muscle dysmorphia (MD), 129, 134

N

Naltrexone treatment, 325–326
Narcissistic personality disorder, 434
Nardil, 220
National Ambulatory Medical Care Survey (NAMCS), 115
National Co-Morbidity Survey, 398
National College Health Assessment (NCHA), 43, 89
National College Health Risk Behavior Survey (NCHRBS), 43
National Commission on Adolescent Health, 158
National Comorbidity Survey, 114, 115, 199
National Counseling Center Directors, 201–202
National Epidemiologic Survey on Alcohol and Related Conditions (NESARC), 41, 116, 118, 294, 296, 299
National Health and Nutrition Examination Survey (NHANES III), 208, 218
National Hospital Ambulatory Medical Care Survey (NHAMCS), 115–116
National Institute of Healthcare Management Foundation, 200
National Institute on Alcohol Abuse and Alcoholism (NIAAA), 52–53, 116, 293
National Latino and Asian American Study, 115, 116

National Longitudinal Alcohol Epidemiologic Survey (NLAES), 294
National Longitudinal Study on Adolescent Health, 104
National Survey of Adolescent and Young Adults: Sexual Health Knowledge, Attitudes, and Experiences, 163
National Survey on Drug Use and Health (NSDUH), 42, 117
Native Americans, 116–117, 208
Negative affective states, 275–276
Negative mood states, 48
Negative reinforcement in drug use, 313–314
Neurobiology
　of body image disturbance, 132–133
　of intimacy, 158–159
　of nicotine dependence, 274–275
　of OCD, 263
Neurochemistry in panic disorder, 236–237
Neurocognition studies, 213–214
Neurodevelopment
　ADHD and, 353
　alcohol disorders and, 301, 304
　of behavioral disorders, 31
　derailment, 68–70
　nature vs. nurture, 66
　nicotine and, 275
　of pre-adult brain, 68
　schizophrenia and, 363–364, 365, 374
　stress and, 70
　of triadic system, 20
　Williams syndrome, 25
Neuroimaging studies, 213, 364
Neuropsychological testing, 356
Neurotransmitter hypothesis, 365
Neurotransmitter systems, 20, 336, 364, 371t. See also Dopamine; Serotonin
"Never-smokers", 278
Nicotine
　dependence, 274–275, 276
　vs. nonnicotine medication, 282–283
　replacement therapies (NRT), 280, 282
　transdermal patch, 278, 282
Nonnicotine medication, 282–283
Nonparaphilic behaviors, 343
Nonpsychotic mental illness, 13
Nonsteroidal anti-inflammatory drug (NSAID), 326
Normative influences, mental health care, 196–197, 196f
Normative male-based trauma, 98, 102
Nunes, Edward V., 310–335

O

Oberstar, Joel V., 352–361
Obsessive-compulsive disorder (OCD)
　with ADHD, 261
　bipolar disorder and, 384
　characteristics of, 258–262, 260t, 261f
　cognitive-behavioral therapy for, 256, 262, 264
　definition of, 435
　depression and, 255
　diagnosis/assessment of, 256–258, 257t
　marijuana use and, 256
　prevalence of, 256
　risk factors of, 262–264
　treatment of, 264–265
Obsessive-compulsive personality disorder (OCPD), 258, 261
Odlaug, Brian L., 231–254
Olanzapine, 371, 371t
Opioid use
　agonist treatment, 324–326, 324t–325t
　dependence on, 316–317
　methylphenidate for, 357
　overdose, 312
Oppositional defiant disorder (ODD), 72
Orbital and medial prefrontal cortex (OMPFC), 24, 29

P

Panic disorder (PD), 215, 231, 236–239
Paranoid personality disorder, 431
Paraphilic behaviors, 343
Parenting/parenthood issues. See also Children/childhood issues; Pregnancy issues
　alcohol use, 300
　attachment theory, 159–160, 185
　connection factor, 104
　delaying, 183
　depression, 216
　early vs. later, 186–187
　emerging adults and, 183–184
　life history theory, 184–185
　"parenting effort", 185
　psychosexual acceleration hypothesis, 185–186
　psychosocial acceleration hypothesis, 187–190
　puberty and, 181, 187–188, 190–191
　as risk-taking reducer, 51
　stress, 146
Pathological gambling, 336–338
PDD. see Pervasive developmental disorders
Peer pressure
　on body image, 130–131
　in risk-taking behaviors, 49–50
　in social skills training, 412
　tobacco use and, 275
Perlick, Deborah A., 195–205
Perry, Bruce, 103
Personality assessments, 53
Personality disorders (PDs). See also Antisocial personality disorder; Obsessive-compulsive disorder
　assessment/diagnosis, 428–430, 428t, 429t
　classification of, 424–425, 425t, 428t
　epidemiology of, 425–427
　etiology of, 427–428
　as schizophrenia, 369
　treatment, 430–431
　types of, 431–435
Personality traits, 47, 300, 301
Pervasive developmental disorder not otherwise specified (PDD-NOS), 407–408, 409
Pervasive developmental disorders (PDD), 72, 369. See also Autistic disorder
　adaptations in, 411
　behavior problems with, 414–417
　communication skills and, 413–414
　developmental trajectory of, 409–410
　diagnostic criteria, 407–408
　environmental influences, 410
　etiology of, 408–409
　intervention therapy for, 409–410
　introduction to, 406
　pharmacology of, 407, 415–417
　physical supports for, 410–411
　school vs. community-based services, 417–418
　social skills training and, 411–413
　visual strategies for, 410
Pharmacological treatments
　antipsychotic medications, 371–372
　for bipolar disorder, 385–387, 385t, 386t
　for compulsive buying, 344
　for drug use disorders, 324–327, 324t–325t
　for eating disorders, 327, 403
　for intermittent explosive disorder, 341
　for pathological gambling, 337
　for personality disorders, 430
　for pervasive developmental disorders, 407, 415–417
　psychostimulants, 356
　for schizophrenia, 370–372, 371t
Piaget, Jean, 66
Picture exchange communication system (PECS), 413–414
Pittsburgh Youth Study (PYS), 10, 13
Pollack, William S., 96–109
Positive affective states, 275–276
Positive reinforcement, 314, 415
Positron emission tomography (PET), 217
Posterolateral orbitofrontal cortex, 29
Posttraumatic stress disorder (PTSD)
　in American Indians, 114
　bipolar disorder and, 383
　in childhood, 70
　diagnosis and treatment, 242–246
　drug use disorders and, 314, 328
　limbic system dysfunctions with, 243
　schizophrenia and, 369
　without treatment, 148
Potenza, Marc N., 3–4, 335–351
Pozdol, Stacie, 406–423
Prairie vole model, 158–159
Prefrontal cortex (PFC)
　anatomy and connectivity, 20, 22, 29
　in fractal triadic model, 30–32, 32f

Index

ontogeny, 29–30
in pre-adult brain, 68
synaptogenesis, 30
Pregnancy issues
  alcohol use, 51, 300
  eating disorder during, 400
  eating disorders, 400
  medication, 217, 221
  parenting, 182, 184
  smoking, 279, 281
  unintentional, 43, 48, 52, 189, 325
Prescription stimulant addiction, 311, 318–319
Primate striatum, 28
Procrastination stressors, 86–87
Prodromal phase of schizophrenia, 365–367, 367f
Project Competence studies, 10–12
Psychiatric disorders, 69, 74–75, 149, 152. See also specific disorders
  age-group variances, 111
  alcohol and, 199
  brain and, 104
  development of, 3–4, 20, 64, 66, 68
  drug use disorders and, 320–321
  marriage and, 172–173
  race variances, 114–115, 117, 120
"Psychic separation", 98
Psychoanalytic stage theory, 6
Psychodynamic psychotherapy, 101, 237–238, 373
Psychosexual acceleration hypothesis, 185–186
Psychosis with bipolar disorder, 383
Psychosocial acceleration hypothesis, 187–190
Psychostimulants, 356, 416
Psychotherapy. See also Cognitive-behavioral therapy; Intervention therapy; Therapeutic interventions
  for compulsive sexual behavior, 343
  for eating disorders, 402–403
  generalized anxiety disorder, 240–242
  for panic disorders, 238
  for pathological gambling, 337–338
  for PTSD, 244
  for social anxiety disorder, 235
PTSD. see Posttraumatic stress disorder
Puberty state, 20, 181, 187–188, 190–191
Pyromania, 342

Q

Quantitative electroencephalograms (qEEGs), 356
Quetiapine, 386
Quit and Win (antismoking) programs, 282

R

Race issues, 44, 113–114
Rasmussen, Steven A., 255–271
Realmuto, George M., 352–361

Recovery phase of schizophrenia, 367–368, 367f
Reese, Hannah E., 126–142
Relapse prevention (RP), 322
Repetitive behaviors, 258
"Reproductive effort" in parenting, 184–185
Research Units on Pediatric Psychopharmacology Autism Network (RUPP), 416
Residual phase of schizophrenia, 367f, 368
Resilience development, 6, 8–14
Restrictive eating, 400, 400t
Reversible inhibitors of monoamine oxidase type A (RIMAs), 234
Reward prediction error, 28
Reward therapy, 281–282
Reynolds, Elizabeth K., 40–63
Risk-taking behaviors, 42–43, 44, 49–51, 301. See also Sexual behavior risks
  with ADHD, 40–41, 47–48
  affective distress and, 48–49
  alcohol use, 41–42, 48
  assessment of, 52
  conduct disorder and, 47–48
  definitions of, 40
  developmental precursors, 47–48
  gambling, 43–44
  genetic influences on, 44–46
  illicit drug use, 42
  integrative models of, 51–52
  neurobehavioral contributors, 46–47
  personality differences and, 47
  prevention of, 52–53
  reduction factors, 51
  understanding, 53–54
Risperidone, 371, 371t, 416
Rogers, Fred, 97
Romantic vs. sexual relationships, 162–165
Rosenthal, Susan L., 158–168

S

Same-sex marriage, 170
Schizoid personality disorder, 431–432
Schizophrenia, 277–278, 365–368, 370
  assessment of, 368, 368t
  childhood-onset, 74, 363
  connectivity hypothesis, 365
  differential diagnosis of, 369
  environmental risks, 364–365
  epidemiology of, 362
  etiology of, 363–364
  gender differences in, 363
  laboratory/imaging findings, 370
  neurotransmitter hypothesis, 365
  pharmacologic treatments, 370–372, 371t
  psychosocial treatments, 372–373
Schizotypical personality disorder, 432
Schore, Alan, 103–104

Second-generation antipsychotic (SGA), 370–371, 372
Secure attachment styles, 159–160
Sedative dependence, 317–318
Selection perspective of marriage, 172–173
Selective serotonin-reuptake inhibitors (SSRIs), 219
Self-construal factor, 118, 119–120
Self-recognition treatment, 301–302
Self-report assessments, 53, 355
Sequenced Treatment Alternatives to Relieve Depression (STAR*D) trial, 208, 215, 218, 220
Serotonin
  anxiety disorders and, 233, 240
  bipolar disorder and, 385
  club drugs and, 319
  in impulse control disorders, 336
  impulse control disorders and, 336
  monoamine oxidase and, 46
  mood regulation and, 133
  personality disorders and, 428
  schizophrenia and, 371
  transporter gene, 20, 46, 211, 353, 385
  triadic node regulation, 20
Serotonin norepinephrine reuptake inhibitors (SNRIs), 219, 234, 238, 241
Serotonin reuptake inhibitors (SSRIs)
  for anxiety disorders, 64, 234, 237, 238, 245
  for body dysmorphic disorder, 134
  for depression, 206, 219, 220
  for eating disorders, 403
  for impulse control disorders, 337
  for OCD, 262, 264–265
  for PDD, 416
  for personality disorders, 433, 435
  for pervasive developmental disorders, 415, 416–417
Severe interpersonal trauma, 144–145
Severe mood dysregulation (SMD), 72
Sexual abuse, 49, 96, 190, 210, 244, 320
Sexual behavior risks, 42–43, 48, 164, 342–343
Sexual maturation, 20, 80, 160
Sexually transmitted diseases (STDs), 44, 52, 164
Sexually transmitted infections (STIs), 158, 164
"Shame-free zones", 104–105
Shame issues, 101–102
Sher, Kenneth J., 292–310
Single-photon emission computed tomography (SPECT), 217
Sinha, Rajita, 143–157
Smith, Anne E., 272–291
Smoking cessation therapies
  behavioral, 281
  contests, 282
  contingency management, 281–282
  interventions, 280–281
  motivational interviewing, 281
  nicotine replacement, 278, 280, 282
  nonnicotine medication, 282–283
  Stages of Change model, 279–280
  treatment considerations, 283

Smoking/tobacco use, 42, 175, 272–273, 275
  epidemiology of, 273
  genetic influences on, 45, 276–277
  marijuana treatment and, 283
  during marriage, 175
  mood and, 275–276
  nicotine dependence, 274–275, 276
  prevention/cessation/treatment, 279–283
  psychiatric comorbidity, 277–279
  Stages of Change model, 279–280
Social anxiety disorder (SAD), 215, 231–235
Social cognitive theory, 160–161
Social skills training, 411–413
Sociocultural features of young adults, 81, 131–132
"Somatic effort" in parenting, 184
Somatoform disorder. see Body dysmorphic disorder
SSRIs. see Serotonin reuptake inhibitors
Stages of Change (SOC) model, 279–280
Stereotypes, 103, 119, 131, 298
Stigma concerns, mental health care, 196f, 197–198
Stress/stressors, 69–70, 70, 149, 152, 276. See also College and/or career stressors
  affective disorders and, 48–49
  alcohol abuse, 143–144
  coping factors for, 149–153
  dopamine and, 47
  drug use disorders and, 314
  of emerging young adulthood, 145–146
  HPA axis and, 48–49, 51
  PTSD and, 70
  substance use and, 148–149
  therapeutic interventions, 151–152
  time-management, 90, 92, 201
  vulnerability factors, 146–147
Striatum
  anatomy and connectivity, 26–28, 26f, 29
  antero-ventral, 133
  development of, 19–20
  dopamine and, 312
  in fractal triadic model, 30–32, 32f
  ontogeny, 28–29
Stuart, Melissa, 406–423
Substance use/abuse, 13, 73, 117–118, 211–212. See also Alcohol use disorder; Drug use disorders
  in emerging/young adulthood, 148–149
  gender distinctions in, 96, 97, 199
  in mental health service utilization, 196f, 199
  psychiatric disorders and, 327–329
  schizophrenia-like symptoms from, 364–365, 369
  tobacco use and, 278
Subsyndromal dependence, 315
Sue, Stanley, 113

Suicide
  with anorexia nervosa, 399
  depression and, 211, 352
  epidemiology of, 208–209
  factors in, 212
  gender distinctions, 97, 102
  ideation, 216, 386
Swann, Alan C., 379–396
Swiezy, Naomi B., 406–423

T

Task Force on Black and Minority Health, 113
Tetrahydrocannibinol (THC), 327
Therapeutic interventions. See also Intervention therapy; Psychotherapy
  cognitive-behavioral therapy, 111, 135–136, 152
  dissonance induction, 136
  group therapy, 244, 434
  humanistic/experiential therapy, 111
  network therapy, 324
  psychodynamic psychotherapy, 101
  against stress, 151–152
Three Center AESOP Study, 362
Thyroid-stimulating hormone (TSH), 217
Thyrotropin-releasing hormone (TRH), 217
Time-management stressors, 90, 92, 201
Tobacco use. see Nicotine; Smoking/tobacco use
Tonic-phasic dopamine theory, 28
Transitional development, 80–93, 300
  competence and resilience, 6, 8–9, 10–12
  developmental tasks and, 6–8
  emerging adulthood, 9–10
  major depressive disorder and, 215–216
  in pervasive developmental disorders, 407
Trauma
  adult development derailment by, 147–148
  depression and, 211
  drug use disorders and, 314
  normative male-based, 98, 102
  OCD and, 263
  severe interpersonal, 144–145
Triadic model of neurodevelopment, 20, 21–22, 21f
Triadic nodes, 3–26, 26–29, 29–30, 30–32
Trichotillomania disorder, 338–339
Tricyclic antidepressants (TCAs), 206, 219, 238, 356
Tryptophan hydroxylase (TPH), 211, 353
"Turning point" opportunities, 10
12-step programs, 302, 321, 323
Twins' studies, 209–210, 262, 364

U

Umberson, Debra, 169–180
Unconditioned responses (UCR), 313
Unconditioned stimuli (UCS), 313
Unipolar depression, 71

V

Valproate treatment, 328
Varenicline Tartrate, 282–283
Variable-focused analyses, 11–12
Venlafaxine (Effexor), 220
Ventromedial prefrontal cortex, 29
Virtual reality (VR) exposure therapy, 244
Virtual response training (VRT), 412
Visual strategies for PDD, 410
Voting Rights Act, 113
Vulnerability factors for stress, 146–147

W

Wellbutrin (bupropion), 220
Wender, Paul, 353
White, Tonya, 362–378
White American youth, 44, 127–128
Wilhelm, Sabine, 126–142
Williams syndrome, 25
Withdrawal cravings, 279
Workplace issues. see Job/workplace issues
World Health Organization (WHO), 206

Y

Yale-Brown Obsessive Compulsive Scale (YBOCS), 258
Yoga practice, 152
Young adults
  ages of, 143
  alcohol use disorder and, 295–298, 296f, 297f
  cannabis use, 211–212
  vs. emerging adulthood, 81–82
  impulse control disorders and, 335–336
  isolation vs. intimacy during, 112
  major depressive disorder and, 215–216
  mortality rates of, 97
  pathological gambling in, 337
  roles/responsibilities of, 144
  romantic relationships of, 163
  sexual behavior of, 164
  substance use of, 148–149
Youth Risk Behavior Surveillance: National College Health Risk Behavior Survey, 52

Z

Zarate, Carlos A., Jr., 206–230
Ziprasidone, 371t, 372
Zyban (bupropion), 282